THE

Occupational

Therapy

Manager

Revised Edition

The American Occupational Therapy Association, Inc.

Disclaimers

"This publication is designed to provide accurate and authoritative information
in regard to the subject matter covered. It is sold or distributed with the understanding that the publisher is not engaged in rendering legal, accounting, or other professional service. If legal advice or other expert assistance is required, the services of a
competent professional person should be sought."

—From the Declaration of Principles jointly adopted by the
   American Bar Association and a Committee of Publishers and Associations

It is the objective of the American Occupational Therapy Association to be a forum
for free expression and interchange of ideas. The opinions and positions expressed
by the contributors to this work are their own and not necessarily those of either the
editors or the American Occupational Therapy Association.

It is expected that the procedures and practices described in this book will be used
only by qualified practitioners in accordance with professional standards and in
compliance with applicable practice statutes. Every effort has been made to assure
that the information presented is accurate and consistent with generally accepted
practices. However, the authors, editor, and publisher cannot accept responsibility for
errors or omissions, or for the consequences of incorrect application of information
by individuals or rehabilitation professionals. No warranty, express or implied, is made
regarding the contents of this text.

AOTA Director of Nonperiodical Publications: Frances E. McCarrey
AOTA Managing Editor of Nonperiodical Publications: Mary C. Fisk
Edited by Margo Johnson
Designed by Carolyn Uhl

Printed in the United States of America

ISBN 1-56900-051-4

Table of Contents

FOREWORD VII
Jeanette Bair, MBA, OTR, FAOTA

ACKNOWLEDGMENTS IX

SECTION 1   INTRODUCTION
1   The Evolution of the Occupational Therapy Delivery System 3
Karen Jacobs, EdD, OTR, CPE, FAOTA

SECTION 2   PLANNING
2   Strategic Planning 51
L. Randy Strickland, EdD, OTR/L, FAOTA
3   Financial Management 63
Nancy Mahon Smith, MBA, OTR, CHE
4   Marketing 101
Tina Shoemaker, MHA, OTR, FAOTA
Carol Wheeler, BSN, RN, CHE
5   The Targeting of Communications 117
Wendy Krupnick, MBA, OTR/L

SECTION 3   ORGANIZING
6   Management Styles, Structures, and Roles 145
Ruth Ann Watkins, MBA, OTR, FAOTA
7   Organizational Effectiveness 163
Patricia Crist, PhD, OTR, FAOTA
8   Management of Rapid Change 191
Sylvia Harlock Kauffman, PhD, OTR, FAOTA

SECTION 4   DIRECTING

9   Team Building and Leadership 213
     Susan C. Robertson, MS, OTR/L, FAOTA

SECTION 5   CONTROLLING

10   Personnel Management 253
     Barbara A. Boyt Schell, PhD, OTR, FAOTA
     John W. Schell, PhD

11   Roles, Relationships, and Career Development 327
     Patricia Crist, PhD, OTR, FAOTA

SECTION 6   EVALUATING

12   Evaluation of Program 395
     PART 1
     Program Evaluation 398
     Christine M. MacDonell, BSOT
     PART 2
     Quality Improvement 411
     Deborah L. Wilkerson, MA
     PART 3
     Documentation of Occupational Therapy Services 424
     Jane Davy Acquaviva, BS, OTR

13   Voluntary Accrediting Agencies 459
     PART 1
     Joint Commission on Accreditation of Healthcare Organizations . .470
     Richard W. Scalenghe, BM, RMT
     PART 2
     CARF, The Rehabilitation Accreditation Commission 485
     Christine M. MacDonell, BSOT
     PART 3
     Accreditation Council on Services for People with Disabilities 494
     Nancy MacRae, MS, OTR/L, FAOTA
     PART 4
     Other Accrediting Agencies Of Interest
     to Occupational Therapy 505

SECTION 7   COMMUNICATING

14   Principles of Communication 511
     Catherine Nielson, MPH, OTR/L, FAOTA

15   Consultation: A Collaborative Approach to Change 533
      Cynthia F. Epstein, MA, OTR, FAOTA
      Evelyn G. Jaffe, MPH, OTR, FAOTA

SECTION 8   PAYMENT, REGULATORY, AND ETHICAL ISSUES

16   Evolving Health Care Systems:
      Payment for Occupational Therapy Services 577
      V. Judith Thomas, MGA
17   State Regulation and Specialty Certification
      of Practitioners 603
      Barbara Winthrop Rose, BSOT, OTR, CVE, CWA, CHT, FAOTA
18   Ethical Dimensions in Occupational Therapy 627
      Karin J. Opacich, MHPE, OTR/L, FAOTA

INDEX 661

Foreword

When AOTA published the first edition of *The Occupational Therapy Manager* in 1985, health care in the United States was beginning to transform in structure, methods and sources of payment, and technology, largely influenced by Medicare's introduction of the prospective payment system and by the advent of the electronic age. Carolyn M. Baum wrote in chapter 1 of the first edition about escalating costs, "vertical systems of care," and "multi-institutional systems." "Managed care" was barely a whisper in conversations of the time. We and others did not know then how far- and deep-reaching the transformation would be.

As AOTA publishes this second edition of *The Occupational Therapy Manager,* the dimensions and the directions of the transformation have become clearer. Karen Jacobs writes in the revised chapter 1 that the provider-driven fee-for-service system many of us knew in our early days of practice is now a payer-driven system and is rapidly becoming a consumer-driven one. "Managed care" is a roar.

L. Randy Strickland, in chapter 2, urges us to look for the opportunities and the threats that this reconfiguring situation presents; also, to examine our strengths and weaknesses. Certainly, opportunities abound for the profession of occupational therapy—in home health care, subacute care, outpatient rehabilitation, education, and business and industry, among others. The chief threats come from the possible deregulation of occupational therapy licensure and certification laws and from a lack of awareness among the public and its decision makers of occupational therapy's contribution to health and wellness. Foremost among the profession's strengths are its enduring emphasis on the whole person and its focus on function as a means of restoring meaning to a person's life. A weakness, particularly apparent as organizational structures flatten and sources of payment shift and consolidate, is insufficient attention to occupational therapy practitioners' competence in management and related disciplines like marketing and evaluation of program.

The Occupational Therapy Manager addresses these subjects. It is a comprehensive, accessible guide for occupational therapy practitioners who aspire to management positions, who already hold such positions, or who now or soon will be constrained simply to "manage"—not just to cope, but to respond wisely, skillfully, and creatively—because of the novelty that surrounds them. Drawing on the knowledge of experts in a wide variety of fields, the book provides overviews of crucial topics and detailed discussions of practical, day-to-day functions.

Nearly every one of the contributors to this edition remarks on the fact that he or she wrote the chapter in the midst of rapid change. Barbara A. Boyt Schell and John W. Schell observe at the conclusion of chapter 10 that the once-traditional configuration of an occupational therapy organization—a department within a hospital or a rehabilitation center—is being superseded by a variety of models. Regardless of model and setting, the Schells contend, the basic principles and strategies of personnel management that they present in their chapter, apply.

We contend the same of *The Occupational Therapy Manager* as a whole. Despite the myriad alterations in health care, the basic principles of management in general—and of occupational therapy management in particular—apply. To provide the highest-quality occupational therapy services in any context, a manager must create a working environment—

1. That is well organized and self-evaluative, yet not bureaucratic.

2. That anticipates and plans for change, then responds effectively when it occurs.

3. That fosters communication within the organization, with outside regulators and payers, and, most important, with clients and potential clients.

Such an environment will attract the most highly skilled professional practitioners.

Jeanette Bair, MBA, OTR, FAOTA
Executive Director
American Occupational Therapy Association

Acknowledgments

Many people contributed to the conceptual development, the selection of content and authors, and the review of manuscripts for this management text. We particularly appreciate the contributions of those who assisted us through the complex process of this edition:

John B. Cox, CAE

Jeanne Luschin, MBA

Johanna Brady, MA, OTR

Penny Kyler-Hutchison, MA, OTR/L, FAOTA

Brena G. Manoly, PhD, OTR

Sarah Hertfelder, MEd, MOT, OTR

Stephanie Hoover, EdD, OTR, FAOTA

Frederick P. Somers

Velma Hart, CAE

Deborah Lieberman, MHSA, OTR/L, FAOTA

SECTION 1

Introduction

Data collected over many years indicate that about three-fourths of occupational therapy practitioners consider direct care to be their primary function and about one-eighth consider it to be their secondary function. Given these high proportions of practitioners involved in direct care, it is understandable that curricula in occupational therapy focus on training for clinical practice.

Yet about one-eighth of registered occupational therapists identify administration as their primary function, and about one-eighth of occupational therapy practitioners identify it as their secondary function. Moreover, every practitioner in today's dynamic health care environment must be a manager of sorts. Cost containment, the flattening of organizations, and utilization tools of managed care, such as case management, have made the individual clinician far more accountable than before for levels of productivity, cost-effectiveness, and outcomes. Knowledge of and competence in good management practices are musts for the contemporary practitioner.

The Occupational Therapy Manager is designed to strengthen and supplement curricula in occupational therapy with a comprehensive introduction to management. It is also intended to be a guide for new, inexperienced managers, explaining the basics of management and pointing them in directions for further study.

The main text of *The Occupational Therapy Manager* has eight sections. The opening chapter, "The Evolution of the Occupational Therapy Delivery System," constitutes section 1 and is introduced here. Separate introductions appear at the beginning of sections 2–8.

Chapter 1 describes the broad context in which occupational therapy organizations operate. It discusses the part that social, economic, and political forces, particularly the federal government, have played in the evolution of the United States health care system. It also explains how health care has changed in recent years: from a hospital-based, physician-centered model to a system in which many kinds of professionals provide care in a variety of settings; from freestanding hospitals to many institutions linked in corporate health networks; and from separate entities to provide care and to pay for it, to organizations in which the provider is also the payer. The chapter goes on to note the dramatic growth in the occupational therapy profession in the last 25 years and to present recent trends in the distribution of personnel. Finally, it looks at the directions in which health care and occupational therapy seem to be headed, driven most forcibly by competition and pressures for cost containment.

The six sections that follow focus on the six primary roles of managers: planning, organizing, directing, controlling, evaluating, and communicating. Each section consists of one or more chapters on the managerial functions encompassed in the particular role. The chapters address both the concepts that underlie the functions and the skills required to carry them out.

The concluding section covers major issues and processes that affect the practice of occupational therapy. The subjects include payment for services, state regulation and specialty certification of practitioners, and ethics.

CHAPTER 1

The Evolution of the Occupational Therapy Delivery System

Karen Jacobs, EdD, OTR/L, CPE, FAOTA

KEY TERMS

Capitation. A fixed, preset amount periodically paid to a provider for each person covered under a contract or a policy for provision of services.

Cross-training. The preparation of a person in one profession to perform skills typically associated with another profession.

Health maintenance organization (HMO). "A prepaid organized delivery system where the organization *and* the primary care physicians assume some financial risk for the care provided to its enrolled members" (Weiner & de Lissovoy, 1993, p. 96).

Indemnity. The standard fee-for-service insurance policies provided by employers, organizations, or individuals. Usually the most expensive type, this insurance covers service from any provider.

Managed care. A synonym for all kinds of integrated delivery systems, in contrast with unmanaged fee-for-service care. Also, "the entire range of utilization control tools that are applied to manage the practices of physicians and others, regardless of the setting in which they practice" (Weiner & de Lissovoy, 1993, p. 97).

This chapter is based in part on "The Evolution of the U.S. Health Care System," by C. M. Baum, 1992, in J. Bair and M. Gray (Eds.), The Occupational Therapy Manager *(Rev. ed., pp. 1–25), Rockville, MD: American Occupational Therapy Association. The occupational therapy students enrolled in professional service management at Boston University, class of 1995, obtained much of the research material for the chapter. The author expresses great appreciation to these future colleagues for their efforts. Copyright ©1992 by the American Occupational Therapy Association, Inc.*

Multiskilled practitioner. A person from one profession who has established competence in specific skills usually associated with another profession.

Preferred provider organization (PPO). An entity that "acts as a broker between the purchaser of care and the provider . . . [C]onsumers have the option of using the 'preferred' providers available within the plan, or not" (Weiner & de Lissovoy, 1993, p. 99).

Karen Jacobs, EdD, OTR/L, CPE, FAOTA, is a clinical assistant professor in the Department of Occupational Therapy at Boston University. Currently the vice-president of AOTA, she served as president of the Massachusetts Association of Occupational Therapy for five years. Her doctorate is from the University of Massachusetts at Lowell.

Occupational therapy has been a part of the United States health care system since the early 1900s. Occupational therapy practitioners are affected by the system's vulnerabilities as well as its strengths. The system is currently shifting from a provider-driven industry to a payer-driven industry. It will eventually become a consumer-driven industry (DeJong & Sutton, 1994). Because of rising costs, a growing emphasis on outcomes and accountability, a lack of services to meet specific needs, an imbalance of services for different populations of the society, and advances in medical technology, the industry has become an object of scrutiny by the government as well as the public. The public expects accessible and affordable health care, viewing it as a right in the same category with education, police protection, and fire protection. The latter are public services supported by a general tax base and offered by public servants. Health care moneys, on the other hand, are generated by business and industry, third-party payers, government subsidies, private fund-raising, and individuals. Moreover, providers of care are independent, licensed practitioners.

In the past, health care in the United States was described in terms of the extent and the characteristics of health problems. Today health care is cast in economic terms. Health care costs rose from $27.1 billion in 1960 to $938.3 billion in 1994. Government spending accounted for $420.2 billion of the 1994 total, most of it for Medicare and Medicaid, but some for public health, veterans' care, military medical services, and state, county, and city medical services (Bodenheimer & Grumbach, 1994; Burner & Waldo, 1995; Clinton, 1994). Table 1-1 and figures 1-1a and 1-1b provide details. This chapter explores different aspects of the United States health care system and the evolution of the occupational therapy delivery system.

THE RIGHT-TO-HEALTH CONCEPT AND ETHICS

The basis for much of the government's involvement in health care is the concept of the right to health. There is reference to the concept in the *Congressional Record* as early as 1796. In the 19th and 20th centuries, it has reappeared at many points. It came to full attention in 1944 in Franklin D. Roosevelt's Economic Bill of Rights (Chapman & Talmedge, 1971). The federal government has intermittently broadened and narrowed its definition of the right to health. The early meaning implied a guarantee of protection to all citizens, regardless of economic or social status, from certain health hazards. Shortly after the turn of the century, the concept took on a noncomprehensive meaning. However, when Roosevelt proclaimed "the right to adequate needed care and the opportunity to achieve and enjoy good health," he was equating it with the most fundamental social and political right guaranteed to every citizen.

Table 1-1: National Health Expenditures, 1960–1994

National Health Expenditures

	Gross Domestic Product (in billions)	Total			Private Funds			Government Funds		
		Amount (in billions)	Per Capita	Percentage of GNP	Amount (in billions)	Per Capita	Percentage of Total	Amount (in billions)	Per Capita	Percentage of Total
1994	$6,735	$938.3	$3,463	13.9	$518.1	$1,912	55.2	$420.2	$1,551	44.8
1993	6,343	884.2	3,299	13.9	496.4	1,852	56.1	387.8	1,447	43.9
1992	6,020	820.3	3,094	13.6	462.9	1,746	56.4	357.5	1,348	43.6
1991	5,725	755.6	2,882	13.2	432.9	1,651	57.3	322.6	1,230	42.7
1990	5,546	696.6	2,686	12.6	410.0	1,581	58.9	286.5	1,105	41.1
1989	5,251	623.9	2,433	11.9	370.7	1,446	59.4	253.2	987	40.6
1987	4,540	506.2	2,013	11.1	298.6	1,187	59.0	207.6	825	41.0
1985	4,039	434.5	1,761	10.8	259.4	1,051	59.7	175.1	709	40.3
1980	2,708	251.1	1,068	9.3	145.8	620	58.1	105.3	448	41.9
1970	1,011	74.3	346	7.4	46.6	217	62.7	27.7	129	37.3
1960	513	27.1	143	5.3	20.5	108	75.5	6.7	35	24.5

Note. *Per capita amounts are based on July 1 Social Security Area population estimates for 1960–90, estimated by the Health Care Financing Administration for 1991–94. From "National Health Expenditure Projections, 1994–2005 [DataView]" (pp. 234–35), by S. T. Burner and D. R. Waldo, 1995, Summer, Health Care Financing Review, 16(4); and "National Health Expenditures, 1993" (p. 280), by K. R. Levit, A. L. Sensenig, C. A. Cowan, H. C. Lazenby, P. A. McDonnell, D. K. Won, L. Sivarajan, J. M. Stiller, C. S. Donham, and M. S. Stewart, 1994, Fall, Health Care Financing Review, 16(1).*

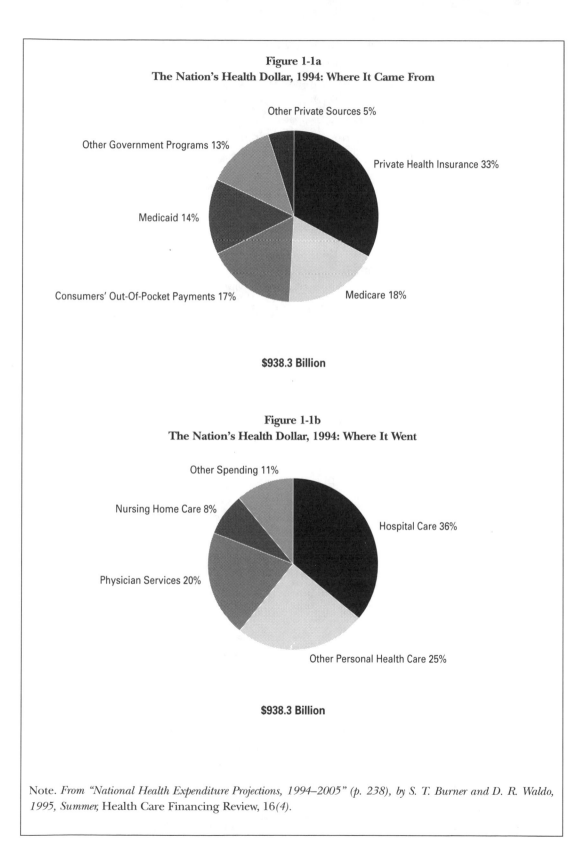

Figure 1-1a
The Nation's Health Dollar, 1994: Where It Came From

Other Private Sources 5%

Other Government Programs 13%

Private Health Insurance 33%

Medicaid 14%

Consumers' Out-Of-Pocket Payments 17%

Medicare 18%

$938.3 Billion

Figure 1-1b
The Nation's Health Dollar, 1994: Where It Went

Other Spending 11%

Nursing Home Care 8%

Hospital Care 36%

Physician Services 20%

Other Personal Health Care 25%

$938.3 Billion

Note. *From "National Health Expenditure Projections, 1994–2005" (p. 238), by S. T. Burner and D. R. Waldo, 1995, Summer,* Health Care Financing Review, 16*(4)*.

Very few political leaders would publicly declare that they do not support a right to health care. However, politicians daily debate the right as the government struggles to balance the budget. Recently a prominent scientific organization put the argument for health care reform in a human rights framework (Chapman, 1993). Whether or not reform goes forward, the framework provides a helpful context for thinking about the right to health care. There are grounds for such a right, the argument goes, in this country's high standard of living and the government's constitutional responsibility to protect the public health. The right would be an assurance of equal access to "basic and adequate health care"—a standard package including preventive, primary, reproductive, and long-term care; most types of acute care; and mental health services (p. vi). The right would be universal; that is, it would inhere in all United States citizens and residents without regard to "financial means, employment status, disabilities, residence, gender, or racial or ethnic background" (p. vii). It would have limits, however:

> The government would provide the security of an entitlement to
> basic health care . . . In exchange, members of society would
> accept a series of obligations: the duty to respect and be sensitive
> to the health care needs of others, responsibility for meeting the
> needs of the most vulnerable and disadvantaged members of soci-
> ety, and individual limits on claims to a reasonable and affordable
> level of health care. (p. vi)

Related to the right-to-health concept is the matter of ethics (see chapter 18, "Ethical Dimensions in Occupational Therapy," for a more complete discussion of this topic). Society, through its laws and systems, tries to clarify moral values in relation to health care. Ethics pertains to society's relationship to the patient or client, the occupational therapy practitioner, and the health care system. It also pertains to the professional relationship between the patient or client and the practitioner, between the patient or client and the health care organization, and between the practitioner and the organization.

Limits may increasingly be placed on health services for moral as well as economic reasons, as ethical issues are raised about the technology available to create, maintain, and prolong life. Although many health care facilities have formal ethics procedures for resolving cases involving these issues, such cases are likely to continue to go before the courts and be matters of national debate for years to come. Further, even persons who use the same reasoning process may arrive at different conclusions based on their value systems (Reitz, 1992).

Occupational therapy practitioners who enter management are likely to encounter ethical dilemmas in their work. They need to develop an understanding of potential conflicts and ways of maintaining their personal ethics while successfully carrying out their roles. Goals such as independence, self-determination, and competency, all seen in the practice of occupational therapy, are based on values and morals (Bloom, 1994). For this reason the American Occupational Therapy Association (AOTA) adopted the *Occupational Therapy Code of Ethics* (see appendix 18-A) stating values, principles, and desirable actions for occupational therapy practitioners.

THE FEDERAL GOVERNMENT'S ROLE IN THE HEALTH CARE SYSTEM

On the grounds of economy, accountability, and consumer protection, the federal government's investment in health care costs demands a public acceptance of responsibility for health services. Historically, however, the federal government has been locked into the role of providing assistance, not control. Since the mid-1940s it has made many significant contributions to the evolving health care system. The following summary of major historical events offers a perspective on these contributions.[1]

CONSTRUCTION OF HEALTH CARE FACILITIES

Little hospital construction occurred during the depression and World War II. In 1944 the American Hospital Association and the United States Public Health Service organized a commission on hospital care to determine the need for hospital facilities. The work of the commission was reflected in the Hospital Survey and Construction Act of 1946, Title VI of the Public Health Service Act. Popularly known as the Hill-Burton Act, this legislation assisted the states in determining their need for hospitals and other health care facilities. Also, it provided grants to states for construction projects. Over the next two decades Congress extended and amended the Hill-Burton Act frequently, expanding its programs to cover diagnostic and treatment centers, chronic disease hospitals, rehabilitation facilities, and nursing homes. In 1964 and again in 1970, Congress earmarked funds for modernization of facilities. The Mental Retardation Facilities Construction Act and the Community Mental Health Centers Act of 1963 provided funding for the construction of facilities for persons with mental retardation and for the construction of community-based mental health centers. Extensions and amendments to this federal legislation continued into the early 1980s.

---

1. *This section is based in part on information from* Health Services in the United States *(2nd rev. ed., pp. 191–218), by F. A. Wilson and D. Neuhauser, 1985, Cambridge, MA: Ballinger.*

The Hill-Burton Act was greatly modified in the National Health Planning and Resources Development Act of 1974. This legislation was especially critical in modernizing health care facilities. Many of the facilities built between 1946 and 1974 were struggling to survive, and their struggle was having a major effect on the total cost of health care. By the mid-1960s new facilities were operational, but too few health professionals were available to staff them. Also, some health facilities were obsolete, requiring nearly $20 billion a year for modernization. Construction costs of facilities increased from $470 million in 1968 to $712 million in 1971. By the early 1970s the federal government began to recognize the need for systems to control and establish meaningful plans for future construction.

HUMAN RESOURCES LEGISLATION

Since the mid-1950s the federal government has had an important role in financing human resources for health. Its first peacetime legislation to support training of health care's human resources was the Health Amendments Act of 1956, benefiting public health personnel and professional and practical nurses. In 1958, Congress established a program of formula grants to schools of public health. Soon to follow was a program of project grants for these and other schools training public health personnel.

The first construction grants for teaching facilities came in 1963, in the Health Professions Educational Assistance Act. Schools of medicine, dentistry, pharmacy, podiatry, nursing, and public health were the eligible recipients. This act also made student loan funds available in medicine, osteopathy, and dentistry. In 1964 the Nurse Training Act provided separate funds for nursing school construction, set aside funds to expand nurse training programs, and established nursing student loan programs. The Health Professions Educational Assistance Amendments of 1965 authorized grants to improve the quality of schools of medicine, dentistry, osteopathy, optometry, and podiatry. The amendments also made scholarship funds available to those schools and to schools of pharmacy.

The first federal funds for support of occupational therapy education came in 1966, with the Allied Health Professions Personnel Training Act. This legislation authorized the award of construction and improvement grants to training centers for allied health professions. It also made advanced traineeships available to allied health professionals. The Health Manpower Act of 1968 extended most of the programs for health and allied health professionals, including those for occupational therapy personnel.

Legislation supporting training in various ways continued into the 1970s (e.g., the Health Training Improvement Act of 1970, the

Comprehensive Health Manpower Training Act of 1971, and the Nurse Training Act of 1975). In the 1970s and the 1980s, however, the federal government began to limit moneys for traineeships. In 1980 the training money for the Allied Health Professions Personnel Training Act was eliminated from the federal budget. From the late 1980s to the early 1990s, the government published a number of reports that documented a shortage of allied health professionals. In 1990, moneys for the Allied Health Professions Personnel Training Act were returned to the federal budget (Elwood, 1991).

HEALTH PLANNING

By the early 1970s the government was acutely aware of the need to control costs. Several major pieces of legislation addressed that need. A 1972 amendment to the Social Security Act created professional standards review organizations. Under this scheme, associations of physicians in a geographic area reviewed professionals' activities and institutions' services to monitor and control both cost and quality. The law made it possible to give hospital utilization review committees the responsibility of carrying out these functions. Also in 1972, Congress enacted legislation giving the secretary the authority to establish limitations on Medicare reimbursements for routine services provided under Part A of Medicare (Hospital Insurance).

Two years later Congress passed the National Health Planning and Resources Development Act to ensure the development of both a national health policy and effective state and area programs of health planning and resource allocation. Under the provisions of this act, each state is divided into health service areas, and health systems agencies are designated to administer them. The agencies have three purposes:

1. To improve the health of area residents

2. To increase the accessibility, the acceptability, the continuity, and the quality of health services

3. To restrain costs and to prevent duplication of health services

In 1982, Congress enacted the Tax Equity and Fiscal Responsibility Act, which, among other provisions, extended the 1972 limits on reimbursements under Medicare to cover ancillary and rehabilitation services. Occupational therapy services are included under this provision.

In April 1983, President Ronald Reagan signed the Social Security Amendments into law, which contained a congressional mandate to alter the way in which health care was subsidized and delivered. The intent of the legislation was to impose further constraints on the level of federal spending for Medicare benefits, particularly for inpatient hospital care.

The law has basically changed the formula for disbursing health care moneys. For decades, health care relied almost exclusively on a hospital-based delivery system. On the basis of a financial formula, the payer (the federal government, an insurance company, or an individual) reimbursed hospitals for the cost of the services that they provided. Under the Medicare prospective payment system (PPS) created by the Social Security Amendments of 1983, the Health Care Financing Administration established a nationwide schedule defining the payment that the government would make for each inpatient stay by a Medicare beneficiary. The level of payment per case is determined by about 500 descriptive categories called *diagnosis-related groups* (DRGs) (*DRG Handbook,* 1994).

The PPS has had a profound effect on the development of the health care industry. It has reduced emphasis on inpatient services and expanded outpatient and community programs. Changes have occurred within both Medicare Part A (Hospital Insurance) and Medicare Part B (Supplementary Medical Insurance), some of which directly affect occupational therapy. In 1986, Congress enacted legislation expanding Medicare coverage of occupational therapy services under Part B to include "services furnished in a skilled-nursing facility (when Part A coverage has been exhausted), in a clinic, [in a] rehabilitation agency, [in a] public health agency, or by an independently practicing therapist" (*Social Security Bulletin,* 1994, p. 94). The effect of the PPS on reimbursement for rehabilitation services becomes very apparent in a comparison of Medicare Part A payments to inpatient hospitals, home health agencies, and skilled nursing facilities before and after introduction of the PPS. In 1983, Medicare paid inpatient hospitals $34.3 billion, home health agencies $1.3 billion, and skilled nursing facilities $.5 billion. In 1993 it paid inpatient hospitals $68.2 billion, about twice the 1983 figure; home health agencies $9.6 billion, about seven times the 1983 figure; and skilled nursing facilities $4.3 billion, about nine times the 1983 figure (*Social Security Bulletin,* 1994).

In 1993, following up on a campaign promise, President Bill Clinton formally introduced a health care reform bill. After many debates, however, the 103rd Congress failed to approve any health care reform bills (Rubin, 1994a & b). Comprehensive reform is now unlikely. Instead, change will probably come under the rubric of insurance reform. The type of reform expected will help persons with medical conditions obtain and keep insurance, making it easier for workers to change jobs without losing coverage (McGinley, 1995).

HUMAN RESOURCES

Providing health care requires a large number of personnel. As table 1-2 indicates, there are close to 200 occupations in health care, including many professions. New ones seem to appear continually because of innovative technology and advances in procedures that require additional specialized skills.

Table 1-2
Health Care Occupations

Field	Primary Title
Administration of health services	Assistant hospital administrator
	Assistant nursing home administrator
	Clinic manager
	Health administrative assistant
	Health agency administrator
	Health agency program representative
	Health care facility surveyor
	Health officer
	Health planner
	Health program analyst
	Health program representative
	Health systems analyst
	Hospital administrator
	Nursing home administrator
Basic sciences in the health field	Anatomist
	Biologist
	Chemist
	Epidemiologist
	Geneticist
	Immunologist
	Microbiologist
	Pathologist
	Pharmacologist
	Physicist
	Physiologist
	Scientist
	Zoologist
Biomedical engineering	Biomedical engineer
	Biomedical engineering aide
	Biomedical engineering technician
	Biomedical engineering technologist
Chiropractic	Chiropractor
Clinical laboratory services	Clinical laboratory assistant
	Clinical laboratory director
	Clinical laboratory scientist
	Clinical laboratory technician
	Clinical laboratory technologist
	Specialist in blood bank technology
Dentistry and allied services	Dental assistant
	Dental hygienist
	Dental laboratory technician
	Dentist

Dietetic and nutritional services	Dietetic assistant
	Dietetic clerical worker
	Dietetic technician
	Dietitian
	Food service worker
	Nutritionist
Economic research in the health field	Health economist
Environmental sanitation	Environmental health aide
	Environmental health technician
	Sanitarian
Food and drug protective services	Food and drug chemist
	Food and drug microbiologist
	Food technician
	Food technologist
	Health inspector
Health and vital statistics	Health demographer
	Health statistician
	Statistical assistant
	Vital record registrar
Health education	Health educator
Health information and communication	Biomedical photographer
	Draftsman
	Health information specialist
	Medical illustrator
	Medical writer
	Poster and display artist
	Science writer
	Technical writer
Library services in the health field	Medical librarian
	Medical library assistant
	Patients' librarian
Medical records	Medical record administrator
	Medical record clerk
	Medical record technician
Medicine and osteopathy	Physician
Midwifery	Lay midwife
	Nurse-midwife
Nursing and related services	Attendant
	Community health nurse
	Home health aide
	Licensed practical nurse
	Licensed vocational nurse
	Nurse-anesthetist
	Nurse-consultant
	Nurse-practitioner
	Nursing aide
	Occupational health nurse
	Orderly
	Quality assurance coordinator
	Registered nurse
	School nurse
	Transplant coordinator
Occupational therapy	Occupational therapist
	Occupational therapy aide
	Occupational therapy assistant
Opticianry	Dispensing optician
	Ophthalmic laboratory technician
	Ophthalmic medical assistant

Optometry	Optometric aide
	Optometric assistant
	Optometric technician
	Optometrist
	Orthoptist
Orthotic and prosthetic technology	Orthotic-prosthetic assistant
	Orthotic-prosthetic technician
	Orthotist
	Prosthetist
Pharmacy	Pharmacist
	Pharmacy aide
	Pharmacy assistant
	Pharmacy technician
Physical education and training	Athletic trainer
	Exercise physiologist
	Physical education instructor
	Physical integration practitioner
Physical therapy	Physical therapist
	Physical therapist aide
	Physical therapist assistant
Physician extenders	Orthop(a)edic physician assistant
	Physician assistant
	Physician extender
	Surgeon assistant
	Urologic(al) physician's assistant
Podiatric medicine	Podiatric assistant
	Podiatrist
Psychology and sociology	Psychologist
	Sociologist
Radiologic technology	Magnetic resonance imaging technologist
	Medical radiation dosimetrist
	Nuclear medicine technician
	Nuclear medicine technologist
	Radiation therapy technician
	Radiation therapy technologist
	Radiologic technician
	Radiologic technologist
Recreational therapy	Recreational therapist
	Recreational therapy aide
	Therapeutic recreational aide
	Therapeutic recreational specialist
	Therapeutic recreational technician
Respiratory therapy	Respiratory therapist
	Respiratory therapy aide
	Respiratory therapy technician
Secretarial and office services	Dental receptionist
	Dental secretary
	Dentist office assistant
	Medical receptionist
	Medical secretary
	Optometric receptionist
	Optometrist office assistant
	Physician's office assistant
Social work	Group work program aide
	Social work aide
	Social work assistant
	Social worker
	Social work technician

Special procedures	Angiogram technologist
	Cardiac catheterization technician
	Computerized tomography scan technician
Specialized rehabilitation services	Art therapist
	Corrective therapist
	Corrective therapy aide
	Dance therapist
	Educational therapist
	Home economist in rehabilitation
	Horticulture therapist
	Industrial therapist
	Manual arts therapist
	Manual arts therapist assistant
	Music therapist
	Orientation and mobility therapist for the blind
Speech pathology and audiology	Audiologist
	Speech pathologist
Veterinary medicine	Animal technician
	Veterinarian
Vocational rehabilitation counseling	Rehabilitation counselor aide
	Vocational rehabilitation counselor
Miscellaneous health services	Acupuncturist
	Cardiopulmonary technician
	Community health aide
	Dialysis technician
	Electrocardiograph technician
	Electroencephalograph technician
	Electroencephalograph technologist
	Emergency medical system manager
	Emergency medical system planner
	Emergency medical technician
	Extracorporeal circulation specialist
	Hypnotherapist
	Medical assistant
	Operating room technician
	Pheresis specialist
	Psychiatric technician

Sources. *Based on information in* The Complete Guide for Occupational Exploration, *edited by M. J. Farr, 1993, Indianapolis: JIST Works; United States Department of Labor, Employment and Training Administration, United States Employment Service,* Dictionary of Occupational Titles *(4th rev. ed.), 1991, Washington, DC: Government Printing Office; and* Health Services in the United States *(2nd rev. ed., pp. 90–92), by F. A. Wilson and D. Neuhauser, 1985, Cambridge, MA: Ballinger.*

ORGANIZATIONS PROVIDING CARE

When people think of the hospital today, they envision a sophisticated facility providing technically advanced procedures to support life and a healthful status. Hospitals, however, were not medically oriented until after the turn of the century. Initially they were facilities for persons who were indigent, and the majority of health care was delivered at home.

From the early 1900s until the early 1970s, most health care was provided and delivered in two facilities, the physician's office and the hospital. Nursing homes were mostly for custodial management, and today's concept of home health care was in its early development.

Modern health care organizations are the result of scientific developments and changes in society. Other facilities are now becoming basic to providing health services to United States citizens (Shepp, 1980). The system includes government, nonprofit, and for-profit facilities (see table 1-3).

Table 1-3
Types of Health Care Organizations

Type of Organization	General Description
Federal government	Hospitals serving disabled veterans
	Hospitals serving the armed forces and the Coast Guard
	Indian Health Service
	Public Health Service hospitals and clinics (including a leprosarium)
	Medical facilities associated with prisons
State government	Infirmaries associated with prisons and reformatories
	Hospitals for persons with mental illness
	State medical school hospitals and clinics
Local government	City hospitals and clinics
	County hospitals and public health clinics
	Rehabilitation facilities
Nonprofit organization	Charity hospitals
	Community hospitals
	Health maintenance organizations (HMOs)
	Home health facilities
	Hospices
	Industrial hospitals and clinics
	Preferred provider organizations (PPOs)
	Private teaching hospitals
	Religious hospitals
	Specialty hospitals
	Surgical centers
	Wellness centers
For-profit organization	Facilities owned by individuals or groups for the care of their own patients or clients
	Investor-owned facilities (hospitals, laboratories, nursing homes, surgical centers, rehabilitation facilities, home health facilities, HMOs, PPOs, and hospices), including corporations and management corporations
	Walk-in medical clinics

Sources. *Based on information in* Health Services in the United States *(2nd rev. ed., pp. 8–16), by F. A. Wilson and D. Neuhauser, 1985, Cambridge, MA: Ballinger; and* A Guide to Health Care Facilities: Personnel and Management *(3rd ed., pp. 16–23), by R. Sloane, 1992, Ann Arbor, MI: Health Administration Press.*

VERTICALLY ORGANIZED HOSPITALS

For years there have been methods of delivering health care services at less cost than that associated with hospitals. Hospitals have been reluctant to support these systems because under the former payment structure, they were paid for the services that they provided to hospitalized persons. The set fees under the PPS now make it economically advantageous for hospitals to move patients with long-term problems out of acute care beds into another type of health care setting as quickly as feasible. Instead of staying in the hospital, patients go to home health care, nursing facilities, hospices, designated subacute care beds, designated rehabilitation beds, designated psychiatric beds, wellness or fitness programs, outpatient surgery, day treatment for the elderly, or outpatient programs. This system has expanded both the importance and the use of the rehabilitation fields and has allowed the hospital to support these fields. Thus most hospitals are now organized in a vertical system as illustrated in figure 1-2.

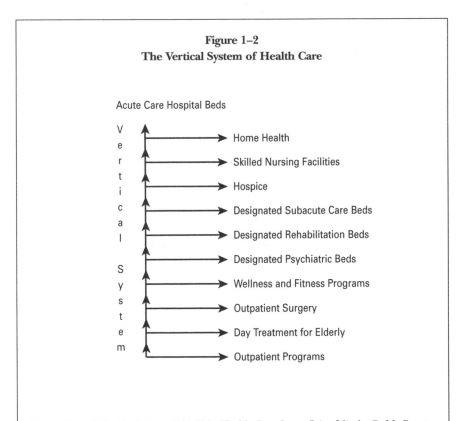

Figure 1–2
The Vertical System of Health Care

Acute Care Hospital Beds

Vertical System

Home Health
Skilled Nursing Facilities
Hospice
Designated Subacute Care Beds
Designated Rehabilitation Beds
Designated Psychiatric Beds
Wellness and Fitness Programs
Outpatient Surgery
Day Treatment for Elderly
Outpatient Programs

Note. *From "The Evolution of the U.S. Health Care System" (p. 21), by C. M. Baum, 1992, in J. Bair and M. Gray (Eds.),* The Occupational Therapy Manager *(Rev. ed.), Rockville, MD: American Occupational Therapy Association. Copyright ©1992 by the American Occupational Therapy Association, Inc.*

This organization serves the hospital well. Patients can be readmitted for necessary procedures. They and their families sense that the hospital is reaching out to meet their needs. Most important, the hospital is able to keep patients in its market by placing them in affiliated systems.

A very skillful economic strategy has created the greatest opportunity in history for rehabilitation. Nearly every one of a hospital's vertical programs requires the rehabilitation profession's skills to be effective. The challenge to the profession is to provide the human resources to staff the programs. Should occupational therapy not have the personnel, other professions will expand their roles to fill the needs.

HEALTH NETWORKS

In the changing society and economy, the freestanding hospital has become vulnerable. This has led to the formation of large health networks linking individual facilities that represent only one of several related corporate activities. The phenomenon is evident in the public sector as well as in the private sector. Since the 1970s many types of multi-institutional systems have developed, with distinct ownership and governance. They have six features in common:

1. Strong financial and organizational management

2. A well-developed market strategy

3. Built-in referral strategies to keep their use high

4. A broad geographical approach

5. An expansive model of service provision, from primary to restorative care, including home health services, ambulatory services, and skilled nursing facilities

6. Shared services for purchasing, billing, maintenance, and marketing

The trend toward large corporate systems taking over facilities with fewer than 100 beds continues in the 1990s. In a 1993 survey the American Hospital Association (1994) found that 50 percent of all hospital systems were owned by for-profit multi-institutional systems. It predicted that the majority of the remaining ones would eventually be linked as multihospital systems. According to the survey, the 18 largest alliances, based on the number of beds, included approximately one-third of the nation's hospitals.

ALTERNATIVE OR INTEGRATED DELIVERY SYSTEMS

Along with vertically organized hospitals and large health networks have come *alternative delivery systems,* more appropriately called *integrated delivery systems* because they "usually involve a significant degree of integration between payer and providers" (Weiner & de Lissovoy, 1993, p. 94). They also entail *managed care*. Some people use this term as a synonym for all kinds of integrated delivery systems, contrasting them with unmanaged fee-for-service care. More recently, however, the term frequently denotes "the entire range of utilization control tools that are applied to manage the practices of physicians and others, regardless of the setting in which they practice" (p. 97). Thus traditional insurers who have introduced various utilization controls are practicing managed care. The types of controls used to manage care include "preadmission certification, mandatory second opinion before surgery, certification of treatment plans for discretionary nonemergency services (such as mental health care), primary care physician gatekeepers, and nonphysician case managers to monitor the care of particular patients" (p. 97).

The two major types of integrated delivery systems operating in today's health care market are health maintenance organizations (HMOs) and preferred provider organizations (PPOs). An *HMO* is "a prepaid organized delivery system where the organization *and* the primary care physicians assume some financial risk for the care provided to its enrolled members" (Weiner & de Lissovoy, 1993, p. 96). Often the physicians in an HMO are periodically paid a *capitation,* that is, a fixed, preset amount for each person covered.

Prepaid health care plans have been around since the early 1900s. They began to multiply in 1973 when the federal government, faced with spiraling health costs, passed the Health Maintenance Organization Act to foster HMOs through loans and grants. In 1971 there were 39 HMOs (*HMO Fact Sheet,* 1985). In 1987 the number peaked at 662 with an enrollment of over 28.5 million. By 1992 the number had decreased to 546; the enrollment, however, had increased to nearly 41.4 million people, or 18.5 percent of the United States population (U.S. Bureau of the Census, 1994). In 1994, HMO membership exceeded over 45 million (Faltermeyer, 1994).

HMOs exist in four basic models (Weiner & de Lissovoy, 1993):

1. A *staff* or *staff-model HMO* is an HMO in which physicians on the staff care for a majority of the persons enrolled. "Although these physicians may be involved in risk-sharing arrangements, a majority of their income usually is derived from a fixed salary" (pp. 100–101).

2. A *group* or *group-model HMO* is an HMO in which "a single large multispecialty group practice is the sole (or major) source of care for [the] HMO's enrollees. The group . . . has an exclusive contract only with the one HMO. Some groups also see fee-for-service or PPO patients; others are not allowed to do so" (p. 96).

3. A *network* or *network-model HMO* is an HMO in which "two or more existing group practices have contracted to care for the majority of patients enrolled in an HMO plan. A network-model HMO sometimes also contracts with individual providers in a fashion similar to an IPA [individual practice association—see number 4]. Providers contracting with this type of HMO are usually free to serve fee-for-service patients as well as those enrolled in other HMOs and PPOs" (pp. 98–99).

4. An *independent* or *individual practice association* (IPA) is an HMO in which "individual physicians (or small group practices) contract to provide care to enrolled members. The primary care physicians may be paid by capitation, or by fee-for-service with a 'withhold' risk-sharing provision. An IPA entity may or may not be legally distinct from the HMO entity with which the member enrolls. Physicians participating in IPAs retain their right to treat non-HMO patients on a fee-for-service basis" (p. 97).

HMOs contribute significantly to lower health care costs because they provide services at little or no charge above the fixed enrollment fee that members pay. Some HMOs are *open ended,* or offer an *open-ended product line.* This arrangement allows members to obtain services from providers outside the HMO's network for additional out-of-pocket fees (e.g., a deductible and coinsurance). It is sometimes called a *point-of-service (POS) plan.* Not exclusively linked to an open-ended HMO, a POS plan "offers the consumer a choice of options at the time he or she seeks services (rather than at the time they [*sic*] choose to enroll in a health plan)" (Weiner & de Lissovoy, 1993, p. 99).

The other type of integrated delivery system, the *PPO,* developed in the 1980s. Typically organized by insurers but sometimes by providers or others (Health Insurance Association of America, 1994), the PPO

> acts as a broker between the purchaser of care and the provider . . . [C]onsumers have the option of using the "preferred" providers available within the plan, or not. Consumers are channeled towards in-plan providers by incentives and disincentives (relating to cost-sharing provisions and benefit coverage). In return for the patient referrals, providers agree that their care will be "managed." Providers are usually paid a discounted fee-for-service payment (e.g., 80 percent of their usual fee) and they do not participate in financial risk sharing. (Weiner & de Lissovoy, 1993, pp. 99–100)

There were 879 PPOs as of December 1992, with an enrollment of about 50.5 million, or 19.5 percent of the United States population (Health Insurance Association of America, 1994).

The concept of managed care has proved so successful in containing costs that many variants of managed care have evolved as large health care organizations and insurance companies compete in the marketplace for new members. As of 1992, more than 60 percent of persons with health insurance were in some form of managed care plan (Brown & Garten, 1994; Loomis, 1994). Enrollment in traditional health insurance plans of the managed indemnity or indemnity type has been steadily falling (Loomis, 1994). *Indemnity,* generally meaning security against loss, refers to the standard fee-for-service insurance policies carried by many employers, organizations, and individuals. Usually the most expensive type, this insurance covers service from any provider.

It is important for HMOs and PPOs to have good prices and high-quality services oriented to wellness and low costs. Occupational therapy products offered in HMOs and PPOs include developmental screenings, education in stress management, arthritis programs, ergonomic consultations, functional capacity evaluations, and hand-related services, among others. Some HMOs and PPOs require home health rehabilitation services. Many are eager to develop contractual relationships for a full scope of rehabilitation services. In HMOs, which require referrals, physicians, nurse-practitioners, and social workers are becoming more oriented to occupational therapy's capacity to help them save money as well as promote health. A rehabilitation organization can develop a business arrangement with an HMO to receive a set amount per month per enrollee.

PUBLIC HEALTH

The medical-industrial complex does not provide all health care services. The American Public Health Association, a voluntary organization of public health professionals, is in its second century of service to the nation. Its activities include the following (Wolman, 1973):

1. Standardization of methods (laboratory and field)

2. Control of communicable diseases

3. Establishment of housing and health criteria

4. Appraisal of health programs

5. Setting of standards for professional education

Members of the American Public Health Association work in public health systems at the local, state, and national levels. The backbone of these systems at the national level is the United States Public Health Service, the oldest agency of the United States Department of Health and Human Services. Established in 1798 as the Marine Hospital Service for the "'care and relief of sick and disabled seamen'" (U.S. Public Health Service, ca. 1988, p. 1), it was first concerned with attending to the health of merchant seamen and preventing epidemics of disease. In the late 19th century, its scope broadened to encompass biomedical research, regulation of biological products in interstate commerce, and studies of environmental hazards. In 1887 it initiated a research program called the Hygienic Laboratory, which became the National Institute (now Institutes) of Health in 1930. Under that institute's auspices, 13 specialty institutes have formed over the years. In 1889, Congress organized the Marine Hospital Service's professional personnel into a quasimilitary corps of physicians under a Surgeon General. The Marine Hospital Service took on the name United States Public Health Service in 1912. In 1946 the Communicable Disease Center, now the Centers for Disease Control and Prevention, was established. The Public Health Service now comprises five agencies: the Alcohol, Drug Abuse, and Mental Health Administration, the Centers for Disease Control and Prevention, the Food and Drug Administration, the Health Resources and Services Administration, and the National Institutes of Health.

For occupational therapy practitioners and support personnel, the public health system represents a critical link to persons who do not use the private health system because of their location or inability to pay. Public health is primarily concerned with preventing disease through public programs, but increasingly it is providing medical care to individual patients through neighborhood health centers. Despite the prevalence of health insurance coverage, by the end of the decade, the number of uninsured Americans will grow from about 37 million to an estimated 55 million, or nearly one in five Americans (Sabo, 1993). Among the uninsured are persons of all ages, incomes, geographic settings, races, and ethnic groups. According to a survey by the Employee Benefit Research Institute (Thompson, 1993), a nonprofit group in Washington, D.C., the young fare worse than the old, and the poor and the middle class worse than the well-to-do. Among adults between the ages of 21 and 24, nearly one in three is without health care coverage. Families with incomes below $15,000 make up a sizable portion of the population without coverage, at 42 percent. Surprisingly, however, families with incomes between $15,000 and $50,000 outnumber the poor. Another startling statistic is that roughly 20 million Americans who are employed are uninsured. Four million of these people work for companies with more than 1,000 employees. The lack of coverage is due to part-time employment status or preexisting health problems. Lack of health coverage among minorities varies. In 1992, 20.1 percent of African-Americans and 32.5 percent of Hispanics were uninsured (U.S. Bureau of the Census, 1994).

The Public Health Service is responsible for a number of programs of great interest to occupational therapy practitioners (see table 1-4). Voluntary organizations and foundations supplement these efforts with a multitude of programs and services (see table 1-5).

Table 1-4
Selected Programs of the United States Public Health Service

Program	Function
Alcohol, Drug Abuse, and Mental Health Administration	
National Institute of Mental Health	Conducts and supports research on mental health, funds training of new researchers, gives technical assistance, and disseminates information
National Institute on Alcohol Abuse and Alcoholism	Conducts and supports research on alcohol abuse, funds training of new researchers, gives technical assistance, and disseminates information
National Institute on Drug Abuse	Conducts and supports research on drug abuse, gives technical assistance, and disseminates information
Centers for Disease Control and Prevention	
National Center for Chronic Disease Prevention and Health Promotion	Prevents death and disability from chronic disease and promotes healthy personal behaviors
National Center for Health Statistics	Monitors health of American people, effect of illness and disability, and factors affecting health and nation's health care system
National Center for Injury Prevention and Control	Prevents and controls nonoccupational injuries
National Center for Prevention Services	Prevents and controls vaccine-preventable diseases, HIV infection, sexually transmitted diseases, tuberculosis, dental diseases, and introduction of diseases from other countries
National Institute for Occupational Safety and Health	Prevents workplace-related injuries, illnesses, and premature death from occupational hazards
Food and Drug Administration	
Center for Devices and Radiological Health	Ensures safety of medical devices
Health Resources and Services Administration	
Bureau of Health Care Delivery and Assistance	Administers programs to ensure availability and provision of health care services in medically underserved areas and to special populations
Bureau of Resources Development	Administers programs for health planning and resource allocation
Bureau of Health Professions	Coordinates, evaluates, and supports development and use of nation's health personnel
National Institutes of Health	
National Library of Medicine	Maintains database on health care
Thirteen specialty institutes	Conduct and support programs of basic and clinical research
Office of the Assistant Secretary for Health	
National Center for Health Services Research and Health Care Technology	Conducts and supports research and demonstrations on availability and provision of health care services

Sources. *Based on information in* Health Services in the United States *(2nd rev. ed., pp. 149–54), by F. A. Wilson and D. Neuhauser, 1985, Cambridge, MA: Ballinger;* CDC: Centers for Disease Control and Prevention *[Fact sheet], by CDC, 1994, May, Atlanta, GA: Author; and* Public Health Service Alcohol, Drug Abuse, and Mental Health Administration, Public Health Service Centers for Disease Control, Public Health Service Food and Drug Administration, Public Health Service Health Resources and Services Administration, Public Health Service National Institutes of Health, *and* The Public Health Service Today *[Fact sheets], by United States Public Health Service, ca. 1988, Bethesda, MD: Author.*

Table 1-5
Public Health Programs

Focus	Organization
Aging	American Aging Association
	American Association for Geriatric Psychiatry
	National Association of Home Health Agencies
Alcoholism	AL-ANON Family Group Headquarters
	American Medical Society on Alcoholism
	Friendly Hand Foundation
Alternative birth	American Association for Maternal and Child Health
	American Nurses Association
	American Society of Child Birth Educators
	Center for Humane Options in Child Birth Experiences
	Society for Obstetric Anesthesia and Perinatology
Arthritis	American Lupus Society
	American Rheumatism Association
	Arthritis Foundation
Battered women	Abused Women's Aid in Crisis
	Feminist Alliance Against Rape
	National Organization for Women
	United Scleroderma Foundation
	Women Against Violence Against Women
	Women in Transition
Blindness, impaired vision	American Association of Ophthalmology
	American Foundation for the Blind
	Better Vision Institute
Burn injuries	American Burn Association
	International Society for Burn Injuries
	Phoenix Society
	Shriner's Hospital for Crippled Children
Cancer	American Association for Cancer Education
	American Cancer Society
	Breast Cancer Advisory Center
	Concern for Dying
	International Association of Cancer Victims and Friends
Cystic fibrosis	Cystic Fibrosis Foundation
	National Genetics Foundation
Deafness, impaired hearing	Acoustical Society of America
	American Deafness and Rehabilitation Association
	Council for Exceptional Children
	Hear Center
	National Association of the Deaf
Drug abuse	Do It Now Foundation
	Families Anonymous
	International Association for Psychiatric Research
	PIL-ANON Family Program
Eye tissue for transplant	Eye Bank Association of America
	Lions Club International

Family planning	Americans United for Life
	Choice
	Family Planning International Assistance
	National Abortion Federation
	Planned Parenthood Federation of America
Genetic services	American Brittle Bone Society
	American Genetic Association of Medicine
	Arthrogryposis Association
	Association for Children with Learning Disabilities
	Muscular Dystrophy Association
	Spina Bifida Association
Hemophilia	American Association of Blood Banks
	National Hemophilia Foundation
Home health care	Home Health Services Association
	National Homecaring Council
Hospice care	American Association of Suicidology
	American Euthanasia Foundation
Mental health	Academy of Psychosomatic Medicine and Services
	American Academy of Child Psychiatry
	American Psychiatric Association
Multiple sclerosis	American Red Cross
	National Multiple Sclerosis Society
Muscular dystrophy	Muscular Dystrophy Association
	Myasthenia Gravis Foundation
	National Ataxia Foundation
Pain	Acupuncture International Association
	American Chiropractic Association
	National Spinal Cord Injury Foundation
Preventive medicine	Healthy America
	International Health Evaluation Association
Rehabilitation	American Association for Rehabilitation Therapy
	American Deafness and Rehabilitation Association
	American Occupational Therapy Association
	American Physical Therapy Association
	National Easter Seal Society
Sickle-cell anemia	National Association for Sickle Cell Disease
Smoking	American Cancer Society
	American Heart Association
	American Lung Association
Spinal cord injury	American Spinal Injury Association
	National Easter Seal Society
	National Spinal Cord Injury Foundation
Sports medicine	American Alliance for Health, Physical Education, Recreation, and Dance
Sudden infant death syndrome	International Council for Infant Survival
	National Sudden Infant Death Syndrome Foundation

Source. *Based on information in* Health Services Directory, *1981, by Anthony T. Kruzas, Detroit, MI: Gale Research.*

THE EVOLUTION OF OCCUPATIONAL THERAPY

Historians of occupational therapy have begun to document the evolution of its theories and concepts of occupation. Christiansen and Baum (1991), Hopkins and Smith (1994), and Quiroga (1995) offer an important complement to the contemporary picture of occupational therapy and should be studied in concert with this chapter.

Trends in the supply and the distribution of occupational therapy practitioners offer another perspective. In regard to supply, the profession swelled by 41,000 between 1970 and 1984—"more than entered the profession in all its previous years combined" (AOTA, 1983–84, p. 17). During the 1970s the growth rate was 9–10 percent per year. In the mid-1980s it slowed to 5 percent, apparently because of a stabilization of output from occupational therapy education programs. The 1990s have seen the growth rate rise to about 7 percent, on average, influenced by an increase in the number of therapists prepared outside the United States (Mindy Hecker, personal communication, December 1995). There have never been more registered occupational therapists (OTRs) or certified occupational therapy assistants (COTAs) in the United States than there were in 1995: 48,736 and 13,087 respectively (AOTA, 1995).

Between 1991 and 1993 the number of graduating occupational therapists grew by 22 percent, and the number of graduating occupational therapy assistants, by 26 percent. In 1992 there were 3,000 new occupational therapists and 1,300 new occupational therapy assistants. These numbers are expected to increase as the more than 185 already accredited education programs for occupational therapists and occupational therapy assistants graduate increasing numbers of students annually, and as new educational programs form across the nation. As of August 1995 there were 257 programs in the accreditation process (including the 185 already accredited, some of which were undergoing review for renewal). A restraint on the growth of these programs might occur, however, because of a shortage of qualified occupational therapy faculty and educational program directors (AOTA, Managers' Notes, August 1995; Silvergleit, 1994).

The dramatic increase in supply has not kept pace with the demand for occupational therapy practitioners. An analysis of the geographic distribution of AOTA members per 100,000 people reveals the most severe shortages of OTRs to be in the Virgin Islands (only 2,000 per 100,000 people, or 2.0%), Puerto Rico (2.3%), West Virginia (4.0%), and Mississippi (5.3%), and the most severe shortages of COTAs to be in Mississippi (0.6%), West Virginia (0.8%), Arkansas (0.8%), Nebraska (0.8%), Kentucky (0.8%), Louisiana (0.9%), Utah (0.9%), and New Mexico (0.9%) (AOTA, 1995).

The growth in the number of occupational therapy practitioners has been accompanied by some changes in the distribution of practitioners across practice settings. Table 1-6 presents data on the numbers and the percentages of OTRs and COTAs in various employment settings at four- or five-year intervals from 1973 through 1990. Data were not available before 1973.

Table 1-6

Primary Employment Settings of OTRs and COTAs, 1973–1990

OTRs

Setting	1973	1977	1982	1986	1990
College, two-year	1.4%	1.2%	0.8%	0.7%	0.6%
College/university, four-year	5.6	4.9	4.1	3.1	3.4
Community mental health center	4.2	4.3	2.4	1.6	1.1
Correctional institution	0.2	0.2	0.1	0.1	—
Day-care center/program	1.4	1.1	1.0	1.1	0.9
General hospital—neonatal intensive care unit	—	—	—	—	0.7
General hospital—psychiatric unit	—	—	—	—	3.5
General hospital—rehabilitation unit	—	—	—	4.2	5.3
General hospital—all other	20.5	19.8	25.3	22.0	15.9
HMO (including PPO/IPA)	0.3	0.2	0.2	0.3	0.4
Home health agency	0.9	2.2	3.8	4.6	3.6
Hospice	—	—	0.0	0.1	0.0
Outpatient clinic (freestanding)	—	—	2.5	2.4	3.7
Pediatric hospital	2.9	2.0	1.6	1.7	1.7
Physician's office	—	—	—	1.1	1.2
Private industry	—	—	0.7	0.5	0.8
Private practice	1.3	2.1	3.5	6.0	7.7
Psychiatric hospital	13.8	11.2	7.4	6.9	4.6
Public health agency	1.6	1.5	0.8	0.9	0.9
Rehabilitation hospital/center	13.4	10.9	8.9	10.5	11.4
Research facility	0.3	0.3	0.4	0.2	0.2
Residential care facility including group home, independent living center	—	4.4	4.2	3.3	2.7
Retirement or senior center	—	—	—	0.2	0.2
School system (including private school)	11.0	14.0	18.3	17.0	18.6
Sheltered workshop	0.7	0.7	0.7	0.4	0.4
Skilled nursing home/intermediate care facility	6.2	7.9	6.0	5.8	6.4
Vocational or prevocational program	0.7	0.5	—	—	—
Voluntary agency (e.g., Easter Seal, United Cerebral Palsy)	—	1.7	1.7	1.4	1.0
Other	14.2	9.4	5.4	3.2	2.5
Total	99.9%	100.0%	99.8%	100.0%	99.9%

COTAs

Setting	1973	1977	1982	1986	1990
College, two-year	0.8%	0.9%	0.6%	0.8%	0.9%
College/university, four-year	0.7	0.6	0.9	0.3	0.3
Community mental health center	4.0	3.5	3.1	3.8	1.7
Correctional institution	0.3	0.2	0.1	0.2	—

Day-care center/program	1.2	2.4	2.0	4.3	1.7
General hospital—neonatal intensive care unit	—	—	—	—	0.1
General hospital—psychiatric unit	—	—	—	—	4.0
General hospital—rehabilitation unit	—	—	—	4.5	5.5
General hospital—all other	15.1	12.7	17.8	14.1	9.4
HMO (including PPO/IPA)	0.7	0.3	0.3	0.2	0.1
Home health agency	0.2	0.4	0.8	1.2	1.5
Hospice	—	—	0.0	0.0	0.0
Outpatient clinic (freestanding)	—	—	1.7	0.9	2.2
Pediatric hospital	1.5	1.2	0.8	0.4	0.7
Physician's office	—	—	—	0.2	0.3
Private industry	1.0	0.5	0.7	—	—
Private practice	0.3	0.4	1.2	1.9	2.7
Psychiatric hospital	22.6	14.3	9.7	8.4	6.6
Public health agency	0.5	0.5	0.3	0.4	0.6
Rehabilitation hospital/center	9.5	11.0	8.4	8.4	10.9
Research facility	0.2	0.3	0.1	0.0	0.2
Residential care facility including group home, independent living center	—	8.5	7.6	7.5	5.9
Retirement or senior center	—	—	—	1.1	0.8
School system (including private school)	3.6	6.2	11.3	14.4	17.0
Sheltered workshop	1.4	0.9	1.9	1.6	1.6
Skilled nursing home/intermediate care facility	22.8	26.1	22.5	20.1	20.1
Vocational or prevocational program	—	—	—	1.6	0.8
Voluntary agency (e.g., Easter Seal, United Cerebral Palsy)	—	0.4	1.2	1.2	1.1
Other	14.7	9.3	6.7	2.3	2.3
Total	100.1%	100.1%	100.0%	100.0%	99.8%

Note. *Missing data are due to changing employment categories on the various administrations of the surveys. Recoding of additional settings from the Other category to existing alternatives may explain the decline in the Other category. For this reason, small differences in the percentages over time should be interpreted with care. The percentages contained in this report, with the exception of the demographic and educational information, represent only the individuals who responded to the AOTA Member Data Survey. They do not include the occupational therapy personnel who chose not to answer and return the survey. From* 1990 Member Data Survey, *by American Occupational Therapy Association, Member Services, 1990, Rockville, MD: Author.*

The data on OTRs reveal the following:

- Moderate to major increases in the percentages in home health agencies, outpatient clinics (freestanding), private practice, and school systems

- Emergence of OTRs in the general hospital settings of neonatal intensive care units, psychiatric units, and rehabilitation units; also in physicians' offices and retirement or senior centers

- A relatively stable percentage in HMOs

- Moderate to major decreases in the percentages in college or university settings, community mental health centers, correctional institutions, day-care centers and programs, psychiatric hospitals, rehabilitation hospitals and centers, residential care facilities, and vocational or prevocational programs

With respect to COTAs, Carr (1993) observes,

> COTAs were trained initially to work in psychiatric hospital practice settings and then in nursing homes and other general medical settings. Many still work in those facilities. The dispersion of COTAs into nontraditional settings came about, not because of training, but because of federal legislation. (p. 26)

There are many similarities between OTRs and COTAs in patterns of distribution across practice settings. COTAs have increased their percentages in the same settings identified earlier for OTRs, have emerged in the same new settings, and have seen their percentages decrease in most of the same settings as OTRs, plus HMOs.

In 1995, 90 percent of OTRs and COTAs were employed, and the future looked good for new graduates. However, the increasing supply of occupational therapy practitioners had yet to meet the increasing demand for occupational therapy services. Therefore it will be important to continue to track changes in the distribution of OTRs and COTAs as a measure of occupational therapy's ability to relate to the changing health care system (Silvergleit, 1994).

SUMMARY OF THE CURRENT HEALTH CARE SYSTEM

Tracing the federal government's role in the evolution of health care shows the current situation in perspective:

- The government built the facilities.
- The government supported training of the human resources.
- The government pays a large portion of health care costs.
- The government supports research.
- The government has been unsuccessful in controlling costs.
- The government is responsible for providing care when persons do not have access to health insurance.

The health care system faces these problems:

- Too many specialized physicians and a geographic maldistribution of physicians in general
- Potential loss of the close relationship between practitioners and patients and clients

- Too many hospital beds
- Too many professionals competing for increasingly limited dollars
- Too few rehabilitation professionals
- More persons with chronic conditions
- An expanding aging population
- The need to find a balance between quality and quantity of life as a result of medical advances

The health care system is at a crossroads. The public and private sectors must deal with these problems. The public is demanding accountability for and outcomes from health care. Where do the system and occupational therapy go from here?

THE FUTURE

Following are some projections of the outcomes of current trends and some opinions about roles and opportunities for occupational therapy practitioners and support personnel relative to them. Every year AOTA publishes *Trends in the Environment,* a summary of important trends, information, and issues in occupational therapy, the general health care field, and society. A valuable adjunct to this chapter, *Trends* can give the occupational therapy manager and practitioner a sense of the health care environment for strategic planning purposes. Table 1-7 provides a sample of the types of trends described in the 1995 edition of *Trends.*

ECONOMICS

Economists continue to influence the delivery of health care. They believe that the constant threat of competition and the daily struggle to protect his or her program may bring out the best in the provider. The health care industry has adopted the concepts and the practices basic to competition, and the government is stimulating competition to control costs. This means that successful programs will flourish and those not able to keep pace in the marketplace will fail. More mergers will occur as health networks are established, and there will be a much greater emphasis on HMOs. A competitive market can be described as a social arrangement whereby life is made difficult for providers so that consumers will have access to reasonably priced services.

Consumers themselves have a direct financial stake in health care. *Copayment* requires them to pay a portion of health care costs out-of-pocket. It will be very important to keep occupational therapy services defined in such a way that consumers as well as third-party payers will be eager to purchase them.

Table 1-7
Types of Trends in the Environment, 1995

Health Care

Within a short period of time, managed care may become the dominant form of health care delivery and financing. Managed care now includes almost any form of coverage that limits enrollees' ability to select their own provider throughout the health care system.

Source: *Hospitals,* April 5, 1993, pp. 18–23

Managed care is affecting the field of mental health. The services for adults, children, and adolescents decreased 2 to 7 percent in hospital inpatient psychiatric settings, said a survey done in 1988–1990. However, there has been an increase in outpatient programs for adolescents and children. Also, more inpatient eating disorder and geriatric programs have been developed.

Source: *AHA News,* May 17, 1993, vol. 29, no. 20

The Congressional Budget Office reported that managed care would leave national health care costs around the same level, but would allow an increase in coverage for Americans.

Source: *The Washington Post,* February 3, 1993

Patient-centered care, which redesigns how hospital resources are used, is becoming more popular at hospitals. The philosophy of patient-centered care involves centering personnel and resources around the patient instead of around specialized departments. Tenets of this type of system include cross-training of professionals, decentralization of services, and work redesign. Collaboration between the professionals is intensified.

Source: *Hospitals,* February 5, 1993, pp. 14–19

Disease and Disability

Americans stated they believed they had a 16 percent chance of becoming disabled for three or more months during their working lives in a Gallup poll. According to Unum Corporation, the actual chances for women are 54 percent and 43 percent for men.

Source: *Wall Street Journal,* date unknown

Eighty percent of people who have borderline high blood pressure could develop conditions over twenty years that lead to heart failure or strokes. Doctors should treat systolic hypertension earlier.

Source: *The Washington Post,* December 23, 1993

The elderly can learn if they are at risk for developing Alzheimer's disease or similar forms of dementia by taking a series of standardized psychological tests.

Source: *The Washington Post,* August 30, 1994

Education

More than 4 percent of students (2.8% males, 5.2% females, 4.3% business, and 6.2% nursing) said that therapy (physical, speech, or occupational) was their probable major field of study.

Source: *Chronicle of Higher Education,* January 13, 1993

ETS allowed disabled students to take the SAT only in March, which did not give these students the same equal opportunity as nondisabled students, and only a limited number of exams were available in large type, on cassette, or in Braille.

Source: *The Washington Post,* April 2, 1994

The following disabilities were found when college students were surveyed: speech .3%, hearing .9%, learning 2.1%, orthopedic 1.1%, health-related 1.5%, partially sighted or blind 2.2%, other 1.5%.

Source: *Chronicle of Higher Education,* January 13, 1993

People are utilizing the ADA laws to fight to get colleges and universities to offer athletic opportunities to students with disabilities since most schools do not do so.

Source: *Chronicle of Higher Education,* May 18, 1994

Society

According to the Employee Benefit Research Institute, almost 39 million Americans were uninsured in 1992. This is more than 15 percent of the population, and the primary reason for this lack of insurance is due to a decline in employer-based coverage.

Source: *AHA News,* February 7, 1994, p. 4

An estimated 10 to 15 percent of all workers are involved for taking care of their aging relatives, which makes elderly care the number one dependent-care issue for employees.

Source: *USA Today,* July 19, 1994

Affordable, quality day-care facilities for children are difficult to find due to the storage of them. More then one-third of children under six are watched by people other than their parents, and a third of those are in unregulated facilities.

Source: *The Washington Post,* March 19, 1993

Less than half of all Americans say they understand the terms HMO network (44%), preferred provider (36%), fee for service (34%), managed care (21%), universal access (19%), and health alliance (14%), which are used in health care.

Source: *USA Today,* August 23, 1994

Trends and Top-10 List

Futurists predict (1) continuation of specializations and computer literacy; (2) higher-level skilled employees will replace lower-level skilled employees in acute care; (3) downsizing will continue; (4) the structure and teamwork in organizations will flatten.

Source: *Hospital & Health Networks,* September 20, 1994, p. 14

Note. *Excerpted from* Trends in the Environment, *compiled by American Occupational Therapy Association, Research Information & Evaluation Department, 1995, January 20, Bethesda, MD: Author. Copyright ©1995 American Occupational Therapy Association, Inc.*

COST CONTAINMENT

Since the early 1980s, medical care items have been increasing 1.9 to 5.6 percentage points more than all items in the Consumer Price Index (U.S. Bureau of the Census, 1994). From 1960 to 1994, expenditures for health care rose from 5.3 percent of the gross domestic product to 13.9 percent (Burner & Waldo, 1995; Levit et al., 1994). The spiraling costs have generated proposals for health care reform and many containment practices, among them, alternatives to inpatient care such as ambulatory or outpatient care; self-insurance; greater emphasis on *utilization review* (that is, independent review of providers' performance to validate quality of care); adherence to DRGs; elimination of redundancy in services; formation of medical service alliances; merger of insurance providers, hospitals, and health care organizations; and the range of utilization control tools known as managed care.

These cost-containment practices, managed care in particular, are having a profound effect on organizational structures and, in turn, on clinical practice. To contain costs and compete successfully for managed care contracts, provider organizations are compressing their structures, cutting their staffs, and reorganizing their way of doing business. In the latter respect they are taking cues from managed care companies' basic expectations:

- Competitive pricing

- Availability of a network/system of care [incorporating the idea of] one-stop shopping [and] a full continuum of care or menu services

- Easy access to all parts of the system . . .

- Seamless transition between all aspects of the system

- Consistent, concise, functionally oriented documentation

- A key contact person for any problems or concerns

(Freda, 1995, p. 1)

Another significant organizational change is the emergence of a new role, *case manager.* "Case management evolved in order to maximize health care expenditures by allocating resources to the most appropriate and effective care" (Fisher, 1995, p. 1). The *external case manager,* an employee of a managed care company, functions as a watch dog or a medical ombudsman, coordinating the care received by the company's members or policyholders, typically the most expensive cases. External case managers are usually registered nurses or social workers (Weiner & de Lissovoy, 1993). They are expected to control the cost of services and the length of services, in the context of the most appropriate outcome (Fisher, 1995). The *internal case manager* functions as a liaison between clinical staff and the external case manager. This person is usually a clinician and frequently a practitioner providing services to the patient whose case he or she is managing. Internal case managers rarely control the cost of services; their role is to explain the need for the services (Fisher, 1995).

The organizational changes necessitated by managed care are having extensive ramifications in clinical practice. First, they have reinforced the trend begun by the PPS toward shorter lengths of stay in hospitals and more provision of services outside the traditional hospital—not just in outpatient facilities and homes, but of late, in day treatment programs and designated subacute care beds. As noted earlier, this shift represents an opportunity for occupational therapy, and for the rehabilitation field in general.

Second, external case managers, not physicians or clinicians, are deciding how much of a specific service a patient will receive. This and other aspects of managed care's increasing presence in the health care marketplace present challenges to clinical practice. Occupational therapy managers and practitioners are finding themselves "negotiating, arguing, and justifying their services" to external case managers (Freda, 1995, p. 1). Moreover, these case managers

> are requiring frequent progress reports for their patients and in many situations will only authorize a small number of sessions at a time. Continuation of clinical services will depend on the actual progress of the patient towards the goals the case manager feels arc appropriate. (p. 1)

The occupational therapy manager or practitioner must strive to understand the external case manager's perspective and responsibility on any given case and collaborate with him or her to ensure that both parties achieve their objectives.

Occupational therapy managers and practitioners are also finding themselves interacting with internal case managers, or taking on the role themselves. In the first instance, again they must collaborate; in the other instance they must learn new skills.

Third, there is a much greater use of aides and technicians in occupational therapy departments because they are less expensive. This includes use of cross-trained, multiskilled aides (see the later section Cross-Training Initiatives). The number of professional staff members relative to the number of nonprofessional staff members is decreasing, and professional staff members are doing more supervising than before. Using COTAs has traditionally been cost-effective. New models of service provision pair an OTR and a COTA to treat a larger caseload than the two can carry working independently; an OTR with an occupational therapy aide to see two or three patients in "individual" sessions; and a COTA with an occupational therapy aide to conduct group sessions. There is also a greater mix of group and individual treatment sessions (Freda, 1995). Another cost-cutting measure to consider is having occupational therapy practitioners teach caregivers (e.g., family members) to carry out certain services that do not call for professional or paraprofessional skills.

The more widespread use of aides and technicians is requiring that managers and practitioners develop statements of appropriate competencies, improve the orientation given to new personnel, and plan and implement inservice training for support personnel already on the job. "Clear, definitive boundaries and role delineation are needed to guarantee quality care" (Freda, 1995, p. 2). Moreover, all the models, old and new, call for careful collaboration among personnel and appropriate supervision by OTRs and COTAs (AOTA, 1995a, 1995b; see also appendix 9-A).

Fourth, in the era of managed care, expectations for documentation are very specific: It must "be timely, [be] integrated for multiple services, be functionally oriented, speak to specific goal attainment, give a specific plan and time line for goal attainment, [and] give a very accurate 'snapshot' of the patient" (Freda, 1995, p. 3). *Critical pathways* or *care maps* have thus become an essential type of record. They are

> an indication of the course of patient treatment on a time line, with an outcome orientation, and with prompts for a multidisciplinary staff to perform certain interventions so that costs are contained and quality, as defined by the consumers, is assured. (Underwood, 1995)

> The pathways/maps give the opportunity to record variances from the expected course of treatment. They also furnish managed care companies [with] very clear information on the product they are considering purchasing and what can be expected in a predetermined length of time. (Freda, 1995, p. 3)

Finally, the increased reliance on aides and technicians is calling for enhancement of practitioners' competence in supervision, particularly the ability to recognize when they should intervene in treatment or reassess a patient's condition. Enhancement of competence in documentation is also imperative.

All this change has significant implications for the occupational therapy manager. First, the manager must be aware that the change is occurring. Then he or she must organize staff members to respond with careful planning, implementation, and evaluation. The competitive market plan guarantees that costs will continue to be the topic of debate in health care provision. On a daily basis, occupational therapy managers and practitioners must be knowledgeable about the realities of cost considerations for both patients and clients and employers. Consumers and insurers will continue to scrutinize the types of diagnoses rendered, the types of treatments and evaluations provided, to whom they are provided, the settings in which they are provided, the duration of treatments, and the effectiveness of treatments in bringing about functional performance. The question will be asked, What can be expected from this expenditure? To provide information on the importance of their services, occupational therapy managers and practitioners must integrate quality improvement concepts into daily activities and document program effectiveness. They must employ standard and reliable measures to show functional changes in the occupational performance of patients and clients. Mere generalizations about occupational performance will not demonstrate the necessity for services.

Chapter 2, "Strategic Planning," and chapter 8, "Management of Rapid Change," offer managers especially helpful information about surveillance and analysis of their environments. Chapter 12, "Evaluation of Program," provides guidance in using program evaluation and quality improvement techniques to determine the effectiveness and the efficiency of clinical procedures. It also explains the elements of timely, functionally oriented documentation specifying short- and long-term goals.

Adjustments must also occur in support systems. Because of the heightened expectations for productivity, practitioners are busier than they were before. To be successful, they need support from the various systems of the organization—for example, adequate space for the increased number of patients whom practitioners must see at the same time and orientation of patients to the new models of service provision (Freda, 1995).

With cost containment as a mandate for the health care industry, the philosophy of wellness is becoming increasingly important to all in the health care equation: consumers, providers, and the federal government. If people stay well, everyone benefits. This emphasis is consistent with occupational therapy's goal of optimal function in occupational performance areas.

INCLUSION OF OCCUPATIONAL THERAPY SERVICES IN MANAGED CARE PLANS

Managers in managed care organizations conduct utilization review. "Utilization review has become the standard method by which payors monitor provider performance" (Foto & Swanson, 1993, p. 123). Managed care systems encourage or require their enrollees to use the selected providers. Unfortunately some managed care organizations and health insurers can and do engage in discriminatory practices that deny consumers access to a variety of health professionals, including occupational therapy practitioners. Some proposals for health care reform would broaden managed care coverage in both enrollment and service. Any reform should prohibit arbitrary exclusion of entire classes or types of professionals from provider panels and networks; it should also require managed care organizations to meet specific criteria ensuring a sufficient number, mix, and distribution of health care providers within their network to meet the diverse needs of consumers and to give consumers the option of choosing a specialist as their gatekeeper within the health plan (Somers & Browne, 1994, p. 3).

Insurance companies and health care providers have consolidated to provide improved managed care ("Blue Shield, Unihealth," 1993). During the last two decades there has been a steady increase in the number of privately insured Americans covered by managed care plans. As of 1992, HMOs or PPOs covered about 40 percent of the United States population (U.S. Bureau of the Census, 1994), and as of 1993, HMOs, PPOs, and POSs held 51 percent of the market among insured people (Health Insurance Association of America, 1994). Financial coverage from HMOs and PPOs, as well as other private group insurance, Medicaid, and Medicare, is accepted by major rehabilitation centers throughout the country. Industry is setting up its own rehabilitation programs to manage catastrophic conditions such as head injury and spinal cord injury. Within 10 years the major rehabilitation organizations may either be linked contractually to the insurance industry or be replaced by facilities directly managed by the insurer.

Occupational therapy managers and practitioners need to prove that their products are both essential and cost-effective to the hospital, the physician, the patient or client, and business and industry. They must pinpoint their area of expertise. Otherwise, consumers may look to other, more cost-effective sources.

COMPETITION

Occupational therapy practitioners and other health care professionals are competing for a shrinking health care dollar. Improving function, which has long been the mission of occupational therapy, is being used by other professionals in documentation as a means to receive third-party payment. Now more than ever, occupational therapy practitioners must know and be able to articulate the unique contributions of the profession. Increasing the public's awareness of the varied services of occupational therapy will aid in marketing those services.

Educating the government is equally important. One way to do this is to write to legislators explaining the mission of occupational therapy and the importance of including it in any comprehensive health care plan (Scott & Somers, 1992).

CROSS-TRAINING INITIATIVES

Cross-training is the preparation of a person in one profession to perform skills typically associated with another profession. A *multiskilled practitioner* is a person from one profession who has established competence in specific skills usually associated with another profession. As indicated earlier, current workforce shortages and economic pressures have precipitated a growing movement by hospitals and other providers to use more aides and other noncredentialed personnel in the provision of services. There are also efforts or proposals to develop cross-training programs, and state hospital associations and others are pressing state legislatures to deregulate practice acts, which apply to health care professionals whom they employ. Initiatives along these lines could range from amendments to practice acts that would relax requirements for supervision of personnel, to proposals for much broader modification of licensure laws, substituting some form of *institutional licensure,* or credentialing of a facility, that would allow the facility's administration to determine necessary staff qualifications and composition. Such efforts would seriously threaten the legal framework that state associations and AOTA have constructed over the last two decades (Somers & Browne, 1994, p. 2).

Occupational Therapy and Cross Training Initiatives, a White Paper published by AOTA, responds to the cross-training initiatives at institutional, local, state, and national levels. It proposes limiting the scope of cross-training to "(a) certified occupational therapy practitioners who are learning skills typically associated with other professions; and (b) certified [occupational therapy] practitioners who are teaching occupational therapy skills to others" (AOTA, Intercommission Council, 1995, p. 1).

ADDITIONAL PAYMENT SOURCES

In the past, rehabilitation organizations and professionals expected payment from medical insurance providers. This will continue to be true for chronic medical problems causing disability. However, other disabling conditions are the result of work, home, and automobile accidents, which are covered by liability insurance. The insurance industry has recognized the cost-benefit potential of comprehensive models of rehabilitation that help a person acquire skills to function at a community level and become employed. This recognition has been the impetus for occupational therapy practitioners to move out of the medical model and provide their products in a variety of environments.

BUSINESS AND INDUSTRY

Work-related injuries in the United States have increased to epidemic proportions in the past decade. In the coming decade, business will spend billions of dollars on medical expenses, disability compensation, and lost productivity. Costs associated with work-related injuries can be controlled through the use of ergonomics and management strategies. *Ergonomics* is "an applied science concerned with designing and arranging things people use so that the people and things interact most efficiently and safely" (*Merriam-Webster's*, 1993, p. 393). "It focuses on the study of work performance with an emphasis on workers' safety and productivity" (Rice, 1995, p. 5). Occupational therapy practitioners are users of ergonomic principles, providing products such as work-site analysis not only to rehabilitate workers with illness or injury but to assist business and industry in organizing and designing the workplace to prevent costly accidents and illnesses. Occupational therapists have been active in designing and implementing work-injury prevention programs in collaboration with managers and employees. Outcomes measures from successful programs can be used as a marketing strategy to validate the efficacy of occupational therapy.

APPLICATION OF TECHNOLOGY

The capability of advanced medical technology to save and extend the lives of persons who have sustained injuries or illnesses such as stroke, traumatic brain injury, and spinal cord injury, has changed the rehabilitation population that occupational therapy personnel serve. To optimize the functional performance of persons with disabilities, occupational therapy practitioners must be competent in using low and high technology and in integrating it into occupational performance (Hammel, 1993).

The rehabilitation field is just beginning to benefit from major technological advances. For example, interactive driving simulators that assess the driving abilities of persons with impairments (from stroke, aging, etc.) and help rehabilitate them have become marketable. Other forms of technology are also being researched to determine which motions contribute to the development of cumulative trauma disorders. This information may prove invaluable for preventive health care in high-risk populations. The use of computer applications, environmental adaptations, and implanted computers to control motions and bodily functions has increased. For example, assistive devices can improve quality of life for persons with a high spinal-cord lesion. Examples of technological devices that enhance a person's ability to communicate and interact with others include software that speeds up keystroke input, devices that convert text to speech, and devices that synthesize speech (Platt & Fraser, 1993).

Occupational therapy managers and practitioners must stay informed about and be involved in research that links technology to occupational performance. One way to do this is to join AOTA's Technology Special Interest Section (TSIS). Another avenue is to use the Internet, a worldwide electronic web that allows for international networking and provides name directories, file archives, databases, and conferencing. This is one developing resource that all occupational therapy practitioners should use.

RECOGNITION FOR OCCUPATIONAL THERAPY IN HEALTH CARE

The strategy in a competitive environment is to streamline efforts and direct them to doing the best job possible. For occupational therapy practitioners, this means helping patients and clients acquire the skills that they need to function at their maximum level and return to a degree of independence with a choice of acceptable options in performing everyday activities. What occupational therapy does must be very visible and easily marketable (see chapter 4, "Marketing"). The profession will have to describe its services as products—for example, driving program, work evaluation, seating and mobility clinic, and life skills program. These labels will make the services easier to understand and will assist purchasers in understanding the results.

Society is demanding accountability for its dollars. What occupational therapy practitioners offer to the health care system is gaining increased recognition for many reasons:

1. The public is more accepting of the roughly 20 percent of Americans who have disabling conditions. AOTA and occupational therapy practitioners were pivotal in passage and implementation of the Americans with Disabilities Act (ADA).

2. Chronic disease affects nearly 20 percent of the American public. The epidemic of AIDS (acquired immunodeficiency syndrome) continues to spread; 45,472 cases were reported in the United States in 1992 (U.S. Bureau of the Census, 1994).

3. Head trauma has become a social problem, and head trauma rehabilitation requires occupational therapy intervention. Every year there are 500,000 hospitalizations due to head injuries, and the annual cost of care per person is $100,000. A method for paying or distributing the cost of care for such people is needed.

4. As the current population ages, occupational therapy practitioners will continue providing programs to increase independence and maintain function in the elderly, thus decreasing the costs of long-term health management. In 1992, persons 65 years old or older constituted 12.6 percent of the nation's population (U.S. Bureau of the Census, 1994).

5. The change to the PPS has raised the consciousness of all providers to the fact that some people do not fit within the norm for care and that society has a responsibility to them.

6. Occupational therapy practitioners have become more active in the workplace because of the increased incidence of cumulative trauma disorders (e.g., carpal tunnel syndrome) and chronic back problems. In 1990 an average of 84 work days per 100 employees was lost because of occupational injury and illness (U.S. Department of Labor, 1993).

7. Wellness and prevention are values inherent in the practice of occupational therapy.

OPPORTUNITY

Over the years the role of occupational therapy has evolved, and even greater change may be imminent. This is a very important time for occupational therapy. With the expansion of home health care organizations, the increased role of skilled nursing facilities as rehabilitation settings for the elderly, the establishment of comprehensive outpatient rehabilitation facilities, and employers' emphasis on returning the injured person to gainful employment, occupational therapy practitioners are in demand. Health care organizations need the profession's services to increase and maintain their market. The profession must respond with confidence that it is giving the people whom it serves the opportunity to gain meaningful lives. The situation is not unlike that when the founders of occupational therapy sought to bring a humanness and a new morality to a system that did not place an acceptable level of effort on supporting human potential.

Occupational therapy's development has not been easy. Participating in the growth and the evolution of an organized, complex system never is. The profession is now ready to assume a responsible role in offering support and direction as that system struggles to be effective. It is critical that occupational therapy practitioners understand why assuming this role is difficult, and know that with specific knowledge and skills, and with a strong commitment to the profession's potential contribution, patients and clients and society as a whole will benefit.

SUMMARY

Because of rising costs, a growing emphasis on outcomes and accountability, a lack of services to meet specific needs, an imbalance of services for different populations of the society, and advances in medical technology, the health care industry has become the object of scrutiny by the government and the public. In the past the health care system was described in terms of health problems. Today health care is cast in economic terms.

Health care costs in 1994 were $983.3 billion, and government's share of the expense was $420.2 billion.

The basis for much of the government's involvement in health care is the concept of the right to health, which has been present in political thought at least since 1796. Related to this concept is the matter of ethics. Limits may increasingly be placed on health services for moral as well as economic reasons, as ethical issues are raised about the technology available to create, maintain, and prolong life.

The federal government has made many significant contributions to health care since the mid-1940s through support of construction of facilities, training of personnel, and planning of health systems. By the early 1970s it was acutely aware of the need to control costs, and several pieces of major legislation followed. A new system of payment for hospital services to Medicare beneficiaries was introduced, which has had a profound effect on the health care field.

Providing health care requires a large number of personnel. There are now close to 200 occupations in health care, including many professions. Also, organizations providing care have diversified greatly. Most hospitals are now organized in a vertical system. The freestanding hospital has become vulnerable. This has led to the formation of large health networks linking individual facilities that represent only one of several related corporate activities. Along with these phenomena have come *integrated delivery systems,* which "usually involve a significant degree of integration between payer and providers" (Weiner & de Lissovoy, 1993, p. 94). They also entail *managed care,* a synonym for all kinds of integrated delivery systems, and also a term used to denote "the entire range of utilization control tools that are applied to manage the practices of physicians and others, regardless of the setting in which they practice" (p. 97). The two major types of integrated delivery systems operating in today's health care market are health maintenance organizations (HMOs) and preferred provider organizations (PPOs).

The medical-industrial complex does not provide all health care services. Public health is primarily concerned with preventing disease through public programs, but increasingly it is providing medical care to individual patients through neighborhood health centers.

Books on the evolution of occupational therapy's theories and concepts provide an important complement to the contemporary picture of the profession. Data on the supply and the distribution of occupational therapy practitioners indicate that the profession continues to expand. However, the growth has not kept pace with the demand. Shortages are evident in certain geographic areas and practice settings.

The health care industry has adopted the concepts and the practices basic to competition, and the government is stimulating competition to control costs. Cost-containment practices, managed care in particular, are having a profound effect on organizational structures and, in turn, on clinical practice.

On a daily basis, occupational therapy managers and practitioners must be knowledgeable about the realities of cost considerations for both patients and clients and employers. To provide information on the importance of their services, occupational therapy managers and practitioners must integrate quality improvement concepts into daily activities and document program effectiveness. They must employ standard and reliable measures to show functional changes in the occupational performance of patients and clients.

This is a very important time for occupational therapy. The profession must respond with confidence that it is giving the people whom it serves the opportunity to gain meaningful lives. The profession is now ready to assume a responsible role in offering support and direction to the health care system.

REFERENCES

Allied Health Professions Personnel Training Act of 1966, Pub. L. No. 89–751, 80 Stat. 1222–1240.

American Hospital Association. (1994). *Guide to the health care field* (1994 ed.). Chicago: Author.

American Occupational Therapy Association. (1995a). Guide for supervision of occupational therapy personnel. *American Journal of Occupational Therapy, 49,* 1027–28.

American Occupational Therapy Association. (1995b). Use of occupational therapy aides in occupational therapy practice [Position paper]. *American Journal of Occupational Therapy, 49,* 1023–25.

American Occupational Therapy Association, Ad Hoc Commission on Occupational Therapy Manpower. (1983–84). *Occupational therapy manpower: A plan for progress.* Rockville, MD: Author.

American Occupational Therapy Association, Intercommission Council. (1995). *White paper: Occupational therapy and cross training initiatives.* Bethesda, MD: Author.

Americans with Disabilities Act of 1990, Pub. L. No. 101–336, 104 Stat. 327.

Bloom, G. (1994). Ethics. In K. Jacobs & M. Logigian (Eds.), *Functions of a manager in occupational therapy* (pp. 51–66). Thorofare, NJ: Slack.

Blue Shield, Unihealth plan giant merger. (1993, June 29). *Los Angeles Times,* p. A1.

Bodenheimer, T., & Grumbach, K. (1994). Paying for health care. *Journal of the American Medical Association, 272,* 634–39.

Brown, R., & Garten, J. (1994). Studies comparing managed care and traditional indemnity plans on the quality of care and patient/client satisfaction with service delivery and cost are ongoing. In *US Industrial Outlook.* Lanham, MD: Berman.

Burner, S. T., & Waldo, D. R. (1995, Summer). National health expenditure projections, 1994–2005 [DataView]. *Health Care Financing Review, 16*(4), 221–42.

Carr, S. (1993). The COTA heritage. In S. Ryan (Ed.), *The certified occupational therapy assistant* (2nd ed., pp. 21–32). Thorofare, NJ: Slack.

Chapman, A. R. (1993). *Exploring a human rights approach to health care reform.* Washington, DC: American Association for the Advancement of Science.

Chapman, B., & Talmedge, J. (1971, January). The evolution of the right to health concept in the United States. *The Pharos,* pp. 30–51.

Christiansen, C., & Baum, C. (Eds.). (1991). *Occupational therapy: Overcoming human performance deficits.* Thorofare, NJ: Slack.

Clinton, W. (1994). *Economic report of the president transmitted to Congress.* Washington, DC: Government Printing Office.

Community Mental Health Centers Act of 1963, Pub. L. No. 88–164, Title II, 77 Stat. 290.

Comprehensive Health Manpower Training Act of 1971, Pub. L. No. 92–157, Title I, §§ 101–110, 85 Stat. 431–461.

DeJong, G., & Sutton, J. (1994, November 23). *REHAB 2000: The evolution of medical rehabilitation in American health care.* Paper presented at the National Rehabilitation Hospital Research Center, Washington, DC.

The DRG handbook: Comparative clinical and financial standards. (1994). Cleveland, OH: HCIA; Baltimore: Ernst & Young.

Elwood, T. (1991). A view from Washington. *Journal of Allied Health, 20,* 47–62.

Faltermeyer, E. (1994, January 10). Health care: More Americans are switching to HMOs. *Fortune, 129,* 14.

Fisher, T. (1995). *The case manager in case management.* Unpublished manuscript, Columbia Healthcare.

Foto, M., & Swanson, G. (1993, August/September). Utilization review and managed care. *Rehab Management* (Marina del Ray, CA: CurAnt Communications), *6,* 123–25.

Freda, M. (1995). *Managed care's impact on delivery of occupational therapy.* Unpublished manuscript.

Hammel, J. (1993). What should occupational therapy practitioners know about technology? *Technology Special Interest Section Newsletter, 3*(3), 1–2.

Health Amendments Act of 1956, Pub. L. No. 84–911, ch. 871, 70 Stat. 923.

Health Insurance Association of America. (1994). *Source book of health insurance data.* Washington, DC: Author.

Health Maintenance Organization Act of 1973, Pub. L. No. 93–222, 87 Stat. 914.

Health Manpower Act of 1968, Pub. L. No. 90–490, 82 Stat. 773.

Health Professions Educational Assistance Act of 1963, Pub. L. No. 88–129, 77 Stat. 164.

Health Professions Educational Assistance Amendments of 1965, Pub. L. No. 89–290, 79 Stat. 1052.

Health Training Improvement Act of 1970, Pub. L. No. 91–519, 84 Stat. 1342.

HMO fact sheet. (1985, April). Bethesda, MD: United States Public Health Service, Office of Health Maintenance Organizations.

Hopkins, H. L., & Smith, H. D. (Eds.). (1994). *Willard and Spackman's Occupational therapy* (8th ed.). Philadelphia: Lippincott.

Hospital Survey and Construction Act of 1946 (Hill-Burton Act), Pub. L. No. 79–725, Title VI of the Public Health Service Act, ch. 958, 60 Stat. 1040.

Levit, K. R., Sensenig, A. L., Cowan, C. A., Lazenby, H. C., McDonnell, P. A., Won, D. K., Sivarajan, L., Stiller, J. M., Donham, C. S., & Stewart, M. S. (1994, Fall). National health expenditures, 1993. *Health Care Financing Review, 16*(1), 247–92.

Loomis, C. (1994, July 11). The real action in healthcare. *Fortune, 130,* 149.

McGinley, L. (1995, January 12). Minor health-care steps, such as reforming insurance, may face hard time in new congress. *Wall Street Journal,* p. A16.

Merriam-Webster's collegiate dictionary (10th ed.). (1993). Springfield, MA: Merriam-Webster.

National Health Planning and Resources Development Act of 1974, Pub. L. No. 93–641, 88 Stat. 2225.

Nurse Training Act of 1964, Pub. L. No. 88–581, 78 Stat. 908.

Nurse Training Act of 1971, Pub. L. No. 92–158, 85 Stat. 465.

Platt, R., & Fraser, M. (1993). Assistive technology in the rehabilitation of patients with high spinal cord lesions. *Paraplegia, 31,* 280–87.

Public Health Service Act of 1944, Pub. L. No. 78–410, ch. 373, 58 Stat. 682.

Quiroga, V. A. M. (1995). *Occupational therapy: The first thirty years, 1900–1930.* Bethesda, MD: American Occupational Therapy Association.

Reitz, S. (1992). Ethical issues in documentation. In J. D. Acquaviva (Ed.), *Effective documentation for occupational therapy* (pp. 219–42). Rockville, MD: American Occupational Therapy Association.

Rice, V. (1995). Ergonomics: An introduction. In K. Jacobs & C. Bettencourt (Eds.), *Ergonomics for therapists* (pp. 3–12). Newton, MA: Butterworth-Heinemann.

Rubin, A. (1994a). Clinton's health-care bill. *Congressional Quarterly, 52,* 492–504.

Rubin, A. (1994b). Uncertainty, deep divisions cloud opening of debate. *Congressional Quarterly, 52,* 2344–53.

Sabo, M. (1993, November 3). House Budget Committee hearing on budget impact of health care revisions. *Federal News Service* (Federal Information Systems Corporation).

Scott, S., & Somers, F. (1992). Orientation to payment. In J. D. Acquaviva (Ed.), *Effective documentation for occupational therapy* (pp. 5–22). Rockville, MD: American Occupational Therapy Association.

Shepp, C. G. (1980). Trends in hospital care. In M. Brown & B. P. McCool (Eds.), *Multi-hospital systems: Strategies for organization and management* (pp. 3–9). Germantown, MD: Aspen Systems.

Silvergleit, I. (1994, September 8). The workforce of the '90s. *OT Week,* pp. 20–24.

Social Security Amendments of 1972, Pub. L. No. 92–603, 86 Stat. 1329.

Social Security Amendments of 1983, Pub. L. No. 98–21, 97 Stat. 65.

Social Security Bulletin, Annual Statistical Supplement. (1994). Washington, DC: Government Printing Office.

Somers, F., & Browne, S. (1994). *Key health care reform issues for 1995 state legislative sessions.* Rockville, MD: American Occupational Therapy Association.

Tax Equity and Fiscal Responsibility Act of 1982, Pub. L. No. 97–248, 96 Stat. 324.

Thompson, R. (1993, March). Uninsured population grows [Employee Benefits Research Institute report]. *Nation's Business, 81,* 58.

Underwood, R. (1995). *Critical pathways: The OT's role* [Disc version of on-line workshop]. Bethesda, MD: American Occupational Therapy Association.

United States Bureau of the Census. (1994, September). *Statistical abstract of the United States* (114th ed.). Washington, DC: Government Printing Office.

United States Department of Labor, Bureau of Labor Statistics. (1993). *Statistical reference index.* Washington, DC: Congressional Information Service.

United States Public Health Service. (ca. 1988). *The Public Health Service: Some historical notes* [PHS Fact Sheet]. Bethesda, MD: Author.

Weiner, J. P., & de Lissovoy, G. (1993, Spring). Razing a Tower of Babel: A taxonomy for managed care and health insurance plans. *Journal of Health Politics, Policy, and Law, 18,* 75–103.

Wilson, F. A., & Neuhauser, D. (1985). *Health services in the United States* (2nd rev. ed.). Cambridge, MA: Ballinger.

Wolman, A. (1973, April). APHA in its first century. *American Journal of Public Health, 63,* 319–21.

SECTION 2

Planning

Section 2, "Planning," consists of four chapters: "Strategic Planning," "Financial Management," "Marketing," and "The Targeting of Communications." Each treats an aspect of the primary function of planning—to articulate a vision, to determine a mission, and to set goals and objectives.

As a concept and as a process, strategic planning (the subject of chapter 2) provides a transition from the broad health care context of section 1/chapter 1 to the narrower context of the occupational therapy organization, taken up in sections 2–8. The chapter describes a four-step process that will help occupational therapy managers analyze trends in the environment and position their organization to respond creatively.

Chapter 3 summarizes developments that have made financial management a central function in health care. It offers a primer on basic accounting, and it explains selected tools of financial management. The chapter also introduces a multitude of concepts and terms that occupational therapy managers must understand in order to function in an era of attention to bottom lines.

Five marketing concepts (product, price, place, promotion, and position) and four marketing processes (organizational assessment, environmental assessment, market analysis, and communications) are the topics of chapter 4. The chapter contrasts the traditional mission-oriented planning cycle of health care organizations with a market-based planning scheme that examines mission in light of the wants and the needs of consumers. Further, the chapter explains marketing's close relationships to strategic planning and community relations.

In chapter 5 the book turns to the subject of community relations, defining community in this context as groups important to the provision of occupational therapy services. The chapter describes the five activities that constitute a communication program. It includes two tables that will aid managers in analyzing their publics and selecting appropriate methods of communication. It also contains a scenario in which an occupational therapy manager recognizes a problem and sets about solving it by using the procedures and the methods described in the chapter.

CHAPTER 2

Strategic Planning

L. Randy Strickland, EdD, OTR/L, FAOTA

KEY TERMS

Mission statement. A setting forth of an organization's purpose, including definition, products, and services.

Situation (SWOT) analysis. An assessment focused on organizational strengths, weaknesses, opportunities, and threats.

Strategic plan. A plan that orients and directs an organization toward the activities that it must accomplish to meet its mission.

Strategic planning. A "managerial process of developing and maintaining a strategic fit between [an] organization's goals [and] resources, and its changing market opportunities" (Kotler & Clarke, 1987, p. 90).

Vision. An ideal, an aim for an organization.

L. Randy Strickland, EdD, OTR/L, FAOTA, is a professor and S. Pearson Auerbach, MD Chair in Occupational Therapy at Spaulding University in Louisville, Kentucky. Formerly he was a regional rehabilitation director for Hillhaven Corporation in Louisville, with administrative responsibility for rehabilitation services and Medicare programs in eight state areas. During his tenure as vice-president of AOTA, he oversaw the organization's strategic planning. Adult education was the focus of his graduate work, taken at North Carolina State University.

I n today's environment the financial or programmatic decisions of the larger organization of which an occupational therapy program is a part often influence the provision of occupational therapy services. To remain or become a successful member of the larger organization, the occupational therapy program must recognize both the opportunities and the challenges that influence its success. All organizations, including their occupational therapy programs, commonly engage in strategic planning. Strategic planning is a key factor in the continued growth and success of any adaptive business, including those offering occupational therapy services. The Sister Kenny Institute in Minneapolis, Minnesota, for example, began as a rehabilitation treatment facility for persons with polio. As polio became less common, the institute redefined its purpose and applied its rehabilitation concepts and programs to the development of a nationally renowned rehabilitation center for varied diagnoses (Kotler & Clarke, 1987). The institute's occupational therapy department was able to reposition itself and contribute to the establishment of highly regarded rehabilitation protocols.

The leaders and the administrators of any organization are typically the driving forces behind the development of the organization's strategic plan. They recognize that the continued success of the organization rests on its ability proactively to anticipate and adapt to change in the economic, political, and social environments. Change in the environment reflects society as a whole. Consideration of environmental changes and internal organizational characteristics creates the opportunity for leaders to translate an organization's purpose into action steps that maximize its competitive stance in an evolving marketplace. Action steps should anticipate future priorities and changes. Hamel and Prahalad (1994), for example, envision a new form of strategy in which

> competition for the future is competition to create and dominate emerging opportunities to stake out new competitive space. Creating the future is more challenging than playing catch up, in that you have to create your own road map. The goal is not simply to benchmark a competitor's products and processes and imitate its methods, but to develop an independent point of view about tomorrow's opportunities and how to exploit them. Path making is a lot more rewarding than bench marking. One doesn't get to the future first by letting someone else blaze the trail. (p. 22)

Assisting an organization in creating its future offers the occupational therapy staff member, manager, or program an opportunity to apply and develop occupational therapy contributions in a systems approach, resulting in internal and external recognition of occupational therapy as a value-added service.

DEFINITIONS

Kotler and Clarke (1987) define *strategic planning* as a "managerial process of developing and maintaining a strategic fit between [an] organization's goals [and] resources, and its changing market opportunities" (p. 90). Strategic planning enables an organization (or a unit within an organization) to develop keen insight into its business operations. Such insight should result in identification of the goals essential for the organization to adapt creatively to both external and internal changes. Proactive strategic planning enhances the opportunity to succeed. Moving beyond the micro-issues of daily managerial activities to the macroview serves a significant value in orienting an organization to the future in all aspects of strategy development.

Strategic planning begins with identification and articulation of a vision. A *vision* is an ideal, an aim for an organization. It goes beyond basic purposes into future scenarios that depict the organization's effectiveness and involvement with its environment at the optimal level. For example, occupational therapy practitioners in school systems have traditionally been involved in K–6 programs. A future scenario for occupational therapy in the school setting might call for intervention programs focused on vocational services for older students, including a transition to the community, thus supporting the school's vision of its students becoming productive citizens. The activities integral to strategic planning stimulate growth and promote a continuous process of assessment, change, and action by the organization. A vision shared by all staff members results in a learning organization, which values the acquisition and the use of new knowledge and skills by its members. A vision clearly defined and understood by an organization's staff members results in attainment of the organization's goals (Senge, 1990).

The preparation of a mission statement follows the development of a vision. Based on the vision, the *mission statement* is a setting forth of the organization's purpose, including definition, products, and services. An organization's mission statement is generally succinct and provides a targeted focus. For example, a nonprofit community reentry program for clients with traumatic brain injury might state its mission as follows:

> XYZ Community Program exists to ensure that our clients return to productive, independent lives in the community. The program provides community-based support services and education to assist the clients in independent living.

This mission statement provides direction without being overly specific. The organization would address more specific plans later in the strategic planning process.

Development or review of a mission statement assists an organization in better using and directing its resources. An appropriately formulated mission statement withstands the test of time and provides for development and initiation of a creative strategic process. Steiner (1979) reinforces the value of the mission statement, asserting,

> Mission statements determine the competitive arena in which a business operates. They determine how resources will be allocated to different demands. They determine the size of the company. They make much easier the task of identifying the opportunities and threats that must be addressed in the planning process. They open up new opportunities, as well as new threats, when changed. They prevent people from "spinning their wheels" in working on strategies and plans that may be considered completely inappropriate by top management. (p. 156)

Creation of a strategic plan follows preparation of a mission statement. A *strategic plan* is a plan that orients and directs an organization toward the activities that it must accomplish to meet its mission. The plan includes goals, objectives, action steps, and an evaluation phase. The organization bases its allocation of financial, physical, and human resources on this plan. The budget of the organization is driven by the plan and should provide adequate funding to meet the plan's goals and objectives.

A well-conceived strategic plan is not a static document filed and reviewed once yearly. It is a flexible tool understood and used throughout the organization. Concise, often limited to a few pages, it provides the basis for communicating the vision, the mission, and the thrust of the organization for a specific time frame. That time frame may be as brief as a year or as long as three to five years.

STEPS IN STRATEGIC PLANNING

The strategic planning process has four basic steps: (1) situation analysis, (2) strategy development, (3) implementation, and (4) evaluation of results.

SITUATION ANALYSIS

Situation analysis is the fundamental step on which the entire strategic planning process rests. This is the time at which the organization's members assess the organization's present position and the areas of concern for the future. Typically described as a *SWOT analysis*, the assessment focuses on organizational strengths, weaknesses, opportunities, and threats (Aldag & Stearns, 1987; Fahey & Randall, 1994). This analysis includes both internal factors and external environmental influences. Identification of key issues forms the basis for development of strategic agendas, which the organization addresses in its strategic plan. This identification phase allows participants to develop understanding and ownership of the organization's present situation as well as its future challenges. Issues may include revenue, program development, community service, sales and marketing, regulatory and legislative developments, and so forth.

The SWOT analysis should involve as many staff members as possible. This is the time to use the organization's most important resource, its employees. Involving staff members provides the occasion for specific discussion regarding the organization and for development of cohesive teams to meet present and future performance demands (Katzenbach & Smith, 1993). Such discussion can be frank and open, with persons being encouraged to express their beliefs regarding both present and future modes of operation.

The situation analysis should have time limits, and it is often advantageous to have a neutral facilitator who is responsible for the process. As with all planning activities, a person should be assigned to record the information obtained. The SWOT analysis should occur at least yearly, through regular departmental meetings or a retreat.

STRATEGY DEVELOPMENT

Step 2, strategy development, involves the prioritization of strategic issues that influence the organization's direction. This is when the organization decides which issues are of greatest importance. Identifying more issues than can be addressed in the prescribed time frame is not uncommon. Prioritization must occur, considering multiple factors: the consumer, finances, program innovation, and market penetration or market share areas (Fahey & Randall, 1994). The organization reviews the information gleaned from the SWOT analysis along with its vision and mission statement to determine the best future course. It establishes general goals (usually three to five) that support the mission. Staff members then review the vision, the mission statement, and the goals and select key measurable objectives. Often these note specific directions for the mission and the goals and provide thrusts for the immediate future. Each objective that undergirds a goal should have at least one strategy or action step for its attainment or support (Aldag & Stearns, 1987).

It is important for the organization to select issues of central concern so that it can be strategically focused (Jacobs, 1994). Activities that are routine in nature should be addressed in the ongoing operating plans of the organization. For example, developing a new outcomes measurement program for outpatients may be a fitting thrust in a strategic plan, whereas ensuring that all outpatient occupational therapy clients are prescreened for insurance coverage may be an appropriate element of an operating plan.

The strategic agenda and related strategies should reflect strategic opportunities. The staff of a developing occupational therapy department in a new rehabilitation center might identify a driving program, community skills/reentry, and injured worker rehabilitation programs as options. In the final analysis the department might be able to undertake only one of these programs in upcoming years. It would then identify a specific objective and strategy related to that program along with an accountable unit or person and a timeline.

IMPLEMENTATION

Implementation of the strategic plan generally corresponds to an organization's business or fiscal year, but may vary according to an organization's practice. The important ingredient is to ensure that all members of the organization have accountability for the plan's use and review (Connors, Smith, & Hickman, 1994). As implementation occurs, staff members should carefully monitor the process and its results. Individuals or units will most likely have responsibility for the implementation of specific strategies that support a key objective.

EVALUATION OF RESULTS

Waiting until year's end to evaluate the success of a strategic plan is not appropriate. The strategic plan, including the vision, the mission statement, the goals and the objectives, and the strategies, should become a daily blueprint for the organization to use in assessing its present and future effectiveness. Members of the organization's units should regularly ask themselves in what activities they have been involved that allow the organization to achieve its strategic objectives. Staff members must view the organization's vision, mission statement, and strategic plan as real and dynamic. Naturally such a process is based on the premise that the organization has selected the most appropriate and measurable strategic objectives to maximize its opportunities for success in both the present and the future. Future is defined as a three- to five-year period. This too is an evolving timeline that the organization must continually reevaluate in the changing environment.

Evaluation of the strategic plan's success should occur regularly. Reports on activities should use the strategic plan, including attainment of its objectives, as part of the measurement process. Similarly the administrators of the organization should regularly use this plan as a part of the management process. All members of the organization should have an opportunity to provide regular feedback regarding the application of the plan's strategies and the identification of new or revised objectives and strategies.

BENEFITS OF STRATEGIC PLANNING

The occupational therapy practitioner may initially ask how he or she can benefit from participation in the strategic planning process. The first and possibly the most important benefit is that the individual practitioner can take ownership of the direction of the organization. By involving its employees in charting present and future activities, an organization empowers them. They realize that they have both the accountability and the authority to help the organization reach new levels of performance and service. The purposes and the goals of the organization can become congruent with those of individual employees through staff participation in strategic planning, particularly in identification of issues and development and implementation of strategies. Employees can assist with their program's strategic planning activities, which will affect the success of the overall strategic plan.

A second benefit of strategic planning is that it gives staff members a broader perspective, helping them think about the organization and its purpose as a whole. No longer can practitioners in health or education environments, or anywhere else, think only of their units. Although the individual occupational therapy practitioner must be concerned with the activities of the occupational therapy unit, he or she must also understand the interrelationship of different aspects of the organization and the effects of that interrelationship on the organization's future viability.

A third benefit is that strategic planning clearly communicates the organization's purpose to its employees and the public. Dissemination of information about vision, mission statement, goals and objectives, and strategies encourages actions that are consistent with the overall strategic plan. The appearance of inconsistency may require reexamination, additional staff communication, and the development of new or revised objectives and strategies.

PITFALLS OF STRATEGIC PLANNING

As previously stated, strategic planning cannot occur only once a year. It is a continuous process, requiring commitment and participation from key administrators and staff members throughout the organization, including occupational therapy managers and practitioners. Assigning the development of a strategic plan to one person or to a small group of persons may result in the development of a document that is neither a dynamic statement nor an important communication and rallying point for the organization's employees. Lippitt (1982) supports total group involvement in planning as essential for organizational renewal. He explains that

> planning—which involves looking ahead—takes us out of the complacency that accompanies seeing things only as they are, not as they might be. It protects us from thinking that this is the final chapter in our career, our personal relationships, let alone that it is obvious that there may be a next chapter. (p. 63)

If planning is closed to widespread participation, the organization will not be as successful as it might be otherwise.

Another pitfall in strategic planning is allowing it to become too complicated. Participants may become so overwhelmed by what is that they can never move on to what might be. Alternatively, in becoming future oriented, staff members may neglect their accountability for present operations. The planning process should provide enough structure to focus on the present and the future throughout the year, not just at one particular time.

Still other pitfalls are allowing too little time for strategic planning or giving it little or no follow through. The process may also suffer from lack of forward-looking, proactive vision. Perhaps the most dreaded outcome is a focus only on the short term (Hamel & Prahalad, 1994).

Any of these pitfalls can sabotage the success of the strategic planning process. The ideal is to allow the organization to succeed and reach new heights previously believed unattainable. To combat sabotage successfully, the entire organization from top down must follow a formal planning process, establish a concise but clearly understood document, and commit itself to review and refine the plan throughout the fiscal year.

A Scenario:
Successful Strategic Planning

Westview Nursing and Rehabilitation Center is a 120-bed skilled nursing facility in Bedford, Indiana. Its Rehabilitation Services Department employs 30 persons, including an occupational therapy staff of 10. The noteworthy point regarding the department is its strategic focus on identifying and implementing programs to meet the community's health care needs. The department has dovetailed its efforts with the facility's overall mission of providing comprehensive health services to community residents and expanding its programs to the community. To ensure growth of the program and the facility, the center established specific objectives and appropriate programmatic strategies.

Over a three-year period the rehabilitation services program has evolved from a contractual part time activity to a large comprehensive department composed of licensed therapists and assistants in occupational, physical, and speech therapy. During the center's strategic planning activities, the rehabilitation director and staff members contributed to an analysis of the total rehabilitation efforts and needs in the facility and the community. In the town of 13,000 there were minimal rehabilitation services and no occupational therapy services.

Through a continuing analysis of community needs and related strategic planning, the number of occupational therapists and occupational therapy assistants has increased from 1 to 10 and is still growing. Of greater importance is the expansion of occupational therapy services to encompass a subacute inpatient unit in the center, a freestanding outpatient clinic focusing on work and sports injuries, contractual services to and management of the community hospital occupational therapy program, and full-time services in the local school district. The Rehabilitation Services Department has recruited, trained, and oriented staff members to the specific demands of each of these settings. Occupational therapy now offers services previously unavailable in the community. Along with the other disciplines in the department, occupational therapy has become known as the community's primary and preferred provider of rehabilitation services.

The facility and its Rehabilitation Services Department have expanded their scope and met previously unfilled or unidentified health needs. The center has significantly enhanced its overall financial profitability while filling an important service niche. Throughout the strategic planning process, administrators have jointly planned with rehabilitation staff members. The administrators and the practitioners feel a sense of ownership, and an underserved community now receives comprehensive services in its own locale.

SUMMARY

All organizations commonly engage in strategic planning. Consideration of environmental changes and internal organizational characteristics creates the opportunity for leaders to translate an organization's purpose into action steps that maximize its competitive stance in an evolving marketplace.

Kotler and Clarke (1987) define *strategic planning* as a "managerial process of developing and maintaining a strategic fit between [an] organization's goals [and] resources, and its changing market opportunities" (p. 90). Strategic planning begins with identification and articulation of a vision. A *vision* is an ideal, an aim for an organization. The preparation of a mission statement follows the development of a vision. Based on the vision, the *mission statement* is a setting forth of the organization's purpose, including definition, products, and services. Creation of a strategic plan follows preparation of a mission statement. A *strategic plan* is a plan that orients and directs an organization toward the activities that it must accomplish to meet its mission. A well-conceived strategic plan is a flexible tool understood and used throughout the organization.

The strategic planning process has four basic steps: (1) situation analysis, (2) strategy development, (3) implementation, and (4) evaluation of results. *Situation analysis* is the fundamental step on which the entire strategic planning process rests. Typically described as a *SWOT analysis*, the assessment focuses on organizational strengths, weaknesses, opportunities, and threats (Aldag & Stearns, 1987; Fahey & Randall, 1994). Step 2, strategy development, involves the prioritization of strategic issues that influence the organization's direction. It is important for the organization to select issues of central concern so that it can be strategically focused (Jacobs, 1994). Implementation of the strategic plan generally corresponds to an organization's business or fiscal year, but may vary according to an organization's practice. The important ingredient is to ensure that all members of the organization have accountability for the plan's use and review (Connors, Smith, & Hickman, 1994). Evaluation of the strategic plan's success should occur regularly. Reports on activities should use the strategic plan, including attainment of its objectives, as part of the measurement process.

The benefits of strategic planning are that the individual practitioner can take ownership of the direction of the organization, that strategic planning gives staff members a broader perspective, and that strategic planning clearly communicates the organization's purpose to its employees and the public. Pitfalls include assigning the development of a strategic plan to one person or to a small group of persons, allowing the plan to become too complicated, and allowing too little time for strategic planning or giving it little or no follow through. The process may also suffer from lack of forward-looking, proactive vision, or from a focus only on the short term (Hamel & Prahalad, 1994).

REFERENCES

Aldag, R. J., & Stearns, T. M. (1987). *Management.* Cincinnati, OH: South-Western.

Connors, R., Smith, T., & Hickman, C. (1994). *The Oz principle: Getting results through individual and organizational accountability.* Englewood Cliffs, NJ: Prentice-Hall.

Fahey, L., & Randall, R. M. (Eds.). (1994). *The portable MBA in strategy.* New York: Wiley.

Hamel, G., & Prahalad, C. K. (1994). *Competing for the future.* Boston: Harvard Business School Press.

Jacobs, R. W. (1994). *Real time strategic change: How to involve an entire organization in fast and far-reaching change.* San Francisco: Berrett-Koehler.

Katzenbach, J. R., & Smith, D. K. (1993). *The wisdom of teams: Creating the high-performance organization.* Boston: Harvard Business School Press.

Kotler, P., & Clarke, R. N. (1987). *Marketing for health care organizations.* Englewood Cliffs, NJ: Prentice-Hall.

Lippitt, G. L. (1982). *Organization renewal: A holistic approach to organization development.* Englewood Cliffs, NJ: Prentice-Hall.

Senge, P. M. (1990). *The fifth discipline: The art and practice of the learning organization.* New York: Doubleday.

Steiner, G. A. (1979). *Strategic planning: What every manager must know.* New York: Free Press.

CHAPTER 3

Financial Management

Nancy Mahon Smith, MBA, OTR, CHE

KEY TERMS

Accounting. The process of collecting, recording, summarizing, analyzing, reporting, and interpreting information about an organization in monetary terms.

Balance sheet. A statement of an organization's assets, liabilities, and net assets, given that assets – liabilities = net assets.

Capital budgeting. The process of planning for expenditures for property, plant, and equipment.

Financial analysis. Assessment of an organization's financial performance through ratio analysis, analysis of key operating indicators, and variance analysis.

Financial forecasting. The process of estimating the future value of a new service, program, or product.

Financial or general accounting. The process of providing financial statements or reports for external use, for example, by government agencies, bankers, and third-party payers.

Financial statement. A statement on an organization's financial position, on changes in that position, or on the results of operations.

Income statement. A statement of revenue and expense flows and net income during a specified period.

This chapter is based in part on "Financial Management," by S. M. Laase, 1992, in J. Bair and M. Gray (Eds.), The Occupational Therapy Manager *(Rev. ed., pp. 83–122), Rockville, MD: American Occupational Therapy Association.*

Management of working capital. Control of working capital (current assets – current liabilities) so that only a small percentage of assets are committed as working capital and therefore unavailable for more productive purposes.

Managerial or management accounting. The process of using information from the financial accounting system and other cost information to prepare reports for specific decision-making purposes internal to the organization.

Nancy Mahon Smith, MBA, OTR, is currently employed by SelectRehab as the director of the Inpatient Rehabilitation Center at Cypress Fairbanks Medical Center, Houston, Texas. At the time she wrote this chapter, she was the vice-president of operations for RehabCare Corporation, responsible for rehabilitation programs in 10 hospitals in the southern United States. She has held a variety of administrative, supervisory, and consulting positions in hospitals, home health agencies, skilled nursing facilities, and ambulatory care settings. Her master's degree is from the University of Baltimore.

This chapter assesses the external financial environment in which health care organizations operate and some internal factors affecting the occupational therapy manager's financial management skills. It then provides an overview of managerial and financial accounting and financial management to address any knowledge or skill deficits that the manager may face.

ASSESSMENT

The assessment focuses chiefly on a review of threats and opportunities in the health care environment. To a lesser extent it identifies the strengths and the weaknesses of the occupational therapy manager in regard to financial management.

THREATS

Three major threats in the health care environment have had a tremendous influence on financial management: rising costs, rapidly changing reimbursement systems, and increased competition.

Rising Costs

As noted in chapter 1, table 1-1, health care expenditures and their share of the gross domestic product (GDP) have been rising at an alarming rate. The Consumer Price Index (CPI) for all items rose 114.9 points, or 388 percent, between 1960 and 1993, while the index of medical care items rose 179.0 points, or 803 percent (U.S. Bureau of the Census, 1994). Table 3-1 shows the growth in various categories of health care expenditures for selected years.

Rapidly Changing Reimbursement Systems

Regulations governing reimbursement for health care and occupational therapy services are continually changing and increasing in complexity. Over the past 20 years, payment for health care services has moved from a charge-based system, through a cost-based system, to a managed system of negotiated discounts, per diems, and case rates, with providers and insurers more closely aligned. Chapter 1, "The Evolution of the Occupational Therapy Delivery System," and chapter 16, "Evolving Health Care Systems: Payment for Occupational Therapy Services," contain more detail on managed care and reimbursement for occupational therapy services.

Increased Competition

Competition manifests itself in a number of ways that are not mutually exclusive and that significantly influence patterns of service provision. On one level there is greater competition for patients. Health care providers in inpatient settings such as acute care general hospitals, specialty units of

Table 3-1
National Health Care Expenditures, 1960–1993

	1960 (in billions)	1970 (in billions)	1980 (in billions)	1990 (in billions)	1993 (in billions)
Total health care expenditures	$27.1	$74.3	$251.1	$696.6	$884.2
Percentage of gross domestic product	5.3%	7.4%	9.3%	12.6%	13.9%
Average annual percentage growth from previous year shown	—	10.6%	12.9%	10.7%	8.3%
Health services and supplies	$25.4	$69.0	$239.4	$672.2	$855.2
Personal health care	23.9	64.8	220.1	612.4	782.5
Hospital care	9.3	28.0	102.7	256.5	326.6
Physician services	5.3	13.6	45.2	140.5	171.2
Dental services	2.0	4.7	13.3	30.4	37.4
Other professional services	0.6	1.4	6.4	36.0	51.2
Home health care	0.0	0.2	1.9	11.1	20.8
Drugs and other medical nondurables	4.2	8.8	21.6	61.2	75.0
Vision products and other medical durables	0.8	2.0	4.5	10.5	12.6
Nursing home care	1.0	4.9	20.5	54.8	69.6
Other personal care	0.7	1.3	4.0	11.4	18.2
Program administration and net cost of private health insurance	1.2	2.8	12.1	38.3	48.0
Government public health activities	0.4	1.4	7.2	21.6	24.7
Research and construction	1.7	5.3	11.6	24.3	29.0

Note. *From "National Health Expenditure Projections, 1994–2005" (p. 236), by S. T. Burner and D. R. Waldo, 1995, Summer,* Health Care Financing Review, 16(4); *and "National Health Expenditures, 1993" (pp. 280–81), by K. R. Levit, A. L. Sensenig, C. A. Cowan, H. C. Lazenby, P. C. McDonnell, D. K. Won, L. Sivarajan, J. M. Stiller, C. S. Donham, and M. S. Stewart, 1994, Fall,* Health Care Financing Review, 16(1).

hospitals and specialty hospitals exempt from Medicare's prospective payment system, and intermediate ·and skilled nursing facilities, compete among themselves for customers. They vie as well with providers in community-based settings such as ambulatory surgery centers, urgent care centers, group and private practice clinics, home health agencies, hospice organizations, rehabilitation agencies, and health promotion/wellness programs. This competition has influenced the volume of patients and the amount of revenue, and has increased certain expenses such as marketing, to affect the financial status of the health care organization.

On another level there is increased competition for scarce resources, including personnel, philanthropic contributions, and capital. Shortages of professional personnel have contributed to increases in labor costs.

With regard to philanthropic contributions and capital, health care organizations are competing not only with one another but with an increasing number of entities outside the health care industry. Changes in tax laws and lending rates have reduced the availability and increased the cost of nonoperating sources of revenue.

OPPORTUNITIES

To address these threats in the external environment, health care financial executives and occupational therapy managers have expanded and further defined their roles and increased their expertise in financial management. This effort has resulted in an improved ability to maximize the value of their organization in congruence with its missions, goals, and objectives.

Evolution of Health Care Financial Management

Over the past 30 years "hospital finance has evolved from a primitive function of bookkeeping/accounting to a role in which it exerts a major influence in the management of hospital assets and the allocation of scarce resources" (Beck, 1980, p. 1).[1] Before Medicare and its requirement for cost reports were introduced in the late 1960s, hospital finance was not very sophisticated and did not need to be. Successful fund-raising drives and philanthropy were prevalent. Hospital administrators raised prices annually. A number of government initiatives, at the federal level with Medicare and Veterans Administration mandates and at the state level with Medicaid, changed this situation. In 1970 the Economic Stabilization Act imposed wage and price controls on health care as well as other industries. In 1977, President Jimmy Carter proposed the Hospital Cost Containment Act. Although it did not pass, it facilitated the American Hospital Association's Voluntary Effort campaign, which urged hospitals to reduce costs and control price increases.

The next federal government proposal, the System of Hospital Uniform Reporting (SHUR), also failed, on the argument that standardizing hospital financial accounting and reporting would be costly and, because of institutional differences, would still not enable comparisons among hospitals. In the meantime many states passed cost-containment and rate-setting legislation. Then in April 1983 the Social Security Amendments, mandating the Medicare prospective payment system (PPS) for hospitals, were signed into law. Since then, reimbursement for hospital capital costs has also shifted to a prospective basis.

---

1. *The historical perspective in this section is based on information from* Basic Hospital Financial Management, *by D. F. Beck, 1980, Rockville, MD: Aspen Systems.*

In regard to community-based care, in 1980, Congress passed legislation expanding Medicare coverage to comprehensive outpatient rehabilitation facilities. More recently it enacted changes in Medicare payment for rehabilitation agencies and home health services, instituted equivalency caps on therapists' salaries, and implemented the Resource Based Relative Value Scale (RBRVS) for reimbursement of physicians. Now, threatened by proposals for increased federal government regulation of reimbursement in the 1990s, private commercial insurers, health care providers, and some states are taking the opportunity to develop their own systems for paying for health care services based on historical costs, per case rates, capitated rates, and other methodologies. The field of health care financial management has evolved to address these changes and to seek opportunities to preserve the efficiency and the effectiveness of health care organizations.

As part of this evolution, health care organizations have further developed and defined their financial management structures and functions. The Financial Executives Institute has categorized functions as follows:

Controllership	Planning for control
	Reporting and interpreting
	Evaluating and consulting
	Administering taxes
	Reporting to government
	Protecting assets
	Appraising economic health
Treasurership	Providing capital
	Maintaining investor relations
	Providing short-term financing
	Providing banking and custody
	Overseeing credits and collections
	Choosing investments
	Providing insurance

(Cleverley, 1992, p. 8)

Table 3-2 illustrates the nature of the planning, reporting, and interpreting activities of the health care organization's financial executive, as well as the close relationships between finance, strategic planning, and marketing. Working in a hospital or a large health care system, the occupational therapy manager may encounter a chief financial officer (CFO),

Table 3-2
Financial Planning in the Strategic Planning Process

Strategic Planning	Financial Planning Tasks and Analyses
Prepare initial mission statement	Develop initial financial goals
Conduct internal analysis	Evaluate financial position against initial goals
	• Rate of return on equity and/or growth in assets
	• Internal sources and uses of capital
Conduct external analysis	Evaluate external financial environment
	• Financial position and objectives of competing and complementary organizations
	• Growth and availability of sources of revenue
	• Growth and availability of external sources of capital
Assess present position	Assess current financial position
	• Comparative financial performance
	• Share of available revenue received
	• Access to and use of available capital
Revise mission statement and develop goals	Revise financial goals
Develop and evaluate alternative strategies	Determine financial impact of alternative strategies
	• On financial goals
	• On use of capital
	To do this—
	• Estimate capital and operating budgets
	• Estimate impact on utilization, revenues, and expenses
Set strategies and objectives	Set financial objectives
	• Determine what movement toward achieving financial goals should occur each year
	• Set targets for acquisition and use of working and long-term capital
Develop contingency plans	Develop financial contingency plan
	• Set financial "trigger points"
	• Determine financial consequences of alternative strategies
	• Investigate alternative sources of working and long-term capital
Develop and implement program and operational plans	Develop program and operational budgets
	• Develop capital budget
	• Evaluate working capital needs
	• Prepare departmental and program budgets
	• Develop financing plan
	• Set rates and estimate reimbursement
Develop evaluation, monitoring, and control system	Establish financial control system
	• Implement management by objectives
	• Determine and evaluate program and departmental budget variances
	• Monitor achievement of financial objectives
	• Monitor capital budgets
Revise and implement contingency plans	Revise financial plan and implement contingency plan
	• Reassess assumptions about external financial environment
	• Evaluate achievement of financial objectives

Note. *From* Strategic Analysis for Hospital Management *(pp. 260–61), by R. Kropf and J. A. Greenberg, 1984, Rockville, MD: Aspen Systems. Copyright ©1984 Aspen Publishers, Inc. Adapted with permission.*

or vice-president of finance, who reports directly to the chief executive officer (CEO), or president. This CFO may have line management responsibilities for patient accounting; patient registration and admissions; medical information systems; computer network systems and data processing; material management and central supply; the controller function, which includes financial reporting, disbursements, and analysis; and risk management. The CFO may also serve in a staff or consultative capacity to the managers of responsibility centers (cost centers). In a small organization the occupational therapy manager may assume some of these controllership and treasurership functions.

Evolution of Occupational Therapy Management

Occupational therapy managers, as financial managers of their areas, have also been challenged by the threats of rising costs, changing reimbursement systems, and increased competition, and are pursuing opportunities to improve their knowledge and skills in financial management. With an overall goal of developing and managing their personnel, operating, and capital budgets consistent with professional standards of quality and their parent organization's objectives, occupational therapy managers may now be responsible for the following:

1. Developing volume and revenue projections for services, consistent with marketing objectives

2. Developing and using effective pricing strategies (including discounts, per diems, capitated rates, and case rates), fee structures, and charging processes

3. Managing the utilization review aspects of the program to meet the organization's expectations regarding contractual allowances, charity care, courtesy allowances, doubtful accounts, costs, and collections

4. Managing payroll and contract labor budgets, and allocating staff in a cost-effective manner consistent with productivity standards

5. Addressing short- and long-term needs for capital for physical plant and equipment, and budgeting actual and depreciated expenses accordingly

6. Budgeting for and managing general and administrative expenses and other operating expenses of the program

7. Meeting projections for earnings, or contributions

STRENGTHS AND WEAKNESSES OF THE OCCUPATIONAL THERAPY MANAGER

The educational preparation of the occupational therapy practitioner provides key skills that are applicable to financial management. Task analysis facilitates cost analysis. Exposure to a wide variety of practice areas enables the occupational therapy practitioner to understand cost shifting along the continuum of care. Training in interpersonal communication skills is also a plus.

A lack of familiarity with the language and the concepts of accounting and finance may be perceived as a weakness of the new manager. The remainder of this chapter addresses this knowledge deficit.

BASIC ACCOUNTING

Accounting is the process of collecting, recording, summarizing, analyzing, reporting, and interpreting information about an organization in monetary terms.[2] The accounting profession makes a further distinction between financial accounting and managerial accounting. *Financial* or *general accounting* provides financial statements or reports for external use, for example, by government agencies, bankers, and third-party payers. These statements must conform to generally accepted accounting principles (GAAP) as specified by the Financial Accounting Standards Board. *Managerial* or *management accounting* uses information from the financial accounting system and other cost information to prepare reports for specific decision-making purposes internal to the organization. These reports assist managers in operating more effectively and efficiently by providing information for decisions regarding financing, resource allocation, productivity, and marketing.

KEY ACCOUNTING CONCEPTS AND TERMS

The occupational therapy manager must have an understanding of the following concepts and terms used in basic and managerial accounting:

> **Entity.** For accounting purposes a business or an organization is an entity capable of taking economic action. An entity is assumed to be a going concern that will continue to function indefinitely.

---

2. *This section is based on information from* Accounting Principles *(Rev. ed.), by R. H. Hermanson, J. D. Edwards, and R. F. Salmonson, 1983, Plano, TX: Business Publications;* Basic Hospital Financial Management, *by D. F. Beck, 1980, Rockville, MD: Aspen Systems;* Finance for the Nonfinancial Manager *(2nd ed.), by H. T. Spiro, 1982, New York: Wiley;* Financial Control in Health Care: A Managerial Perspective, *by D. W. Young, 1984, Homewood, IL: Dow Jones–Irwin;* The Financial Management of Hospitals *(8th ed.), by H. J. Berman, S. F. Kukla, and L. E. Weeks, 1994, Ann Arbor, MI: Health Administration Press; and* Hospital Finance: A Comprehensive Case Approach, *by J. L. Bolandis, 1982, Rockville, MD: Aspen Systems.*

Transactions. Accounting records and reports must include all transactions of an entity so that financial statements accurately reflect the entity's financial condition. Summarizing transactions is an acceptable practice. To the extent possible, accounting transactions should be based on objectively determined facts (e.g., documents).

Cost valuation. An item's historical cost, or the price paid to acquire it, is the basis for its valuation as an asset or a liability. This is in contrast to its replacement cost or market value.

Double entry, or duality. Every transaction requires at least two entries, one on the debit side and one on the credit side. Debit entries must balance credit entries.

Conservatism. When opinion and judgment are used in valuing assets or estimating income, conservative estimates should be made. For example, at year's end, accountants generally use the lower-of-cost-or-market-value rule when valuing inventory, such as splinting supplies, even though replacement cost might be higher because of price increases.

Consistency. Consistent accounting techniques, such as using the same method to compute depreciation on equipment, should be followed so that current accounting reports can be compared with those of prior years. This does not preclude changes to improve or update accounting principles; prior years' reports can be restated to reflect these changes.

Full disclosure. Accounting reports must accurately and completely reflect significant data. They should include and clearly state information that could influence the decisions of the users of financial statements.

Materiality. Accounting reports should reflect significant activities so that the effort and the cost of recording them are justified. Materiality depends on the relative amount of a transaction, its importance to the total operation, and the effects of its exclusion (e.g., the exclusion's leading to incorrect or misleading conclusions). For example, a plastic goniometer may have a useful life of greater than one year; however, the cost of capitalizing it is not justifiable, and failing to capitalize it has no effect on an overall financial analysis of the organization.

Accrual basis of accounting. Generally accepted accounting principles require that financial statements be prepared on an *accrual basis* rather than on a cash basis. Revenue, deductions from revenue, and losses are recorded in the period in which they are realized (earned), and expenses are recorded in the period in which they are incurred, regardless of the flow of cash. This permits an accurate assessment of net income, or excess of revenue over expenses, for each accounting period.

Revenue. The *revenue* of a health care organization consists mainly of the value of all the services rendered to patients. Revenue is identified by the organizational unit (typically a department) that produced it.

Deductions from revenue. *Deductions from revenue* that result in payment of less than full charges may be due to *contractual allowances,* differences between rates billed to a third-party payer such as Medicare, and amounts received from that payer because of a prior contractual agreement; or *courtesy allowances,* such as discounts for employees or physicians. *Doubtful account allowances* (from bad debts, i.e., accounts billed but not collectible) also reduce gross revenue but may be reported as an expense. *Charity allowances,* charges for the care of charity patients, may be described in a footnote to a financial statement, but the care is not considered a deduction from revenue because payment was never expected (Cleverley, 1992).

Expenses. *Expenses* are expired costs that have been incurred in exchange for a good or a service. Expenses are charged to the organizational unit that incurred them.

Matching of revenues and expenses. Expenses related to a particular good or service are matched against revenues derived from it in each accounting period. Also, deductions from revenue are matched against gross revenue. This enables each organizational unit to evaluate its performance and to plan and control its activities more effectively.

Capital assets. Acquisitions or improvements that cost over a certain amount and have an expected life of more than one or two years are *capital assets.* These include buildings, fixed and major movable equipment, land, and land improvements. All except land may be depreciated.

Depreciation. *Depreciation* is a technique used to allocate a portion of the original cost of a capital asset as an expense to each year of the asset's useful life, in order to match revenues with expenses better. Three methods of depreciation are used: straight line, sum-of-years' digits, and double declining balance. The latter two are often referred to as *accelerated depreciation* because a higher allocation of costs is taken in the early years. Depreciation is usually *booked;* it does not involve an outflow of cash. However, third-party payer requirements or incentives cause many health care organizations to *fund* depreciation, that is, to transfer cash to a restricted account.

Fund accounting. *Fund accounting* requires an organization to segregate its resources, obligations, and capital balances into separate accounts, or *funds,* based on legal restrictions and administrative and organizational requirements. Each fund has its particular purpose (e.g., plant expansion) and its own self-balancing accounting records (i.e., debits equaling credits). Interfund transfers are handled as if they involved separate entities. An organization's financial statements generally do not show individual fund accounts. However, changes appear in the statement of changes in fund balances (see Other Financial Statements, later in this chapter).

Fund accounting is common in government and not-for-profit organizations. There are two basic types of funds: unrestricted and donor restricted. A not-for-profit organization's *unrestricted fund,* often called the *general* or *operating fund,* is used to account for the resources, the obligations, and the capital of day-to-day operations. *Donor-restricted funds,* which may be temporarily or permanently restricted by the donor, may be categorized as endowment funds (generally held to generate income), plant replacement and expansion funds, and specific-purpose funds (such as a fund for research).

Chart of accounts. A *chart of accounts* is a listing of the titles of all asset, liability, capital, expense, and revenue accounts, each with a corresponding numeric code. Its purpose is to facilitate the recording and the reporting of financial information about an organization. Financial reports may be generated by individual organizational units, called *responsibility centers* (or *cost* or *revenue centers*), such as an occupational therapy department, as well as by functional areas such as a comprehensive rehabilitation program that includes occupational therapy, physical therapy, and speech pathology. Each responsibility center incurs similar expenses, which are recorded in such subaccounts as salaries and wages, employee benefits, professional fees, medical and surgical supplies, nonmedical and nonsurgical supplies (e.g., office supplies), purchased services (e.g., biomedical repair services), utilities, other direct expenses, depreciation, and rent. The accounts are collectively referred to as the *ledger.*

Forms of business organization. Businesses may be established as single proprietorships, partnerships, or corporations. A *single* or *sole proprietorship* is a business owned by one person and often managed by him or her. For accounting purposes it is an entity separate from the personal financial activities of the owner; however, there is no legal distinction between the business and the owner in regard to personal liability for business debts. An example is an occupational therapy practitioner who organizes a small private consulting business as a single proprietorship, obtains an employer (tax) identification number, and reports revenue, expenses, and business income or loss on Schedule C of his or her tax return, Internal Revenue Service Form 1040.

A *partnership* is a business owned by two or more persons associated as partners, and often managed by them. The partnership agreement should specify the investment and the duties of each partner, and the means of dividing the earnings or the losses each year and the assets on the withdrawal or the death of a partner. Some private practices in occupational therapy are organized as limited partnerships in which two or more persons have contributed capital for start-up.

A *corporation* is a business owned by one or an unlimited number of persons and incorporated under state law. Persons other than the owners often manage a corporation. Ownership is divided into shares of stock; owners are called *stockholders*. The corporation is a separate legal entity from its owners, with limited liability in regard to debts and with an unlimited life that may continue after the death of the original owners. Transfer of ownership is easy through transfer of shares of stock. Examples of publicly traded corporations are national firms that provide hospital or therapy services. They are incorporated under the laws of the state in which their home office is based or under the laws of another state (because it may have more liberal incorporation laws or better tax benefits); owned by numerous stockholders, with stock publicly traded on one of the stock exchanges; and managed by a chief executive officer and a board of directors. An example of a privately held corporation is a provider of outpatient occupational and hand therapy services with one or several clinic locations that is incorporated under Texas law; owned by one or several stockholders, with its stock privately held by these persons and not listed or available for purchase through a stock exchange; and managed by the founding occupational therapy practitioner. An example of a not-for-profit corporation is a hospital that is affiliated with a tax-exempt religious organization or a government entity.

FINANCIAL STATEMENTS

Financial accounting provides statements on an organization's financial position, on changes in that position, and on the results of operations (*profitability*).[3] The occupational therapy manager must understand the preceding accounting terms and concepts to be able to read and interpret the types of statements generated: the balance sheet, the income statement, and, to a lesser extent, the statement of cash flows and the statement of owners' equity or the statement of changes in fund balances.

All financial statements are prepared using data from the same accounting system and are therefore interrelated. Financial statements measure either levels (financial status on a particular date) or flows (changes in financial activity occurring during a specified period). The balance sheet is a level statement that reports the status of each account of the organization on a particular date. The income statement is a flow statement that shows the movement of revenue and expenses into and out of the organization during a specified period, usually 12 months. The statement of cash flows, also a flow statement, summarizes all the balance sheet changes arising from the flow of cash into and out of the organization during a specified period, usually 12 months. The statement of owners' equity and the statement of changes in fund balances are also flow statements. Annual reports are prepared using the organization's fiscal year, which may or may not correspond to the calendar year or to the organization's Medicare cost-reporting year.

The numbers that are entered on a balance sheet and an income statement are the results of numerous accounting transactions. These transactions can be illustrated using *T-accounts* (so-called because they look like the letter *T*), with debits shown on the left side, credits on the right side, and the name of the account written across the top of the T (see figure 3-1a). An increase in assets is entered on the left side, a reduction in assets on the right side. Likewise, an increase in liabilities and fund balance (or equity) is entered on the right side, a decrease on the left side. Therefore a debit (abbreviated *Dr.*) represents either an increase in an asset account or a decrease in a liability or fund balance (or equity) account. A credit

3. *This section is based on information from* Accounting: A Management Approach *(7th ed.), by G. Shillinglaw and Philip E. Meyer, 1983, Homewood, IL: Irwin;* Accounting Principles *(Rev. ed.), by R. H. Hermanson, J. D. Edwards, and R. F. Salmonson, 1983, Plano, TX: Business Publications;* Essentials of Health Care Finance *(3rd ed.), by W. O. Cleverley, 1992, Gaithersburg, MD: Aspen Publishers;* Finance for the Nonfinancial Manager *(2nd ed.), by H. T. Spiro, 1982, New York: Wiley;* Financial Control in Health Care: A Managerial Perspective, *by D. W. Young, 1984, Homewood, IL: Dow Jones–Irwin; and* Hospital Finance: A Comprehensive Case Approach, *by J. L. Bolandis, 1982, Rockville, MD: Aspen Systems.*

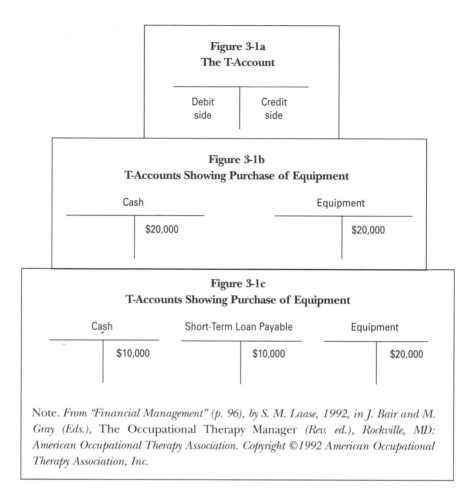

Figure 3-1a
The T-Account

| Debit side | Credit side |

Figure 3-1b
T-Accounts Showing Purchase of Equipment

Cash   Equipment

$20,000 $20,000

Figure 3-1c
T-Accounts Showing Purchase of Equipment

Cash   Short-Term Loan Payable   Equipment

$10,000 $10,000 $20,000

Note. *From "Financial Management" (p. 96), by S. M. Laase, 1992, in J. Bair and M. Gray (Eds.),* The Occupational Therapy Manager *(Rev. ed.), Rockville, MD: American Occupational Therapy Association. Copyright ©1992 American Occupational Therapy Association, Inc.*

(abbreviated *Cr.*) represents either a decrease in an asset account or an increase in a liability or fund balance (or equity) account.

For example, an organization purchases a $20,000 piece of equipment with cash. Figure 3-1b illustrates how the T-accounts reflect this transaction: Equipment is debited and cash is credited. If the organization finances the purchase with $10,000 in cash and a $10,000 short-term loan, the effect on the relevant T-accounts is as shown in figure 3-1c: Equipment is debited and cash and short-term loan payable is credited. In both these transactions the total dollar value of debits equals the total dollar value of credits. Each accounting transaction involves at least one debit entry and one credit entry. These two elements characterize *double-entry bookkeeping.*

The accountant documents, or *journalizes,* transactions in chronological order in a journal. Each journal entry directs the posting of the specific dollar amount to the correct account. Computerized financial accounting systems facilitate *cross-indexing,* or numbering, of journal entries and ledger accounts to trace recorded transactions from ledger to journal, or journal to ledger. An occupational therapy manager of a responsibility center in a hospital may receive a monthly summary of the center's ledger accounts and journal entries to control and evaluate financial performance better.

THE BALANCE SHEET

The *balance sheet* is a statement of an organization's assets, liabilities, and net assets, given that assets – liabilities = net assets. In for-profit corporations the net assets are considered owners' or stockholders' equity or interest. In not-for-profit corporations the net assets are considered fund balances. The date on the balance sheet is the last day of the period covered by the income statement. Often prior years' figures for the same date are included for comparative purposes.

Figure 3-2
Sample Not-for-Profit Hospital

Balance Sheet
December 31, 1995
(in thousands of dollars)

Assets			Liabilities and Fund Balance	
Current Assets			**Current Liabilities**	
Cash		$ 900	Accounts payable	$ 300
Accounts receivable			Accrued liabilities	100
Patient accounts	1,250		Short-term loan payable	500
Other	50		Mortgage payable, current	200
		1,300		
Inventories		50	**Total current liabilities**	1,100
Prepaid expenses		100		
			Long-Term Liabilities	
Total current assets		2,350	Mortgage payable, long-term	2,800
Assets Whose Use Is Limited			**Total Liabilities**	3,900
to Capital Improvements		50		
			Fund Balance	4,000
Property, Plant, and Equipment				
Land and buildings	6,000			
Equipment	2,000			
		8,000		
Less accumulated depreciation		2,500		
Property, plant, and				
equipment (net)		5,500		
Total Assets		$7,900	**Total Liabilities and Fund Balance**	$7,900

Note. *Adapted from "Financial Management" (p. 97), by S. M. Laase, 1992, in J. Bair and M. Gray (Eds.),* The Occupational Therapy Manager *(Rev. ed.), Rockville, MD: American Occupational Therapy Association. Copyright ©1992 American Occupational Therapy Association, Inc.*

Figure 3-2 illustrates the format and some representative accounts on the balance sheet of a not-for-profit organization, in this case a hospital. As the name implies, there is a basic accounting equation: assets = liabilities + fund balance (or equity). Usually assets are presented on the left side of the balance sheet, liabilities and fund balance (or equity) on the right. Assets are financed either by sources outside the organization (that is, liabilities) or by the organization itself (that is, fund balance or equity).

Current assets are those that an organization expects to convert into cash within a year. Current asset accounts include cash, short-term investments, accounts receivable, inventories, and prepaid expenses. *Cash* represents funds on hand in cash and in savings and checking accounts. Cash and *short-term investments* (e.g., certificates of deposit, government securities, and other temporary marketable securities) are sometimes combined into one account as *cash equivalents*. *Accounts receivable* represent the amounts due from customers for prior services or goods. In the health care industry, patients represent the bulk of accounts receivable. In figure 3-2 the net amount of patient accounts receivable is shown; it is derived from gross accounts receivable minus contractual allowances and courtesy allowances. The other accounts receivable balance in the example reflects medical office building rents due. *Inventories* include medical, surgical, nonmedical, and nonsurgical supplies. *Prepaid expenses* are expenditures for future services, such as liability insurance premiums and equipment lease payments.

Assets whose use is limited include funds set aside by directive of the governing board for specific purposes such as payment of malpractice costs, capital improvements, or debt repayment. In figure 3-2 the hospital board has restricted $50,000 for a building campaign.

Property, plant, and equipment, sometimes called *fixed assets,* represent permanent capital assets of an organization. In figure 3-2 they are shown at their historical, or acquisition cost, less *accumulated depreciation.* Net fixed assets are shown at $5.5 million, their *book value.* Other assets and intangibles, such as goodwill, may be included here. *Goodwill* is the excess of cost over net assets acquired, as in the case of a premium price paid to obtain a satellite outpatient clinic in anticipation of future high revenue from that location.

Current liabilities are obligations that an organization must pay within one year. Current liability accounts include accounts payable, accrued liabilities, notes payable, current maturities of long-term debt, and income taxes payable. *Accounts payable* represent the amount an organization is obligated to pay for the goods and the services it has received. In figure 3-2 the hospital has been charged for, but has not yet paid, invoices totaling $300,000 for a variety of supplies and services. *Accrued liabilities*, or *accrued expenses*, are obligations that result from prior operations, such as vacation pay, employee benefits (including pension and health plan costs), rent, insurance, and interest. *Notes payable* include short-term loan obligations. *Current maturities of long-term debt* represent the amount of principal, not the total amount of payment (principal and interest), that will be paid on long-term debt within the year. In figure 3-2 this category is represented by mortgage payable, current. For-profit companies would include liabilities for income taxes payable under current liabilities. These are not shown in figure 3-2 because the hospital in the example, a not-for-profit corporation as described in Section 501(c)(3) of the Internal Revenue Service code, is exempt from federal income taxes. An organization's *working capital* is its current assets minus its current liabilities.

Long-term or *noncurrent liabilities* are obligations that extend longer than one year. They include mortgages, bonds, capitalized lease payments, and estimated malpractice claim costs.

Fund balance represents the difference between assets and liabilities. Increases in this account ordinarily result from *contributions* or *earnings*. Not-for-profit organizations usually do not make a distinction. The fund balance consists of the excess of revenue over expenses, from the income statement (see figure 3-3), and donated funds (endowments, grants, etc.). In for-profit organizations, *equity* accounts include retained earnings, common stock, preferred stock, and paid-in capital. The *retained earnings* account contains the after-tax earnings of prior years, minus dividends paid. The other equity accounts reflect contributions. Fund balance or equity is not synonymous with or related to cash available. In most cases the cash balance will be much less than the fund balance.

THE INCOME STATEMENT

The *income statement* shows revenue and expense flows and net income during a specified period. That is, it explains how an organization's financial position changed through operations. For-profit organizations may also call this statement a *profit-and-loss* or *earnings statement*. Not-for-profit organizations may refer to it as a *statement of revenue and expenses*. Such organizations call net income *excess of revenue over expenses*, or *surplus* (or *deficit*).

The accounting conventions governing the recognition and the matching of revenues and expenses are used in preparing the income statement. Only resource inflows (revenues) and resource outflows (expenses) are shown. Exchanges in types of assets, or between assets and liabilities, are not reflected. For example, collection of an accounts receivable is an exchange of an accounts receivable asset for a cash asset.

Payment of a short-term loan is an exchange of a reduction in a cash asset for a reduction in a short-term loan payable liability. These transactions are reflected in the balance sheet.

Figure 3-3 illustrates a representative income statement of a not-for-profit hospital. In hospitals, *operating revenue* comes from two sources: (1) care of patients and (2) other services that occur in providing care to patients—for example, cafeteria, gift shop, and pharmacy sales to employees, patients, and visitors; silver recycling sales; parking fees from employees and visitors; revenue from educational programs; and medical office building and other rent. The corresponding accounts for these two sources are gross patient revenue and other operating revenue. The *gross patient revenue* account shows inpatient and outpatient revenue. *Deductions from revenue* (e.g., contractual allowances) are subtracted from gross

---

Figure 3-3
Sample Not-for-Profit Hospital

Income Statement
For the Year Ended December 31, 1995
(in thousands of dollars)

Operating Revenue		
Gross patient revenue		
Inpatient	$1,400	
Outpatient	900	
		$2,300
Deductions from revenue		200
Net patient revenue		2,100
Other operating revenue		300
Total operating revenue		2,400
Operating Expenses		
Salaries, wages, and benefits	1,400	
Supplies	300	
Depreciation	160	
Interest	40	
Other	100	
Total operating expenses		2,000
Income (loss) from operations		400
Nonoperating Revenue		
Contributions	40	
Investment income	100	
Total nonoperating revenue		150
Excess of Revenue over Expenses		$ 550

Note. *Adapted from "Financial Management" (p. 99), by S. M. Laase, 1992, in J. Bair and M. Gray (Eds.),* The Occupational Therapy Manager *(Rev. ed.), Rockville, MD: American Occupational Therapy Association. Copyright ©1992 American Occupational Therapy Association, Inc.*

patient revenue to yield *net patient revenue*. *Other operating revenue* is added to net patient revenue to obtain *total operating revenue*. Merchandising businesses such as durable medical equipment suppliers that acquire goods for resale to customers use a classified income statement that separates revenue and expenses into operating and nonoperating items. *Sales revenue* would be the primary source of operating revenue listed on their income statement. *Cost of goods sold* would be documented separately.

Operating expenses consist of assets that are consumed and liabilities that are increased in the provision of services related to organizational operations. In figure 3-3 the hospital has reported its expenses by type of expenditure. Other organizations may report expenses by type of responsibility center, such as patient care services and general and administrative services. Merchandising businesses include selling expenses as operating expenses. The difference between total operating revenue and *total operating expenses* indicates the hospital's *income* (or *loss*) *from operations*.

Nonoperating revenue (or *nonoperating gain*) is derived from activities that are not related to care of patients and normal hospital operations. Figure 3-3 shows two sources: *contributions* and *investment income* (interest or earnings generated from endowment or general funds). The contributions are unrestricted. Restricted contributions are taken directly into the fund balance because they are not freely available to finance operations. Gains or losses on disposal of capital items, and rental of facilities not used in operations, are other sources of nonoperating revenue.

The income from operations plus *total nonoperating revenue* equals the *excess of revenue over expenses*. The hospital in figure 3-3 shows a surplus of $550,000. The mission of a not-for-profit corporation does not allow excess revenues to be distributed to owners, so the hospital will reinvest excess revenues for replacement of facilities and equipment and expansion of services, and record them in the fund balance on the balance sheet. If this were a for-profit organization, it would expense income taxes, showing the resultant net earnings (or loss) on the income statement and recording them in the owners' equity section of the balance sheet. Distribution of excess revenues to the owners, as earnings per share, would also be shown on the income statement.

OTHER FINANCIAL STATEMENTS

Although they are of considerable importance to the individual responsible for the controllership and treasurership functions of an organization, the additional financial statements known as the statement of cash flows, and the statement of owners' equity or the statement of changes in fund balances, are not routinely used by the occupational therapy manager.

The *statement of cash flows* summarizes the receipt and the disbursement of cash. It measures an organization's ability to meet short-term cash needs. Sources of cash flowing from operations, investments, and financing activities are tracked.

Net assets are reported on separate financial statements that differ between for-profit and not-for-profit companies. For-profit companies use the *statement of owners'* or *stockholders' equity*, sometimes called the *statement of retained earnings*, which provides details regarding classes and shares of stock, earnings, and stock dividends. Not-for-profit companies use the *statement of changes in fund balances* to track the flows into and between donor-restricted and unrestricted funds during the year.

FINANCIAL MANAGEMENT

This section addresses selected financial management concepts and techniques that occupational therapy managers will find helpful: financial forecasting, analysis of financial statements, capital budgeting, and management of working capital.[4] The references listed at the end of the chapter offer information on other areas of financial management, such as leasing, long-term debt and stock, acquisitions and mergers, and bankruptcy and reorganization.

FINANCIAL FORECASTING

Translating a plan for a new service, program, or product into numbers involves *financial forecasting*, the process of estimating the future value of that new service, program, or product. A *pro forma*, or projected statement of the expected results of each course of action, with the sales or revenue forecast and the forecast of funds required or expenses, is used. Table 3-3 provides an example of the major steps in the development of a forecast for a new product line.

In a similar fashion, but on a different scale, organizations engage in a type of forecasting called *budgeting*, in which they translate their plans for a given period into financial terms. An organization's master budget may

4. *This section is based on information from* Cost Accounting: A Managerial Emphasis *(5th ed.), by C. T. Horngren, 1982, Englewood Cliffs, NJ: Prentice-Hall;* Cost Accounting for Health Care Organizations: Concepts and Applications, *by S. A. Finkler, 1994, Gaithersburg, MD: Aspen Publishers;* Essentials of Health Care Finance *(3rd ed.), by W. O. Cleverley, 1992, Gaithersburg, MD: Aspen Publishers;* Financial Control in Health Care: A Managerial Perspective, *by D. W. Young, 1984, Homewood, IL: Dow Jones–Irwin; and* Management Accounting for Healthcare Organizations *(Rev. ed.), by J. D. Suver and B. R. Neumann, 1985, Oak Brook, IL: Healthcare Financial Management Association, and Chicago: Pluribus Press.*

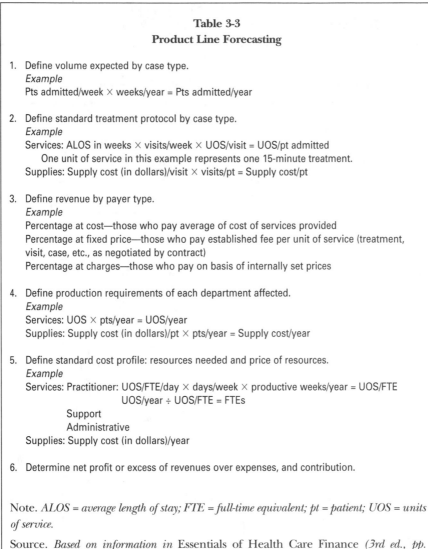

Table 3-3
Product Line Forecasting

1. Define volume expected by case type.
   Example
   Pts admitted/week × weeks/year = Pts admitted/year

2. Define standard treatment protocol by case type.
   Example
   Services: ALOS in weeks × visits/week × UOS/visit = UOS/pt admitted
       One unit of service in this example represents one 15-minute treatment.
   Supplies: Supply cost (in dollars)/visit × visits/pt = Supply cost/pt

3. Define revenue by payer type.
   Example
   Percentage at cost—those who pay average of cost of services provided
   Percentage at fixed price—those who pay established fee per unit of service (treatment,
   visit, case, etc., as negotiated by contract)
   Percentage at charges—those who pay on basis of internally set prices

4. Define production requirements of each department affected.
   Example
   Services: UOS × pts/year = UOS/year
   Supplies: Supply cost (in dollars)/pt × pts/year = Supply cost/year

5. Define standard cost profile: resources needed and price of resources.
   Example
   Services: Practitioner: UOS/FTE/day × days/week × productive weeks/year = UOS/FTE
                           UOS/year ÷ UOS/FTE = FTEs
           Support
           Administrative
   Supplies: Supply cost (in dollars)/year

6. Determine net profit or excess of revenues over expenses, and contribution.

Note. *ALOS = average length of stay; FTE = full-time equivalent; pt = patient; UOS = units
of service.*

Source. *Based on information in* Essentials of Health Care Finance *(3rd ed., pp.
253–56), by W. O. Cleverley, 1992, Gaithersburg, MD: Aspen Publishers.*

consist of the operating budget, which is the pro forma or projected statement of revenue and expenses, the capital budget, and the cash budget. Each organization has its own process for developing its budget. Table 3-4 provides an example of the major steps in the budget cycle. The financial executive responsible for the controllership function is usually responsible for coordinating the preparation of the budget. The entire process may take three to six months to complete (Esmond, 1982). The period for which the budget is developed is usually 12 months. Occupational therapy managers generally prepare operating budgets for their responsibility centers and contribute information for the preparation of the organization's capital budget, which is discussed in the next section.

Table 3-4
The Budgeting Process

Planning	Long-range planning
	• Approve organizational strategy
	• Approve operating plan
Budgeting	Development of budget format and guidelines
	• Prepare economic forecasts (e.g., inflation factors, new developments that may affect organization, and impending government regulations)
	• Determine budget format and timetable
	• Establish preliminary assumptions regarding rate increases and net income requirements
	Distribution of approved budget package, including assumptions, forms, schedules, and historical data
	Communication: general and technical budget meetings with line management; technical assistance when necessary
	Forecasting of volume (e.g., patient days, outpatient visits, and responsibility center activity levels)
	Preparation of preliminary revenue budget, personnel budget, operating expense budget (including budgets for new and expanded programs)
	Holding of departmental budget hearings
	Preparation of tentative operating budget (containing projections of revenue, expenses, contractual allowances, doubtful account allowances, vacancy allowances, depreciation, interest expense, and insurance)
	• Determine desired net income, salary increases, and rate increases
	• Approve new programs, and new and upgraded positions
	Approval of budget, first by budget committee, then by full governing board
Monitoring and controlling	Distribution and implementation of approved budget with regular feedback

Note. *From "Financial Management" (p. 117), by S. M. Laase, 1992, in J. Bair and M. Gray (Eds.),* The Occupational Therapy Manager *(Rev. ed.), Rockville, MD: American Occupational Therapy Association. Copyright ©1992 American Occupational Therapy Association, Inc.*

Key Forecasting Concepts and Terms

A familiarity with the following concepts and terms will enable the occupational therapy manager to collaborate with the financial executive in developing financial pro formas and budgets. The strong emphasis on cost accounting and cost concepts reflects the current trend toward increased scrutiny and management of costs in the changing health care environment.

Cost accounting. *Cost accounting* is a subset of accounting that measures, as accurately and as efficiently as possible, the resources used to produce a particular good or service, and then classifies, summarizes, and interprets that information to facilitate decision making regarding establishment of prices and pricing policies, negotiation of reimbursement contracts with third-party payers, maximization of revenue, preparation of flexible budgets, monitoring of productivity and efficiency, preparation of reports for external groups such as hospital associations and government agencies, and strategic planning.

Responsibility centers. *Responsibility centers* are the "smallest segments of activity or areas of responsibility for which costs are accumulated" (Horngren, 1982, p. 967). Also called *cost centers,* they are considered *revenue-producing centers* if they generate incremental reimbursement for the incremental services they render, such as in occupational therapy, or *non-revenue-producing service centers* if they do not generate incremental reimbursement for the incremental services they render, such as in housekeeping. These distinctions are fading, however, as reimbursement moves away from charge-based systems.

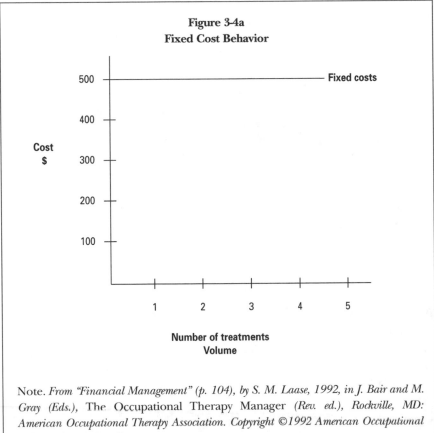

Figure 3-4a
Fixed Cost Behavior

Note. *From "Financial Management" (p. 104), by S. M. Laase, 1992, in J. Bair and M. Gray (Eds.),* The Occupational Therapy Manager *(Rev. ed.), Rockville, MD: American Occupational Therapy Association. Copyright ©1992 American Occupational Therapy Association, Inc.*

Cost finding. *Cost finding* is the process of allocating the costs of the non-revenue-producing service centers to one another and to the revenue-producing centers on the basis of statistical data that measure the amount of service rendered. Cost finding enables an organization to identify the full costs (direct and allocated indirect) of operating each revenue-producing center.

Cost classifications. Costs can be classified in four ways: by their traceability to the object being costed (i.e., direct or indirect), by their behavior in response to volume of output (i.e., fixed, variable, semifixed, or semivariable), by their controllability by management (i.e., controllable or uncontrollable), and by their relevance in decision making (i.e., sunk, discretionary, avoidable, incremental, or opportunity).

Direct costs are those that are clearly traceable to one product or responsibility center. Examples in an occupational therapy unit are staff members' salaries and medical supplies used in treatment. *Indirect costs* are those that are not clearly identified with one product or center. Examples are the costs of security and housekeeping for common areas. Indirect costs may be assigned to responsibility centers as equitably as possible, such as by square feet or on the basis of results of a time study.

Fixed costs are those that remain at the same level for a given period despite variations in volume, that is, in number of units of service rendered. Examples are depreciation, insurance on assets, rent, and the administrator's salary. Figure 3-4a shows fixed cost behavior. Total fixed costs do not change with volume. However, as the volume increases, the average fixed cost per patient, or unit of service decreases. Figure 3-4b illustrates how fixed costs are divided among a greater number of units of service as volume increases. This concept has ramifications for pricing.

Variable costs change in direct proportion to changes in volume. If the number of treatments increases by 5 percent, then variable costs, such as those for supplies, will also increase by 5 percent. The steeper the slope of the line, the greater the variable costs per unit. See figure 3-5.

Semifixed costs change in response to variations in volume, but not proportionally. Salary expense for supervisors is an example of semifixed costs. Supervisors may be added at intervals as staff increases warrant, for example, one for every five to seven therapists. These costs are also called *step costs,* referring to the nature of their cost curve, as seen in figure 3-6. Semifixed costs can be considered variable or fixed, depending on the size of the steps and the volume.

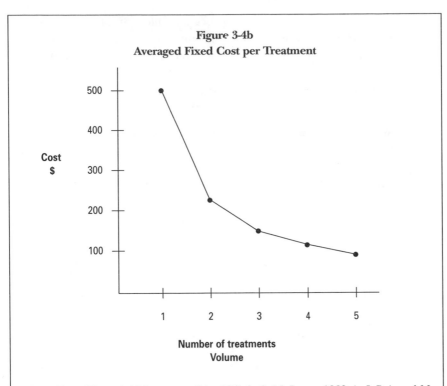

Figure 3-4b
Averaged Fixed Cost per Treatment

Note. *From "Financial Management" (p. 104), by S. M. Laase, 1992, in J. Bair and M. Gray (Eds.),* The Occupational Therapy Manager *(Rev. ed.), Rockville, MD: American Occupational Therapy Association. Copyright ©1992 American Occupational Therapy Association, Inc.*

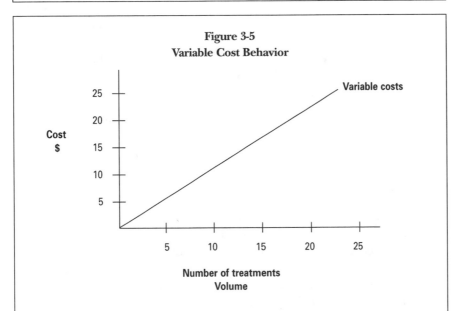

Figure 3-5
Variable Cost Behavior

Note. *From "Financial Management" (p. 105), by S. M. Laase, 1992, in J. Bair and M. Gray (Eds.),* The Occupational Therapy Manager *(Rev. ed.), Rockville, MD: American Occupational Therapy Association. Copyright ©1992 American Occupational Therapy Association, Inc.*

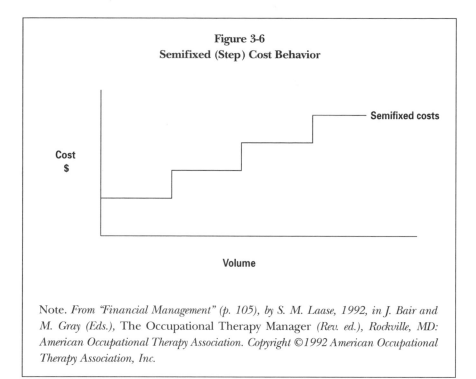

Figure 3-6
Semifixed (Step) Cost Behavior

Cost
$

Semifixed costs

Volume

Note. *From "Financial Management" (p. 105), by S. M. Laase, 1992, in J. Bair and M. Gray (Eds.),* The Occupational Therapy Manager *(Rev. ed.), Rockville, MD: American Occupational Therapy Association. Copyright ©1992 American Occupational Therapy Association, Inc.*

Semivariable costs are costs that have both fixed and variable elements. Utilities, for example, have a basic monthly minimum charge (fixed), plus additional charges that are directly proportional to the number of units used (variable). Figure 3-7 illustrates the semivariable cost curve. Figure 3-8 depicts the total cost for a department or program, which consists of all fixed, variable, direct, and indirect costs.

Controllable costs are those over which a manager has a reasonable measure of influence. Examples include nonmedical supplies for the unit. *Uncontrollable costs* are those that are associated with a unit but over which the manager has little or no control. Once capital expenditures are made, associated depreciation is an uncontrollable cost.

Sunk costs represent those that are not affected by the decision under consideration because they have already been incurred. For example, the book value of an asset is a sunk cost. *Discretionary costs* are a category of fixed costs that are fixed by management but can be changed in different reporting periods, such as asset insurance, legal and audit fees, and research expenses. *Avoidable costs* are those that will be affected by the outcome of a decision. They can be eliminated or saved if an activity is discontinued or a volume reduced. Sunk costs are not avoidable. *Incremental costs* are the

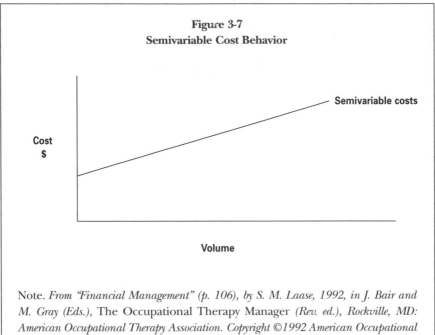

Figure 3-7
Semivariable Cost Behavior

Note. *From "Financial Management" (p. 106), by S. M. Laase, 1992, in J. Bair and* M. Gray *(Eds.),* The Occupational Therapy Manager *(Rev. ed.), Rockville, MD:* American Occupational Therapy Association. Copyright ©1992 American Occupational Therapy Association, Inc.

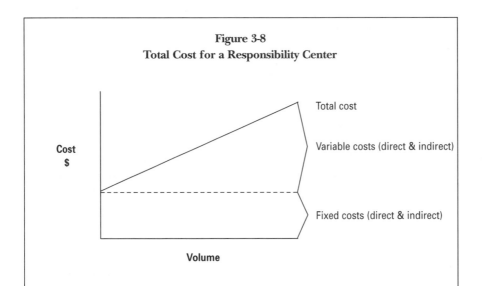

Figure 3-8
Total Cost for a Responsibility Center

Note. *From "Financial Management" (p. 106), by S. M. Laase, 1992, in J. Bair and* M. Gray *(Eds.),* The Occupational Therapy Manager *(Rev. ed.), Rockville, MD:* American Occupational Therapy Association. Copyright ©1992 American Occupational Therapy Association, Inc.

changes in total costs resulting from a new activity or an increase in volume. *Opportunity cost* is the value of the best alternative use of a limited resource that is foregone by its use in a particular way.

Ratio of cost to charges. *Ratio of cost to charges* compares charges from patients' bills with costs by applying the ratio of the organization's costs to its charges.

Overhead. *Overhead* is any cost of doing business other than the direct cost associated with the production of outputs (goods or services).

Break-even analysis. *Break-even analysis,* also called *cost-volume-profit analysis,* determines the level of volume needed to make profit equal zero and revenue equal cost. It is computed as follows:

Fixed cost ÷ (Rate − Variable cost) = Break-even volume in units

"In health care, because revenue is subject to payer mix, adjustments are made for cost payers, fixed-price payers, and charge payers to find the average price paid so that volume and break-even can be estimated more accurately" (Cleverley, 1992, p. 232).

Contribution margin. *Contribution margin* is "the amount by which the price per unit of service exceeds its variable cost" (Finkler, 1994, p. 694). The terms *contribution* and *contribution margin* are also used on a larger scale to quantify profitability of operations, or operating margin, by dividing net operating income by total revenue (see Ratio Analysis, later in this chapter).

Budgeting philosophies. Budgeting philosophies are approaches to budgeting. Common ones are *incremental budgeting,* in which the expense budget is based on last year's costs plus an inflation factor, and *zero-base budgeting,* in which all expenditures are examined and justified.

ANALYSIS OF FINANCIAL STATEMENTS

Financial analysis consists of assessing an organization's financial performance through ratio analysis and analysis of key operating indicators, comparing the results with industry norms and tracking trends over time. Variance analysis is used to compare actual results with the budget.

Ratio Analysis

Financial statements generate important data that can be analyzed using quantitative methods known as *ratios* to look at critical areas of financial management: liquidity, profitability, asset management, debt management, and market value. In health care management, emphasis is placed on certain *liquidity ratios,* such as the current ratio and the days-in-accounts-receivable ratio, and certain *profitability ratios,* such as the total

---

Table 3-5
Commonly Used Financial Ratios

Liquidity Ratios

Current	Current assets ÷ Current liabilities
Days in pt AR	Receivables ÷ Revenue/day
	or
	Net pt AR ÷ Average daily net pt revenue
	or
	Net pt AR ÷ Net pt revenue/day

Profitability Ratios

Total margin	Excess of revenues over expenses ÷ Total revenue
	or
	Net profit after taxes ÷ Total revenue
Operating margin	Net operating income ÷ Total revenue
Operating margin, price level adjusted (to reflect depreciation and to examine ability to replace fixed assets)	(Operating income + Depreciation – Price level depreciation) ÷ Total revenue
Return on equity	Net profit after taxes ÷ Equity
	or
	Excess of revenue over expenses ÷ Fund balance

Note. *AR = accounts receivable; pt = patient.*

Source. *Based on information in* Essentials of Health Care Finance *(3rd ed., pp. 136–37, 149–53), by W. O. Cleverley, 1992, Gaithersburg, MD: Aspen Publishers; and* Financial Management Theory and Practice *(2nd ed., p. 201), by E. F. Brigham, 1979, Hinsdale, IL: Dryden Press.*

---

margin ratio and the operating margin ratio. Table 3-5 illustrates the methods of calculating selected ratios. Managers can identify strengths and weaknesses of their organization, and favorable and unfavorable trends in its performance, by comparing the organization's ratios with industry norms and with its own ratios over time. Normative industry data can be obtained from the Financial Analysis Service of the Healthcare Financial Management Association.

Analysis of Key Operating Indicators

Health care organizations identify and track key operating indicators, primarily for internal uses. Common indicators that they track include the following:

Occupancy—by percentage of licensed beds filled

Average daily census (ADC)—by number of patients

Average length of stay (ALOS)—in days; may be adjusted for case mix

Net price per discharge—in dollars; may be adjusted for case mix

Cost per discharge—in dollars; may be adjusted for case mix

Nursing cost per patient day—in dollars

Ancillary (such as occupational therapy) cost per unit of servic— in dollars

Inpatient man-hours per discharge—in hours; may be adjusted for case mix

Full-time equivalents (FTEs) per occupied bed—in FTEs; also reported as employees per occupied bed (EPOB) or man-hours per patient day (MH ppd)

Average salary per FTE—in dollars; also reported as wages per man-hour

Net price per outpatient visit—in dollars; also reported as average charge per visit

Cost per outpatient visit—in dollars

Outpatient man-hours per visit—in hours

Outpatient revenue—by percentage of total in- and out-patient revenue

Commercial mix—by percentage of patients with commercial (nongovernmental) insurance; further broken down by managed care mix

Medicare mix—by percentage of patients with Medicare as their primary insurance coverage

Occupational therapy managers must be knowledgeable about and supportive of their organization's goals and objectives in regard to the key operating indicators that they select for monitoring. As with ratios, normative industry data are available for some operating indicators so that managers may compare these aspects of their organization's performance with industry benchmarks. Temporal analysis may also be conducted by comparing the past value of an operating indicator with its current number, again to identify favorable and unfavorable trends.

Variance Analysis

A comparison of budgeted and actual revenues and expenses is also routinely performed at all levels of health care organizations. The occupational therapy manager, as a responsibility center manager, should perform and be prepared to document and submit for review, a variance report for all subaccounts with unfavorable (U) variances between budgeted and actual numbers. Variances in expenses may be due to the following:

Price—a higher or lower price or rate paid for inputs or resources consumed, such as salaries or craft supplies

Quantity—more or fewer resources consumed per unit of activity; a change in efficiency, such as with a new, inexperienced practitioner

Worked versus paid hours, or productive versus nonproductive hours; further, nonproductive nonworked hours (sick leave, vacation, or holiday) versus nonproductive worked hours (administration or training) versus productive worked hours

Volume—more or fewer units of activity; a change in center workload

Acuity—the amount that spending differed from expectations because of the severity of patients' illnesses

Revenue variances may be due to the following:

Market size—a greater or smaller number, or volume, of patients in the community than expected

Market share—a greater or smaller percentage of the share of the market of total community patients served

Patient mix—a difference in the mix of diagnoses among patients

Price—a difference in actual prices charged or actual receipts expected, rather than gross charges, based on the rates various payers are willing to pay

Corrective actions should be planned as part of the variance analysis and report.

CAPITAL BUDGETING

Capital budgeting focuses on planning for expenditures for property, plant, and equipment. An earlier section of this chapter discusses classifying assets as capital based on useful life and cost, and the meaning of the term fixed assets. As with an operating budget, each organization has its own process for developing a capital budget. Table 3-6 provides an example of the major steps in the development of a capital budget. Many organizations initiate the capital budgeting process before they initiate the operating budget process. The capital budgeting process uses forms or worksheets developed to highlight key information needed to evaluate the merits of each expenditure. It may involve forecasting for periods in excess of one year.

Table 3-6
The Capital Budgeting Process

Idea generation	
Data gathering: summaries of proposals or descriptions of proposed expenditures from requesting managers	Identify possible alternatives.
	• Make or buy?
	• Purchase, finance, or lease?
	• Self-operate or contract?
	• Obtain from which manufacturer?
	Identify resources currently available.
	Identify costs.
	• Quotes?
	• Shipping?
	• Installation and renovation?
	• Specialized training?
	• Other costs over project's life cycle?
	Identify and classify benefits.
	• For operational continuity or financial benefit?
	• Quantitative and qualitative benefits?
	• Replacement to maintain current business?
	• Replacement to reduce costs?
	• Expansion of existing products or markets?
	• Expansion into new markets or products?
	• For safety or regulatory reasons?
	• For other reasons, such as employee retention?
	Review prior performance.
	• What is reliability of manager's previous forecasts?
	• What is organization's experience with similar proposals?
	Estimate risk.
	• What proportion represents fixed or sunk costs?
	• What is project's sensitivity to volume fluctuations?
Financial analysis	Estimate expected cash flow.
	Review riskiness of projected cash flow.
	Select and apply appropriate formula[a] to determine actual cost of capital and discounted cash flows, to allow comparisons between asset's value to firm and its cost.
	Assess effect on value of organization.
Decision making	Determine whether governing board approval is needed.
	Establish timetable.
Postcompletion audit	Compare actual results with those predicted in request.
	Explain variances.

Source. *Based on information in* Essentials of Health Care Finance *(3rd ed., pp. 369–75), by W. O. Cleverley, 1992, Gaithersburg, MD: Aspen Publishers; and* Financial Management Theory and Practice *(2nd ed., p. 353), by E. F. Brigham, 1979, Hinsdale, IL: Dryden Press.*

a. Different methods, such as computation of net present value, payback period, internal rate of return, profitability index, and equivalent annual cost, may be used. See sources in note for more detail.

MANAGEMENT OF WORKING CAPITAL

Working capital, defined in the discussion of the balance sheet as current assets minus current liabilities, should be carefully controlled so that only a small percentage of assets are committed as working capital and therefore unavailable for more productive purposes. Key points in management of cash on hand, marketable securities, accounts receivable, inventories, and current liabilities are noted here.

Cash on Hand

An organization needs a certain level of cash on hand to conduct transactions; to cover itself in case of unpredictable fluctuations in inflows and outflows; to speculate, such as to take advantage of a bargain price on supplies; and to maintain a minimum balance in a bank account to avoid paying service fees. Many responsibility centers use a petty cash account to facilitate conducting small transactions. They hold receipts until they generate sufficient expense to make accounting for the transaction cost-effective. They then make journal entries to debit the appropriate account, such as nonmedical supplies, for the aggregate amount when they balance the petty cash account on a periodic basis. Large organizations may use a formal cash budget, which is a statement showing the organization's projected cash inflows and outflows over a specified period.

Marketable Securities

An organization may hold short-term marketable securities such as certificates of deposit to finance seasonal or cyclical operations, to meet an upcoming financial requirement such as construction, or when it has just sold stocks or bonds. The person responsible for the treasurership functions of the organization manages the investment of the marketable securities.

Accounts Receivable

Prudent management of accounts receivable, to shorten the time it takes to convert accounts receivable to cash, and to minimize lost charges and uncollectible amounts, can have a significant influence on the profitability of an organization by allowing for the investment of surplus funds. The occupational therapy manager can help reduce the cash conversion cycle in the following ways:

- By obtaining required insurance and eligibility information before initiating services
- By ensuring that charges are posted in a timely manner
- By ensuring that medical record documentation is completed in a timely manner to allow for completion of charts on discharged patients

- By settling outpatient accounts at discharge or departure
- By setting up a system to respond quickly to requests for further documentation from third-party payers

An understanding of some additional accounts receivable terms and concepts may be helpful to the occupational therapy manager:

Lockbox plan. Under a *lockbox plan,* an organization's customers send payments directly to a post office box, from which an intermediary bank may pick them up, clear the checks, and wire the funds to the organization's bank; or the organization's bank itself may pick up the checks.

Credit terms. *Credit terms* are terms of payment of an invoice. They may include a discount as an incentive for prompt payment. For example, the credit terms "2/10, net 30" on an invoice mean that the vendor will give a 2-percent discount if the bill is paid within 10 days and that if the buyer does not take the discount, the vendor requires full payment in 30 days. "Net 60" means that the vendor offers no discount and expects full payment in 60 days.

Aging schedule. An *aging schedule* breaks down accounts receivable according to how long they have been outstanding.

Inventories

Inventories are another category of current assets requiring careful management. Inventories can be conceptualized as *safety stock,* which is held for unusual occurrences, and *working stock.* Quantitative techniques, such as the Economic Ordering Quantity (EOQ) model, exist to help organizations determine their optimal level of inventory of safety and working stock and the optimal number of orders to place each year. Some organizations use the Just In Time approach to inventory management, which strives for minimal inventories. In the determination of optimal level of inventory, the organization must balance two kinds of costs: (1) the cost of tying its capital up in inventory, incurring related costs, such as storage, inspection, insurance, and property taxes, and risking a decrease in value due to depreciation, obsolescence, or loss; against (2) the costs of running short, resulting in loss of customer goodwill, loss of sales, and disruption of service, and the costs of placing frequent orders, incurring more shipping and handling costs while losing quantity discounts.

Current Liabilities

As for the current liabilities side of the balance sheet, an understanding of short-term credit may be helpful to the occupational therapy manager. Four types of short-term credit may be available: (1) *accounts payable,* conceptualized as trade credit obtained by delaying payment (and as a result, forfeiting discounts for prompt payment); (2) *accrued liabilities,* such as accrued wages and accrued income and Social Security taxes; (3) *commercial bank loans,* shown on the balance sheet as notes payable, with interest scaled from the prime rate up; and (4) *commercial paper,* consisting of unsecured promissory notes, which are available only to large organizations. An organization may also raise funds by pledging or selling (*factoring*) accounts receivable.

SUMMARY

Three major threats in the health care industry have had a tremendous influence on financial management: rising health care costs, rapidly changing reimbursement systems, and greater competition among providers for patients and scarce resources. All three developments have brought about great pressures and numerous measures in the public and private sectors to contain costs.

To address these threats, health care financial executives and occupational therapy managers have expanded and further defined their roles and increased their expertise in financial management. The educational preparation of the occupational therapy practitioner provides key skills that are applicable to financial management. A lack of familiarity with the language and the concepts of accounting and finance may be perceived as a weakness of the new manager.

Accounting is the process of collecting, recording, summarizing, analyzing, reporting, and interpreting information about an organization in monetary terms. *Financial accounting* provides financial statements for external use, whereas *managerial accounting* provides reports for internal decision making. The occupational therapy manager must have an understanding of many concepts and terms used in basic and managerial accounting: entity, transactions, cost valuation, double entry, conservatism, consistency, full disclosure, materiality, accrual basis of accounting, revenue, deductions from revenue, expenses, matching of revenue and expenses, capital assets, depreciation, fund accounting, chart of accounts, and forms of business organization.

Financial statements measure either levels (financial status on a particular date) or flows (changes in financial activity occurring during a specified period). The balance sheet is a level statement that reports the status of each account of the organization on a particular date. The income statement is a flow statement that shows the movement of revenue and expenses into and out of the organization during a specified period, usually 12 months. The statement of cash flows, also a flow statement, summarizes all the balance sheet changes arising from the flow of cash into and out of the organization during a specified period, usually 12 months.

The major components of a balance sheet are current assets (cash, short-term investments, accounts receivable, inventories, and prepaid expenses); assets whose use is limited; property, plant, and equipment, less accumulated depreciation; current liabilities (accounts payable, accrued liaibilities, notes payable, and current maturities of long-term debt); long-term liabilities (e.g., mortgages, capitalized lease payments, and estimated malpractice claim costs); and fund balance or, in for-profit organizations, equity. An income statement reports operating revenue (gross patient revenue and other operating revenue), operating expenses, nonoperating revenue (e.g., contributions and investment income), and excess of revenue over expenses. The statement of cash flows summarizes the receipt and the disbursement of cash.

Occupational therapy managers will find several financial management concepts and techniques helpful: financial forecasting, analysis of financial statements, capital budgeting, and management of working capital. Translating a plan for a new service, program, or product into numbers involves financial forecasting, the process of estimating the future value of that new service, program, or product. Financial analysis consists of assessing an organization's financial performance through ratio analysis and analysis of key operating indicators, comparing the results with industry norms and tracking trends over time. Variance analysis is used to compare actual results with the budget. Capital budgeting focuses on planning for expenditures for property, plant, and equipment. Management of working capital calls for careful control so that only a small percentage of assets are committed as working capital and therefore unavailable for more productive purposes.

REFERENCES

Beck, D. F. (1980). *Basic hospital financial management.* Rockville, MD: Aspen Systems.

Berman, H. J., Kukla, S. F., & Weeks, L. E. (1994). *The financial management of hospitals* (8th ed.). Ann Arbor, MI: Health Administration Press.

Cleverley, W. O. (1992). *Essentials of health care finance* (3rd ed.). Gaithersburg, MD: Aspen Publishers.

Economic Stabilization Act of 1970, Pub. L. No. 91–379, 84 Stat. 799.

Esmond, T. H., Jr. (1982). *Budgeting procedures for hospitals* (1982 ed.). Chicago: American Hospital Association.

Finkler, S. A. (1994). *Cost accounting for health care organizations.* Gaithersburg, MD: Aspen Publishers.

Hermanson, R. H., Edwards, J. D., & Salmonson, R. F. (1983). *Accounting principles* (Rev. ed.). Plano, TX: Business Publications.

Horngren, C. T. (1982). *Cost accounting: A managerial emphasis* (5th ed.). Englewood Cliffs, NJ: Prentice-Hall.

Social Security Amendments of 1983, Pub. L. No. 98–281, 97 Stat. 65.

United States Bureau of the Census. (1994, September). *Statistical abstract of the United States* (114th ed.). Washington, DC: Government Printing Office.

ADDITIONAL RESOURCES

Tracy, J. A. (1994). *How to read a financial report* (4th ed.). New York: Wiley.

CHAPTER 4

Marketing

Tina Shoemaker, MHA, OTR, CHE
Carol Wheeler, BSN, RN, CHE

KEY TERMS

Environmental assessment. An organization's reexamination of the patient population to be served and the mode and the location of service delivery, with the aim of answering the question, What business are we in?

Market analysis. An organization's use of information identified in organizational and environmental assessments to define a market and determine if its perception of the wants and the needs of the market is valid.

Marketing. "A social and managerial process by which individuals and groups obtain what they need and want through creating and exchanging products and values with others" (Kotler & Armstrong, 1991, p. 5).

Marketing management. "The analysis, planning, implementation, and control of programs designed to create, build, and maintain beneficial exchanges with target buyers for the purpose of achieving organizational objectives" (Kotler & Armstrong, 1991, p. 10).

Organizational assessment. An organization's reevaluation of its effectiveness relative to the patient population, the community, and the health care system itself.

Place. The method of distributing a product to a target market, or the means of giving the target market access to a product.

Position. The place that a product holds among similar products in the marketplace.

Price. "The financial, physical, and psychological costs to people of doing business with you" (MacStravic, 1980, p. 11).

Product. "Anything that can be offered to a market for attention, acquisition, use, or consumption and that might satisfy a need or want" (Kotler & Armstrong, 1991, p. 7).

Promotion. All attempts to make a product visible and desirable to a target market or a segment of that market.

Target market. Of all the persons or organizations that a marketer could influence, the portion, or segment, that the marketer wishes to influence.

Tina Shoemaker, MHA, OTR, CHE, is a senior consultant with Rural Health Consultants, an organization based in Lawrence, Kansas, that assists communities in restructuring their health care systems. Formerly she served as a regional vice-president for Stormont-Vail Enterprises, Inc., a proprietary health services management company affiliated with Stormont-Vail Regional Medical Center in Topeka, Kansas. She earned her master's degree at the University of Minnesota and her occupational therapy degree at the University of Kansas.

Carol Wheeler, BSN, RN, CHE, is the vice-president for regional operations for Stormont-Vail Regional Medical Center in Topeka, Kansas. She supervises the operations of various business ventures, including the management of rural hospitals, home health and hospice care, various outpatient services, pharmacies, management information systems, and a physician billing service. She has completed two-and-a-half years of graduate work toward a master's degree in health administration at the University of Minnesota.

Marketing has become as commonplace as strategic planning, financial management, and community (public) relations in health care organizations. To compete in the American health care system of this decade and the next, occupational therapy managers and practitioners must be familiar with concepts of marketing and their successful application. This chapter reviews marketing concepts and applications in the context of occupational therapy services.

Marketing as a function is accepted in the health care organization, but its place in the structure and its relationship to other, similar functions are not consistent across organizations of similar size and scope. Many persons in the health care setting confuse marketing with strategic planning or community relations because the outcomes of these functions seem to be the same as the outcomes of marketing. This confusion is not unlike that which occurs between occupational therapy and physical therapy, or occupational therapy and social work. The outcomes seem to be the same in terms of increased function of the patient, but the process that is applied through the disciplines is different.

Just as occupational therapy can be described as a system of knowledge and skills applied within a framework of theory, marketing is a system for operational planning from an information base. An organization gathers and analyzes the information through a disciplined study of the needs of the patients (customers), physicians (referral sources), administrators (the source of an occupational therapy organization's or program's funding), and reimbursers (the source of the larger organization's funding). These four groups are referred to as *target markets*. Of all the persons or organizations that a marketer could influence, the target market is the portion, or segment, that the marketer wishes to influence.

A DEFINITION OF MARKETING

Kotler and Armstrong (1991) define *marketing* as "a social and managerial process by which individuals and groups obtain what they need and want through creating and exchanging products and values with others" (p. 5). Building on this description, they define *marketing management* as "demand management," or "the analysis, planning, implementation, and control of programs designed to create, build, and maintain beneficial exchanges with target buyers for the purpose of achieving organizational objectives" (p. 10). These definitions reveal marketing to be a function that results in the development of a product or a service designed to appeal to particular customers or groups of customers with similar needs. Traditionally, health care and other nonprofit or charitable organizations developed their products or services based on what they thought the customer ought to want relative to their own plans for the organization.

With increasing competition in the health care system, they have been compelled to organize products or services in terms of what will be most appealing to the customer.

ESSENTIAL CONCEPTS OF MARKETING

Traditionally, marketing theory has focused on four key concepts, classically called the four P's of market plan development: product, price, place, and promotion. In addition, the concept of position is essential to the application and the implementation of marketing theory. An understanding of these basic concepts provides a base on which to build a specific market plan.

PRODUCT

The concept of product underlies the entire marketing effort. A *product* is defined as "anything that can be offered to a market for attention, acquisition, use, or consumption and that might satisfy a need or want" (Kotler & Armstrong, 1991, p. 7). In health care a product is most commonly a service that can be provided to a patient directly, or indirectly through other organizations. The target market is often thought to be the patient, but more frequently it may be the physician or the organization to which the patient looks for care and therapy decisions.

The concept of product line development provides for the grouping of products with like attributes, often around a core attribute such as a body system, a disease entity, or a disability type. Currently, products are being organized around the diagnosis-related group (DRG). Many payment systems use DRGs to classify patients by the amount of health care resources that they and their providers consume during an illness.

As an occupational therapy organization develops an idea for a product, it should try to answer several questions:

1. What is the product to be marketed?

2. What attributes of this product will the patient desire?

3. What benefits will be derived by the provider for developing and marketing the product?

4. What will be the basis for the exchange?

An example of a product is pediatric developmental assessment. The attribute sought by the patient is an assessment outcome and information or recommendations for therapeutic intervention. The benefits to be derived by the provider are referrals for therapy and an increase in the number of referrals for assessment relative to the total done in the area (that is, an increase in the organization's market share). The basis for the exchange is that the parties trade something of value: The patient gives cooperation and payment for services; the practitioner offers expertise and advice.

PRICE

Generally speaking, *price* is the value of the monetary exchange that occurs when a product is purchased. It may be that simple. However, other factors should be considered. MacStravic (1980) defines price as "the financial, physical, and psychological costs to people of doing business with you" (p. 11). Often forgotten in determining pricing strategies is the idea of psychological costs. For example, a parent may find it difficult to seek a pediatric developmental assessment if he or she is not psychologically ready to accept the possibility of an abnormal finding.

Pricing strategies should take into consideration not only the financial, physical, and psychological aspects of a product or a service, but also its competition and its fair market value. Decisions to price a service under its actual cost may be valid if an organization can expect the low price to attract consumers who will also buy other products of the organization. Such a product is called a *loss leader.* For example, an organization may price pediatric developmental assessment below its actual cost if the organization judges that the revenue from treatment of children found to have abnormalities will offset any shortfall in the revenue from assessment and increase the likelihood that the family will seek other services from the organization. Other pricing considerations include third-party payment practices and rates, current charges for similar services offered by the organization or the program, and the desired profit margin.

PLACE

The concept of *place* is easily understood as a matter of distribution or access—that is, the method of distributing a product to a target market, or the means of giving the target market access to a product. The following questions related to place might be asked during development of the pediatric developmental assessment service:

1. How will the service be offered (e.g., in the hospital, in an outpatient clinic, or in a school)?

2. When will the service be provided (i.e., what days of the week and what hours of the day)?

3. How will the patient gain access to the service (e.g., by referral from a physician, a nurse, a counselor, a social worker, or a parent, or by self-referral)?

4. Who will be eligible for the service?

5. How long will an assessment take?

6. On what basis will testing be done (i.e., inpatient or outpatient)?

7. If the service will be available to both inpatients and outpatients, how will the way in which it is delivered differ?

8. Are there physical or psychological obstacles that will impede access to the service (e.g., inadequate parking space, an inconvenient location, or long waiting periods)?

Answering questions like these will assist the provider in developing a product to which the target market can easily gain access.

PROMOTION

Promotion is the concept that most people commonly associate with marketing. It is just one aspect of marketing, however. *Promotion* is defined as all attempts to make a product visible and desirable to a target market or a segment of that market. It may include, but is not limited to, the following:

1. Advertising through newspapers and other print media, radio, television, billboards, and brochures

2. Personal contact by a representative of the organization or the person providing the service, through health fairs, shopping center displays, and presentations at meetings of parent-teacher organizations and in other settings frequented by the target market

3. Atmospherics, a method used to affect the environment so as to produce a specific emotional response in the target market (Lauback & Rand, 1980)—for example, showing a film on developmental disabilities at a parent-teacher organization meeting

4. Bonuses, incentives, discounts, and the development of some tangible reward system to encourage use of the product

Promotional campaigns are often unsuccessful if they are only conducted once; they should be repeated at appropriate intervals. Promotion makes a product more visible to the market.

POSITION

The final concept, *position,* refers to the place that a product holds among similar products in the marketplace. A product changes position as it takes on attributes that set it apart from other products. The design of a product, and in some ways the promotion of it, should be based on these qualities. For example, the pediatric developmental assessment may be the only such service currently available, or it may differ from others in that the parent participates in testing procedures.

A TRADITIONAL PLANNING CYCLE

A comparison of traditional and market-based planning cycles reveals the effect that marketing orientation has on an organization (Berkowitz & Flexner, 1978). In a traditional planning cycle, illustrated in figure 4-1, an organization considers its mission or purpose before it plans its operations, or sets its goals. Once the organization adopts its goals for a given period (usually one to three years), it develops specific strategies or objectives that become the basis for implementation of services, new programs, and actual delivery of care to the patient. In the evaluation phase of a traditional planning model, the organization reviews its programs and services to determine its success in implementing its mission. This is an important point, for this model provides no assurance that the organization considers the wants and the needs of the patient in evaluating its work. The mission statements of most human service organizations express a commitment to serve the needs of the patient. An organization can overlook these needs if its programs are not designed around them.

A MARKET-BASED PLANNING CYCLE

In figure 4-2, marketing information is the central process that drives the cycle. The components of marketing information are organizational assessment, environmental assessment, market analysis, and communications. These components create an information flow that interacts with and enriches the traditional model.

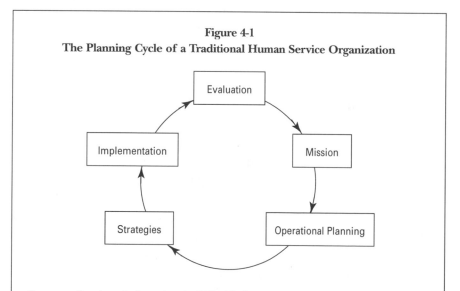

Figure 4-1
The Planning Cycle of a Traditional Human Service Organization

Sources. *Based on information in "The Marketing Audit: A Tool for Health Service Organizations," by E. N. Berkowitz and W. A. Flexner, 1978, Fall,* Health Care Management Review, *pp. 52–53; and "How Hospital Marketing and Planning Relate," by G. Stuehler, Jr., 1980, May 1,* Hospitals, *pp. 96–99.*

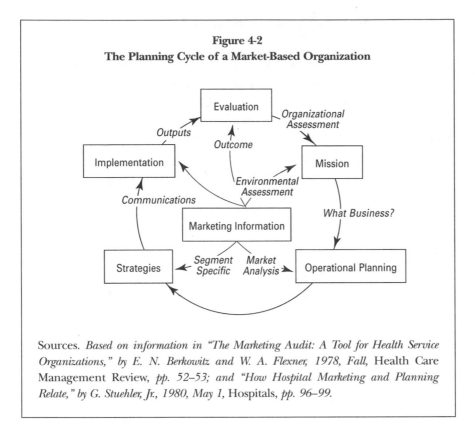

Figure 4-2
The Planning Cycle of a Market-Based Organization

Sources. *Based on information in "The Marketing Audit: A Tool for Health Service Organizations," by E. N. Berkowitz and W. A. Flexner, 1978, Fall,* Health Care Management Review, *pp. 52–53; and "How Hospital Marketing and Planning Relate," by G. Stuehler, Jr., 1980, May 1,* Hospitals, *pp. 96–99.*

In market-based planning, it is essential to understand (1) what was, (2) what is, and (3) what could be. To provide a base for product development, the organizational and environmental assessments conducted at the beginning of a planning cycle should address these three points.

ORGANIZATIONAL ASSESSMENT

Many organizations are rethinking their missions in light of rapidly changing systems of payment for services and the increase in competition from both health care organizations and non-health-care organizations entering the health care business. Hospitals in particular are becoming health service corporations or human service organizations to broaden the scope of services that they provide and to position themselves more effectively. In this reevaluation, called *organizational assessment,* the organization looks at its effectiveness relative to the patient population, the community, and the health care system at large. Effectiveness in the years ahead will be determined by the quality of care as well as the quality of management of the complex systems needed to provide that care.

An occupational therapy organization can obtain much of the information that it needs for an organizational assessment from its records. Table 4-1 outlines a variety of other data sources available for this research.

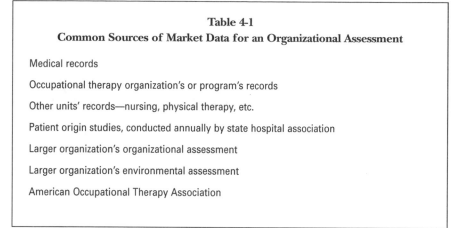

Table 4-1
Common Sources of Market Data for an Organizational Assessment

Medical records

Occupational therapy organization's or program's records

Other units' records—nursing, physical therapy, etc.

Patient origin studies, conducted annually by state hospital association

Larger organization's organizational assessment

Larger organization's environmental assessment

American Occupational Therapy Association

Olson (1983) describes a sample market audit (a type of organizational assessment) by an occupational therapy department.

ENVIRONMENTAL ASSESSMENT

In considering their missions, health care organizations are asking themselves the question, What business are we in? Answering the question usually results in a reexamination of the patient population to be served and the mode and the location of service delivery. This involves a systematic *environmental assessment*. At this point the disciplines of marketing and strategic planning merge. The role of strategic planning is to affirm and challenge the mission of the organization, to identify future directions, and to establish a context for future development. Chapter 2 discusses this function in greater depth.

Environmental assessment involves a review of the characteristics (demographics) of the organization's current patients and those of other providers: age, sex, diagnosis, location of treatment (inpatient versus outpatient), referring physician, length of hospital stays, cost of care, and so forth. The assessment includes a history of change that may have occurred for groups of patients with similar characteristics, and projections of what may happen with certain patient groups based on population changes or new technology.

As part of the environmental assessment, the organization also studies physicians' characteristics, such as type of specialty, number, age, productivity, and referral patterns. It should take both a historical and a prospective view in determining whether to recruit a certain type of physician. Another important variable is the physician's use of resources—for example, how extensively he or she draws on ancillary services such as occupational therapy and how long his or her patients tend to be hospitalized.

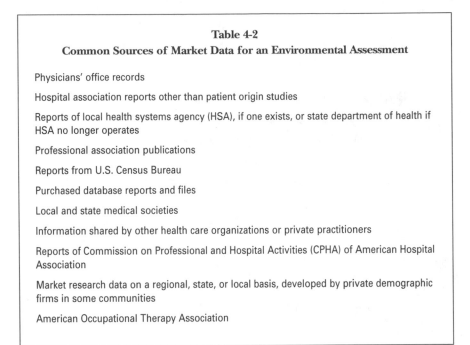

Table 4-2
Common Sources of Market Data for an Environmental Assessment

Physicians' office records

Hospital association reports other than patient origin studies

Reports of local health systems agency (HSA), if one exists, or state department of health if HSA no longer operates

Professional association publications

Reports from U.S. Census Bureau

Purchased database reports and files

Local and state medical societies

Information shared by other health care organizations or private practitioners

Reports of Commission on Professional and Hospital Activities (CPHA) of American Hospital Association

Market research data on a regional, state, or local basis, developed by private demographic firms in some communities

American Occupational Therapy Association

Environmental assessment gives the organization a sense of what the market is like for its products or services. The assessment also begins to define how the organization can position itself through operational planning, or goal setting, to be most effective in its environment. Table 4-2 lists some common sources of data for an environmental assessment.

MARKET ANALYSIS

Market analysis uses information identified in the organizational and environmental assessments to define the market and determine if the organization's perception of the wants and the needs of the market is valid. This is generally done through some form of survey conducted by the organization or by contract with a market research firm. In the survey process the organization asks randomly selected members of the target market about their wants and needs and their preferences in seeking satisfaction of those needs.

Through market analysis the organization determines (1) whom it will serve, (2) how it will organize its services, (3) how it can group potential consumers with similar needs, and (4) what is unique about its services or products. The organization determines whom it will serve on the basis of its mission and the information it has obtained in the environmental assessment.

How it will serve those people depends on how their needs are clustered with similar needs of others. The clustering of people with similar needs is called *segmentation of the market*. The marketer looks for what people have in common, to which he or she can appeal with a particular product or service. Traditionally, occupational therapy practitioners have clustered their patients in categories like pediatrics, physical disabilities, cardiac conditions, and learning disabilities. These categories describe needs around which treatment programs are designed. In categorizing patients this way, by their needs as presumed from their clinical disability, occupational therapy practitioners are segmenting a market. The market in this example is all the persons in need of occupational therapy services. A segment of that overall market is cardiac patients.

The next step in market analysis is categorizing services to meet the needs of a segmented market, or developing a product line. The changing reimbursement system and other economic forces are making it increasingly difficult for human service organizations to offer all things to all people. If there is not sufficient demand for specialized services, consumers and purchasers may abandon them or obtain them by contract from another organization. By evaluating its product lines, or the array of services it provides, and comparing these with the potential for services, the organization positions itself in the marketplace.

Occupational therapy managers should be aware of the type of planning cycle that their organization uses and the personnel who are involved in organizational and environmental assessment and market analysis. In most large organizations an occupational therapy manager is unlikely to participate at this level of planning. However, for the occupational therapy organization or program to serve the patients it has identified as a target market, the occupational therapy manager must ensure that information about that target market is included in the planning process. Thus information should flow upward to the larger organization's decision makers and planners.

Decision makers and planners should, in turn, make information available to the occupational therapy organization or program, to aid it in developing effective market plans and promotional activities specific to its segments of the market. It is through department- or program-level planning that a large organization conceives and carries out implementation strategies. At this stage the manager and the staff design new programs, evaluate programs with poor performance records, and make changes in program operation to improve cost-effectiveness.

From the marketing information assembled in the organizational and environmental assessments and the market analysis, an organization develops a market plan by applying the four P's with a view to the position it wants to achieve. Figure 4-3 describes the information flow resulting in a database for a market plan.

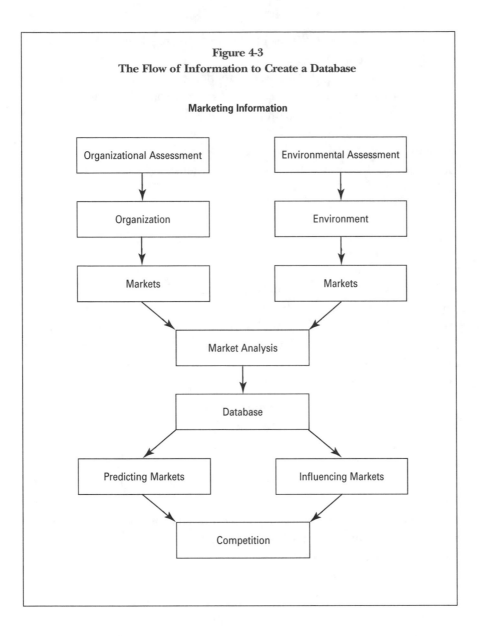

Figure 4-3
The Flow of Information to Create a Database

MARKETING COMMUNICATIONS

An organization generates marketing communications between strategy (or objective) development and implementation. *Marketing communications* include advertising, promotions (unpaid placement of information in the media), and education of those who can assist the organization in marketing its product.

At this stage, marketing overlaps with community relations. The role of community relations is to communicate the values of the organization to the community it serves. A detailed discussion of this aspect of marketing appears in chapter 5, "The Targeting of Communications."

An organization measures the outputs, or the results, of implementing its market plan in terms of the number of members of key segments whom it serves and the positive or negative financial effect of the programs and the services that it offers. It includes these components in the evaluation of its offerings and in the measure of the quality of its services. They serve as the basis for organizational assessment, which begins the planning cycle once again.

Throughout the planning cycle the role of marketing is to validate the mission of an organization in relation to the people and the organizations it will serve. Basic to that role is the organization's understanding and balancing its own wants and needs with those of the target market. This is the beneficial exchange referred to in Kotler's definition of marketing. It involves offering something of value (a service) for consideration by a target market (a desired customer), who will offer something of value (cooperation, payment, support) in return.

A Scenario: The Marketing of a Pediatric Developmental Assessment

Having identified children at risk for developmental delay as a target of its pediatric market, an occupational therapy organization chooses to market a pediatric developmental assessment.

To develop a plan to attract this population, the organization first undertakes an organizational assessment, seeking information to help it understand its past relationship with the pediatric population—what was. It examines data on previous programs that it has provided for children and the response of patients, parents, and referral sources. With these former consumers it attempts to identify wants and needs, psychographic information (e.g., perceptions and feelings about the programs), and demographic data (age, sex, zip code, etc.).

Next the organization begins an environmental assessment, an investigation of what is and what could be. It explores the market for its service among the portion of the pediatric population that it has not served before. Working with population data for its locale, it estimates the number of children at risk. It also investigates the target market being seen for developmental assessment by the competition—nurses, physical therapists, and other occupational therapy organizations.

The organization also assesses government regulations that will affect the assessment program, the program's social impact, and its effect on other providers. Further, the organization studies the competition—available services that are similar, their design, and their position in the marketplace.

By surveying a randomly selected portion of a potential target market, the organization seeks feedback from potential patients, from physicians, and from others who might refer patients for an assessment. It designs separate surveys for parents of children at risk, physicians (in family practice, pediatrics, neurology, and internal medicine), and other potential referrers, such as social workers. By separating the surveys the organization learns the following:

From the Parents

- Their perceptions of the organization—why they would or would not obtain services from the assessment program and whether they think they could afford the services

- Their knowledge of the program

- Convenience issues—what time of day they would want the assessment, in what setting, and so forth

From Physicians and Others

- Their knowledge of the assessment program

- Their perceptions of occupational therapy as an acceptable intervention for developmental delay

- Their willingness or inclination to refer patients

- The information that they would want from an assessment

The occupational therapy organization uses the survey information to design the program and a communications plan to support it.

The organization is now ready to position itself in the market. First, the organization asks itself whether it is unique in the community in providing the pediatric developmental assessment or whether the assessment has unique attributes that should attract the target market. Finding neither characteristic to be the case, the organization attempts to influence the behavior of the market by enhancing its product through price, place, and promotion.

CONCLUSION

Marketing is a process of applying information based on assumptions about the behavior of the organization doing the marketing, the consumer of products, and the environment in which marketing exchanges take place. This chapter has identified concepts and terminology used in marketing health care services. The concepts are fairly straightforward, but their application is complex. Skills in applying marketing theory and concepts are gained through experience based on the ability to analyze available data and make decisions. The occupational therapy manager must understand the importance of the database on which marketing decisions are made. Advanced study of business theory, finance, statistics, and organizational design is recommended before occupational therapy managers apply marketing theory without the help of a marketing professional.

SUMMARY

Marketing is a system for operational planning from an information base. An organization gathers and analyzes the information through a disciplined study of the needs of patients, physicians, administrators, and reimbursers. These four groups are referred to as *target markets*. Of all the persons or organizations that a marketer could influence, the target market is the portion, or segment, that the marketer wishes to influence.

Kotler and Armstrong (1991) define *marketing* as "a social and managerial process by which individuals and groups obtain what they need and want through creating and exchanging products and values with others" (p. 5). Building on this description, they define *marketing management* as "demand management," or "the analysis, planning, implementation, and control of programs designed to create, build, and maintain beneficial exchanges with target buyers for the purpose of achieving organizational objectives" (p. 10).

A market plan is based on five key concepts: (1) *product,* "anything that can be offered to a market for attention, acquisition, use, or consumption and that might satisfy a need or want" (Kotler & Armstrong, 1991, p. 7); (2) *price,* "the financial, physical, and psychological costs to people of doing business with you" (MacStravic, 1980, p. 11); (3) *place,* the method of distributing a product to a target market, or the means of giving the target market access to a product; (4) *promotion,* all the attempts to make a product visible and desirable to a target market; and (5) *position,* a product's place among similar products in the marketplace.

A comparison of traditional and market-based planning cycles reveals the effect that marketing orientation has on an organization. In the evaluation phase of a traditional planning model, an organization reviews its programs and services to determine its success in implementing its mission. This model provides no assurance that the organization considers the wants and the needs of the patient in evaluating its work. In market-based planning, it is essential for an organization to understand (1) what was, (2) what is, and (3) what could be. An organization first undertakes an *organizational assessment,* in which it looks at its effectiveness relative to the patient population, the community, and the health care system. The organization then performs an *environmental assessment,* in which it asks,

What business are we in? Answering the question usually results in a re-examination of the patient population to be served and the mode and the location of service delivery. At this point the disciplines of marketing and strategic planning merge.

A market analysis follows. Through such an analysis an organization defines (a) whom it will serve, (b) how it will organize its services, (c) how it can group potential consumers with similar needs, and (d) what is unique about its services or products.

Communications, the fourth component of marketing information, includes advertising, promotions, and education. Marketing and community relations overlap at this stage.

Marketing concepts are fairly straightforward, but their application is complex. Advanced study of business theory, finance, statistics, and organizational design is recommended before occupational therapy managers apply marketing theory without the help of a marketing professional.

REFERENCES

Berkowitz, E. N., & Flexner, W. A. (1978, Fall). The marketing audit: A tool for health service organizations. *Health Care Management Review,* pp. 51–57.

Kotler, P., & Armstrong, G. (1991). *Principles of marketing* (5th ed.). Englewood Cliffs, NJ: Prentice-Hall.

Lauback, P. B., & Rand, R. (1980, May 19–21). *Marketing management for health care executives.* Seminar conducted by the American College of Hospital Administrators, Wichita, KS.

MacStravic, R. E. S. (1980). *Marketing by objectives for hospitals.* Germantown, MD: Aspen Systems.

Olson, T. S. (1983). Health care marketing. In H. L. Hopkins & H. D. Smith (Eds.), *Willard and Spackman's Occupational therapy* (6th ed., pp. 848–54). Philadelphia: Lippincott.

ADDITIONAL RESOURCES

Kotler, P., & Andreasen, A. R. (1996). *Strategic marketing for nonprofit organizations* (5th ed.). Englewood Cliffs, NJ: Prentice-Hall.

Levitt, T. (1986). *The marketing imagination* (Expanded ed.). New York: Free Press.

CHAPTER 5

The Targeting
of Communications

Wendy Krupnick, MBA, OTR/L

KEY TERMS

Communication. A two-way process involving both the sending and the receiving of messages.

Communication vehicle. A method for transmitting a message.

Decoding. Deciphering the content of a message according to one's own experiences.

Encoding. Putting a message into words that are meaningful to the receiver.

Noise. Extraneous factors that hinder reception of a message.

Segmentation. Division of target groups into smaller publics by similar characteristics or attributes.

Target groups. Audiences of people currently or potentially important to the provision of occupational therapy services.

Wendy Krupnick, MBA, OTR/L, is an assistant professor and the fieldwork coordinator at The Sage Colleges. Earlier she worked in communications for over 10 years, serving as director of public affairs for AOTA and as a communications consultant to several nonprofit associations, among other positions. She earned her MBA in marketing at George Washington University.

One of the many roles of the occupational therapy manager is to ensure that the occupational therapy organization is productive and provides services of quality. Another, less tangible role is to increase other health care professionals' understanding of occupational therapy services. The kind of information relayed to, and the relationships established with, members of the health care team affect the reputation of the occupational therapy organization. To further these relationships and to influence health care professionals positively, occupational therapy practitioners should present accurate, timely, and relevant information on a regular basis.

As professionals within a large health care system, occupational therapy practitioners must be able to assess their audience and adjust their message for particular target groups. Demands on the profession in the present health care environment require the ability to communicate effectively with a diverse number of groups, including health care providers, administrators, third-party payers, patients and clients, and families, all of whom have different needs, levels of understanding, and interests.

Marketing experts Kotler and Andreasen (1991) stress that

> influencing behavior is largely a matter of *communication*. It is a matter of *informing* target audiences about the alternatives for action, the positive consequences of choosing a particular one, and the motivations for acting (and often *continuing* to act) in a particular way. (p. 506).

The key to successful communication, then, is being able to inform and motivate an audience to act. Communication is a two-way process involving both the sending and the receiving of messages. Delivering information in a form that is meaningful to the target audience is one-half of the equation. Taking steps to ensure that the message is received as intended, including ensuring that it promotes a positive response, is the other half.

The following scenario serves to introduce some communication terminology and strategies:

> The county fire department chiefs initiate a telephone solicitation to raise funds to support a county training facility. The group informs residents that the community needs to pool funds to train volunteer firefighters because the funding for individual communities' training facilities has been cut. A personal message delivered by firefighters affiliated with neighborhood fire districts helps motivate people to contribute.

Successful communication involves four essential components: (1) a sender, (2) a receiver, (3) a message, and (4) a response. The communication process just described begins with a *sender,* the county fire department chiefs, who want to convey a message relating the county fire department's need for funds, to a *receiver,* the homeowners whom local fire districts serve. The underlying message is that training will be available to all firefighters, including those who belong to the fire district serving the homeowner being contacted. In the communication literature this is referred to as *encoding,* that is, putting a message (the need for funds) into words that will be meaningful to the receiver. In the example the *communication vehicle* for transmitting the encoded message is telephone solicitation. Homeowners receive the message and begin *decoding,* or deciphering the content according to their own experiences. The content that they receive may not be the content that the solicitor intends because of individual differences and interpretations. Perhaps the solicitor chooses the wrong wording, or reads the solicitation aloud and does not seem credible. Maybe one homeowner recently contributed to the fund drive of a local fire district whose message was similar to the county's; maybe another homeowner, unhappy with frequent telephone solicitations, declines to take the call. These extraneous factors, or *noise,* hinder reception of the message. Noise can occur anywhere on the communication chain, interfering with encoding, transmitting, decoding, or response. The sender must therefore seek feedback from the receiver regarding the communication.

The literature (Engel, Warshaw, & Kinnear, 1991; Kotler & Andreasen, 1991) defines the communication process as follows:

1. The sender formulates the intended message.

2. The sender encodes the intended message, or translates it into language (verbal, nonverbal, visual).

3. The sender transmits the message through a communication vehicle.

4. The receiver decodes the content.

5. Having received the message, the receiver retains only the parts of it that are memorable or relevant.

6. The receiver responds.

7. The sender solicits feedback to determine the effectiveness of the message or the contact.

Given the many points on the communication chain at which breakdown of the intended message can occur, content must be as relevant as possible to the receiver or the target group to reduce the potential for messages being lost, ignored, or misinterpreted.

DEVELOPMENT OF A COMMUNICATION PROGRAM

Like the communication process, an effective communication program also follows a sequence of activities, which provides direction to individual efforts: (1) identification of communication objectives, (2) definition of target groups, (3) definition of the message, (4) selection of communication methods, and (5) implementation and evaluation of the communication program (Kotler & Andreasen, 1991).

IDENTIFICATION OF COMMUNICATION OBJECTIVES

Occupational therapy managers can clarify their communication objectives by asking themselves, What is my purpose in contacting this particular group—to seek awareness of the profession, an increase in referrals, more funding, larger space, or name recognition? What action do I want the audience to take as a result of the communication? Following are examples of objectives:

- To educate potential consumer groups A, B, and C about occupational therapy services, in order to increase the breadth of demand for services or increase the quantity of services delivered by x percent

- To inform current patients and clients about the benefits of occupational therapy, in order to increase their participation in occupational therapy and make family members aware of its value

- To increase the number of referrals from department A to the outpatient clinic by x percent over the next year

- To improve reimbursements from third-party payers by x percent for y types of services or patients and clients

- To develop a pool of x qualified therapists to fill staff vacancies

- To reward and motivate employees

- To generate administrative support or increase the pool of referral sources for a new treatment specialty (e.g., work hardening, pediatric services, or community-living-skills groups) by signing x contracts for service

DEFINITION OF TARGET GROUPS

Once the occupational therapy manager has set communication objectives, he or she identifies *target groups,* or audiences of people currently or potentially important to the provision of occupational therapy services. The manager further segments these groups into *targets,* or smaller publics, by demographic or behavioral characteristics, funding potential, service specialty, or a meaningful attribute such as potential user. Topor

(1988) suggests thinking of the behavior or the reaction of target markets to services as an aid in identifying particular groups: What is the group's point of view? Why would its members be interested in occupational therapy? Is the message a new idea or an updating of the group's information? Each target should consist of homogeneous segments of the larger group; that is, members of a target should share particular characteristics or attributes. This segmentation accomplishes two purposes: It forces occupational therapy practitioners to acknowledge that they cannot be all things to all people, and it allows them to structure a message to meet the unique information needs of each target (Topor, 1988). According to Kotler and Clarke (1987), all organizations eventually discover that they cannot reach all consumers and must identify which groups they can most effectively serve. Occupational therapy practitioners should analyze their work environments to determine what occupational therapy services are provided and which target groups could benefit from these services (Topor, 1988). They should view the services as the users perceive the services; that is, practitioners should describe the characteristics of the services from the perspective of each of the key target groups (Topor, 1988).

For example, to increase referrals within a teaching hospital, an occupational therapy manager would divide the hospital's primary referral sources into distinct groupings: staff physicians, and other health care providers who may influence referral for services, such as discharge planners, nurses, and physical therapists. The manager would further divide the audience of physicians into specialty areas such as cardiologists, orthopedists, pediatricians, and physiatrists. Each group has specific information needs and concerns that can be addressed in different ways. Pediatricians, for example, need to know why occupational therapy practitioners work with children, which children may benefit from occupational therapy intervention, and what outcomes they can expect given the recommended frequency of treatment. Discharge planners may need to know what effect occupational therapy can have on patients' abilities to function in their living environments, which types of patients occupational therapy practitioners generally treat in this particular hospital setting, when therapy should be introduced, and how therapy may influence patients' lengths of stay in the hospital.

Because people listen to and perceive information selectively, communicating successfully depends on presenting the right message to the right public (Engel, Warshaw, & Kinnear, 1991). Identifying publics is one of the first tasks to be completed, and recognizing the need to communicate differently to each public is part of the second task. The communicator must determine who the audience is and what the audience needs to know to take action. The communicator's goal is to provide target groups with relevant information in order to elicit a desired response—for example, to stimulate an awareness of the role of occupational therapy. The communicator can greatly enhance his or her efforts by using a variety of media and repeating the message frequently. Lastly, the communicator must establish a feedback mechanism so that he or she can measure the audience's response to the message (Kotler & Clarke, 1987).

Sample target groups are patients and clients, referral sources, administrators, hospital or facility employees, third-party payers, principals and school personnel, and legislators and other public officials:

Patients and clients can be segmented into two groups: current and potential. Current patients and clients need to know why they are receiving occupational therapy and what it can help them accomplish. Members of the community, or potential patients and clients, need consumer information on specific areas of occupational therapy practice, such as helping patients or clients return home after a stroke, teaching energy conservation and joint protection techniques to persons with arthritis, helping children with developmental disabilities make friends or learn hobbies, and teaching community-living skills to persons with mental illness.

Referral sources need to know how occupational therapy can help effect the early recovery of specific patients and clients. This target group might include physicians, administrators of preferred provider organizations, other health care team members in a hospital or a health care facility, or third-party payers. These audiences should be helped to understand why timely occupational therapy consultation and treatment are beneficial and what the expected outcomes are. Often overlooked are fellow colleagues in neighboring departments. Contact in treatment team meetings with nurses and physical therapists can generate referrals for patients and clients who previously might not have received care. Studies conducted by Professional Research Consultants in Omaha, Nebraska, show that referring physicians consider the frequency of communication about the referred patient important in selecting hospitals (White & Christensen, 1990). Given this emphasis on communication, follow-up with referral sources on the progress of patients and clients is an excellent way of furthering the relationship and reinforcing the awareness of the role of occupational therapy.

Administrators, who are concerned with revenue, need statistics on the length of stay, the cost of service, the quantity of treatment, and the capability of occupational therapy to generate income. These persons are not always aware of the role of occupational therapy or the scope of services that the practitioner can offer. Messages to this group might include information about the kinds of treatments that current patients and clients are receiving or the opportunity to serve potential patients and clients with new technologies and services.

Hospital or facility employees are often the greatest conduit of information to patients and clients because of their direct and frequent contact with that population. Occupational therapy managers and practitioners can increase consumers' awareness of occupational therapy manyfold by providing employees with appropriate information about the location of the department, the purpose of occupational therapy, and the types of treatments offered (such as strategies to improve self-care; activities to increase strength and endurance; and techniques to help persons manage anger, time, or work interactions, or cope with stress).

Third-party payers work with information about the cost-effectiveness of occupational therapy and its record in reducing the number of readmissions or reducing the need for additional, more expensive services.

Principals and school personnel should be made aware of how occupational therapy can help children with special needs perform better in the school environment and how occupational therapy practitioners can support teachers in their efforts to teach children with special needs in their classrooms.

Legislators and other public officials who influence legislation and regulations affecting occupational therapy are an important target group. These officials should be made aware that occupational therapy helps return people to work and to independent living, thus reducing their dependence on public funds and increasing their contributions to society.

In sum, one of the primary reasons for segmenting audiences into groups is to deliver a message that focuses on each group's needs and interests. By first identifying who the prospective audience is and what its interests or concerns involve, the communicator can begin to define the benefits of the service for that particular group (Kotler & Roberto, 1989).

DEFINITION OF THE MESSAGE

Defining the message to meet communication objectives takes planning and the ability to break a service into its component parts—a natural extension of activity analysis and therefore second nature to occupational therapy practitioners. Daniel A. Nimer (cited in Wager, 1988), a marketing consultant and the president of DNA Group, Inc., in Northbrook, Illinois, cautions that a message should not leave the receiver questioning the content with a "So what?" or a "Who cares?" The most creatively crafted message is useless if it reaches a group that either is not motivated to act or is indifferent to the content. The message should focus on the benefits of occupational therapy services to that target group and include other information to move the target group to action.

Kotler and Andreasen (1991) have identified two approaches that can be applied to occupational therapy. One approach is to work with representatives of the target groups to define how they view occupational therapy, what benefits they perceive, and what services they particularly appreciate. The other approach is to meet with key representatives of the organization or the institution and hold a brainstorming session to produce ideas. For example:

> The manager of an occupational therapy department in a hospital is interested in increasing the number of referrals for occupational therapy. She notes that several types of patients could benefit from occupational therapy but are not being referred, and that some referrals come right before a patient is scheduled for discharge.

To help develop a message, the manager can meet with referral groups, collect data through a questionnaire distributed to all departments, or brainstorm the issue with selected members of referral groups and departments. Ultimately the manager has to convince several groups within the hospital system that patients and referral sources would benefit from occupational therapy. The success of the plan depends on what is said, to whom, and when.

> After collecting information from key groups on why referrals are low, the manager in the example begins to *package,* or strategically put together, information to strengthen her position. The department's statistics on use are helpful at this stage, that is, the number of patients evaluated, the number treated, the number on waiting lists, the number discharged to home health, and so forth.

The information that the manager wants from other health care professionals includes their perception of what occupational therapy practitioners do, their opinion of how well it is done, the kinds of patients that they did or did not refer for occupational therapy, the lengths of stay of those persons, and readmission rates. Analysis of the data should result in identification of the problem and its cause, and contribute to development of a sound strategy to address the pertinent issues. In this example, needing to determine the reason for low referrals, the manager should consider whether lack of information about the types of patients who are treated in occupational therapy is contributing to the problem.

The challenge to managers is to convey specific information to several groups so that the result is overwhelming support of their position. The message must address the targets' needs, the value that people place on the goals set in occupational therapy, and their willingness to work with occupational therapy staff members in establishing mutually beneficial relationships. In fact, according to Wager (1988), communication should not only provide information, but contribute to the development of positive relationships.

Information should be presented in a manner that is convincing to the particular group being addressed. In other words, it is important to demonstrate to referral sources how occupational therapy interventions are beneficial: to the nursing team that occupational therapy assists patients in becoming independent in self-care; to hospital administrators that occupational therapy helps in the early discharge of patients and can continue in the home setting; and finally, to all, that occupational therapy is a necessary and specialized intervention that contributes to a person's quality of life.

In general, to develop a particular message for a target group, it is helpful to think about the five Ws identified in journalism: who, what, when, where, and why:

1. *Who* is this group; how is it defined?

2. *What* information or action does the group want from occupational therapy practitioners?

3. *When* should the group act (is this a contact for immediate referral, or is the information to be stored and retrieved at a later date)?

4. *Where* should the group go for services?

5. *Why* should the group listen to the message, or how can it benefit from services?

Table 5-1 presents analyses of three publics in terms of these questions.

SELECTION OF COMMUNICATION METHODS

Communication between occupational therapy practitioners and other members of the health care system is critical to the growth and the acceptance of the profession. By exchanging information and ideas with other groups and by increasing their visibility within both the organization and the community, occupational therapy practitioners gain the exposure that is necessary for achieving understanding, awareness, and respect.

Selecting the appropriate method of communication largely depends on the message and the public. Communication may be formal, as in letters and reports, or informal, as in displays and conversation. Every method has its positive and negative characteristics. An occupational therapy manager should choose the method that best suits his or her needs.

Regardless of the method selected, to ensure that the message is received as intended, the sender must repeat it frequently (Wager, 1988). Further, to increase the likelihood that the message will be received as intended, the sender should use a combination of approaches. Many avenues of communication are open to occupational therapy practitioners. Sometimes an informal telephone call will suit their needs. A

Table 5-1

Development of the Occupational Therapy Message

Who is group?	Referral sources, segmented by specialty affiliation	Patients and clients, segmented by age group, treatment orientation, illness or injury, or other descriptive category	Reimbursers
What information does group want?	Functional outcomes Current treatment methods Communication regarding person's progress Cost of treatment Length of treatment	Benefits of treatment Expectations of therapy Treatment descriptions and goals Identification of support groups and resources Accessible and cost-effective treatment Methods for coping with pain, fear, and disabling conditions Methods for actively participating in life activities	Functional outcomes Cost-benefits of treatment Length of treatment
When should group act?	On change in person's health status, behavior, or developmental stage that results in loss of functional ability or independence At diagnosis After surgical procedure	When functional independence is affected at home, school, or work When developmental delays are experienced When mobility is impaired When emotional difficulties interfere with daily living	On change in person's health status, behavior, or developmental stage that results in loss of functional ability or independence At diagnosis After surgical procedure
Where should group go for services?	Occupational therapy department in hospital, freestanding clinic, or rehabilitation center Home health service School system Private practice in occupational therapy Corporate health department	Personal physician or health provider for occupational therapy referral Occupational therapy department in hospital, freestanding clinic, or rehabilitation center Home health service School system Private practice in occupational therapy Corporate health department	Occupational therapy department in hospital, freestanding clinic, or rehabilitation center Home health service School system Private practice in occupational therapy Corporate health department
Why should group seek occupational therapy?	It improves independence. It leads to productive living. It promotes engagement in life tasks. It helps people adapt to life changes after illness or injury. It teaches energy conservation and work simplification to reduce injury and stress to body.	It teaches people how to do for themselves. It helps people return to work after injury. It helps people adapt to life changes after illness or injury. It teaches energy conservation and work simplification to reduce injury and stress to body.	It reduces long-term dependency on health care system. It teaches people how to do for themselves. It helps people return to work after injury. It is cost-effective.

telephone call provides immediate feedback, although the message may be easily forgotten. Contact by letter is more formal and furnishes written documentation of the communication. However, it does not allow for immediate feedback, nor does it ensure that the message was actually delivered to the person for whom it was intended.

Table 5-2 categorizes the most frequently used communication methods and indicates their various uses. Some methods are effective in reaching target audiences, whereas others are useful for distributing general information.

Internal Communication

Internal communication generally refers to communication among people within an organization. It can take place over lunch, at an exercise class, on the way to a meeting, or in the parking lot. Interactions at such moments help build support systems and are often more influential than external communications. These support systems can also be tapped during communications with other target groups, either as references or for testimonials and the like. The image of an occupational therapy unit in a large organization depends on the effectiveness of its internal communications. For example, with effective internal communications, other staff members, including the receptionist, would know something as simple, yet vital, as the location of the occupational therapy unit.

The staff members of an educational or health care organization have many commonalities. Thus numerous opportunities are available to build rapport, share information, and educate others about the world of occupational therapy.

Internal Communication Methods

An organization's employee newsletter. An employee newsletter provides many opportunities for sharing information about occupational therapy with colleagues. Such a newsletter is distributed to all staff, from support to technical to professional. Consequently information must be general in nature, have major public appeal, and be interesting to read. The idea is to attract attention to occupational therapy programs in order to improve awareness of occupational therapy services. For example, an article might describe occupational therapy in terms of clients' successes, new equipment or services, new staff members and their unique backgrounds or specialties, clinical activities, or available inservice materials. Pictures of staff members engaged in activities with clients might be included. Help in writing or placing articles can usually be obtained from an organization's public relations or personnel department, whichever group is responsible for employee relations.

Table 5-2
Sample Checklist for Assessing Communication Methods

	General Occupational Therapy Information	Information about Specific Occupational Therapy Service	Teaching Opportunity	Public Information/ Awareness	Personal Contact
Types of Internal Communication					
Organization's employee newsletter	X	X		X	
Organization open house	X	X		X	X
Inservice training, seminars, workshops		X	X	X	X
Progress notes, memos, reports		X		X	
Case conferences		X	X		X
Participation in activities sponsored by organization	X	X		X	X
Types of External Communication					
Organization's community newsletter	X	X		X	
Annual reports	X	X		X	
Community/ daily newspapers	X	X		X	
Direct mail		X		X	
Seminars/ workshops		X	X	X	X
Health fairs and exhibits	X	X		X	X
Scholarly articles		X	X	X	
Participation in community, charitable, and religious organizations (newsletters, fund-raisers, volunteer programs)	X	X		X	X
Guest speeches at community programs	X	X	X	X	X
Presentations at professional conferences		X	X	X	
Speakers' bureau	X	X	X	X	X
Personal visits	X	X	X	X	X

An organization open house. An open house is another way to display the whys and the hows of occupational therapy. The audience will include persons passing by who stop because the occupational therapy display has caught their eye. They may be staff or patients and clients and their family members, depending on the location of the event (e.g., a public cafeteria versus the occupational therapy department, which is more oriented toward staff members). Once people have stopped, more detailed information can be offered. An open house provides personal contact and allows information exchange. Some excellent methods of describing occupational therapy include posters depicting occupational therapy practice, statistics on the kinds of patients and clients treated by occupational therapy practitioners, and displays of treatment modalities and equipment complete with explanations on why particular activities were selected. To attract the most attention, information should be simple, be in lay terms, be presented in a professional manner, and have a visual component.

Inservice training, seminars, and workshops. Continuing education programs allow specific information on occupational therapy to be delivered to a target group. Occupational therapy practitioners can volunteer to present a topic and invite persons who would benefit from and be interested in the information. Topics can range from occupational therapy evaluations for persons with mental illness to the care and the treatment of persons with hand and wrist injuries. Presenters should tailor their topic to the audience's needs and design the presentation to educate participants on the benefits of occupational therapy to the audience's patients and clients. In this way, presenters can be assured of the audience's attention and can more thoroughly cover a topic. Advanced preparation and time are required, but once materials are collected, the program can be repeated, and modified, for different audiences.

Progress notes, memos, and reports. These types of communication tools also provide information about occupational therapy to those who read them. Progress notes should be concise and descriptive so that the reader understands the purpose, the method, and the results of the occupational therapy intervention. Ideally written after each treatment, they should, over time, serve to document change in a patient's or client's condition. Memos should be short and have a clear objective—for example, responding to a request, confirming a meeting, outlining the results of a meeting, informing people about new staff and practice hours, or announcing new services. One way of reinforcing referrals is to send referral sources a brief note informing them of their patient's or client's progress. The follow-up note is also a good tool for developing and sustaining satisfaction in patients and clients.

Reports are good tools for making the administration aware of occupational therapy services. For instance, a manager might write a report about the growth of the occupational therapy unit over the previous six months or about the outcomes of an occupational therapy inservice program for teachers. Reports should always begin with an introductory paragraph and then proceed to specific information. Content might cover the number of referrals received each month, the types of referrals in relation to the length of treatment, and the revenue generated by the program versus the cost of services (e.g., staff salaries, equipment). The report should conclude with a summary of the essential points for people to remember. These might include a statement identifying occupational therapy as one of the important factors in reducing readmission rates or further disability.

Case conferences. In case conferences, occupational therapy practitioners report on patients' or clients' progress more comprehensively than they do in progress notes. These conferences provide opportunities to describe occupational therapy principles to other health care personnel and to members of the patient's or client's family, and to educate them about occupational therapy's benefits.

Participation in activities sponsored by the organization. One way of getting recognition for an occupational therapy unit is to participate in volunteer efforts sponsored by the organization, such as fund drives, talent shows, and community service projects. Working with others provides an opportunity for informal dialogue. People assume different roles and relate to one another as peers collaborating on a task. Conversation can turn to occupational therapy's relationship to the project or its role in the organization. Either way this informal method will make a lasting impression because of the personal contact.

External Communication

Contact with persons outside an organization is defined as *external communication*. Some of the characteristics associated with internal communication apply to external communication. One of the main differences can be a focus on the profession of occupational therapy rather than on an occupational therapy organization or unit. Many opportunities are available for influencing people's perceptions and generally raising the public's awareness of the existence and the need for occupational therapy. Through external communication the profession can be promoted in the community.

External Communication Methods

An organization's community newsletter. This publication is distributed to people who reside within an organization's service area. Included are current and potential patients and clients, members of the business community, educators, community leaders, and general residents of the community. Just like the information in an organization's employee newsletter, the information in this publication must be general in order to appeal to its diverse audiences. These audiences relate best to stories about people or to information that may be personally useful, such as parenting hints, screening information for school-age children, or tips on dealing with holiday stress. One method of ensuring the inclusion of a story on occupational therapy is to know the market, that is, to determine who the primary consumers of occupational therapy are in the community and to write a story aimed at them or their families. With the current competition among health care providers increasing, a multitude of newsletters are reaching consumers' mail boxes. Periodic feature stories about occupational therapy will go a long way toward name recognition and awareness of occupational therapy services.

An organization may produce other publications targeted at the community, such as information brochures about services and announcements about community education opportunities. Practitioners can volunteer to present consumer information in these publications about an area of occupational therapy practice, such as learning disabilities, stroke, or stress management. This will enhance both the organization's and occupational therapy's image in the community.

Annual reports. Such reports provide opportunities to highlight an organization's strengths. An annual report can record the past, interpret the present, and project the future. It can identify trends and reinforce an organization's image. An annual report is distributed to many publics, most often to representatives of the community. The manager should make sure that occupational therapy is mentioned in it, either by picture and caption or by written paragraph. The report provides an opportunity to highlight new equipment, services, clubs (such as a stroke club for patients and their families), and so forth.

Community and daily newspapers. Community newspapers have the highest readership of all newspapers. More people read more of the information in community newspapers than the information in major city and daily newspapers. Community newspapers are also locally oriented; therefore their staff members are eager to print information about local people and businesses. Particulars about activities to which the public is invited (such as open houses and health fairs in malls) should be provided to these papers. Additionally, they should be notified about staff changes and promotions, and occupational therapy practitioners' presentations at conferences and seminars. Community and daily newspapers feature stories on businesses, organizations, and service programs. They are ideal for reporting stories on exceptional success with patients and clients. Through this medium, occupational therapy practices and purposes can be described in a way that easily captures the public's interest. The style or health editors of community newspapers and many daily papers are generally interested in printing information about health, fitness, leisure, coping strategies, and so forth, and they often describe personal and professional community resources that can assist people in dealing with contemporary living. More information on contacting the media is available in *Promoting the Profession: A Resource Guide for Marketing and Publicizing Occupational Therapy* (Carleton, 1993).

Direct mail. This is targeted distribution of information via the mail. For example, if a department plans to expand its occupational therapy services to include evaluation and treatment of children with learning disabilities, it might distribute information about the new service to the persons who are likely to make referrals. The direct mail piece could be in the form of a letter, a fact sheet, or a brochure. Target groups might be guidance counselors, pediatricians, social workers, special education teachers, parents of children with learning disabilities, and so forth. Direct mail ensures that a message is received by the people who are most likely to act on the information.

Seminars and workshops. Continuing education programs offered to community residents provide increased visibility for occupational therapy. Every time that the profession appears in the public eye means additional exposure. Occupational therapy staff members should customize workshops to the needs of the community and to their own areas of expertise. If the community has a large elderly population, a seminar on maintaining the elderly in the community would be appropriate. If the major work in the community is human services (as opposed to industry), a workshop on stress might be conducted. Parenting workshops might be presented through the local health department, the YMCA/YWCA, adult education programs, or the educational offerings of health maintenance organizations (HMOs). Such presentations not only bring occupational therapy to the public's attention; they strengthen occupational therapy's public image and enhance the credibility of the occupational therapy practitioner as an expert health care provider (Sanchez, 1988).

Health fairs and exhibits. These are excellent means of providing general information about occupational therapy to consumers. Occupational therapy practitioners can team up with other health care professionals in their own or another organization, or plan their own exhibit. Contracting with a mall to display information on occupational therapy is a good way of recruiting people for the profession or demonstrating the diverse areas of occupational therapy practice. Adaptive devices, splinting supplies, sensory stimulation materials, crafts, and testing equipment make for interesting displays. Exhibits should be of interest to the people who visit a mall on a weekend afternoon, mainly parents and young families, teenagers, and older adults. The goal, once again, is general exposure to raise people's consciousness.

Scholarly articles. An important way to generate professional exposure for occupational therapy is to publish scholarly articles in the journals of other professions. The content of the article should be geared to the readership of the journal. For example, to educate teachers on the role of occupational therapy in the evaluation and the treatment of children with developmental delays, a staff occupational therapist might submit a paper to a journal published by the Council for Exceptional Children. Similarly, to inform psychiatrists about the role of occupational therapy in mental health, a therapist might submit a paper to a journal published by the American Psychiatric Association. The *Journal of Rehabilitation* is a good placement for articles on occupational therapy program development and research. The idea is to reach a specialized group and present specialized information.

Participation in community, charitable, and religious organizations. Community, charitable, and religious organizations consist of persons whose special interest is to support the group's cause. These persons represent some of the community's interests and are potential occupational therapy patients and clients or referral sources. Occupational therapy practitioners who participate in these organizations have a unique opportunity to establish valuable contacts and promote the profession. The contacts they make could result in improved access to the media, inclusion in other groups' long-range plans, and coverage for occupational therapy. Occupational therapy practitioners could benefit from recognition as understanding and enthusiastic members of the community who will align themselves with a beneficial cause. References to occupational therapy should not be self-serving; rather, practitioners should portray the profession as fulfilling a health care need.

Guest speeches at community programs. This is another method of increasing occupational therapy's visibility. Practitioners can speak at programs offered by hospital groups, senior citizen centers, youth organizations, political gatherings, and the county or state health department, and to groups concerned with education. Timely topics are wellness and illness prevention, safety in the home, occupational therapy in home health, and day care for the elderly. Promoting independence in the elderly, another possible topic, is becoming an important concern in every community as the older population grows and health care funds shrink. Occupational therapy speakers could also guide families in choosing a nursing home, suggest ways of adapting the home environment to promote safety and independence, or offer help in understanding the psychological changes accompanying aging. The importance of early treatment for learning disabilities could generate such topics as when a child needs professional help, how children learn, and how parents can tell if children are developing normally.

Presentations at professional conferences. Presentations at the conferences of other professional groups, such as the American Public Health Association, Hospital and Community Psychiatry, and the Group Health Association of America (the trade organization for HMOs), are another means of promoting occupational therapy. In these contexts it is helpful to provide fact sheets and written materials as handouts. All materials should include information on where to obtain occupational therapy evaluations and treatment.

Speakers' bureau. By developing and promoting a roster of speakers, a state or local occupational therapy association can reach and influence a variety of audiences and help establish an image of occupational therapy as a profession with competence in a wide range of practice areas. As an organization of occupational therapy professionals, the state or local association already has the necessary ingredients for a successful speakers' bureau. The task is to identify speakers and topics through the association's newsletter and professional network. In choosing the persons to be included in the bureau, the association should seek dynamic public speakers who have the skills and the interest to relate material to consumers. Professional competence does not necessarily make a person a good public speaker; someone who cannot tailor information to a non-health-profession audience may leave listeners confused.

A plan for promoting a speakers' bureau should include contact with civic, religious, and fraternal organizations that welcome suggestions for speakers. The plan should also specify contact with support groups, such as those for people recovering from strokes and heart attacks, for families of persons with mental illness, and for parents of children with special needs. The local chamber of commerce can often provide lists of organizations in the community. Schools, colleges, and parent-teacher organizations, as well as radio corporations with programs that attract particular audiences, should be among the groups and the agencies that are informed about the speakers' bureau.

Personal visits. With some publics, one-to-one communication is essential. For example, occupational therapy practitioners should pay personal calls on legislators and other public officials to be certain that they have sufficient information to make favorable decisions on issues of concern to the profession and its consumers. Slide-tape shows, fact sheets, brochures, and a promotion piece such as an occupational therapy calendar can help practitioners make points during and even after such visits. Timely features in the broadcast and print media can also influence public officials' understanding of occupational therapy.

IMPLEMENTATION AND EVALUATION OF THE COMMUNICATION PROGRAM

Before an occupational therapy organization implements communication activities, it should conduct a complete review of its objectives in relation to target groups, messages, and communication methods, analyzing how well each component of the program can meet the objectives, and making adjustments as necessary. For example, if the communication goal is to increase referrals to a work hardening program, is an open house that features pictures of practitioners working with children or frail clients appropriate? A communication program has greater potential for success if its components are coordinated.

As stated previously, using a variety of communication methods increases the likelihood that the message will be received. Additionally, the message must be repeated with some frequency to compete with the abundance of information delivered daily via telephone, newspaper, television, radio, mail, and advertisements.

After the communication program is implemented, it should be evaluated for effectiveness. Comparing results measured over a specified period with the original objectives will indicate whether or not the program has been successful. The more measurable the objective—such as "a 10-percent increase in referrals to the hand clinic over six months"— the easier the analysis of results.

Although it is always good to meet objectives, sometimes one learns more when objectives are not met. A step-by-step review of the communication program to identify the causes for the shortfall should be conducted. Factors to consider include unrealistic expectations for the number of referrals; too short a time period for evaluation; an unclear message; too much noise; poor choices of communication methods; or wrong target group. Engel, Warshaw, and Kinnear (1991) stress that a postmortem appraisal is an important component of the communication process.

A Scenario:
Development and Implementation
of a Communication Program

Following is an example of a situation that could benefit from a communication program:

> The manager of an occupational therapy department has discovered that the number of referrals to the department and the number of treatment hours per client have declined as a result of early discharges and changing patterns of payment for services.

DEFINITION OF SPECIFIC OBJECTIVES

In the scenario the occupational therapy manager has identified a particular concern; now she must set a specific goal.

> Through investigation and analysis the manager determines that developing and providing home health services will increase the demand for occupational therapy and add to the department's revenues. These services will also compensate for the decrease in referrals and treatment hours brought on by early discharges and changing patterns of payment for services. The objective of the program will be to maintain the continuity of follow-up care, which will aid in improving the rate of recovery and decrease hospital readmissions. The manager sets a goal of 10 home health referrals per month, or 120 per year.

PREPARATION OF A COMMUNICATION PLAN

The department must now develop a plan for reaching the goal. The communication objective is to disseminate information to referral sources so that they are aware of the benefits of occupational therapy treatment for clients whom they serve and so that they increase their referrals to occupational therapy. As discussed earlier, the remaining steps include definition of target groups, definition of the message, selection of appropriate communication methods, and implementation and evaluation of the communication program.

Definition of Target Groups

> The department defines its target groups as physicians, social workers, nurses, hospital discharge planners, community agencies, support groups, religious groups, senior citizen centers, community media, the county medical society, and other health organizations. It segments the physicians further into specialty areas: cardiologists, orthopedists, and physiatrists.

Definition of the Message

The message to each group should address *who* can be served in a home health setting; *what* types of services will be provided; *when* the treatment should be provided (e.g., immediately on discharge for approximately *x* weeks); *where* the treatment will be provided, if applicable; and *why* occupational therapy treatment will be effective.

> The department's message to cardiologists states that persons recovering from stroke can make greater progress toward independence through training in self-care and activities of daily living in their homes. Assistance in coping in their own unique kitchens, bathrooms, and living spaces, the message continues, will help these persons continue the progress that they have begun in the hospital. The treatment should start immediately on discharge and terminate when the client shows a satisfactory level of safety and judgment, usually within a prescribed number of sessions, the message suggests.
>
> To substantiate the merits of this service, the message cites the results of studies describing the link between occupational therapy home health services and injury prevention, social networking, and quality of life after stroke. A study by Radomski (1995), the message points out, has demonstrated that a person's quality of life after stroke is affected by both the amount of physical restoration that he or she achieves and emotional factors such as the person's ability to socialize, perform social roles, and feel socially confident. Occupational therapy practitioners, the message continues, are uniquely positioned to address these issues with the client and the family. They can provide information, identify resources, and co-lead educational or support groups to meet the social-emotional needs of persons who have experienced stroke.

Selection of Communication Methods

The manner in which the department provides information will influence the success of the plan. The department should tailor the information to what each audience wants and needs to know.

Whenever a new service is instituted, it should be kicked off with an open house. This provides a good opportunity to introduce guests to, or refamiliarize them with, occupational therapy. If the correct people are invited, such as physicians, administrators, and discharge planners, the open house will provide personal contact with potential referral sources. Printed information about the service should be made available. This can be done with inexpensive fact sheets that address the who, what, when, where, and why in a clear and attractive format.

The department schedules an open house. Further, the manager arranges an inservice session for the hospital's Cardiac Care Department. She also plans a direct mailing to local cardiologists. Department staff members prepare printed fact sheets geared to health care professionals, consumers, and family members, and make the sheets available to physicians and their patients and families.

Recognizing that the home health service is newsworthy, the manager arranges for its announcement in the hospital's community newsletter and in local newspapers. Further, she seeks speaking engagements for staff members of the new service through the local health department, the local library, the local chamber of commerce, and community health groups and clubs. Staff members post printed information on community bulletin boards, in libraries, and in the waiting areas of health care facilities. The manager obtains a list of physicians in the community from the county medical society and sends a direct mail piece to them. Various other facilities such as subacute care hospitals that might benefit from occupational therapy home health services are contacted.

The final plan should take timetables and budgets into consideration. A realistic schedule for completing activities, gathering materials, and assigning responsibilities should be included.

IMPLEMENTATION

Once the organization has contacted potential referral sources, it should recontact them and follow up with additional information.

Soon after its initial contact with various referral sources, the occupational therapy department follows up with letters repeating the home health service's hours, costs, and therapy components. Enclosed with the letter is a brief description of the types of clients who have been treated recently, to encourage similar referrals.

After a source has made a referral and a practitioner has completed an initial evaluation, the organization should keep the referral source informed of significant progress. To accomplish this, the practitioner might document progress on a form headed with the organization's name, address, telephone number, and hours.

EVALUATION

To determine the success of its communication plan, an organization must evaluate its promotional activities. All referral sources should be asked how they heard of the new service. This information will assist not only in evaluating the effectiveness of the communication outreach but also in planning subsequent communication efforts.

The plan should be reviewed after there has been ample time to implement it. Usually six months later is a reasonable time for assessment. The overall evaluation will help to fine-tune goals and activities. Activities that were ineffective should be eliminated, and those that gave positive results should be repeated.

> On the first visit to new clients, staff members of the home health service routinely ask the clients who referred them to the service. The department then contacts the referrers directly to ascertain the source of their information—an inservice presentation, an article in the hospital's newsletter, word of mouth, direct contact from an occupational therapy practitioner, and so on. The aim is to determine who the primary referral sources are and which communication tools are the most effective.
>
> About six months after the introduction of the service, the manager reviews the results: Has the department achieved its overall goal of 10 referrals per month? Is its timetable realistic? Have any unanticipated problems developed? Has the program led to unexpected benefits?

SUMMARY

Demands on the profession in the present health care environment require the ability to communicate effectively with a diverse number of groups, including health care providers, administrators, third-party payers, patients and clients, and families, all of whom have different needs, levels of understanding, and interests. Communication is a two-way process involving both the sending and the receiving of messages. Successful communication involves four essential components: (1) a sender, (2) a receiver, (3) a message, and (4) a response. The process itself entails seven steps: (1) The sender formulates the message; (2) the sender *encodes* the message, or puts it into words that will be meaningful to the receiver; (3) the sender transmits the message, using a *communication vehicle*, or method; (4) the receiver *decodes* the content, or deciphers it according to his or her own experiences; (5) the receiver retains only the memorable or relevant parts of the message; (6) the receiver responds; and (7) the sender solicits feedback to determine the effectiveness of the message or the contact.

An effective communication program follows a sequence of activities: (1) identification of communication objectives, (2) definition of target groups, (3) definition of the message, (4) selection of communication methods, and (5) implementation and evaluation of the communication program.

Occupational therapy managers can clarify their communication objectives by asking themselves, What is my purpose in contacting this particular group?

To ensure that a message is heard, the occupational therapy manager identifies *target groups,* or audiences of people currently or potentially important to the provision of occupational therapy services. The manager further segments these groups into *targets,* or smaller publics, by particular characteristics or attributes. This allows the manager to structure a message to meet the unique information needs of each target (Topor, 1988). Sample target groups (and targets within them) are patients and clients (potential and current), referral sources (physicians, administrators of preferred provider organizations, other health care team members in a hospital or a health care facility, or third-party payers), administrators, hospital or facility employees, third-party payers, principals and school personnel, and legislators and other public officials.

The message should focus on the benefits of occupational therapy services to a particular target group and include other information to move the target group to action. In general, to develop a particular message for a target group, it is helpful to think about the five Ws identified in journalism: (1) *Who* is the group? (2) *What* information or action does it want? (3) *When* should it act? (4) *Where* should it go for services? (5) *Why* should it listen to the message?

Selecting the appropriate method of communication largely depends on the message and the public. An occupational therapy manager should choose the method that best suits his or her needs. *Internal communication* generally refers to communication among people within an organization. Methods include an organization's employee newsletter, open houses, inservice programs, progress notes, memos, reports, case conferences, and participation in activities sponsored by the organization. Contact with persons outside an organization is defined as *external communication.* Among the methods in this category are an organization's community newsletter, annual reports, community and daily newspapers, direct mail, seminars and workshops, health fairs and exhibits, scholarly articles, participation in local organizations, guest speeches at community programs, presentations at professional conferences, a speakers' bureau, and personal visits.

Once the organization has contacted its target audiences, it should recontact them and follow up with additional information. After the communication program is implemented, it should be evaluated for effectiveness.

REFERENCES

Carleton, S. (Ed.). (1993). *Promoting the profession: A resource guide for marketing and publicizing occupational therapy.* Rockville, MD: American Occupational Therapy Association.

Engel, J. F., Warshaw, M. R., & Kinnear, T. C. (1991). *Promotional strategy: Managing the marketing communications process* (7th ed.). Homewood, IL: Irwin.

Kotler, P., & Andreasen, A. R. (1991). *Strategic marketing for nonprofit organizations* (4th ed.). Englewood Cliffs, NJ: Prentice-Hall.

Kotler, P., & Clarke, R. N. (1987). *Marketing for health care organizations.* Englewood Cliffs, NJ: Prentice-Hall.

Kotler, P., & Roberto, E. L. (1989). *Social marketing: Strategies for changing public behavior.* New York: Free Press.

Radomski, M. V. (1995). There is more to life than putting on your pants. *American Journal of Occupational Therapy, 49,* 487–90.

Sanchez, P. M. (1988). How to promote clinical services ethically and effectively. *Health Marketing Quarterly, 5,* 43–61.

Topor, R. S. (1988). *Your personal guide to marketing a nonprofit organization.* Washington, DC: Council for Advancement and Support of Education.

Wager, R. J. (1988). Approach the community as more than one public. *Provider, 14*(6), 8–10.

White, D., & Christensen, M. (1990). Marketers hone their skills to reach target markets. *Hospitals, 64*(15), 62–66.

ADDITIONAL RESOURCES

Cravens, D. W. (1991). *Strategic marketing* (3rd ed.). Homewood, IL: Irwin.

Fischer, C. A., & Schwartz, C. A. (Eds.). (1996). *Encyclopedia of associations,* vol. 1, *National organizations of the United States* (30th ed.). Detroit: Gale Research.

Lesly, P. (Ed.). (1991). *Lesly's handbook of public relations and communications* (4th ed.). New York: AMACOM.

MacStravic, R. S. (1985). Word-of-mouth communications in health care marketing. *Health Progress, 66*(8), 25–29.

MacStravic, R. S. (1987). Presenting the right evidence. *Health Progress, 68*(7), 55–60.

MacStravic, R. S. (1989). Market administration in health care delivery. *Health Care Management Review, 14*(1), 41–48.

Ristino, R. J. (1989). Public relations marketing: Applying public relations techniques to the marketing mix. *Health Care Management Review, 14*(2), 79–85.

Scott, S. J., & Acquaviva, J. D. (1985). *Lobbying for health care: A guidebook for professionals and associations.* Rockville, MD: American Occupational Therapy Association.

Organizing

Three chapters constitute section 3, which focuses on the manager's role as an organizer. The role encompasses activities aimed at creating and maintaining a formal structure for accomplishing tasks. Chapter 6, "Management Styles, Structures, and Roles," discusses traditional and contemporary theories of management and the effect of organizational climate on employees' motivation. It stresses the powerful influence of a manager's style and the important effects of organizational structure. Because of their effectiveness, participative management and the attendant skill of consensus building receive special attention.

The interaction between an organization and its environment is the subject of chapter 7. The chapter portrays organizations as open systems that receive input from the environment, transform the input into output, and use feedback to modify themselves. Further, it relates systems thinking to new concepts and approaches like continuous quality improvement and learning organizations.

Chapter 8, "Management of Rapid Change," focuses on the challenge of organizing when change is engulfing the organization. Persons manage change in four phases, the chapter explains: generating awareness, letting go, creating, and integrating the creation into the whole. The extensive discussion of research on change is well balanced with guidelines and techniques for managing change and with examples of implementation.

CHAPTER 6

Management Styles, Structures, and Roles

Ruth Ann Watkins, MBA, OTR, FAOTA

KEY TERMS

Management. Getting work done through other people.

Management style. A characteristic way of performing the role of manager.

Organizational climate. "A set of properties of the work environment that is assumed to be a major force in influencing the behavior of employees on the job" (Hamner & Organ, 1978, p. 278).

Organizational structure. The pattern in which administrative, functional, and power elements are arranged in an organization.

Role. An "organized set of behaviors expected of an individual in a specific position" (Gibson, Ivancevich, & Donnelly, 1994, p. 325).

Ruth Ann Watkins, MBA, OTR, FAOTA, is the president of Out & About, Inc., a private company providing services for elderly persons. In 34 years as a professional, she has held a succession of management positions, from supervisor to president. She did her graduate work in business administration at the University of Chicago.

M *anagement* is getting work done through other people. This chapter discusses theories of organization and motivation and the ways in which management styles, organizational structure, and roles affect the attainment of objectives through the work of others.

THEORIES OF ORGANIZATION

The theories that have influenced the ways in which people manage have changed over the years, as have the roles of the manager. Also, the worker and the meaning of work have changed. Historically the *classical school* of organization was the first formalized approach to management. Authoritarian in nature, it "emphasizes the need for well-established lines of authority equal to responsibility" (Morse & Lorsch, 1970, p. 61). Principles of management that have evolved from this school include the scientific, administrative (or classical management), human relations, behavioral science, and management science (or quantitative) approaches. The *scientific approach* emphasizes "job analysis, financial incentives and the separation of managerial tasks from performance tasks" (Mescon, Albert, & Khedouri, 1988, p. 43). The *administrative approach* "concentrates on division of the organization by major functions, structuring the organization in relation to authority, and managing employees" (p. 45). The *human relations approach* relies on human relations techniques such as "more effective supervision, employee counseling and giving workers more opportunities to communicate on the job" (Mescon, Albert, & Khedouri, 1988, p. 46). The basis of the *behavioral science approach* is its emphasis on "applying behavioral science concepts to the design and management of organizations," with the results being improved individual and organizational effectiveness (p. 47). The *management science approach* uses models to quantify the variables of a problem, allowing managers to "objectively define and compare relationships among them" (p. 48).

Remnants of the classical school are still in existence in some settings. The current emphasis on efficiency, productivity, and cost reduction, and the trend toward specialization are conducive to a resurgence of an authoritarian approach.

Such a resurgence, however, would not be congruent with today's worker and the modern meaning of work, which reflect an opposite approach most commonly referred to as *participative management,* a "concept of managing that encourages employees' participation in decision making and matters that affect their job" (Gibson, Ivancevich, & Donnelly, 1994, p. 171). Workers' involvement in decision making is considered desirable and essential to high motivation. Balancing workers' needs and desires to be involved in decisions that affect their work environment with the needs and the goals of the organization requires great skill on the part of today's manager.

Also separate from the classical school and its offshoots is the *process approach,* which considers management "a process because the work of attaining objectives through others is not a one-time act but an ongoing series of interrelated activities. These activities are referred to as management functions" (Mescon, Albert, & Khedouri, 1988, p. 48).

In these turbulent times of revolutionary change in health care, a manager must be able to determine how the parts of the system in which he or she works are interrelated and how they are influenced by external systems. A helpful approach in this regard, of fairly recent origin, is *systems thinking* as applied to organizational management. "Systems thinking is a conceptual framework, a body of knowledge and tools that has been developed over the past fifty years, to make full patterns clearer, and to help us see how to change them effectively" (Senge, 1990, p. 7). It looks at all the parts of an organization, the internal and external events that affect the organization, and the relationships between the parts and the events.

Mescon, Albert, and Khedouri (1988) compare, from a systems perspective, the structure of an organization to a mobile. When one piece is touched, it causes all the other pieces to move, to a greater or lesser extent. They do not all move instantaneously, but they continue to move over time, depending on where and how hard the mobile was touched. Chapter 7, "Organizational Effectiveness," discusses systems theory in detail.

Senge (1990) has advanced the theory of a *learning organization,* which is based on systems thinking. It "invests in improving quality thinking, the capacity for reflection and team learning and the ability to develop shared visions and shared understandings of complex business issues" (p. 289).

Another recent approach that is based on systems theory but takes into consideration the different types of effective responses required because of the complexity of different situations is the *contingency approach.* It

> extends the practical application of systems theory by identifying major internal and external variables that affect the organization. Because it holds that concepts or techniques must be appropriate to the specific situation at hand, the contingency approach is often called situational thinking. In the situational perspective there is no "best way to manage." (Mescon, Albert, & Khedouri, 1988, p. 63)

THEORIES OF MOTIVATION

Underlying the different management approaches have been various theories of motivation. Gibson, Ivancevich, and Donnelly (1994) classify theories of motivation as content theories or process theories. Content theories focus on factors within the person that affect behavior but can only be inferred. Process theories describe, explain, and analyze how behavior is affected. Table 6-1 provides a managerial perspective on the more widely cited content and process theories of motivation.

Table 6-1
A Managerial Perspective on Content and Process Theories of Motivation

Theoretical Base	Theoretical Explanation	Founders of the Theories	Managerial Application
Content	Focuses on factors within the person that energize, direct, sustain, and stop behavior. These factors can only be inferred.	**Maslow**—five-level need hierarchy. **Alderfer**—three-level hierarchy (ERG). **Herzberg**—two major factors called hygiene-motivators. **McClelland**—three learned needs acquired from the culture: achievement, affiliation, and power.	Managers need to be aware of differences in needs, desires, and goals because each individual is unique in many ways.
Process	Describes, explains, and analyzes how behavior is energized, directed, sustained, and stopped.	**Vroom**—an expectancy theory of choices. **Skinner**—reinforcement theory concerned with the learning that occurs as a consequence of behavior. **Adams**—equity theory based on comparisons that individuals make. **Locke**—goal-setting theory that conscious goals and intentions are the determinants of behavior.	Managers need to understand the *process* of motivation and how individuals make choices based on preferences, rewards, and accomplishments.

Note. *From* Organizations: Behavior, Structure, Processes *(8th ed., p. 149), by J. L. Gibson, J. M. Ivancevich, and J. H. Donnelly, Jr., 1994, Burr Ridge, IL: Irwin. Copyright 1994 by Richard D. Irwin Publishers. Reprinted with permission.*

Maslow (1954) hypothesizes that there exists a *hierarchy of needs,* with five levels. At the lowest level are the physiological needs, such as the needs for nourishment, shelter, and relief from pain. The highest level of need is for self-actualization, or fulfillment of oneself by "maximizing the use of abilities, skills and potentials" (Gibson, Ivancevich, & Donnelly, 1994, p. 148).

Herzberg (1966) offers a *motivation-hygiene model,* which identifies two kinds of factors that influence employees' motivation: satisfiers and dissatisfiers. Satisfiers, or motivation factors, are such variables as the work itself, opportunity for advancement, and recognition. Dissatisfiers, or hygiene factors, are variables like salary and quality of supervision, which will result in discontent among employees if the factors are absent in the workplace.

McGregor (1960) has developed *Theory X* and *Theory Y,* which describe the assumptions about human motivation that are the basis for the concepts of authoritarian and participative management. Theory X assumes that people dislike work; that they must be directed, controlled, and coerced; and that they are primarily motivated by money. Theory Y assumes that people have an intrinsic interest in their work, that they desire to be self-directing and to seek responsibility, and that motivators include participation in establishing goals and solving problems that affect the organization.

Morse and Lorsch (1970) have proposed the *contingency theory,* which contends that "the proper 'fit' among task, organization, and people seems to develop strong 'competence motivation' in individuals regardless of organizational style" (p. 61). Sense of competence is a continuing motivator; when a person achieves one competence goal, he or she sets a new, higher one.

THE EFFECT OF ORGANIZATIONAL CLIMATE ON MOTIVATION

In recent years, increased attention has been given to the environment of an organization and its influence on the motivation and the self-esteem of workers. Organizational environment is also referred to as *organizational climate* or *organizational culture.* Hamner and Organ (1978) define *climate* as a

> set of properties of the work environment that is assumed to be a major force in influencing the behavior of employees on the job. These properties include the size, structure, leadership patterns, interpersonal relationships, systems complexity, goal direction and communication patterns of the organization. (p. 278)

The physical location, the demographics of clients, and the types of services provided also affect organizational climate. The type and the characteristics of an organization, in turn, influence the roles, the responsibilities, and the behaviors of its employees.

The reengineering and the downsizing of organizations that began in the late 1980s have directly affected the climate of companies experiencing them. They have also indirectly affected the climates of other organizations.

Organizational Characteristics

Morse and Lorsch (1970) group organizational characteristics into two sets of factors: formal and climate. *Formal characteristics* include the "pattern of formal relationships and duties as signified by organizational charts and job manuals, patterns of formal rules, procedures, control and measurement systems, time dimensions incorporated in formal practices and goal dimensions incorporated in formal practices" (p. 63). The goals of an organization reflect what it is trying to achieve and become. The policies indicate how the goals are to be attained and how employees are to behave in order to contribute to the achievement of the goals. Staff members should be informed of the goals of the organization for which they work and should have a working knowledge of its policies and procedures. Several management experts believe that every person who works in a company, regardless of position, must understand the business.

Climate characteristics are the subjective perceptions and orientations that employees have developed about their organizational setting. These include the character of superior-subordinate and colleague-colleague relationships, top executives' management style, structural orientation, distribution of influence, and time and goal orientation (Morse & Lorsch, 1970).

Organizations have traditionally been hierarchical in nature, but they are changing and so are workers. The workforce is much more diverse culturally, ethnically, and racially, as well as in language skills and educational levels. Across cultures, employees' needs, values, work styles, and work ethics may differ.

The characteristics of a health care organization that used to make it unique in comparison with a business organization are rapidly blurring. The countrywide move to managed care and capitation of payment for health care, and the development of local, regional, and national networks of health care delivery systems, are radically changing organizational structure and climate. Performance used to mean something quite different to persons who provided services and persons who received them than it does today or will tomorrow.

Hamner and Organ (1978) conclude that the "traditional hierarchical system of organization breeds a climate of fear and mistrust, which reduces management effectiveness" (p. 279). To build an organizational climate that encourages achievement, management must focus on "an approach that offers warmth and support to each individual, communicating organizational goals and standards but not attempting to control the means of reaching those goals and standards" (p. 279).

In *The Art of Japanese Management,* Pascale and Athos (1982) report on a study in which they compared Japanese and American management practices. They conclude that the "best firms linked their purposes and ways of realizing them to human values as well as economic measures like profit and efficiency" (p. 332). Pascale and Athos refer to seven "levers:" superordinate goals, strategy, structure, systems, staff, style, and skills. The successful managers were able to integrate these significant levers into the fabric of the organization.

A manager must develop an atmosphere that motivates staff members to work toward the achievement of the organization's goals and at the same time to satisfy their own needs for a sense of accomplishment, competence, recognition, appreciation, and "winning." Toffler (1980) and others have pointed out that the new worker seeks meaning in his or her work, along with financial rewards. People vary in the values, the needs, and the skills that they bring to the workplace, and in their manner of responding to identical organizational environments.

MANAGEMENT STYLES

The type of climate that a manager creates for staff members and the way in which he or she organizes work, communicates as both a sender and a receiver, and motivates employees, are influenced by the organization and the workers. A manager's behaviors are also a function of his or her own needs, goals, motives, abilities, values, and biases. All these factors contribute to a manager's *style,* or characteristic way of performing the role of manager. "Style is what other people say it is" (Pascale & Athos, 1982, p. 277). Metzger (1988) and others have pointed out that the manager's leadership style has the single greatest effect on a group's productivity and growth.

Several leadership styles are discussed in the following sections. Others exist in the literature and in practice.

COLLABORATIVE VERSUS COMPETITIVE STYLES

Many managers underestimate the powerful influence that their behavior has on staff members. A manager's behavior is a strong form of symbolic communication. Staff members look to the manager for cues about what behavior is expected, how to perform it, and what the consequences of it will be. For example, if a manager works closely with his or her peers in other areas of the organization, seeks their counsel, treats them as respected colleagues, and deals with conflict openly, the manager will convey to his or her staff members the message that collaborative relationships are expected. Such a management style can be categorized as *collaborative*. A collaborative style facilitates working relationships among staff. An organization that values teamwork and promotes it in direct care invites a collaborative style.

On the other hand, if a manager rarely meets with peers except in meetings called by a superior, plans programs in a hands-off manner, and refers to other departments in demeaning ways, he or she will convey the message that competition is to be the flavor of working relationships. Such a *competitive* style does not fit in a setting in which teamwork is expected. It creates an atmosphere of conflict for staff members, who are torn between the behavior their manager expects and the behavior their teammates expect. Conversely, a manager whose style is collaborative will not fit in an organization that values and rewards competitive behavior.

SITUATION MANAGEMENT

The range of problems facing a manager is so great that one habitual set of responses or alternatives is inadequate. A manager must be able to perceive differences—among people, circumstances, motives, assumptions, and physical and technological realities (Metzger, 1988)—and tailor his or her style of action to fit the situation. For staff members to trust a manager, however, they must feel comfortable in predicting how the manager will behave in various situations.

The key to effective situation management is understanding how to define a situation for others. Once a manager has defined a situation in a certain way, people will continue to see it that way. Badaracco and Ellsworth (1989) argue that

> managers . . . should approach dilemmas with preconceived biases toward handling them in certain ways. The rationale for these prejudices is a quest for integrity, an effort that is at once moral, philosophical, and practical—for it strives to achieve coherence among a manager's daily actions, personal values, and basic aims for his or her organization. (p. 4)

The manager should be aware of his or her biases, needs, values, personal vision, and behavior in various situations. (For a detailed discussion of ethics in management, see chapter 18, "Ethical Dimensions in Occupational Therapy.")

OTHER MANAGEMENT STYLES

Gibson, Ivancevich, and Donnelly (1994) describe four types of managerial styles, referred to as *types A, B, C,* and *D,* based on how managers use exposure and feedback. *Exposure* is "the process that the self uses to increase the information known to others"; it "is termed exposure because it sometimes leaves the self in a vulnerable position" (p. 586). *Feedback* is "dependent on the active cooperation of others . . . [W]hen the self doesn't know or understand, more effective communications can be developed through feedback from those who do know" (p. 586). Type A managers are autocratic, exhibiting anxiety and hostility, and appearing aloof and cold. They do not use exposure or feedback. Type Bs are interested in developing relationships with subordinates and use feedback, but are unable to express feelings and ideas; therefore staff members have a difficult time knowing what type B managers really think. On the other hand, type C managers use exposure because they are interested not in the ideas and the feelings of others, but in their "own sense of importance and prestige" (p. 587). Type Ds balance exposing their own feelings and ideas and obtaining feedback. Gibson, Ivancevich, and Donnelly consider type Ds to have the most effective style of management.

Badaracco and Ellsworth (1989) discuss three leadership styles: political, directive, and value driven. They compare the styles in relation to philosophy of management, underlying theories of motivation, approach to managing change, use of power and delegation of authority, use of consensus and teamwork, style of decision making, and use of communication tools and techniques. For example, political leaders "act in non-threatening ways" (p. 33) and "keep goals general and flexible, and sometimes vague" (p. 27). Directive leaders, through "hands-on involvement and enthusiastic enforcement of high standards, make the meaning of personal commitment and the desired actions clear to subordinates" (p. 47). Value-driven leaders, "because they seek opportunities to build and defend values, . . . develop a wide range of informal relations with others" and "use these personal dealings with others . . . to show their commitment to their companies' values" (p. 86).

Gibson, Ivancevich, and Donnelly (1994) discuss several other forms of leadership, such as the charismatic type. They point out that some research has been done and articles have appeared on these leadership styles, but current research findings are not sufficient to support them. (For more discussion of leadership styles, see chapter 9, "Team Building and Leadership.")

ORGANIZATIONAL STRUCTURE

Economic factors have been a major force behind changes in the areas in which occupational therapy practitioners work and in the structures of the corresponding organizations. Technological factors are also necessitating change, as well as providing the tools to alter organizational structures.

Organizational structure refers to the pattern in which administrative, functional, and power elements are arranged in an organization. The formal structure that a manager creates is an important ingredient in influencing the behavior of staff members on the job and accomplishing the goals of the organization. The formal structure provides a framework for dividing work, developing specific job functions, and making task assignments. It also establishes lines of authority, working relationships among staff members, and systems of communication. Whether a manager is dealing with a newly created unit or a well-established, perhaps entrenched one, he or she is working within the structure of the organization.

The size of work groups, the tasks to be done, the roles that staff members take, the resources available, the expectations of the leadership of the organization, and consumers' expectations influence the structure that the manager develops. Frequently occupational therapy managers find themselves in the middle, between their subordinates and the administration, the administration and the physicians, or the administration and the governing board. This is particularly true of managers working in hospitals.

A manager of a private practice responsible for staff members who are contracted out to various work settings, such as outpatient clinics, extended-care facilities, and school districts, must develop structures that accommodate flexible scheduling, quality control, and communication with staff members as well as with the organizations that have purchased staff members' services. Some of the structures will be similar to those of an occupational therapy department that is located within a community hospital, but others will be different because of the nature of the private practice setting and the organizational structures of the various work sites served.

Occupational therapy managers who work in internally integrated regional health systems that offer multiple levels of care, from acute to home health and hospice, must develop infrastructures that facilitate clinical decision making and provision of treatment as patients move along the continuum of care. Such structures must be coordinated with the structures of other units within the organization, including other health care units and support services like medical records. In such a system, examples of structures that eliminate redundancies and improve the use of resources are a centralized database, standardized client records, and standardized evaluations.

Although the use of teams to provide treatment has been in existence in rehabilitation and mental health settings for many years, the use of various types of teams is a growing innovation in organizing work. Senge

(1990) believes that "teams, not individuals, are the fundamental learning unit in modern organizations" and that "when teams are truly learning, not only are they producing extraordinary results but the individual members are growing more rapidly than could have occurred otherwise" (p. 10).

Dumaine (1994) identifies five of the most common teams:

1. *Problem-solving teams,* which consist of knowledge workers who come together to solve a specific problem, then disperse

2. *Management teams,* which consist of managers from various departments or functions who coordinate work among teams

3. *Work teams,* which are groups of people who do the daily work

4. *Virtual teams,* which are a new type of work team in which "members talk by computer, flying in and out as needed, and take turns as leaders" (p. 87)

5. *Quality-circle teams,* which consist of workers and supervisors who "meet intermittently to air workplace problems" (p. 87)

A stroke team is an example of a work team.

WORK AND ROLE DEMANDS

As mentioned earlier, in creating or changing a structure, a manager must consider the tasks to be performed by a group. If a manager is responsible for several groups of occupational therapy personnel who provide services to different areas of the organization, he or she must consider the commonalities as well as the differences in work and role demands placed on staff members. The manager has to decide whether to centralize or decentralize authority and responsibility in relation to staff assignments. For example, he or she must consider whether to delegate more authority to a work group that is physically located in another building, such as in an outpatient clinic or an extended-care facility, than to a work group that is on the same site as the manager.

The transformations in health care and society; higher expectations from patients and clients, employers, and employees; and a more diverse, more educated work group call for a structure that accommodates rapid change and features involvement, participation, and commitment of the employee. In addition, the structure must allow the manager to maintain a balance between the entrenched ideals that health care is a right and that patients and clients should receive care regardless of ability to pay, and the financial resources of the patient or client and the organization. Organizational systems that enhance efficiency, effectiveness, productivity, and accountability must be built.

PARTICIPATIVE MANAGEMENT AND CONSENSUS BUILDING

Studies have shown that successful managers use participative management. This approach is complex but effective. It emphasizes joint problem solving and decision making by some or all persons who are relevant to the problem (Metzger, 1988). The skill of building consensus is key to this form of management. Staff members must come to a consensus on what the real problem is in a specific situation and how they will solve it. The manager's role is to be an active listener, paying close attention to reservations and doubts, encouraging expression of different views, and dealing with conflicts openly and candidly. The manager must be willing to accept a solution that is different from the one that he or she favors.

The manager must define the framework within which staff members can make a consensus decision. For example, if the board of a hospital decides that the facility will provide services seven days a week, a manager should bring staff members together and build consensus on how to implement the decision, not on whether to implement it. In such a situation the manager will most likely have to spend time providing information so that staff members understand the reason for the decision and its relationship to organizational goals. The manager will also have to deal with staff members' feelings because such a change will affect their work and personal lives. These feelings should be acknowledged and discussed on an individual as well as a group basis. Providing staff members with an opportunity to express their feelings and participate in decision making will help establish group ownership of the implementation plan.

According to Metzger (1988), tasks that are performed through cooperation rather than competition are more efficiently accomplished. Ad hoc committees, focus groups, peer reviews, and recognition of individual and group efforts are methods that a manager can use to facilitate participative management. The astute manager will surround himself or herself with competent people and let them do their jobs. He or she will also involve staff members in setting performance standards that deal with quality and productivity, and in developing departmental or program procedures. Job descriptions should reflect tasks and responsibilities, including participation in identifying problems and helping to find solutions. Kanter (1982) has found that "companies that produced the most entrepreneurs have cultures that encourage collaboration and teamwork." Such companies also have complex structures that link people in multiple ways and help them go beyond the confines of their defined jobs to do "what needs to be done" (p. 102).

To lead teams, managers must also be skilled in conflict resolution. "Conflict resolution occurs when the reasons for a conflict are eliminated" (Schermerhorn, Hunt, & Osborn, 1994, p. 599). Conflict that prevents individuals or groups from working together constructively is harmful in an organization. There are many ways to pursue conflict management. The important goal is for the manager to "achieve or set the stage for true conflict resolution" (p. 599). Chapter 9, "Team Building and Leadership," addresses conflict resolution in more detail.

COMMUNICATION

An effective communication system is basic to successful management. The communication process is complicated because so many different messages are being conveyed and each person interprets them differently. The amount and the type of experience that an individual practitioner has affects the ways in which he or she interprets messages. Chapter 14, "Principles of Communication," addresses communication in detail.

ROLES AND RESPONSIBILITIES

As stated at the beginning of this chapter, the roles of managers have changed over the years. Dramatic, global change is the environment in which today's managers operate. The "loads of information and communication needed for wealth production" have resulted in "powershifts" with the workforce (Toffler, 1990, p. 210).

> What is happening is that the knowledge load, and more important, the decision load, are being redistributed. In a continual cycle of learning, unlearning, and relearning, workers need to master new techniques, adapt to new organizational forms, and come up with new ideas. (p. 211)

To function in such an environment, managers must be prepared to adapt instantly. Further, they must feel comfortable in a wide range of organizational structures and roles, and in sharing decision-making power with staff members.

ROLES

Role refers to an "organized set of behaviors expected of an individual in a specific position" (Gibson, Ivancevich, & Donnelly, 1994, p. 325). The manager has many roles, as well as explicit and implicit responsibilities. These change from situation to situation and task to task. Whether a manager is a director, a supervisor, or an administrator, an important role he or she plays is that of liaison between his or her staff members and other centers of authority in the organization. The manager also represents the administration to the employees as the interpreter of the organization's policies and the implementer of its programs. A manager achieves real power through a network of satisfactory relationships (Metzger, 1988) built on personal contact, negotiation, support, shared goals and values, and trust. Well-developed interpersonal skills are necessary to develop such relationships.

The occupational therapy manager also fills the roles of professional, leader, coach, counselor, decision maker, trainer, supervisor, supervisee, facilitator, mediator, group member, visionary, planner, and change agent. In today's climate he or she must be a risk taker as well. According to Michael Hammer, there will be few managerial jobs in the future, and those that will exist will "'have three flavors: [The first is] a process owner, . . . a work engineer, who's concerned about how we go about filling work orders, designing products. The second is coach—teaching, developing people, . . . [and] the third kind is the leader, who primarily motivates— creates an environment where people get it done'"(as quoted in Lancaster, 1995, p. B1).

Role modeling is a powerful tool. With it the manager can encourage self-rewarding behaviors among staff members and achievement of competence goals. The manager who conveys the message that employees are an organization's most important asset will be effective at motivating staff members and engendering trust. (For more discussion of roles, see chapter 7, "Organizational Effectiveness.")

EXPLICIT RESPONSIBILITIES

Explicit responsibilities refers to responsibilities that are visible, tangible, quantifiable, and measurable. Explicit responsibilities that accompany managers' roles include making decisions, providing feedback, communicating effectively, motivating staff members, securing resources, managing conflict, collaborating, and attaining organizational goals. A review of recent advertisements for occupational therapy manager positions indicates some new explicit responsibilities, not required a few years ago—for example, marketing, doing strategic planning, negotiating contracts, and managing staff members across multiple facilities. (For more discussion of managers' responsibilities, see chapter 9, "Team Building and Leadership," and chapter 14, "Principles of Communication.")

Many factors affect which explicit responsibilities receive a manager's attention at any given time. Intradepartmental conflicts may result from a manager's attending to one responsibility to the exclusion of another. For example, top management may require an occupational therapy manager to participate in the organization's strategic planning process. This may put the occupational therapy department's plans for securing additional resources on hold. Department staff members may feel that the manager is not meeting her explicit responsibilities. The manager, however, may think that the delay is not significant nor an abdication of an explicit responsibility.

A reality of management is that managers and the persons whom they manage sometimes do not see eye to eye on what workers want most (Metzger, 1988). However, managers do make assumptions about how their actions influence the performance and the satisfaction of their subordinates. The validity of their perceptions is based on their previous experience, their value systems, the information they receive, and the method by which they process it. These factors influence how managers execute their explicit responsibilities.

IMPLICIT RESPONSIBILITIES

Implicit responsibilities refers to responsibilities that are expected, though not expressed. Such responsibilities are subtle and intangible, but vital to integrity and leadership. The implicit responsibilities of the managerial role include being trustworthy and possessing and fostering integrity. Also implied is a subordination of one's own and staff members' interests to organizational goals. This can create a conflict for the manager, and great skill is required to maintain a climate that integrates the needs and the interests of staff members with the values and the goals of the organization.

Badaracco and Ellsworth (1989) point out that "people care personally about the intangibles and the way they are resolved." The way in which managers deal with the intangibles of situations "can influence how much trust others are willing to place in them" (p. 197).

SUMMARY

The theories that have influenced the ways in which people manage have changed over the years, as have the roles of the manager. Also, the worker and the meaning of work have changed. The classical school of organization, authoritarian in nature, was the first formalized approach to management. From it several other management approaches have evolved: scientific, administrative, human relations, behavioral science, and management science. Today's worker and the modern meaning of work reflect a nonauthoritarian approach known as participative management. Other management approaches of recent vintage are the process approach, systems thinking, the learning organization, and the contingency approach.

Underlying the different management approaches have been various theories of motivation—for example, Maslow's (1954) hierarchy of needs, Herzberg's (1966) motivation-hygiene model, McGregor's (1960) Theory X and Theory Y, and Morse and Lorsch's (1970) contingency theory. In recent years, increased attention has been given to organizational climate and its influence on the motivation and the self-esteem of workers. An organization's climate is characterized by the subjective perceptions and orientations that employees have developed about the setting.

Organizations have traditionally been hierarchical in nature, but they are changing and so are workers. The "traditional hierarchical system . . . breeds a climate of fear and mistrust." Management must focus on "an approach that offers warmth and support to each individual" (Hamner & Organ, 1978, p. 279).

Many managers underestimate the powerful influence that their behavior has on staff members. For example, through their actions, managers can communicate that they expect collaborative relationships. The range of problems facing a manager is so great that one habitual set of responses or alternatives is inadequate. The key to effective situation management is understanding how to define a situation for others. The manager must also have an understanding of self—that is, his or her values, biases, and needs, and what he or she knows and does not know. Managers of today and tomorrow must be committed to continual learning.

The formal structure that a manager creates is an important ingredient in influencing staff members' behavior and accomplishing organizational goals. The size of work groups, their tasks, staff members' roles, available resources, and top management's and consumers' expectations influence the structure that the manager develops. The transformations in health care and society; higher expectations from patients and clients, employers, and employees; and a more diverse, more educated work group call for a structure that accommodates rapid change and features involvement, participation, and commitment of the employee. Also, systems that enhance efficiency, effectiveness, productivity, and accountability must be built. Successful managers use participative management, which emphasizes joint problem solving and decision making. Tasks are more efficiently accomplished when they are performed through cooperation rather than competition.

The manager has many roles, among them, liaison between his or her staff members and other centers of authority in the organization. A manager achieves real power through a network of satisfactory relationships.

Explicit responsibilities of the manager are making decisions, providing feedback, communicating effectively, motivating staff members, securing resources, managing conflict, collaborating, attaining organizational goals, marketing, doing strategic planning, negotiating contracts, managing staff members across multiple facilities, and more. Implicit responsibilities include being trustworthy, possessing and fostering integrity, and subordinating staff members' and the manager's own interests to organizational goals.

REFERENCES

Badaracco, J. L., Jr., & Ellsworth, R. R. (1989). *Leadership and the quest for integrity.* Boston: Harvard Business School Press.

Dumaine, B. (1994, September 5). The trouble with teams. *Fortune,* pp. 86–88, 90, 92.

Gibson, J. L., Ivancevich, J. M., & Donnelly, J. H., Jr. (1994). *Organizations: Behavior, structure, processes* (8th ed.). Burr Ridge, IL: Irwin.

Hamner, W., & Organ, D. W. (1978). *Organizational behavior: An applied psychological approach.* Plano, TX: Business Publications.

Herzberg, F. (1966). *Work and the nature of man.* New York: Thomas Y. Crowell.

Kanter, R. M. (1982, July-August). The middle manager as innovator. *Harvard Business Review,* pp. 95–105.

Lancaster, H. (1995, January 24). Managers beware: You're not ready for tomorrow's jobs. *Wall Street Journal,* p. B1.

Maslow, A. (1954). *Motivation and personality.* New York: Harper & Row.

McGregor, D. (1960). *The human side of enterprise.* New York: McGraw-Hill.

Mescon, M. H., Albert, M., & Khedouri, F. (1988). *Management: Individual and organizational effectiveness* (3rd ed.). New York: Harper & Row.

Metzger, N. (1988). *The health care supervisor's handbook* (3rd ed.). Rockville, MD: Aspen Publishers.

Morse, J. J., & Lorsch, J. W. (1970, May-June). Beyond Theory Y. *Harvard Business Review,* pp. 61–68.

Pascale, R. T., & Athos, A. G. (1982). *The art of Japanese management: Applications for American executives.* New York: Warner.

Schermerhorn, J. R., Jr., Hunt, J. G., & Osborn, R. N. (1994). *Managing organizational behavior* (5th ed.). New York: Wiley.

Senge, P. M. (1990). *The fifth discipline: The art and practice of the learning organization.* New York: Doubleday.

Toffler, A. (1980). *The third wave.* New York: Morrow.

Toffler, A. (1990). *Powershift: Knowledge, wealth, and violence at the edge of the 21st century.* New York: Bantam.

ADDITIONAL RESOURCES

Caminiti, S. (1995, February 20). What team leaders need to know. *Fortune,* pp. 93, 98, 100.

Hammer, M., & Champy, J. (1993). *Reengineering the corporation.* New York: Harper Collins.

Hammonds, K. H., Kevin, K., & Thurston, K. (1994, October 17). The new world of work. *Business Week,* pp. 76–87.

Kennedy, M. M. (1984). Negotiate for cooperation and support. *Hospital Manager, 14*(6), 1–2.

Klein, J. A. (1984, September-October). Why supervisors resist employee involvement. *Harvard Business Review,* pp. 87–95.

Knox, T. A. (1984). Hospital manager role demanding more complex skills. *Hospital Manager, 14*(4), 3–4.

Peacock, N. (1994, October 17). Techno convert: Never met a computer I didn't like. *Business Week,* pp. 100–102.

Peters, T. J., & Waterman, R. H., Jr. (1982). *In search of excellence: Lessons from America's best-run companies.* New York: Harper & Row.

Saseen, J. A., Neff, R., Hattangadi, S., & Sansoni, S. (1994, October 17). The winds of change blow everywhere. *Business Week,* pp. 92–93.

Schwartz, K. B. (1984). Balancing objectives of efficient and effective occupational therapy practice. *American Journal of Occupational Therapy, 38,* 198–200.

Wysocki, B., Jr. (1984, September 11). The chief's personality can have a big impact—for better or worse. *Wall Street Journal,* pp. 1, 16.

CHAPTER 7

Organizational Effectiveness

Patricia Crist, PhD, OTR, FAOTA

KEY TERMS

Continuous quality improvement (CQI). A new way to evaluate the performance of health care systems, its primary objective being to meet the needs of both external customers and internal customers (employees) by designing processes that improve operational effectiveness and reduce costs; in business, called *total quality management* (TQM).

Cycles of events. Continuous patterns of activity among components of a system, having four important qualities: interdependency among components; complementarity in relation to a shared goal; repetition as activities are enacted more than once; and predictability (Wheatley, 1992).

Effectiveness. Management to attain goals.

Efficiency. Management to minimize the cost of resources.

Integrated system, organized delivery system. A seamless network of interdependent organizations linked to accomplish a common goal and typically located in one geographic region.

Learning organization. An approach based in systems thinking that integrates humans' natural motivation for learning into the management of organizations, and focuses on processes within systems, not products.

Management. The process of getting other people to complete activities efficiently and effectively (Robbins, 1994).

Management level. A hierarchical differentiation of authority within an organization: *first-line*, usually involving direction of a specific aspect of work; *middle*, typically involving oversight of a department or a collection of specific services; and *top*, frequently involving oversight of a major function of the organization.

Management role. A common set of behaviors based on the objective of the work task that a manager is overseeing or directing.

Mission. A specific purpose for a subcomponent of a system.

Norm. A general expectation of all people who occupy a given role.

Organization. "A systematic arrangement of people in order to accomplish specific purposes" (Robbins, 1994, p. 3).

Organizational effectiveness. An organization's performance within a system.

Process approach. Working with people in organized groups to get work done (Koontz, 1964), through four functions: planning, organizing, leading, and controlling.

Role. "A set of behavior patterns expected of someone occupying a given position in a social unit" (Robbins, 1994, p. 445).

System. A set of interdependent and interrelated parts arranged in a manner that produces a unified whole (Robbins, 1994).

Systems approach, systems thinking, systems theory. An approach to management that posits two basic types of systems: open and closed. *Open systems* are in continuing relationship with their environment to maintain life. *Closed systems* are not connected to their environment.

Total quality management (TQM). See *continuous quality improvement* (CQI).

Values. Basic convictions about what should and should not be done, based on what is declared to be right or wrong.

Patricia Crist, PhD, OTR, FAOTA, is a professor and the chair of the Department of Occupational Therapy at Duquesne University. A manager herself, she chaired the AOTA task force that developed "Occupational Therapy Roles" and has taught and written on the topics of roles, systems, and fieldwork. Her doctorate is from the University of Northern Colorado.

Over the past several decades, health care managers, third-party payers, and policy analysts have increasingly become interested in the efficiency and the effectiveness of organizations. The outcome has been development, implementation, and evaluation of organized health care delivery systems. The traditional system of health care consisted primarily of a collection of independent institutions with minimal communication or coordination among them. Each was a system unto itself, a minisystem. Now health care innovation is embracing organizational forms capable of meeting the many challenges of the emerging health care environment (Devers et al., 1994):

1. An aging population
2. Increased numbers of persons with chronic illness or lifelong disability
3. Cost containment
4. Rapid advances in medical technology
5. Exponential growth in the types of health care providers, along with geographic maldistribution and inadequate numbers of certain personnel

The minisystems of yesterday are linking to form a limited number of coordinated megasystems providing clinically and fiscally responsible services for a defined population.

With the rapid reform occurring in health care in the 1990s, occupational therapy managers will increasingly be compelled to plan and implement services that are valued, necessary, and cost-effective within a coordinated system of care. Trends such as product lines, critical pathways, patient-focused care, managed care, transitional services, skilled care, and competitive advantage are all outcomes of the new alignments. Understanding the concepts behind a systems approach to management will assist occupational therapy managers in making decisions about planning, organizing, leading, and controlling occupational therapy services. This chapter provides insight into the systems approach to management.

THE LIVES OF MANAGERS

Occupational therapy managers work in organizations—community centers, rehabilitation facilities, school districts, industrial plants, hospitals, and more—and their lives as managers are defined by those organizations. An organization is "a systematic arrangement of people in order to accomplish specific purposes" (Robbins, 1994, p. 3). Every organization has distinct purposes, which are expressed in terms of goals, and every organization is composed of people operating within a systematic structure. The function of a manager is to direct the work-related activities of others to achieve an organization's goals.

MANAGEMENT, EFFICIENCY, AND EFFECTIVENESS

Management is the process of getting other people to complete activities efficiently and effectively (Robbins, 1994). *Efficiency* is management to minimize the cost of resources. It addresses "the relationship between inputs and outputs" (p. 5): either more output for the same input or the same output for less input. For example, efficiency means increasing the number of contact hours with patients while maintaining the number of staff members, or maintaining the number of contact hours with patients while decreasing the number of staff members. *Effectiveness* is management to attain goals. Completing goal-directed activities is important to an organization. For example, an occupational therapy program develops goals to provide a higher percentage of consumers with services.

Efficiency and effectiveness are related: Efficiency is a means to an end; the end reflects effectiveness. For instance, to increase the percentage of patients receiving occupational therapy services, while containing program costs, the program manager of a rehabilitation unit may hire eight certified occupational therapy assistants (COTAs) and assign two each to the four registered occupational therapists (OTRs) already on the staff, to form teams for each rehabilitation program in the unit. An organization may be efficient, but not effective. Because a manager must use resources wisely to accomplish organizational goals and objectives, a manager cannot be effective unless he or she is efficient. A good manager organizes work so that it is both efficient and effective. A poor manager may use resources efficiently, but not meet the goals of the organization (good efficiency, poor effectiveness), or may mismanage resources and achieve goals poorly (poor efficiency, poor effectiveness).

MANAGEMENT LEVELS

Organizations typically include *management levels*. A *first-line manager* or a *supervisor* is the lowest level of manager; he or she usually directs a specific aspect of work. For example, the person in an occupational therapy department who oversees fieldwork education or manages a specific service such as hand therapy, pediatrics, or adolescent psychiatry, is a first-line manager or a supervisor. A *middle manager* typically oversees a department or a collection of specific services; he or she might have the role of occupational therapy department chief, director of rehabilitation services, district manager, or, on a campus, dean, program director, or department chair. A *top manager* is near or at the top of an organization. Frequently he or she is a strategic planner, overseeing a major function of the organization. Top managers' roles are vice-president, president, chair of the board, chief operating officer (COO), and chief executive officer (CEO).

Authority within an organization increases as one moves up management levels. As illustrated in figure 7-1, the majority of managers are first-line managers in the hierarchy.

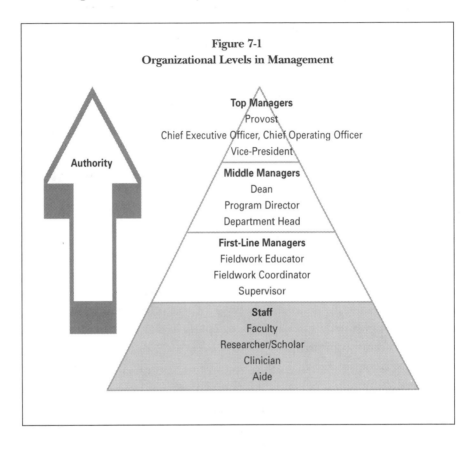

Figure 7-1
Organizational Levels in Management

Authority

Top Managers
Provost
Chief Executive Officer, Chief Operating Officer
Vice-President

Middle Managers
Dean
Program Director
Department Head

First-Line Managers
Fieldwork Educator
Fieldwork Coordinator
Supervisor

Staff
Faculty
Researcher/Scholar
Clinician
Aide

Career mobility may include movement up the managerial ladder. In a clinic the role sequence might be manager of the hand program, coordinator of outpatient services, director of occupational therapy services, director of rehabilitation services, then vice-president of patient services. In education the managerial journey might include fieldwork coordinator, faculty department chair, dean, provost, then president.

Good managers work for their money (Robbins, 1994). Supply and demand determine salaries, but upper-level managers report extended work hours: Top managers average 57.0 hours of work per week at the office and another 10.5 hours at home, middle managers 50.0 and 7.0 hours respectively. Thus middle and top managers spend roughly 40 to 65 percent more time working than 40-hour-per-week employees do.

MANAGEMENT ROLES

In today's health care environment, occupational therapy managers still attend to local organizational issues. Now more than ever, however, they must attend to linkages among organizations that either provide resources or use their services. Managers coordinate the provision of services using a variety of management roles. A *management role* is a common set of behaviors based on the objective of the work task that a manager is overseeing or directing. Following the first careful study of chief executive officers, Mintzberg (1973, 1977) categorized management roles as follows:

1. *Interpersonal roles:* ceremonious or symbolic behaviors, such as being a figurehead, a leader, and a liaison

2. *Informational roles:* information-handling activities, such as being a spokesperson, a monitor, and a disseminator

3. *Decisional roles:* choice-making acts, such as being an entrepreneur, a disturbance handler, a resource allocator, and a negotiator

This germinal study revealed that, contrary to popular belief, managers have little time to reflect or to process information systematically before making decisions, because of numerous interruptions, engagement in a large number of varied, unsystematic activities of short duration, and multiple role expectations. Regardless of management level, life as a manager includes frequent intermixing of the roles just identified. To execute them, Mintzberg concluded, the preferred style among managers is verbal communication.

Mintzberg's study warrants replication in today's health care environment. The information age coupled with reimbursement issues has markedly increased managers' responsibilities for preparing reports and written documentation to demonstrate their organization's efficiency and effectiveness. Potential conflict or role dissatisfaction may result if managers cannot balance their preference for verbal communication with the demands of their job.

AVERAGE, SUCCESSFUL, AND EFFECTIVE MANAGERS

Doing well as a manager involves more than performing the activities of specific roles. Luthans, Rosenkrantz, and Hennessey (1985) and Luthans, Hodgetts, and Rosenkrantz (1988) studied managers' allocation of time among four activities:

1. *Traditional management:* planning, decision making, and controlling

2. *Communication:* processing paperwork and exchanging routine information

3. *Human resource management:* staffing, training, motivating, managing conflict, and disciplining

4. *Networking:* socializing, politicking, and interacting with outsiders

On this basis they differentiated three types of managers: average, successful, and effective. As table 7-1 shows, the three types allocate their time differently to the four activities. Average or typical managers engage mostly in traditional management (32% of their time) and communication (29% of their time). Overall, they distribute their time fairly evenly across the four activities. Effective managers, defined by the quantity and the quality of their performance as well as the commitment and the satisfaction of their subordinates, spend much of their time communicating (44%). Overall, they invest themselves heavily in the internal operations of the organization. Successful managers, defined by speed of promotion in the organization, involve themselves mostly in networking (48% of their time), significantly reducing their attention to internal operations. These findings clearly refute the assumption that promotion is based on performance: It is related to social and political skills too.

Mintzberg's (1973, 1977) findings about verbal communication are interesting in light of this more recent information. Communication obviously remains important; it is always first or second in percentage of time allocated, regardless of the type of manager.

Table 7-1
Time Allocated to Management Activities by Average, Effective, and Successful Managers

	Average	Managers Effective	Successful
Traditional management	32%	19%	13%
Communication	29	44	28
Human resource management	20	26	11
Networking	19	11	48

Source. *Based on information in* Real Managers, *by F. Luthans, R. M. Hodgetts, and S. A. Rosenkrantz, 1988, Cambridge, MA: Ballinger.*

The life of a manager includes not only a diversity of roles and related task performances, but also choices about implementation of management activities. Given that the life of a manager occurs within an organization, management in occupational therapy must reflect the context in which an occupational therapy manager performs. Management in its simplest form reflects the mission and the goals of an organization. However, this perspective limits information and resources for the effective management of resources and work. An occupational therapy manager must understand the interaction between the organization and the environment. This understanding is based on *systems theory*, which a manager applies through systems thinking. *Systems thinking* can help occupational therapy managers make more effective and efficient choices and decisions.

THE ORIGINS OF SYSTEMS THEORY

Systems theory was conceived by Ludwig von Bertalanffy in the 1920s and early 1930s. A biologist, von Bertalanffy (1968) used chemistry and physics to demonstrate that both biological and social structures were open systems. He theorized that *open systems* were in continuing relationship with their environment to maintain life. If input from the environment ceased, then disorganization and even death of the organism resulted. Further, von Bertalanffy hypothesized that *closed systems* were not connected to their environment, that is, not responsive to environmental pressures or needs. The resulting activity was static and noninteractive.

Von Bertalanffy's work in biology influenced beliefs about the management of organizations. As the field of management matured in the 1960s, two approaches emerged: the process approach and the systems approach. Each brought existing, diverse perspectives on management into a unified framework. Both survive today as viable concepts for designing, studying, and influencing organizations, and as models of effective management.

THE PROCESS APPROACH

In the early 1960s the *process approach*—working with people in organized groups to get work done—emerged (Koontz, 1964). In this approach, managers perform four functions: planning, organizing, leading, and controlling. As seen in figure 7-2, these functions occur sequentially, and the process is continuous and circular.

The four functions provide an organizing theme for popular textbooks and management seminars even today (Robbins, 1994). Managers perform these functions to achieve the stated purposes of their organization. *Planning* involves defining goals, establishing a strategy, and developing plans to coordinate work activities. *Organizing* entails determining

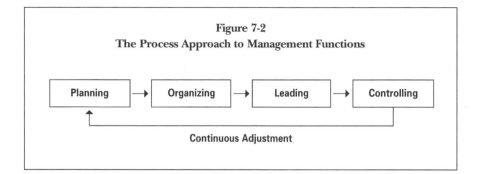

Figure 7-2
The Process Approach to Management Functions

Planning → Organizing → Leading → Controlling

Continuous Adjustment

structure to identify which tasks will be done, who will do them, how the tasks will be grouped, who will report to whom, and who will make decisions. *Leading* includes motivating workers, directing or coordinating others, using effective communication channels, and resolving conflicts. *Controlling* means monitoring work to ensure implementation and accomplishment of objectives and their related activities, or correction of objectives when significant deviations occur.

Occupational therapy managers today use the process approach to describe their roles. A manager's job description or annual performance objectives may reflect the four functions just identified in such statements as the following:

1. Plan a high-quality, community-based program for persons with head injuries to assist them in making a smooth transition from the hospital to the community

2. Implement an organizational structure that clearly defines the roles of rehabilitation staff members and indicates the lines of communication

3. Coordinate the effective, efficient use of therapists, assistants, and aides in the department

4. Monitor the budget to ensure that revenue exceeds expenses and costs on a monthly basis

Earlier this chapter discusses levels of management. As illustrated in table 7-2, managers at all levels within an organization perform the four management functions. The significant difference is the amount of time that they allocate to each function. Additionally the content of the functions differs. For example, a first-level manager in occupational therapy oversees individual jobs, a middle manager designs working service-delivery departments, and an occupational therapy practitioner at a top management level plans organizations.

Table 7-2
Time Allocated to Management Functions by Organizational Level

	First-Line	Managers Middle	Top
Planning	15%	18%	28%
Organizing	24	33	36
Leading	51	36	22
Controlling	10	13	14

Source. *Based on information in "The Job(s) of Management" (p. 103), by T. A. Mahoney, T. H. Jerdee, and S. J. Carroll, 1965,* Industrial Relations, 4(2).

The four functions describe major internal management tasks. A structure such as the systems approach is needed to relate these functions to a broader context, to help an organization respond to external or environmental factors that influence it and its components.

THE SYSTEMS APPROACH

The *systems approach* to management, frequently referred to as *systems theory,* emerged in the mid-1960s as a beneficial method of analyzing and influencing the operation of organizations. A *system* is a set of interdependent and interrelated parts arranged in a manner that produces a unified whole (Robbins, 1994). Occupational therapy practitioners are familiar with systems such as the human body, biological equilibrium, and communities. A system has four components: input, a transformation process, output, and feedback. Figure 7-3 illustrates a system. The human body consists of numerous interdependent, interrelated parts and subsystems that take in food and water (input), digest and absorb essential nutrients that the body needs (transformation), and use this transformed nourishment to create new body parts, energy, or waste (output). The body thrives if the system operates effectively; it becomes dysfunctional if the input, the output, or the feedback is not beneficial.

These four components are also the basis of the systems approach to management. As explained earlier, there are two basic types of systems: closed and open. An open system is in constant, dynamic interaction with its environment. In health care and business, organizations are viewed as open systems.

For example, with the advent of health care reform in the mid-1990s, major health care systems are emerging or transforming themselves to control costs and provide efficient services to consumers. Physicians' offices,

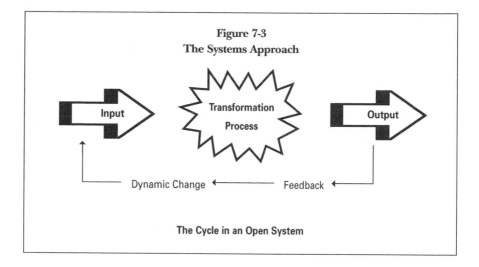

Figure 7-3
The Systems Approach

Input

Transformation
Process

Output

Dynamic Change ← Feedback ←

The Cycle in an Open System

outpatient services, rehabilitation centers, nursing homes, and hospitals are forming health care provider systems to address the needs of their consumers. These are open systems: Staff, facilities, capital, and equipment provide *input* to the health care system. The system *transforms* the inputs into *outputs,* such as interdisciplinary staff, coordinated services, product lines, and critical pathways. The success of this system depends on beneficial interaction with the environment, that is, with the groups and the institutions dependent on it: consumers, insurance providers, government agencies, and so forth. The system must provide continuing, cost-efficient, high-quality services to respond to environmental demands such as consumer satisfaction and profits, both of which either allow the system to continue or force it to dissolve. Consumer satisfaction and profits are forms of *feedback* that modify the organization of the system. Figure 7-4 illustrates the organization of a simple health care system.

The parts of an open health care system become interdependent because of reliance on the environment to provide inputs and to use system outputs appropriately; this synergy leads to an organization that is coordinated to achieve goals and provide useful products for the system. As a result, effective organizations engage in some type of strategic planning to provide the best organizational structure. This planning identifies and engages opportunities and market niches that will give the organization a competitive advantage. Thus many topics discussed elsewhere in this book (see chapter 2, "Strategic Planning," and chapter 4, "Marketing") are relevant to developing effective open systems.

The process approach, then, offers the methods for transforming input into viable output, and systems thinking places these management approaches in a context that makes work in an organization a viable

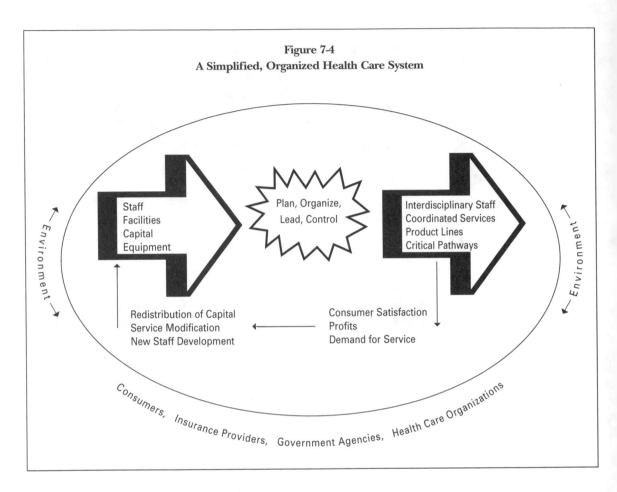

Figure 7-4
A Simplified, Organized Health Care System

response to environmental needs. For example, the manager of an occupational therapy clinic can be effective at getting work done and creating high-quality services using the process approach. However, if he or she does not give attention to environmental issues, using a systems perspective, the program may falter because of a lack of resources to offer specific services or to address consumer and health-related needs.

ORGANIZATIONS AS SYSTEMS

The interrelated goals and objectives of a system are the motivation or the energy for action.[1] As stated earlier, a system consists of multiple smaller systems or organizations with similar interests. Although a systems perspective can be applied to a variety of systems (technological ones, biological ones, etc.), this chapter confines discussion to systems thinking

---

1. *This section is based in part on "A Systems Approach to Management" by W. E. Scott, 1992, in J. Bair and M. Gray (Eds.),* The Occupational Therapy Manager *(Rev. ed. pp. 153–56), Bethesda, MD: American Occupational Therapy Association. Copyright ©1992 by the American Occupational Therapy Association, Inc.*

in organizational management. Each subcomponent of a system identifies a *mission,* or a specific purpose for itself. A *mission statement* is a carefully written declaration that guides the business activity of an organization, including staffing, resource allocation, programming, and products.

In a system a mission statement of a specific organization identifies the transformational processes that it uses to provide outcomes or resources needed by the system. For example, the mission of a community mental health center as part of mental health services offered by a county government might be to provide community-based housing, vocational rehabilitation, and long-term support groups (transformational processes) in order to maintain persons with chronic mental health problems in the community (outcomes) and reduce the need for use of institutional care (resources). An occupational therapy manager in this mental health center would have to match his or her unit's services to the organization's mission. The center's mission might place a higher value on training persons in work activities than on training persons in self-care. On the other hand, center staff members might recognize that their more severely involved consumers are using time and resources dysfunctionally, and ask the occupational therapy manager to develop a community reentry program for independent living to address this problem. Thus managers operationalize the mission of the organization to meet the system's expectations; that is, they transform input into viable outcomes and resources.

SYSTEMS AS CYCLES OF EVENTS

Mission statements articulate a specific organizational objective for each component of the system. An analogous system is the human body. Each of the body parts has a specific form and function—in other words, a mission. The body parts are interrelated and organized to perform specific tasks; for example, heart-lung interactions oxygenate blood. Patterns of activity among body parts are repeatable and predictable, providing homeostasis as well as responding to stress through standard alterations in system function.

Just like the parts of a human system, the components of an organized social system are structured to support continuous patterns of activity: Output from one component becomes input to another, and so on. This patterned activity among components, frequently referred to as *cycles of events,* has four important qualities:

1. *Interdependency* among components of the system
2. *Complementarity* in relation to a shared goal
3. *Repetition* as activities are enacted more than once
4. *Predictability,* which provides stability

(Wheatley, 1992)

In social systems, cycles of events are important because they are the energy that drives productivity. These qualities and cycles of a system can be readily identified—for example, the human system, ingesting and using food as it passes through the body; the college system, moving a student from application to admission to registration and then to graduation; and the occupational therapy program, advancing a consumer from referral to evaluation to treatment to discharge. Systems become more complex by increasing the number of connections or interdependencies among their components. The outputs from one component create energy or input for another component: the ability of the human body to perform work, the employability of college graduates, or the occupational therapy consumer's capacity to return to work after rehabilitation. Thus a cycle of events is under way, and form facilitates function.

CONTROL

Preserving these valued patterns of activity, or functions, within a sociobiological system or organization is desirable and essential. Also, efficiency in operation of these patterns leads to more effective results. Thus control becomes important in management. More specifically, controlling the energy that supports sociobiological system operations becomes the focus. In social organizations, people transform energy into products. People must be motivated to stay in an organization and perform certain work roles because the organization depends on their productivity. Staffing an occupational therapy department in a rehabilitation center to provide reliable, high-quality services is central to effective management.

Unlike body parts, which do not make choices to come and go, employees in organizations do. So a system must create motivation to perform work, especially predictable rather than spontaneous work. Spontaneity, variability, and instability reduce the efficiency of a system. Management strategies to control variance in human performance are integral to the effectiveness of a system. Thus activities and resources that support social control—such as strategic planning; shared values, missions, and vision; policies and procedures; recognition of performance; and quality management—are keys to system operations. All of these are discussed elsewhere in this book (see chapter 2, "Strategic Planning," chapter 6, "Management Styles, Structures, and Roles," and chapter 10, "Personnel Management").

SYSTEM INTEGRATION

Control in social organizations relies on formal rules and directives describing expectations for acceptable and unacceptable behavior. Organizational behavior is achieved through three interrelated factors for social integration: roles, norms, and values (Katz & Kahn, 1978).

A *role* is "a set of behavior patterns expected of someone occupying a given position in a social unit" (Robbins, 1994, p. 445). Roles are interdependent within and across persons. For example, a faculty member in occupational therapy is typically also a practitioner, a professional leader, and a researcher. A clinician might perform the roles of practitioner, fieldwork educator, and supervisor. For academic programs in occupational therapy to function, there are faculty members, fieldwork coordinators, and program directors. For occupational therapy clinics to operate, persons must fill the roles of staff members, supervisors, fieldwork educators, and administrators. A manager might be a professional leader, a peer educator, a practitioner, and a clinical researcher. The functional interdependence of roles ties people together and provides the foundation for the operation of a system. In education this functional interdependence between two systems is exemplified in the roles of fieldwork educator (in the clinic environment) and fieldwork coordinator (in the academic environment). These two roles, each in different organizations, perform as system *integrationists* in the preparation of entry-level practitioners. (For more information about roles, see chapter 11, "Roles, Relationships, and Career Development.")

Norms support conformity in performance, which facilitates system control. *Norms* are general expectations of all people who occupy a given role. The fact that persons in an organization share norms provides cohesiveness and predictability in performance; the norms pressure people to behave and perform in particular ways. Norms regarding use of resources, work performance, social interactions, and output expectations are part of an organization. In occupational therapy, norms dictate activities such as contact hours with patients, absenteeism, dress, documentation, supervision, and even use of fringe benefits such as holidays and continuing education. Norms are frequently delineated in an organization's policies and procedures manual.

Values are used to justify roles and norms and are the basis for expressing aspirations (Katz & Kahn, 1978). *Values* are basic convictions about what should and should not be done, based on what is declared to be right or wrong. Values that influence system operation are both individual and organizational in nature and promote ethical behavior. For example, when occupational therapy staff members value the psychosocial aspects of treatment, roles and norms will convert these aspirations into action. Managers will not consider the lack of reimbursement for psychosocial aspects an excuse. Instead, they will create ways of weaving these aspects into therapy without harming efficiency or reimbursement. Better yet, managers will initiate outcome studies to document the effectiveness of the new program or become advocates with their reimbursement systems to meet the needs of consumers better.

A SYSTEMS APPROACH TO ORGANIZATIONAL EFFECTIVENESS

Clearly, understanding systems and their workings is essential for occupational therapy managers. With the rapid realignment of the health care system, good managers must manage information and make decisions in the context of overseeing their immediate environment in relation to its purpose within a system. The major advantage of the systems approach is that it discourages management from looking for immediate results at the expense of future successes (Robbins, 1994). As a result, evaluation of an organization's performance within a system—that is, evaluation of *organizational effectiveness*—should occur in order for an organization to be responsive and adaptable. Regular assessment provides information regarding productivity, efficiency, quality of output or services, employees' and customers' satisfaction, stability, predictability, and flexibility.

EXAMINATION OF SYSTEM INTEGRATION

Three methods can be used to assess systems: the organizational goals approach, conceptualized by Strasser, Eveland, Cummins, Deniston, and Romani (1981); the systems approach to organizational effectiveness, proposed by Churchman (1981); and the integrated systems approach, described by Devers et al. (1994).

The Organizational Goals Approach

Strasser et al.'s (1981) organizational goals approach assesses an organization's effectiveness in accomplishing its goals. The phrase "attention to the bottom line" originated in this approach. The bottom line in an occupational therapy program might be returning patients to their home or job, providing therapy efficiently, or graduating students for entry-level practice. This approach makes sense because organizations are created to meet specific goals. However, to use this approach in assessing integrated systems, a manager must evaluate goal setting and attainment in light of long- not short-term goals, and long-term goals must reflect environmental expectations and needs for the product being produced. As applied to systems theory, the organizational goals approach may fall short in providing information regarding a system's effectiveness.

The Systems Approach to Organizational Effectiveness

Churchman's (1981) systems approach suggests examining the five coordinated parts of a system necessary to accomplish a given set of goals: objectives, environment, resources, component activities, and management.

1. *Objectives.* Goals and objectives are the motivation behind a system. The objectives of a system should be specific and

measurable in order to assess how a system is doing. They should focus on the output of the system.

2. *Environment.* In systems theory the environment surrounds, or in effect determines, the organization's objectives. The environment is evaluated to assess external demands influencing system operations. External demands include required inputs for operation as well as availability of outputs for use by others. This "energy exchange" between the environment and an organization fine-tunes the latter for survival.

3. *Resources.* A system needs resources to do its work and to convert output into an advantage. Resources in social organizations include, but are not limited to, people, capital, employees' motivation and competence, and even the location of the operation. Assessment includes both the use of current resources and the loss of opportunities because resources are deployed elsewhere. Management information systems support these activities in most organizations.

4. *Component activities.* Managers use two methods to describe the parts of a system: (1) organizational charts, which present groupings, and (2) missions, which reflect work relationships and transcend lines of authority. In Churchman's approach, the latter component is salient. Analyzing missions enables a manager to estimate the worth of an activity to the total system.

5. *Management.* Efficient and effective management includes planning, organizing, leading, and controlling, as already discussed under The Process Approach. The systems approach uses these processes to transform input into viable output. Managers must assess how plans are being carried out as well as why follow-through may be lacking. In this assessment, managers must elicit feedback in order continually to adjust performance to meet organizational goals, and in order to be ever mindful of factors motivating employees' performance.

The Integrated Systems Approach

Devers et al. (1994) present a method for assessing the organized, vertically integrated delivery systems for health care delivery that are rapidly emerging today. An *organized delivery system* is a seamless network of interdependent organizations (e.g., an ambulatory care clinic, a physicians' group, a hospital, a nursing home, and a home health agency) linked to accomplish a common goal (e.g., provision of continuous long-term care to persons with a particular chronic illness or disability). They are typically located in one geographic region; thus consumers can move easily among them. An organized delivery system is not a hospital or rehabilitation program chain. Health care leaders purport this seamless network of coordinated organizations to be more efficient and effective for the consumer than individual health care agencies. Projections envision only three or four managed care systems serving the country's largest cities, instead of a large array of independent organizations. In some regions of the United States, there may be only one option. In the future, health care systems, not organizations, will compete for a share of the market.

An integrated systems approach to assessing organizational effectiveness focuses on more than just the internal processes of an organization or simply goal attainment within an organization. It focuses on outcome measures of the interaction among the organizations that are part of the vertically organized health care delivery system. Three types of assessment emerge: functional integration, physician-system integration, and clinical integration (Devers et al., 1994):

1. *Functional integration* is the extent to which key support functions and activities (such as financial management, human resources, information management, quality improvement, strategic planning, and marketing) are coordinated across units. (p. 10).

2. *Physician-system integration* is the extent to which physicians benefit economically through their affiliation with the system, are committed to using the system, and have substantial administrative involvement with the system. (p. 10).

3. *Clinical integration* is the extent to which patient services are coordinated across various functions, activities, and operating units of a system. Six major dimensions of clinical integration [are] examined including: (1) clinical protocol development; (2) medical records; (3) clinical outcomes data collection and utilization; (4) clinical programming and planning efforts; (5) shared clinical support services; and (6) shared clinical service lines. (p. 14)

In functional integration the focus is on how functions and activities are synchronized or standardized among the various units of a system. The degree to which the same approaches, policies, and practices are used across the various units reflects effectiveness in the integrated system.

Physician-system integration reflects the historical medical model. As health care delivery is transformed, the authoritative control of physicians will also change. Physicians' services are very expensive. To reduce or contain costs, other providers who can perform these services will emerge to deliver specific health care and related accountability to the integrated health system. Thus physician-system integration will either disappear or be replaced by a focus on other professional groupings or even interdisciplinary specialist teams.

Clinical integration currently depends on leadership from physicians in developing the new systems. However, as other health care professions demonstrate their efficiency and effectiveness through outcome studies, and their willingness to be providers within the new systems, their leadership in developing treatment protocols will become evident.

As can be seen in this section of the chapter, health care has become more complex, and evaluation measures to determine effectiveness have also been modified. Assessments of organizational effectiveness initially focused only on organizational goals. Attention gradually turned to an organization's relative contribution to a larger system. Now health care professionals are developing methods to study *system effectiveness,* which again expands the meaning of organizational effectiveness. Occupational therapy managers would be wise to create services that relate to system integration. Occupational therapy organizations that can create seamless operations will be sought. For example, developing evaluations that support or even reliably predict patients' movement through the health care system may be more important than conducting evaluations that are specific to one organization or that generate information not easily transferred. Regardless of the method used to assess organizational effectiveness, the manager should view the outcomes as learning experiences that help him or her modify or adapt the organization's operations and processes and create a better fit within the system.

SYSTEM CHANGE

Just as body systems seek homeostasis, so do systems as organizations. At first glance this analogy would mean that once in operation, the system is seemingly static, not dynamic as described earlier in this chapter. The reality is quite the contrary. An effective system is responsive, adaptable, and self-renewing (Wheatley, 1992). Process and outcome are equally important factors in determining organizational effectiveness. A systems approach to organizational effectiveness reflects several factors relevant to long-term survival. As an organizational system changes, attention to these factors is essential.

1. Market share

2. Stability of earnings

3. Employee absenteeism and turnover rates

4. Growth in research and development expenditures

5. Level of internal conflict

6. Degree of employee satisfaction

7. Clarity of internal communications

(Robbins, 1994, p. 583)

INTEGRATED HEALTH SYSTEMS

The realignment evident today in health care, frequently referred to as *reengineering*, is reorganizing providers into *integrated systems* or *organized delivery systems* to be more efficient and effective. Vertically organized, integrated systems consist of a network of organizations that provide a coordinated continuum of services for a defined population (Devers et al., 1994). The integrated system is responsible for the clinical and fiscal health status of the defined population and is frequently aligned with a specific insurance provider if it is not one itself.

As this transition to managed care and organized delivery systems evolves, managers will need outcome measures to assess the extent to which the new systems are fulfilling their goals and contributing to the health care mission. Current reengineering is focusing on acute care. To satisfy consumers, the focus must broaden to other health care fields, such as rehabilitation and long-term care. Challenges in creating this new system include realigning entrepreneurial interests within each organization that participates in the integrated system and addressing the lack of incentives for achieving systemwide objectives (Devers et al., 1994). Ultimately the challenge will be to develop systemwide assessments that provide information about comparability and compatibility among the various units of a system, instead of the traditional evaluations of individual units. With the rapid changes in health care, focus on the process rather than the outcomes will make systems adaptable and may ultimately ensure their survival.

To implement and monitor change in integrated systems, managers have sought a new approach to improving health care organizations. *Quality assurance* (QA) has not proved adequate for guiding systemwide problem-solving functions because it focuses on benefits or outcomes, not process. Quality assurance examines employees' level of performance in relation to organizational goals. An employee's failure to reach a desired level of performance might be related to problems in the system or external causes, neither of which are addressed by QA processes (Kritchevsky & Simmons, 1991). In current thinking, QA is regarded negatively as a process that deals with internal symptoms; the causes that actually inhibit health care delivery at its best go undetected (Lopresti & Whetstone, 1993).

TOTAL QUALITY MANAGEMENT AND CONTINUOUS QUALITY IMPROVEMENT

As a result of the inadequacy of QA, *total quality management* (TQM) and *continuous quality improvement* (CQI; also called *quality improvement,* QI) are touted as new ways to evaluate the performance of health care systems. The primary objective of TQM and CQI is to meet the needs of both external customers, those who purchase goods and services, and internal customers, the employees, by designing processes that improve operational effectiveness and reduce costs (Gillem, 1988). TQM is frequently used in business; CQI is health care's version of TQM. According to Deming ("Adopting Deming's Ideas," 1990), 94 percent of all errors are attributable to the system, not to employees. TQM and CQI approaches to evaluating the performance of a system are continuous processes, not events. The focus is not only on inspection to achieve quality, but on the constant improvement of process.

For these approaches to effect systemwide change, several factors must be in place: embracing of the TQM or CQI vision by all entities in the system; empowerment of workers to improve work processes; implementation of TQM training to provide qualified leadership; putting of quality, not quantity, first as the measure of performance; focus on teamwork; and provision of professional development for all employees ("Adopting Deming's Ideas," 1990). In full operation TQM and CQI provide a process for perpetual adaptation of a system because they create information, primarily statistics and visual representations of a system's quality. (For more information, see chapter 12, "Evaluation of Program.")

LEARNING ORGANIZATIONS

Learning organizations is the new buzzword in organizational management. This approach, based in systems thinking, integrates humans' natural motivation for learning into the management of organizations. Learning organizations focus on processes within systems, not products. Thus the challenge is not to be solely product oriented as suggested by QA, but to create organizations that are process oriented by using reflection, inquiry, and experimentation. Shared vision replaces control in organizations, and managers become facilitators of team learning.

Learning organizations reflect six activities or disciplines, according to Senge (1990): systems thinking, personal mastery, shared vision, mental models, team learning, and dialogue.

SYSTEMS THINKING

Senge (1990) incorporates the body of knowledge on systems thinking into understanding the operation of a learning organization. The structure of systems influences behaviors. However, instead of structure determining work behaviors, this approach advocates that systems leverage work processes to create new behaviors in workers. This thinking must go beyond employees' immediate work responsibility or role to include a systemwide reflection.

PERSONAL MASTERY

Personal mastery means competence, expertise, or proficiency. Typically this mastery supports the ability to dominate others who have less competence. Senge (1990) advocates a different view:

> Personal mastery is the discipline of continually clarifying and deepening our personal vision, of focusing our energies, of developing patience, and of seeing reality objectively. (p. 7)

Personal mastery is the cornerstone of an organization's capacity to learn. Thus a learning organization focuses on the professional development of its workers.

SHARED VISION

Building a *shared vision* means developing the capacity of the members of an organization to hold a common picture of the future. This must be genuine vision that encourages people to learn and excel. A shared vision cannot be a top-down management mandate or the words of a charismatic leader. It must grow from the people and foster genuine commitment and enrollment, not simple compliance. Vision statements as used in TQM can become cookbooks, even endpoints, instead of the guidance provided by dynamic principles and practices expressed in a genuinely shared vision.

MENTAL MODELS

Mental models are preconceived notions about how things work in the world and how people take actions based on these notions. Deeply ingrained, mental models support generalized patterns of expectations or behaviors. For example, mental models preset employees' expectations about what will occur at a staff meeting, even to who will say what and for what reason. Although mental models provide predictability, they also block learning and innovation because no inquiry into doing things differently is present. In working in a learning organization, members use *inward mirrors* to reflect on their own mental models. This organizational reflection must be a balance between inquiry and advocacy, with people expressing their thoughts effectively while being open to influence by others.

TEAM LEARNING

Team learning is essential, for teams, not individuals, are the fundamental unit in an organization. The goal of the team is to develop interaction patterns that facilitate dialogue among team members instead of using patterns of communication that undermine effective learning. Senge (1990) calls this "genuinely thinking together." Managers know the benefits when staff members work together. Managers also know the exponential possibilities created when a team has goals, rather than individuals having goals and protecting their turf.

In learning organizations, team learning has several important characteristics:

1. Examining one another's assumptions, even suspending assumptions

2. Showing regard for one another as colleagues and working collaboratively

3. Searching for innovative, coordinated actions through insightful thinking about complex issues

4. Listening for deep meaning, challenging mental models and patterns of interaction, and showing genuine concern during dialogue among participants

(Senge, 1990)

Practicing the characteristics of team learning will help occupational therapy managers and practitioners develop competencies that they can use to facilitate systems thinking.

DIALOGUE

The last discipline that Senge (1990) advocates for a learning organization is the promotion of dialogue to solve problems and to communicate information. *Dialogue* is the process used during team learning to facilitate systems thinking, development and implementation of shared visions, and examination of mental models. Senge differentiates dialogue from discussion. Discussion is superficial and self-investing, used only to protect or defend individual territory. The term has roots in words like *concussion* and *percussion,* suggesting "a heaving of ideas back and forth in a winner-takes-all competition" (p. 10). In discussion, views are presented and defended, whereas in dialogue, different views are presented as a means of discovering a new view. In dialogue the flow of meaning is important. Discussion results in decisions; dialogue results in exploration of complex issues. Frequently teams are accustomed to making decisions, or to discussing but leaving the final decision to the manager. They have to embrace and consciously develop the skill of dialogue.

Review of Senge's notion will offer the occupational therapy manager tools to facilitate systems thinking and provide an approach not fixed to end products but to development of a flexible, responsive organization. In a learning organization, attention to roles and organizational structure is secondary to creating relationships that provide smooth, efficient operation and responsiveness.

SUMMARY

Understanding the concepts behind a systems approach to management will assist occupational therapy managers in making decisions. An *organization* is "a systematic arrangement of people in order to accomplish specific purposes" (Robbins, 1994, p. 3). The function of a manager is to direct the work-related activities of others to achieve an organization's goals. *Management* is the process of getting other people to complete activities efficiently and effectively (Robbins, 1994). *Efficiency* is management to minimize the cost of resources. *Effectiveness* is management to attain goals. Efficiency is a means to an end; the end reflects effectiveness.

Organizations typically include *management levels*. A *first-line manager* or a *supervisor* is the lowest level of manager; he or she usually directs a specific aspect of work. A *middle manager* typically oversees a department or a collection of specific services. A *top manager* is near or at the top of an organization, frequently overseeing a major function of the organization.

Managers coordinate the provision of services using a variety of management roles. A *management role* is a common set of behaviors based on the objective of the work task. Mintzberg (1973, 1977) categorized management roles as interpersonal, informational, and decisional. Life as a manager includes frequent intermixing of these roles. To execute them, the preferred style among managers is verbal communication.

By studying managers' allocation of time among traditional management, communication, human resource management, and networking, researchers have differentiated three types of managers: average, successful, and effective. Average managers engage mostly in traditional management and communication, effective managers in communication, and successful managers in networking.

An occupational therapy manager must understand the interaction between the organization and the environment. As the field of management matured in the 1960s, two approaches emerged: the process approach and the systems approach. In the *process approach*—working with people in organized groups to get work done—managers perform four functions: planning, organizing, leading, and controlling. *Planning* involves defining goals, establishing a strategy, and developing plans. *Organizing* entails determining structure. *Leading* includes motivating, directing, and coordinating others. *Controlling* means monitoring work.

The four functions describe major internal management tasks. A structure such as the *systems approach* is needed to relate these functions to a broader context. A *system* is a set of interdependent and interrelated parts arranged in a manner that produces a unified whole (Robbins, 1994). A system has four components: input, a transformation process, output, and feedback. There are two basic types of systems: *closed,* or not connected to the environment; and *open,* or in continuing relationship with the environment. In health care and business, organizations are viewed as open systems. The interrelated goals and objectives of a system are the motivation or the energy for action. Each subcomponent of a system identifies a *mission,* or a specific purpose for itself. Managers operationalize the mission to meet the system's expectations; that is, they transform input into viable outcomes and resources.

The components of an organized social system are structured to support continuous patterns of activity, frequently referred to as *cycles of events.* Cycles of events are the energy that drives productivity. In social organizations, people transform energy into products. People must be motivated to stay in an organization and perform certain work roles. Management strategies to control variance in human performance are integral to the effectiveness of a system. Thus activities and resources that support social control are keys to system operations.

Organizational behavior is achieved through three interrelated factors for social integration: roles, norms, and values (Katz & Kahn, 1978). A *role* is "a set of behavior patterns expected of someone occupying a given position in a social unit" (Robbins, 1994, p. 445). Roles are interdependent within and across persons. This ties people together and provides the foundation for the operation of a system. *Norms,* which are general expectations of all people who occupy a given role, support conformity in performance, which facilitates system control. *Values*—basic convictions about what should and should not be done—are used to justify roles and norms and are the basis for expressing aspirations (Katz & Kahn, 1978).

Evaluation of *organizational effectiveness* should occur in order for an organization to be responsive and adaptable. Three methods can be used to assess systems: (1) the organizational goals approach, which assesses an organization's effectiveness in accomplishing its goals; (2) the systems approach to organizational effectiveness, which suggests examining the five coordinated parts of a system necessary to accomplish a given set of goals (objectives, environment, resources, component activities, and management); and (3) the integrated systems approach, which focuses on functional integration, physician-system integration, and clinical integration.

Attention to seven factors is essential to long-term survival of a system: "market share, stability of earnings, employee absenteeism and turnover rates, growth in research and development expenditures, level of internal conflict, degree of employee satisfaction, [and] clarity of internal communications" (Robbins, 1994, p. 583).

The realignment evident today in health care is reorganizing providers into *integrated systems* or *organized delivery systems* to be more efficient and effective. These are networks of organizations that provide a coordinated continuum of services for a defined population (Devers et al., 1994). To implement and monitor change in integrated systems, managers have sought a new approach, *total quality management* (TQM) or *continuous quality improvement* (CQI). The focus is not only on inspection to achieve quality, but on improvement of process. In full operation TQM and CQI provide a process for perpetual adaptation of a system.

Learning organizations, an approach based in systems thinking, integrates humans' natural motivation for learning into the management of organizations. Learning organizations focus on processes within systems, not products. Learning organizations reflect six activities or disciplines, according to Senge (1990): systems thinking, personal mastery, shared vision, mental models, team learning, and dialogue.

REFERENCES

Adopting Deming's quality improvement ideas: A case study [Quality Watch]. (1990, July). *Hospitals, 43,* 58–60.

Churchman, C. W. (1981). *The systems approach.* New York: Dell.

Devers, K. J., Shortell, S. M., Gillies, R. R., Anderson, D. A., Mitchell, J. B., & Erickson, K. L. M. (1994). Implementing organized delivery systems: An integration scorecard. *Health Care Manager Review, 19,* 7–20.

Gillem, T. R. (1988). Deming's 14 points and hospital quality: Responding to the consumer's demand for the best value health care. *Journal of Nursing Quality Assurance, 2,* 70–78.

Katz, D., & Kahn, R. L. (1978). *The social psychology of organizations* (2nd ed.). New York: Wiley.

Koontz, H. (Ed.). (1964). *Toward a unified theory of management.* New York: McGraw-Hill.

Kritchevsky, S. B., & Simmons, B. P. (1991). Continuous quality improvement: Concepts and applications for physical care. *Journal of the American Medical Association, 266,* 1817–25.

Lopresti, J., & Whetstone, W. R. (1993). Total quality management: Doing things right. *Nursing Management, 24*(1), 34–36.

Luthans, F., Hodgetts, R. M., & Rosenkrantz, S. A. (1988). *Real managers.* Cambridge, MA: Ballinger.

Luthans, F., Rosenkrantz, S. A., & Hennessey, H. W. (1985). What do successful managers really do? *Journal of Applied Behavioral Science, 21,* 255–70.

Mintzberg, H. (1973). *The nature of managerial work.* New York: Harper & Row.

Mintzberg, H. (1977). Folklore and fact. *Harvard Business Review, 66,* 32–35.

Robbins, S. P. (1994). *Management* (4th ed.). Englewood Cliffs, NJ: Prentice-Hall.

Senge, P. M. (1990) *The fifth discipline: The art and practice of the learning organization.* New York: Doubleday.

Strasser, S., Eveland, J. D., Cummins, G., Deniston, O. L., & Romani, J. H. (1981). Conceptualizing the goals and systems models of organizational effectiveness: Implications for comparative evaluation research. *Journal of Management Studies, 18,* 332–40.

von Bertalanffy, L. (1968). *General systems theory: Foundations, development, application.* New York: Braziller.

Wheatley, M. J. (1992). *Leadership and the new science: Learning about organizations from an orderly universe.* San Francisco: Berrett-Koehler.

CHAPTER 8

Management of Rapid Change

Sylvia Harlock Kauffman, PhD, OTR, FAOTA

KEY TERMS

Capability analysis. An assessment of personal and organizational capability of undertaking a needed change, including information, people, resources, support, and infrastructure.

Change. "The passing from one place, state, form, or phase to another" (*Random House Dictionary*, 1987, p. 344).

Creating. The third phase in managing change: visioning, enlisting and maintaining commitment, ensuring authority and assuming responsibility, planning creatively and thoroughly, allocating necessary resources, and managing interpersonal dynamics efficiently and effectively.

Generating awareness. The first phase in managing change: personal-professional surveillance, clinical practice surveillance, organizational surveillance, consumer and market surveillance, environmental surveillance, and a capability analysis.

Innovation. "Something new or different introduced; . . . the act of innovating: introduction of new things or methods" (*Random House Dictionary*, 1987, p. 984).

Integrating. The fourth phase in managing change: developing systems to monitor implementation and consistently initiating corrective action until the changes become habitual and part of the framework of daily operations.

Letting go. The second phase in managing change: identifying kinds of resistance to change and selecting methods for managing them.

> **Surveillance.** Monitoring to increase awareness of the opportunity or the need for change and to help identify the nature and the timing of the change needed.
>
> **Visioning.** Articulating the direction that change should take and sketching a general image of the future.

"When we choose to see the world in new ways we literally change the world that is there for us to see."

● ●

(Clarke, 1994, p. 48)

Sylvia Harlock Kauffman, PhD, OTR, FAOTA, is the manager of occupational therapy and physical therapy, Tahoma District, Group Health Cooperative of Puget Sound, in Tacoma, Washington. She has over 30 years of clinical and administrative experience. Before assuming her current position, she was the administrator for rehabilitation services at St. Joseph Medical Center in Tacoma. Her doctorate, awarded by the University of Washington, is in communications.

Change is inevitable. As individuals grow and age, they change. The work groups, the organizations, and the cultural systems of which they are a part change. The body of knowledge and the technology in their professional fields expand and change. The pace of change itself is accelerating. This chapter describes the process of change and provides concepts and tools for managing oneself and others in a time of rapid change.

The occupational therapy manager and practitioner have experienced more changes in the past 10 years than in any previous decade in the history of the profession. Two to three times as many textbooks and journal articles pertaining to occupational therapy practice have been published in the past decade than were published in all prior ones. The number and the content of them reflect a significant expansion in the body of knowledge of the field and increasing specialization. Advances in assessment and treatment approaches, in equipment and tools, and in assistive technology are making it possible to help patients and clients achieve ever greater levels of functional performance and independence. To be effective, the occupational therapy manager and practitioner must keep up-to-date with changes and developments in the field.

The health care delivery system in which the occupational therapy manager and practitioner work is also undergoing dramatic change. Advances in medicine have made it possible to do more for patients and clients. The payment systems have in general supported the delivery of more care. However, the accelerating cost, the variety of delivery system and payment structures, and decision making by individual consumers have also generated a host of limitations to universal access to care. The current delivery system is fragmented, inefficient, and disproportionately biased in support of emergency and illness care over health maintenance and illness or injury prevention. The goals of health care reform are to make effective health care services affordable and accessible to as many people as possible and to promote the long-term health and functioning of the population. There is hot debate about the best ways to accomplish these goals. There is even hot debate about whether the goals are desired by all. Moreover, the various approaches to reform have major effects on the opportunity for occupational therapy practitioners to continue to serve effectively patients and clients who need and can benefit from their services. Occupational therapy practitioners must actively participate in efforts to educate consumers and to change the health care delivery system in ways that meet the needs of persons with temporary or permanent physical or mental disability.

Similar expansions in knowledge and technology are occurring in the fields of management and organizational development, including new concepts and tools for managing change. In today's environment, occupational therapy managers must understand the process of change, know themselves, and acquire the skills to manage change effectively.

THE PROCESS OF CHANGE

Change means "the passing from one place, state, form, or phase to another" (*Random House Dictionary,* 1987, p. 344). It is a process. In that process something dies or is lost as something else is created or added. Change, as used in this chapter, is akin to *innovation,* "something new or different introduced; . . . the act of innovating: introduction of new things or methods" (*Random House Dictionary,* 1987, p. 984).

> Innovation refers to the process of bringing any new, problem solving ideas into use. Ideas for reorganizing, cutting costs, putting in new budgeting systems, improving communications, or assembling products in teams are also innovations. Innovation is the generation, acceptance, and implementation of new ideas, processes, products or services. It can thus occur in any part of a corporation, and it can involve creative use as well as original invention. Application and implementation are central to this definition; it involves the capacity to change or adapt. (Kanter, 1983, pp. 20–21).

Managing change involves four phases: (1) generating awareness, (2) letting go, (3) creating, and (4) integrating the new creation into the whole. A time of rapid change is characterized by simultaneous change on many fronts and by rapid movement through the four phases of change. Change is not inherently unidirectional; the pendulum may swing back and forth and sideways. One never truly repeats the past, however.

Even during times of rapid change, there will be continuity in some aspects of a person's self, job, profession, personal life, and interpersonal relationships. The key to a person's achieving his or her highest level of effectiveness is maintaining a harmony between change and continuity that fits him or her (Burns, 1993; Herman, 1994). Having the knowledge and the skills to manage change effectively will enable occupational therapy managers and practitioners to incorporate a high proportion of change within that harmony for both themselves and their staff members.

In the sections that follow, the four phases of change are discussed in turn as if they were sequential phases. In reality, however, change is more disordered than that. Phases overlap and different persons may themselves be in different phases at a given point.

GENERATING AWARENESS

Becoming aware of the opportunity or the need for change is the first phase in managing change. Occupational therapy managers and practitioners should engage in several kinds of *surveillance,* or monitoring, to increase their awareness of the opportunity or the need for change and to help identify the nature and the timing of the change needed. The areas that they should regularly survey and question include the following:

1. Their personal-professional values, goals, satisfaction, and stress levels, taking into account interdependencies with significant others in their lives; and their professional opportunities

2. Their current assumptions and ways of doing things on the job, including their personal performance

3. Clinical practice trends and developments in occupational therapy

4. Clinical practice trends and developments in related fields

5. Trends, opportunities, and threats in the organizations in which they work

6. Consumers' knowledge, satisfaction, and expectations, particularly in regard to occupational therapy

7. Trends in the political, economic, business, and regulatory environments that have potential influence on them, including both opportunities and threats

8. Their own and their organization's capability to respond to the opportunities and the need for change

Personal-Professional Surveillance

Many tools are available in the marketplace for assessing personal values, goals, satisfaction, and stress levels (Bolles, 1994; Herman, 1994; Sinetar, 1987). These tools can help managers and practitioners attend to the physical, emotional, cognitive, and spiritual aspects of their lives; assess their professional opportunities; and evaluate the strengths and the weaknesses in their own performance. Both annual and symptom-driven checkups of personal and professional status and goals are recommended.

Herman (1994), in his book *A Force of Ones,* offers his readers some exercises and a questionnaire on personal strategy and tactics for "stepping off the treadmill" and taking a fresh, focused look at what they are doing and how they are doing it (pp. 111–26). Conway (1994) has designed methods to help people identify opportunities for improvement in their efficiency and effectiveness, as well as methods to help them actually accomplish that improvement. Occupational therapy managers and practitioners should continually spend a small percentage of their time on surveillance activities such as these.

Clinical Practice Surveillance

Occupational therapy managers and practitioners can track clinical practice trends and developments in occupational therapy through regular scanning and reading of occupational therapy literature; attendance at local, state, and national continuing education meetings and conferences; informal contacts with their peers; and participation in study groups, inservice programs, or occupational therapy research projects. All occupational therapy practitioners, especially managers, should regularly engage in these surveillance activities.

The tracking of trends and developments in related fields is difficult for occupational therapy managers and practitioners to accomplish alone. However, they should all periodically seek information about the trends in other fields through involvement in multidisciplinary professional networks, attendance at multidisciplinary or other professions' conferences, reviews of journals, attendance at inservice presentations by representatives of other professions, and participation in multidisciplinary projects.

Organizational Surveillance

The current shift in large organizations is toward a flat, interactive structure (Wall, Solum, & Sobol, 1992). Formal and informal networks across departments and programs in an organization are encouraged, as are matrix reporting relationships. More frequent communication is also urged. Such structures and processes increase the opportunity for gathering information about what is going on in an organization for all levels of employees, including front-line occupational therapy practitioners. The information gathered by any one person, however, may be incomplete. Managers and practitioners should use the openness of communication responsibly by verifying information before responding to it and before passing it along. The advance warning about an opportunity or a need for change is worth the effort to process the information appropriately.

Consumer and Market Surveillance

Occupational therapy has many consumers—patients and clients, families, referral sources, payers, and legislators, to name a few. Some of these consumers speak a common language with occupational therapy managers and practitioners. Some do not. It is becoming increasingly important to find out the expectations of all these consumer groups, in their language (Fournies, 1994). Occupational therapy managers and practitioners must increase their surveillance of the expectations and the satisfactions of their consumer groups. These groups will have increasing power in the next decade and beyond in determining how limited resources will be spent. Occupational therapy managers and practitioners must help them become aware of what occupational therapy is, how occupational therapy can potentially benefit them, and what they can real-istically expect from occupational therapy. Occupational therapy man-agers and practitioners in turn must know more about the expectations, the knowledge base, and the perceptions of these consumer groups in order to plan strategies for influencing them. This surveillance must take place continuously in all interactions with these consumers, whether the interactions are through care of patients and clients, written documen-tation, meetings, letters, projects, focus groups, surveys, organizations for persons with disabilities, or informal contacts. "Never ignore the rumblings of dissatisfaction from customers; they indicate not only criti-cism but the opportunity and direction of change" (Clarke, 1994, p. 9). As a rule, occupational therapy managers and practitioners underuse these surveillance opportunities in comparison with their counterparts in more market-oriented professions.

Environmental Surveillance

Tracking trends in the political, economic, business, and regulatory envi-ronments that have potential effect on occupational therapy is becoming increasingly difficult. The pace of change in all these realms is increasing, and many health care organizations are decreasing their support for mid-level managers, including occupational therapy managers. Yet tracking and influencing such trends is extremely important, for as Clarke (1994) puts it, the rules are written in these arenas.

One option is for occupational therapy managers to provide more support to their professional organizations to carry out these surveillance activities. Another is for them to join coalitions with organizations of relat-ed professions and organizations representing persons with disabilities (or organizations with similar objectives), in order to leverage resources and influence. Managers must not simply delegate surveillance, strategizing, and action responsibilities to their professional organizations, however. They must request constant feedback and keep sufficiently informed themselves to provide policy and strategy direction and support to their organizations.

All these surveillance activities help managers and practitioners iden-tify opportunities or needs for change and gain a general sense of the type of change needed. As Clarke (1994) states,

> The starting point for change is not organizational navel-gazing; rather it is looking outward to the major "stakeholders" in the business and identifying what is changing and how it will impact on you. It means identifying the few important trends and issues to which your organization (profession/program) is particularly vulnerable. (p. 2)

Capability Analysis

A final area in which assessment must occur before change begins is capability of undertaking the needed change. Capability involves information (data, technical knowledge, political intelligence), people (skills, expertise, experience, numbers), resources (funds, materials, space, time), support (endorsement, backing, legitimacy), and infrastructure (organizational structure, communication system, procedures) (Clarke, 1994; Kanter, 1983). This capability analysis applies to each occupational therapy practitioner as well as to the occupational therapy manager and the organization as a whole.

LETTING GO

Change can begin only when one is willing to let go of what is. Even if the occupational therapy manager or practitioner believes that change is desirable, that it is accomplishable, and that he or she has the energy to invest in it, there will be resistance. If the manager or the practitioner doubts any of those three propositions, there will be greater resistance (Burns, 1993; Clarke, 1994). Table 8-1 identifies typical kinds of resistance and methods for managing them. The sections that follow discuss the various methods.

Visioning

Visioning refers to articulating the direction that change should take and sketching a general image of the future. For example:

- The occupational therapy service will be cost-effective, will be consumer driven, and will assist persons with functional limitations in achieving productive lives at work and at home.

- The occupational therapy team will be flexible and productive, and team members will be mutually supportive.

- The occupational therapy documentation system will be efficient, be user-friendly, meet regulatory requirements, and help consumers understand the benefits of occupational therapy.

- The legislature will pass legislation requiring all health care insurers to offer no less than a standard benefit package, and occupational therapy will be included in the standard benefit package.

These four examples of vision statements address the service as a whole, team building, documentation systems, and access to health care, respectively. Each is a potential focus of change. Vision statements highlight key characteristics; they direct attention to certain qualities or outcomes of performance. They do not alone provide a blueprint for change, however. They help reduce fear of the unknown and ambiguity by focusing discussion on and involvement in an assessment of performance in

Table 8-1
Kinds of Resistance to Change and Methods for Managing Them

Kind of Resistance	Method for Managing
Fear of unknown	Visioning
Uncertainty	Communicating
Ambiguity	Involving
Ignorance of why change	Explaining
is desirable or necessary	Selling
	Structuring involvement in surveillance
Known, accepted routines	Inspiring
Force of habit	Modeling
Inertia	
Investment, pride in what is, in past	Grieving
accomplishments	
Loss of meaningful relationships	
Loss of satisfying functional activities	
Loss of power	Communicating
Lack of control	Involving
Fear of failure due to perceived personal lack	Supporting
of capability	Counseling
Fear of failure due to perceived incomplete	Providing training
commitment of others	Providing resources
Exhaustion	Designing incremental change
Perception that payoff will not be worth effort	Providing additional resources
	Relaxing productivity expectations
	Rewarding, rewarding, rewarding

relation to the vision and by stimulating awareness of opportunities for change and improvement. Such participatory assessment and brainstorming redirect free-form anxiety into creative problem solving and strategizing. Vision statements are deceptively simple. Deletion or addition of a word in one of the sample vision statements, for example, will change the focus or the scope.

An organization may create visions in response to what-if possibilities or in response to environmental trends. Visions that reflect employees' core personal values are likely to be meaningful and to serve as a driving force for change. Visions that reflect values about which employees are neutral or to which they are opposed are likely to be less influential or to generate active resistance. The skillful occupational therapy manager will assess the values of those responsible for creating and implementing change and will create visions that take those values into account. For example, the manager may recognize that to price services competitively, the organization must introduce cost reductions; nonetheless, it must maintain acceptable levels of quality of care and access to care.

Explaining

Those who first perceive the need for change are in the position of explaining and selling their beliefs and rationale to others. Clarke (1994) recommends widespread involvement of line staff members and mid-level managers in surveillance so that there is a common base of experience and understanding on which to build when the time comes to initiate change:

> The more people that can be involved in the external business realities of customer and competitors, the more they will "smell the smoke and feel the fire." Rather than telling people why the change, it's a question of involving people in discovering the need for change themselves. (Clarke, 1994, p. 87)

In the absence of widespread attention to surveillance, a manager must expend extra time and effort to create awareness and justify a need for change before developing and launching the blueprint for change. If occupational therapy practitioners do not understand and internalize the opportunity or the need for change, their commitment and follow-through will be low and the change ineffective.

Inspiring

Changing takes energy. Continuing in accepted routines, doing things from force of habit, is easier. Inspirational messages, enthusiasm, and modeling from leaders and others committed to the change often help overcome the inertia of habit. To maintain momentum throughout the change effort, the occupational therapy manager must inspire humor and provide recognition and other rewards for performance that facilitates change and supports staff members.

Grieving

Even if a change is positive, losses occur. There may be significant invest-ment and pride in what is, in past accomplishments. It is not that those accomplishments were wrong; it may just be that new circumstances require a change. There may be losses in positive relationships and in satisfying functional activities secondary to change. Acknowledging these losses formally and informally is important. Farewell parties serve a pur-pose; so do parties to burn old forms. They facilitate letting go. Opportunities to talk informally about losses are important as well. However, there also needs to be closure on grieving and an expectation of moving on.

Communicating and Involving

In times of change, open, frequent, two-way communication is especially important. The best way to counter resistance due to perceived loss of power and control is to involve people in exploring the validity of their perceptions and in planning and implementing changes. The manager must structure the involvement within participatory boundaries to make it manageable. Clarke (1994) provides suggestions for structuring such participation. Leaders and co-workers must accept criticism and must reframe negative, defensive, blaming communications into problems to be resolved.

Designing Incremental Change

Burnout is a real threat to successful change. Leaders should be sensitive to the fact that change requires an expenditure of energy, introducing it in manageable quantities to avoid burnout and discouragement in the long run. In times of rapid change, managers must monitor for signs of burnout and strive to protect work units from unrealistic expectations. Implementation of plans for change should address the availability of additional, temporary personnel or training resources, and temporary relaxation of productivity expectations to balance the costs of implementing change. Rewards and recognition contribute to the perception that the extra effort is worthwhile and appreciated.

CREATING

For a change effort to be successful, managers must pay careful and sufficient attention to the creating phase. Key components of this phase include visioning, enlisting and maintaining commitment, ensuring authority and assuming responsibility, planning creatively and thoroughly, allocating necessary resources, and managing interpersonal dynamics efficiently and effectively.

Visioning

The leaders of a change effort must have and communicate a vision, but be open to others fleshing it out and translating it into an implementation plan.

> The process of change begins with "what-ifing," hypothesizing and inventing new possibilities, from which one can look back at the past situation and as a result start to shift from the predictable past to a possible future . . . Getting people aboard with change means giving them a destination they want to go to and then spending lots of time painting a picture of what it will be like when they arrive. (Clarke, 1994, p. 125)

As stated earlier, the leaders must also select visions reflecting values that are consistent with the values of the persons who will be responsible for designing and implementing change.

Enlisting and Maintaining Commitment

To enlist and maintain the commitment of the persons crucial to the implementation and the continuing support of a change, a manager must communicate, communicate, communicate. He or she must make clear to each consumer group, in terms that it values, the benefits of the change. For example:

- Increased productivity will benefit occupational therapy practitioners by ensuring job and salary retention.

- Increased productivity will benefit patients and clients and their families by reducing costs and thereby ensuring continued availability of the service.

- The organization will manage the increase in productivity in such a way that occupational therapy practitioners will still be able to provide quality service within normal work hours.

Communication must be two-way, soliciting the concerns of and the benefits desired by key audiences in order to address them appropriately. Change often involves trade-offs in desired benefits. Frequent communication helps clarify the trade-offs and identify the choices that people are most willing to support. Frequent communication also enables the proponents of change to build and reinforce their case.

Ensuring Authority and Assuming Responsibility

Any change effort, no matter how large or small, must have a sponsor and a leader. The sponsor provides authority and resources (money, people, time, equipment, and help) for the change effort and coordinates it with other components of the organization to prevent duplication, ensure consistency, obtain support, and remove organizational roadblocks, as appropriate. The leader owns the problem and manages the creation and the implementation of the blueprint for change. All persons who are potentially affected by the change are responsible for providing input. All of them, or representatives whom they select, may participate in generating creative, efficient, and workable strategies for accomplishing the needed change (Conway, 1994).

Planning Creatively and Thoroughly

Effective change, or innovation, requires creative thinking:

> I found that the entrepreneurial spirit producing innovation is associated with a particular way of approaching problems that I

call "integrative": the willingness to move beyond received wisdom, to combine ideas from unconnected sources, to embrace change as an opportunity to test limits. To see problems integratively is to see them as wholes, related to larger wholes, and thus challenging established practices—rather than walling off a piece of experience and preventing it from being touched or affected by any new experience. (Kanter, 1983, p. 27)

DeBono (1982, 1992) presents several useful exercises for developing skills in creative thinking. Leaders of change efforts should use strategies that foster creative brainstorming in the initial stages of developing plans for implementing change. Examples include writing scenarios, using metaphors, and portraying problems as pictures rather than words (Clarke, 1994). Leaders should not move too quickly to strategy selection; they should allow time for generation and analysis of options.

Planning should be detailed enough to give clear direction to those who must implement a plan, and to enable occupational therapy practitioners to visualize and anticipate consequences. The following plan and questions about consequences offer an example:

The unit will accomplish a 10-percent increase in productivity by—

1. Changing documentation from daily SOAP [subjective observation, objective findings, assessment, plan] notes, to a daily checklist and weekly SOAP notes with additional SOAP noting for exceptional circumstances; or to exception-based charting in relation to a standardized clinical care pathway.

   - What effect will this have on physicians' and other team members' knowledge of patients' progress and care planning?

   - What effect will this have on the needs of payers and the need for legal documentation?

   - What must be created or included in a checklist or a clinical care pathway?

2. Planning and using cancellation and no-show times more productively.

   - For what should that time be used?

   - Who is responsible for generating plans for use of that time?

   - What changes in documentation of time are needed to track effective use?

   - How much cancellation and no-show time can be used effectively?

3. Developing and implementing strategies to reduce cancellation and no-show time.

- Should double booking or overlapping of patients' schedules be initiated? What would be the effect on other team members' efficiency, on the satisfaction of patients and their families, on outcomes for patients, and on quality of care?

- Should patients be called to remind them of appointments? All patients? Patients who have one cancellation or one no-show? Are secretarial resources available or needed to implement this? At what cost?

4. Reassigning caseloads when the volume of patients varies above or below certain levels (a certain number of patients or visits).

- Are on-call therapists available for peak volumes?

- Can or should therapists be cut in periods of low volume?

- What would be the effect on quality of care? How would this be measured and verified?

- What would be the effect on staff satisfaction? On staff retention?

- How does the proposed pattern compare with staffing patterns in comparable facilities in the local area?

This scenario by no means addresses all the options and issues. It does, however, begin to illustrate the level of detail and complexity of issues that a manager may need to address in developing a blueprint for change. Timing is also a key element in planning, and it depends on willingness, motivation, and capability to implement the change. "Just as timing is the secret of great theatre so it is the secret of successful change" (Clarke, 1994, p. 178).

Allocating Necessary Resources

Change may require new learning and involve initial inefficiency as new habits and routines are established, unpredicted bugs worked through, and new technologies and equipment incorporated. The manager must ensure the availability of the resources (time, money, equipment, training assistance, and relaxation of productivity expectations) needed to implement change if the effort is to succeed and if the commitment of those responsible for implementing change is to be maintained.

Managing Interpersonal Dynamics Efficiently and Effectively

Individuals implement change (Wall, Solum, & Sobol, 1992). They can be assisted to change through directing, coaching, supporting, training, rewarding, and implementing consequences if they do not. Successful change often involves effective use of teamwork.

> [A] requirement for empowering people to reach for a future different from the past is respect for the individuals in the organization. For people to trust one another in areas of uncertainty where outcomes are not yet known, they need to respect the competence of the other. (Kanter, 1983, p. 34)

The leaders and the implementers of change must be very skilled in managing individual relationships and group dynamics.

INTEGRATING

Integrating the new structures, processes, and outcomes into standard operating procedures is the final step in accomplishing a change. Integrating requires developing systems to monitor implementation and consistently initiating corrective action until the changes become habitual and part of the framework of daily operations. It may require rewriting descriptions of organizational structure, operating procedures, job descriptions, and performance standards. Integrating also involves evaluating whether the change has accomplished the outcomes and the vision expected. The literature on continuous quality improvement offers good descriptions of tools for evaluating the effectiveness of change or improvement efforts (Conway, 1994).

In times of rapid change a manager may neglect the integration phase. To do so, however, is to risk the initial investment, and perhaps more crucial, to risk credibility with and commitment of occupational therapy practitioners for the next change effort.

CHANGING EXPECTATIONS OF OCCUPATIONAL THERAPY MANAGERS AND PRACTITIONERS

Organizations are responding to the diversity and the pace of change (Naisbitt & Aburdene, 1990; Toffler, 1990), becoming more consumer oriented, more flexible, more rapidly responsive, flatter and more fluid in structure, and more innovative. Constant change has become an expected part of daily operations.

OCCUPATIONAL THERAPY MANAGERS

Managers in turn are expected to function as effective leaders, with primary emphasis on establishing direction, aligning people, and motivating and inspiring their staff members (Kotter, 1990). Managers need to grow continually, to develop, and to empower their employees. They are the orchestrators of skilled workforces, not the heroes or the regulators of the status quo. Managers must be expert strategists. Kissler (1991) identifies

11 skills that managers must exhibit to implement strategic options:

1. Market and consumer understanding

2. Strategic thinking

3. Leadership

4. Business and financial acumen

5. Interpersonal relations

6. Group development

7. Diagnosis

8. Work innovation

9. Self-management

10. Business communications

11. Technological know-how

How will the occupational therapy manager learn and acquire these skills? Self-selection plays a part. Continual investment in learning, both on and off the job, plays an even more important part.

OCCUPATIONAL THERAPY PRACTITIONERS

Occupational therapy practitioners are being asked to change in many of the same ways. They must be market and consumer oriented, have good interpersonal and teamwork skills, be flexible, be innovative, be conversant with new technology, take responsibility for themselves, keep up-to-date on clinical practice changes and developments in occupational therapy, and, most important, continually learn, adapt, and grow. Herman (1994) states,

> Managers cannot really empower groups to be inventive or courageous, to confront tough issues rather than avoid them, or to choose courses of action that are unfamiliar and uncomfortable to individual group members. Only individuals can see beyond conventionally popular views, depart from consensus and stand for an unpopular position, generate a personal, driving vision that will inspire others to take a new direction, or risk resources and personal reputation to achieve a vision. And managers cannot compel individuals to be empowered; individuals have to empower themselves. (p. xiv)

SUMMARY

Change is inevitable, and the pace of change itself is accelerating. To be effective, occupational therapy managers and practitioners must keep up-to-date with changes and developments in the field. Moreover, in today's environment, occupational therapy managers must understand the process of change, know themselves, and acquire the skills to manage change effectively.

Change means "the passing from one place, state, form, or phase to another" (*Random House Dictionary,* 1987, p. 344). Change is akin to *innovation,* "something new or different introduced; . . . the act of innovating: introduction of new things or methods" (*Random House Dictionary,* 1987, p. 984).

Managing change involves four intertwined phases: (1) generating awareness, (2) letting go, (3) creating, and (4) integrating the new creation into the whole.

To maintain their awareness of the opportunity or the need for change, occupational therapy managers and practitioners should engage in constant *surveillance,* or monitoring, in the following areas: personal-professional values, goals, satisfaction, and performance; trends and developments in occupational therapy; trends and developments in related fields; trends, opportunities, and threats in the organizations in which they work; consumers' knowledge, satisfaction, and expectations; and trends in the political, economic, business, and regulatory environments that have potential influence on them, including both opportunities and threats. Managers and practitioners should couple this awareness with a *capability analysis,* an analysis of their own and their organization's capability to respond to the opportunities and the need for change.

Change can begin only when one is willing to let go of what is. There will be resistance to change. Key methods for managing different types of resistance include *visioning,* or articulating the direction that change should take and sketching a general image of the future; explaining, selling, and structuring involvement in surveillance; inspiring and modeling; grieving; communicating, involving, supporting, counseling, training, and providing resources; and designing change in incremental steps, providing additional resources, relaxing productivity standards, and rewarding.

Key components of the creating phase include visioning, enlisting and maintaining commitment, ensuring authority and assuming responsibility, planning creatively and thoroughly, allocating necessary resources, and managing interpersonal dynamics efficiently and effectively. Communication must be two-way, soliciting the concerns of and the benefits desired by key audiences. Any change effort must have a sponsor and a leader. The sponsor provides authority, resources, and coordination. The leader manages the creation and the implementation of the blueprint for change. All persons who are potentially affected by the change are responsible for providing input. Planning should be detailed enough to give clear direction to those who must implement a plan, and to enable occupational therapy practitioners to visualize and anticipate conse-quences. The manager must ensure the availability of the resources needed to implement change. Individuals can be assisted to change through directing, coaching, supporting, training, rewarding, and imple-menting consequences if they do not. Successful change often involves effective use of teamwork.

The final phase involves integrating the new structures, processes, and outcomes into standard operating procedures. This requires developing systems to monitor implementation and consistently initiating corrective action until the changes become habitual and part of the framework of daily operations. In times of rapid change a manager should be careful not to neglect the integration phase.

Organizations are responding to the diversity and the pace of change. They expect managers to function as effective leaders. Managers need to grow continually, to develop, and to empower their employees. They must be expert strategists. Kissler (1991) identifies 11 skills that managers must exhibit to implement strategic options: (1) market and consumer under-standing, (2) strategic thinking, (3) leadership, (4) business and financial acumen, (5) interpersonal relations, (6) group development, (7) diagno-sis, (8) work innovation, (9) self-management, (10) business communica-tions, and (11) technological know-how.

To be effective in today's era of rapid change, occupational therapy practitioners must be market and consumer oriented, have good inter-personal and teamwork skills, be flexible, be innovative, be conversant with new technology, take responsibility for themselves, keep up-to-date on clinical practice changes and developments, and, most important, con-tinually learn, adapt, and grow.

REFERENCES

Bolles, R. N. (1994). *The 1994 what color is your parachute?* Berkeley, CA: Ten Speed Press.

Burns, R. (1993). *Managing people in changing times: Coping with change in the workplace. A practical guide.* St. Leonards, Australia: Allen & Unwin Pty.

Clarke, L. (1994). *The essence of change.* Hemel Hempstead, England: Prentice-Hall International.

Conway, W. (1994). *Winning the war on waste: Changing the way we work.* Nashua, NH: Conway Quality.

DeBono, E. (1982). *Lateral thinking for management.* New York: Penguin.

DeBono, E. (1992). *Sur/petition.* New York: McQuaig Group and Harper Collins.

Fournies, F. F. (1994). *Why customers don't do what you want them to do—and what to do about it.* New York: McGraw-Hill.

Herman, S. M. (1994). *A force of ones.* San Francisco: Jossey-Bass.

Kanter, R. M. (1983). *The change masters: Innovation and entrepreneurship in the American corporation.* New York: Simon & Schuster.

Kissler, G. D. (1991). *The change riders: Managing the power of change.* Reading, MA: Addison-Wesley.

Kotter, J. P. (1990). *A force for change: How leadership differs from management.* New York: Free Press.

Naisbitt, J., & Aburdene, P. (1990). *Megatrends 2000.* New York: Morrow.

The Random House dictionary of the English language (2nd unabridged ed.). (1987). New York: Random House.

Sinetar, M. (1987). *Do what you love, the money will follow.* New York: Dell.

Toffler, A. (1990). *Powershift: Knowledge, wealth, and violence at the edge of the 21st century.* New York: Bantam.

Wall, B., Solum, R. S., & Sobol, M. R. (1992). *The visionary leader: From mission statement to a thriving organization, here's your blueprint for building an inspired, cohesive customer-oriented team.* Rocklin, CA: Prima.

SECTION 4

Directing

In the directing role the manager is concerned with motivating and stimulating staff and promoting morale and job satisfaction. Chapter 9, the sole component of this section, takes a cue from the increasing reliance on teams in health care and connects the concepts of teamwork and leadership. It identifies effective behaviors of team members, leaders, and managers. It also discusses supervision and mentoring as managerial processes and tools. The extensive list of references and resources at the end of the chapter will prove valuable to the occupational therapy manager.

CHAPTER 9

Team Building and Leadership

Susan C. Robertson, MS, OTR/L, FAOTA

KEY TERMS

Leadership. An observable, learnable set of practices that "enable others to act" (Kouzes & Posner, 1987, p. xvii).

Management. Planning, organizing, controlling, and directing the activities of an organization to achieve desired outcomes.

Mentoring. The development of personal and professional skills in a less experienced person (Robertson, 1992).

Supervision. "A process in which two or more people participate in a joint effort to promote, establish, maintain, and/or elevate a level of performance and service; . . . a mutual undertaking between the supervisor and the supervisee that fosters growth and development; assures appropriate utilization of training and potential; encourages creativity and innovation; and provides guidance, support, encouragement, and respect while working toward a goal" (AOTA, 1995, p. 1027).

Team. A group of equally important people collaborating, developing cooperative goals, and building trusting relationships to achieve shared goals (Kouzes & Posner, 1987).

Vision. "An ideal and unique image of the future" (Kouzes & Posner, 1987, p. 85).

Susan C. Robertson, MS, OTR/L, FAOTA, is currently a senior occupational therapist at the National Institutes of Health and a doctoral student in human development at the University of Maryland. Earlier she served as manager of the TriAlliance project, Interdisciplinary Team Development. The author of Find a Mentor or Be One, she has conducted many workshops on team building and mentoring. She earned her master's degree in occupational therapy administration and education at San Jose State University.

Are leaders born or made? Many great minds have addressed this question, and the answer is not clear. Some maintain that leadership is natural, that leaders are born with the temperament and the innate ability to influence other people. Others hold that leaders learn the attitudes and the behaviors that encourage followership. Most experts agree, though, that leadership is at least in part learned, so everyone can acquire the knowledge, the behaviors, and the attitudes necessary to become a leader as well as to strengthen the effectiveness of the leaders whom they follow.

Leadership and followership are characteristics of persons who are able to achieve their goals as they work in groups. These topics are relevant to every occupational therapy practitioner, particularly in today's climate of health reform. Throughout their careers, all occupational therapy practitioners will have many opportunities to take on a variety of leadership roles and to serve in various team roles. Successful team members and leaders take a broad look at their roles. They extend their relationships to include those who are influenced by them and those whom they influence. Being a good follower as well as a collaborative leader strengthens their ability to achieve valued outcomes. Being a strong leader, a sensitive team member, and a skilled manager contributes to the role of the occupational therapy practitioner in the health care marketplace.

This chapter defines teamwork and leadership and puts them in the context of occupational therapy practice. It describes the contributions of leaders and managers, supervisors and mentors. Topics are organized around the following questions:

- What is a team, and what kinds of teamwork and leadership roles exist in occupational therapy practice?
- What is the relationship between teamwork and leadership?
- What are behaviors of effective team members?
- What are behaviors of effective leaders?
- What is the relationship between leadership and management?
- What are behaviors of effective managers?
- What are supervision and mentoring?

TEAMS, TEAMWORK, AND LEADERSHIP IN OCCUPATIONAL THERAPY

A *team* is a group of equally important people collaborating, developing cooperative goals, and building trusting relationships to achieve those goals (Kouzes & Posner, 1987). The settings in which occupational therapy practitioners work and the roles that they take on in practice, education, and research involve them in many teams. Most obvious are the teams in the workplace—professional colleagues who work together to improve a person's ability to cope with illness or impairment. Occupational therapy practitioners in other settings work on teams that may include people skilled in curriculum design and research, for example; teams can vary, including people from very different areas of expertise.

Leadership is an observable, learnable set of practices that "enable others to act" (Kouzes & Posner, 1987, p. xvii), and contrary to the notion that there is only one assigned leader, enabling is a skill that several team members may contribute. Leadership encompasses many facilitative behaviors that ensure team productivity.

The next three sections define typical teams in occupational therapy. They also identify the common leadership responsibilities of occupational therapy managers.

PRACTICE

At the clinical level, occupational therapy practitioners form teams with consumers—the persons seeking occupational therapy services and their family and caregivers. Practitioners also participate in interdisciplinary and interagency teams to provide efficient, high-quality services. The occupational therapy manager is often responsible for both managing and providing direct service, so he or she must juggle priorities to be a contributing member of the team providing service.

Managers in clinical settings ensure that adequate staff are present and prepared to provide services, that needed equipment has been budgeted, and that space is available for all forms of treatment. Managers and their clinical team collaborate to develop policies that guide the sharing of treatment space, the allocation of funds for continuing education, and the communication of program needs, usually through the annual budget process. Managers work with facility administrators and fiscal officers, equipment providers, support staff, and building maintenance staff. Managers assume both leadership and team roles within their organization to gather resources for providing optimal care in a timely fashion.

Occupational therapy managers set the climate for teamwork; they model effective team interactions with their subordinates as well as with their superiors. Managers ensure that all parts of the team function to their best ability. Managers in practice settings are most effective using strong leadership and team-building skills.

EDUCATION

Occupational therapy educators, whether in academic or fieldwork settings, form a number of significant teams. Foremost among these teams are those that educators form with their students. Fieldwork educators must also be team players with their students' academic faculty to ensure a positive fieldwork experience. University and college faculty are responsible to education program administrators, who form another branch of the team that ensures high-quality education. On yet another level, academic and fieldwork faculty are a part of AOTA's Commission on Education, the profession's team specializing in occupational therapy education policy and programming.

Managers may take on leadership roles in education as chairs of educational programs, as directors of clinical education programs, and as fieldwork coordinators for education programs. In many practice settings, managers oversee their department's clinical education program. They collaborate with their clinical team on the number and the specialization of fieldwork placements to be offered each year. They provide resources for staff development, especially refinement of supervisory skills, and they create educational opportunities for both fieldwork supervisors and students. Clinical and academic educators in the profession need strong team and leadership skills.

RESEARCH

Researchers also take on team and leadership roles in the profession. Occupational therapy practitioners engaged in research with human subjects form teams with the persons providing data and as well as with other researchers or data collectors. Researchers rely on teamwork with project administrators who supply or monitor funds as well as those who manage staff members, subjects, materials and supplies, and hardware and software for data analysis. By publishing research outcomes, researchers lead the profession in clarifying and validating practice.

Managers oversee the research activities of department staff and conduct their own studies. Motivating staff members to become involved, building research capabilities, and maintaining the efficacy of research are essential roles of occupational therapy managers. Researchers are most effective with a broad repertoire of team and leadership skills.

TYPES OF TEAMS

Team members may be peers or managers or consumers, and may be from different levels in an organization's hierarchy. A team may mix peers and managers; peers and consumers; peers, managers, and consumers; and so forth. Not only is it possible for practitioners to form successful teams with their supervisors and subordinates, but such teams have the potential to be highly rewarding. What successful and rewarding teamwork requires is an understanding of the various types of teams and the roles that members of these teams must assume in order for the group to function effectively and efficiently. In addition, successful teamwork requires flexibility among team members so that they can voluntarily take on unassigned roles to help the group function.

According to the American Congress of Rehabilitation Medicine's *Guide to Interdisciplinary Practice in Rehabilitation Settings* (1992), in *multidisciplinary teams,* a member's primary allegiance is to his or her discipline. Although several disciplines may be represented, each person is responsible for acting in behalf of his or her discipline as the team addresses issues of interest to the group. Consequently the team members may tend to protect their discipline's perspectives, sometimes at the expense of achieving the group's goals. For example, an occupational therapy manager in a multidisciplinary team meeting to negotiate the budget would be likely to protect allocations to the occupational therapy department. Members of multidisciplinary teams may distrust and misunderstand persons representing other disciplines.

In this sense, multidisciplinary teams may be less effective and efficient than interdisciplinary teams. *Interdisciplinary teams* are considered highly desirable in today's health system (American Congress of Rehabilitation Medicine, 1992). Membership encompasses representatives from all groups that the product and the process of a team may influence. For example, an interdisciplinary team to develop an outpatient program for persons with chronic mental illness would include consumers, service providers, administrators, and the like. Interdisciplinary teams are goal directed, not bound by discipline-specific roles and functions, and better able to assign the talents of individuals to achieve the group's goals. On interdisciplinary teams, members use group process skills effectively. They engage in collaborative identification of problems and generation of solutions; they share responsibility for the group effort (American Congress of Rehabilitation Medicine, 1992).

Transdisciplinary teams maintain the characteristics of interdisciplinary teams, but go a step further. Team members may support and enhance programs and activities of other disciplines in an effort to provide the most cost-effective, timely, efficient service (American Congress of Rehabilitation Medicine, 1992). In managed care, for example, during a home visit a transdisciplinary employee might collect data on a patient's food intake, adjust a foot splint, check on crutch walking, install a shower bench, and instruct the patient in the safe use of the bench.

Although many organizations have historically functioned with multidisciplinary teams, health care trends point to greater use of interdisciplinary and transdisciplinary teams. Whatever types of teams an organization uses, the ability to contribute as a team member and a leader becomes a core skill for emerging and experienced managers in the health systems of today and tomorrow.

TEAMWORK AND LEADERSHIP

A few words are in order about the relationship between teamwork and leadership. In the past, authors have often written about team building and leadership as distinct topics. Recent literature, though, draws connections between these two functions.

An enticing volume by Lundy (1986/1991), *Lead, Follow, or Get Out of the Way,* highlights the goal of "participative leadership" (p. 8). The book defines a *leader* as a person who has followers, not subordinates. To engender commitment to goals, strong leaders "inspire others to help themselves and the group" delineate goals and evaluate progress by involving colleagues in planning and decision making (p. 100).

For participative management to succeed, all members of a team must take on leadership roles and behaviors, and leaders must be part of the team. At times the designated leader is not the real leader; any one of a team's members can assume leadership behaviors. Some forms of group behavior, such as brainstorming, enable team members to create a vision, building it with the ideas of each person. Although many consider creating a vision to be a leader's role, any member of a team can assume that role.

Because the formation and the endurance of teams are pivotal, every person's contribution of both team and leader behaviors is needed. Understanding what leader behaviors would resolve a dilemma or facilitate a decision enables anyone on the team to contribute a leadership function. Further, an effective leader can take on various team-member characteristics and behaviors to maximize the group's function. Team members can help a leader lead, and a leader can help people be strong team players. The interplay among individuals in a dynamic, collaborative environment is the key to great management.

To tease out the behaviors of team members and leaders, this chapter presents them as two sets of skills. However, they are the ends of a continuum. Every person on a team should be skilled in using both sets of behaviors.

BEHAVIORS OF EFFECTIVE TEAM MEMBERS

Being an effective team member requires a combination of attitudes and skills. Knowledge of group process is the basis of being a contributing team member. Being aware of roles that help or hinder a group in functioning is important; being able to choose one of those roles at a given time for the benefit of the group is critical to productive teamwork. Beyond knowledge, though, the give-and-take of cooperation, an adherence to the overriding goal of the group, a willingness to function in less-glamorous roles when the group needs them, and a sensitivity to one's own needs as they play out in the group process—all these abilities depend on a person's attitude about teamwork.

TEAM SKILLS

The literature on effective team behaviors is extensive, but full of consistency across authors. The most frequently cited attributes, culled from publications that appear in References and Additional Resources, are as follows:

Interpersonal Characteristics

Trustful and caring of others

Skilled in communication and interpersonal relations

Given to strong informal relationships

Aware of others

Rewarding of others' efforts

Cooperative in decision making

Constructive in resolution of conflict

Able to confront poor performance in self and others

Friendly, open

Empathic

Collaborative

Able to function interdependently

Intellectual/Cognitive Characteristics

Global in perspective yet able to attend to details

Outcome oriented

Organized

Oriented to problem solving

Flexible

Positive in thought

Personality Characteristics

Competent and self-confident

Able to assume responsibility

Self-aware

Ready to assume clear roles

Committed

Observing of high standards

Comfortable initiating change

Equality minded

Fortunately, occupational therapy education provides a strong foundation on which to build team skills. Working in groups throughout the educational process; forming teams with classmates, faculty, and supervisors to learn and practice the skills and the techniques of occupational therapy; and maximizing therapeutic use of self in interpersonal relations—all these are examples of the fundamental skills that collaborative team players use. The key is recognizing these parts of educational experiences and capitalizing on them in each professional role.

The abilities to work in groups, to take on roles that enable others to function optimally, and to communicate with people from diverse backgrounds are critical elements of teamwork. Occupational therapy practitioners begin to develop these abilities as they enter the profession. Increasing sophistication in coordinating the work of several people for a common goal comes with experiences in group work. Young practitioners should position themselves to be part of many different kinds of teams and to take on different roles. By assessing their experiences, determining what enables them to succeed, and identifying what limits them, they can learn how to make their best contributions to a team and build their self-confidence in teamwork.

Given that different kinds of team experiences are important, what configurations might a practitioner seek? Blake, Mouton, and Allen (1981/1987) describe five patterns possible in teams:

1. "One alone": each person working alone

2. "One to one": two persons working together part of the time

3. "One to some": several but not all persons tackling a problem

4. "One to all": persons working alone, touching base occasionally

5. "All to one": all persons helping one person strengthen his or her effectiveness as a team member

(p. 10)

Selecting the pattern of relationship suitable for the moment may initially be the responsibility of the team leader, but people may informally shape teams as they tackle the issues before them. With each of these styles, Blake, Mouton, and Allen (1981/1987) recommend that effective team building include "focus on the *real* issues, skillful use of group process to ensure even participation among team members, avoidance of self-delusion, dependency on the team rather than outside sources to solve problems, active and participative team roles, effort directed to an expected outcome, integration of content and process, and a sense of out-reach" (p. 189).

Each team pattern is valuable in the evolution of a team. Like developing human beings, teams go through identifiable stages. Synthesizing relevant literature on the stages of team development, Jones (1992) and Miller (1992) have suggested the following levels:

1. *Getting started:* Newly formed teams use more formal patterns of interaction than well-established ones do. Seeking information about the group's task, getting to know other team members, understanding each person's commitment to the goal and his or her values and standards of quality, and defining the parameters of the problem to be addressed as well as interpersonal boundaries—these are the developmental tasks at the first stage of team evolution. In this period, building trust is fundamental to the future of the team. The group designs early plans for implementing the shared goals of its members, and it identifies the contributions that each team member can make to achieving the team's vision.

2. *Truly beginning:* At this stage of development, less formality begins to characterize interpersonal interactions. With candid assessments of its progress toward desired results, the group begins to establish priorities. Because conflict is common in this stage, teams often decide how to handle communication and feedback and how to make decisions. The culture of the group emerges, values become more defined, and the roles and the responsibilities of each team member are challenged and reevaluated. As this stage draws to a close, the team has articulated a goal-driven plan compatible with realistic implementation strategies.

3. *Designing the plan:* With practiced strategies for negotiating among team members, the group tackles the question of how best to achieve its goals. It delineates very specific action steps, and it links timelines and deadlines with assignment of responsibility for parts of the plan to various team members. Roles are often clarified and shifted as the talents of each team member become more apparent. The team is able to look outward, to seek resources for accomplishing action steps, and to persuade others to endorse its activities.

4. *Doing:* Carrying out implementation strategies is the team's focus at this stage. The goal becomes overriding; the group is driven to achieve its purpose. High commitment, solid trust among team members, flexibility and respect for individual differences, less

conflict, and more evenly shared leadership are the characteristics of teams able to achieve their goals fully. Often the team is able to achieve even more than it initially intended.

Strong teams help each member function at every stage of development. At each stage of evolution the group faces the following tasks: What is needed to help nudge a group to decision making? How might everyone's input be facilitated? What might help redirect a dissatisfied person to influence the group positively? How these questions are handled varies at different developmental levels, just as parents' responses to their children's behavior differ at various ages. The expert team member anticipates group evolution and adjusts his or her contributions to foster healthy team development.

If team building is integral to goal achievement, then leaders' roles and responsibilities must support creative, targeted, healthy team development. The next section examines the contributions that leaders can make to a team's ability to achieve its valued goals.

BEHAVIORS OF EFFECTIVE LEADERS

There are hundreds of articles and books about leadership—what it is and what it is not. Each one is valuable, offering a nuance to a very rich and complex topic. Reading about leadership as much as possible will help a manager advance along the career continuum.

A highly recommended book is DePree's (1989) *Leadership Is an Art.* Especially convincing is DePree's view of leadership as stewardship. The leader owes several things to the institution:

Assets (in material products and fiscal security) . . .

Legacy (a value system that guides people in the organization) . . .

Future leadership (identification and nurturing of future leaders) . . .

A sense of quality (definitions of caring and commitment in interpersonal relationships) . . .

Maturity (self-worth, belonging, responsibility, expectancy, accountability, and equality) . . .

Rationality (trust, dignity, self-fulfillment, and freedom and space).

(pp. 11–17)

Stewardship highlights the collaborative nature of leadership, based on the dynamic relationships that leaders form with their organization and their followers.

In *The Leadership Challenge: How to Get Extraordinary Things Done in Organizations,* Kouzes and Posner (1987) synthesize the characteristics of leaders, providing a useful organizational framework. Followers expect great leaders to be "honest, competent, forward-looking, and inspiring" (p. 16). These characteristics form the basis of leadership practices. Leadership practices incorporate behavioral commitments that leaders make to their organization. The next five sections briefly describe five leadership practices identified by Kouzes and Posner: (1) challenging the process; (2) inspiring a shared vision; (3) enabling others to act; (4) modeling the way; and (5) encouraging the heart.

CHALLENGING THE PROCESS

Leaders search for opportunities and then "experiment and take risks" (Kouzes & Posner, 1987, p. 29). "Question authority"; "Move from the status quo"; "Life is an adventure"; "Fix what you find broken"; "Go where no man before has gone": All these "phrases for living" reflect this first leadership practice. Leaders are people who "search out opportunities and step into the unknown. They take risks, innovate, experiment, and treat mistakes as learning opportunities. Leaders stay prepared to meet challenges . . . [They] break free of daily routines, foster psychological hardiness, and set up little experiments" (Grady, 1992, IX-5).

Leaders are vulnerable, open, and responsive to trends in the environment. They anticipate the need for change by involving themselves with communities, both geographical and professional. By synthesizing domestic and international life events and evaluating the potential effect of those events on daily life, they see the need for different ways of thinking about and doing activities that have become routine.

As the health system in America flexes and remolds itself, occupational therapy practitioners must also change. Professional leaders capable of envisioning the interrelationships of the whole person with the expanded context of health promotion and wellness must emerge. The leaders that the profession nurtures will challenge traditional health practices, experiment with innovative practice models, and enmesh themselves and the profession in learning how best to provide needed health and rehabilitation services. Occupational therapy leaders will challenge the process.

INSPIRING A SHARED VISION

Leaders envision the future and enlist others (Kouzes & Posner, 1987). A vision is "an ideal and unique image of the future" (p. 85). A leader creates a clear vision that compels others to act. This hallmark of leadership places the person with a passionate view of where the organization is going in a position to inspire others to be as passionate in achieving it.

> You have to know where you're going, to be able to state it clearly
> and concisely—and you have to care about it passionately. That all

> adds up to vision, the concise statement/picture of where the company and its people are heading, and why they should be proud of it. (Peters & Austin, 1985/1986, p. 334)

A guiding vision unites people in a common goal and rewards them for accomplishing tasks that implement the vision or part of it. The excitement and the pride of ordering tasks, the dedication to analyzing mistakes and improving procedures, and the commitment to a common purpose are heightened by a leader who is able to communicate expressively and help others define their unique orientation to the future (Kouzes & Posner, 1987).

Tichy and Devanna (1990) discuss the process of creating a vision. An organization's vision includes two parts: "(1) a conceptual model and . . . (2) emotional appeal" (p. 130). Compelling visions are meaningful because they not only articulate the purpose of the organization but do so in a way that motivates people. Because vision is about change, it requires that people reexamine basic assumptions, values, and beliefs and modify them in order to move in a new direction. A motivating vision enables people to "visualize themselves in the future organization" (p. 132), in the political system influenced by those in power, in the social system's expected relationship patterns, and in the cultural system with its values, norms, and habits.

Occupational therapy needs people who synthesize the past, anticipate future trends, and communicate these persuasively to others in the profession, in the health arena, and in communities at large. The profession needs leaders who believe in the fundamental basis of occupational therapy, who intuitively navigate the profession through continuous changes, and who can see the common meaning in these changes for health and education and for all segments of the profession. Such leaders are capable of inspiring a shared vision.

ENABLING OTHERS TO ACT

Leaders foster collaboration and strengthen others (Kouzes & Posner, 1987). Leaders must understand motivation in order to build the human resources to achieve common goals. Manz and Sims (1989) suggest that effective leaders establish commitment to excellence by enabling people to motivate themselves: "Leaders successfully influence the way people influence themselves" (p. 7). Group interaction is a cornerstone of enacting a vision. Leaders foster cooperation on important aspects of the task and involve people in identification of problems, generation of solutions, and evaluation of the effects of implementation.

"One of the most important things [a leader] can give others is hope, with direction, encouragement, and believability" (Ziglar, 1985/1986,

p. 219). Feinberg and Levenstein (1985) describe the transforming leader as striving for personal growth in others. Some guidelines for doing this include "show[ing] a personal interest in individual progress . . . ; build[ing] charismatic relationships . . . ; encourag[ing] other people to shine . . . ; provid[ing] psychological support . . . ; ask[ing] questions . . . ; [and] keep[ing] people informed" (pp. 116–18).

To enable others to act, leaders influence situations. Cohen (1990) describes four basic strategies of influencing: "persuasion, negotiation, involvement, and direction" (p. 57). *Persuasion* is using logic to convince people. It involves the leader's giving a good reason for his or her request and emphasizing the worthiness of the cause or the personal/professional need. *Negotiation* involves collaborating with others, coming to a solution with which both leader and followers agree, "compromising, and exchanging something" so that both parties are satisfied and committed to the goal (p. 61). Effective use of *involvement* is facilitated by sharing information and enabling group members to solve problems together and engage as a team in reaching goals. Although it requires some time, fostering a sense of ownership among team members increases involvement. *Direction* is giving orders without discussion. It is a strategy to be used sparingly—when urgency is needed or when the requested action is not desirable to the individual but essential for the organization.

Enabling others succeeds when the leader and the team members cooperate, resolving conflicts as they arise. A number of possible outcomes of a conflict help guide the patterns of interaction between people in conflict:

1. "Win-win": All parties agree with the solution and commit themselves to it; conflict is viewed as collaboration to achieve a better solution.

2. "Win-lose": One party wins, the other loses; conflict is viewed as competition.

3. "Lose-win": One party loses, the other wins; conflict results in one person giving in, pleasing or appeasing others.

4. "Lose-lose": Both parties lose; in adversarial conflict there is a tone of vindictiveness, revenge.

5. "Win": One person wins, but without the desire to see another person lose; conflict is seen as every person for himself or herself.

6. "Win-win or no deal": The parties are not able to arrive at a win-win solution, so they call off the deal, agreeing to disagree; conflict is an opportunity to search for a solution agreeable to both parties, but if none emerges, it is better to call the deal off.

(Covey, 1989/1990, pp. 205–34)

Striving for win-win solutions is optimal and fundamental. Leaders interested in common gain have integrity and maturity and use self-awareness, creativity, morality, conscience, and free choice in relationships. With these characteristics, leaders build trusting relationships based on high levels of risk taking and consideration of others. They develop agreements after cooperatively defining the desired results, the operating guidelines, the resources available to accomplish shared goals, the standards of accountability, and the anticipated consequences (Covey, 1989/1990).

MODELING THE WAY

Leaders set examples and plan small wins (Kouzes & Posner, 1987). They create a set of beliefs, a culture within which a group operates. The culture, the behaviors acceptable to and expected by the group, must be consistent with the leader's vision. A leader who espouses delegation, group planning, and consensus decision making must support these views with his or her actions.

Schein (1985) suggests that there are several approaches to "embedding culture" and reinforcing it. What the leader thinks and how he or she behaves establish a conceptual framework for others. Followers use several indicators to determine a person's real values, motivators, and beliefs:

1. What leaders pay attention to, measure, and control;

2. Leader reactions to critical incidents and organizational crises;

3. Deliberate role modeling, teaching, and coaching by leaders;

4. Criteria for allocation of rewards and status;

5. Criteria for recruitment, selection, promotion, retirement, and excommunication.

(pp. 224–25)

At the start of creating a vision, leaders must consistently act on their beliefs to form a structure and procedural guidelines in line with the vision. An organization's culture remains intact when leaders' behaviors are consistent with the organization's structure, systems, standard operating procedures, design of physical space, and formal statements about mission, philosophy, and goals (Schein, 1985).

Organizations that promote a culture of participative management need to build in structures to foster real participation. For example, quality circles can create productive teams within an organization. "Possibility teams identify strengths, imagine ways to make possibilities reality, and build on the power of combined resources in the organization" (Batten, 1989, p. 100). Leaders can make a vision reality by showing others a positive perspective, one that includes the contributions of different views.

ENCOURAGING THE HEART

Leaders recognize individual contributions and celebrate accomplishments (Kouzes & Posner, 1987). People will give their all for a competent leader. Without reward, however, that level of commitment will fade, so it becomes imperative to understand what each person on a team finds rewarding. Some people value quiet written notes of appreciation. Others relish group acknowledgment—a lunch with the team, flowers from the group, an afternoon of golf.

Motivating people to believe in the team, to want to be part of the group despite the challenges, and to strive for excellence has a twofold foundation. One part of it is honoring how each individual's work improves the program or refines the product. The other part is identifying how the coordinated efforts of the entire team move it toward achieving collective goals.

Sensitivity to what it takes for each person to play his or her part helps the leader identify the timing of rewards. Understanding when team commitment has resulted in sacrifices in other life responsibilities for each person is also important. Knowing each member as a person enables the leader to create ways to acknowledge the synergy of the team.

Leadership practices like those discussed in this chapter help people understand the characteristics of good leaders. There are many ideas about what makes an effective leader; table 9-1 presents those of three authors.

Despite the attempts to reduce leadership to a set of learnable attributes, "there are no pure types of leadership" (Cribben, 1981, p. 47). What often occurs, however, is that a leader selects a characteristic pattern of behavior. Some leaders are able to persuade others to behave as the manager intended, to do the job to the manager's satisfaction. They may come across as "bureaucrats, zealots, Machiavellis, missionaries, climbers, exploiters, temporizers, and glad-handers" (pp. 36–37). On the other hand, effective leadership enables people to address the manager's intentions while satisfying their own needs. Leaders may not always be popular and consistently successful, yet they may be effective. Effective leaders are "the entrepreneur, the corporateur, the developer, the craftsperson, the integrator, and the gamesman" (pp. 41–42). The challenge is to balance one's choice of styles and to select styles that work.

LEADERSHIP AND MANAGEMENT

Organizations need both leadership and management, and people need to have both leadership and management skills. How do these functions differ? Leadership has historically included the ability to manage imple-

Table 9-1
Characteristics of a Leader: Three Perspectives

Bennis (1989)	DePree (1989)	Nanus (1989)
Guiding vision—clear idea and strength to persist	Has consistent and dependable integrity	*Roles*
		Direction-setter
Passion—passion for promises of life, hope, love of and inspiration to others	Cherishes heterogeneity and diversity	Change agent
	Searches out competence	Spokesperson
	Is open to contrary opinion	Coach
	Communicates easily at all levels	*Skills*
Integrity—self-knowledge, candor, and maturity	Understands concept of equity and consistently advocates it	Farsightedness
		Mastery of interdependence
Trust—earning cooperation from co-workers	Leads through serving	Anticipatory learning
	Is vulnerable to skills and talents of others	High integrity
Curiosity and daring—risk-taking, learning from errors and adversity		Organization design
	Is intimate with organization and its work	Initiative
	Is able to see broad picture	Mastery of change to shape future
	Is spokesperson and diplomat	
	Can be tribal storyteller	
	Tells why rather than how	

Sources. *Based on information in* On Becoming a Leader *(pp. 39–41), by W. Bennis, 1989, Reading, MA: Addison-Wesley;* Leadership Is an Art *(pp. 131–32), by M. DePree, 1989, New York: Dell; and* The Leader's Edge: The Seven Keys to Leadership in a Turbulent World *(pp. 81–98), by B. Nanus, 1989, Chicago: Contemporary Books.*

mentation of a vision. In today's organizational world, however, the roles and the functions of leaders and managers have become more distinct.

"Managers push and direct. Leaders pull and expect" (Batten, 1989, p. 2). Leaders are the people who create guiding visions. "Leaders organize activities for change, reshape current practices to adapt to environmental change" (Grady, 1992, IX-1). The clear distinction between leadership and management is the "distinction between getting others to do and getting others to want to do" (Kouzes & Posner, 1987, p. 27).

Within the boundaries of the leader's vision, managers create a structure that enacts that vision. Managers plan activities especially designed to help the organization meet its goals. Managers organize people and activities, detailing how various parts of the organization will link with one another and identifying lines of authority and responsibility. Managers control an organization through product evaluation, employee evaluation, and fiscal accountability. Managers direct the flow of information, the timing of outcomes, and the interrelationships of productivity from the organization's units.

Table 9-2 presents distinguishing characteristics of leaders and managers. The leader appears to have the more desirable attributes, but the manager's qualities may also be just what is needed at a particular time. The important message is that both sets of skills are necessary to achieve goals. The person who is looking far into the future can have difficulty keeping an eye on the present. The person who does things right may also be doing the right thing. The leader needs a competent manager, and the manager needs an inspired and inspiring leader. Cultivating both sets of skills will enhance a person's flexibility, the range of his or her influence, and the timeliness of his or her targeted plans and strategies.

The entire system for producing services is the responsibility of top management. The larger the system needed to produce a product or a service, the greater the number of people who will be found in upper management positions; small companies have one top manager. Leaders may be found throughout an organization.

Leaders help the team define a shared goal. Managers plan how to implement the goal, then delegate responsibility for completing a task to others in the organization. They also delegate *authority* for making decisions or allocating resources to complete the task. Those in authority have power to ensure that the task is completed within the highest-quality standards. Both leaders and managers empower others to act.

Table 9-2
Distinguishing Characteristics of a Leader and a Manager

Leader	Manager
Innovates	Administers
Is an original	Is a copy
Develops	Maintains
Focuses on people	Focuses on systems and structure
Inspires trust	Relies on control
Has long-range perspective	Has short-range view
Asks what and why	Asks how and when
Has eye on horizon	Has eye on bottom line
Originates	Imitates
Challenges status quo	Accepts status quo
Is own person	Is classic good soldier
Does right thing	Does things right

Note. *From* On Becoming a Leader *(p. 45), by W. Bennis, 1989, Reading, MA: Addison-Wesley. Copyright ©1989 by Warren Bennis, Inc. Adapted by permission of Warren Bennis, Inc., Santa Monica, CA, and Addison-Wesley Publishing Company, Inc.*

POWER

A word about power is in order. Power is *not* a dirty word. Bothwell (1983) attributes the origin of the concept to a Greek word meaning "to be able to." Power is necessary to make things happen; it creates change and produces results. It can be a positive influence rather than a negative controlling force. Power is the ability to influence events strongly. Power is not control, but the ability to clarify expectations and develop intrinsic motivation (Batten, 1989).

Knowing how power works is a critical skill for both leaders and followers, managers and subordinates. Some key sources of power are these:

1. "Legitimate power": Persons in positions of authority in an organization (e.g., department managers) have legitimate power, "delegated to [them] by members of the organization" through design of and adherence to a formal organizational hierarchy.

2. "Reward power": Formal rewards may be "bonuses, . . . transfers, or high grades"; informal rewards may be notes of appreciation or spoken thank you's.

3. "Coercive power": Formal punishment, used by persons in authority, may include firing, demotion, or expulsion. Informal punishment, used by peers, subordinates, or superiors, may entail ostracism, being the subject of gossip, deprivation, threats, or criticism. "Research has shown that informal rewards are used less often than formal rewards, yet are more effective."

4. "Referent power": This source of power is given by followers who look up to a leader. It may or may not be linked to a position in an organization.

5. "Expertise": Doing something extremely well tends to result in being followed.

6. "Respect": When people have high regard for a person for what he or she has accomplished, they give that person power.

7. "Liking" as a way to empower oneself: Meeting the needs of others often creates followers.

8. "Charisma": Personal magnetism can draw followers to a leader. Charisma can be expanded by caring for others, communicating caring, succeeding in desired endeavors, and having strong convictions.

9. "Possession of knowledge": This source provides understanding and reasoning that can result in expertise.

10. Ability to "communicate one's knowledge": Through teaching, writing, public speaking, and selling, a person can attract a group of followers.

11. "Control and dissemination of information": This is a different form of power, to be distinguished from wisdom, expertise, or communication skills.

(Bothwell, 1983, pp. 153–61)

Both leaders and managers are most effective when they understand what power is and learn how to use it constructively. They can use power for self-gain, but using it respectfully for the good of the organization builds trust and collaboration among all members of the team. Power, in fact, is essential if the organization intends to accomplish its objectives.

DECISION MAKING

Just as leaders and managers must become comfortable with different types of power, so must they build their ability to make decisions—numerous, highly varied ones, daily. What is important is the ability to understand the ramifications of a decision, consider several alternatives, efficiently decide, and thoughtfully communicate the decision.

Decision making is a critical skill of both leaders and managers. Whether defining what the essential vision of an organization is or planning how to allocate funds for projects that help the organization meet its goals, people make decisions, both consciously and unconsciously. The stakes become higher as the decisions that need to be made affect more people, use more resources, or change the direction of the organization. Further, every team member influences decision making individually and as part of the team. How specific decisions are made can make or break, and shape, both the process and the product of a team.

Some decisions are the sole responsibility of the manager. The decision to hire or to fire an employee is one that an occupational therapy manager typically makes. Other decisions are the province of higher-level managers; the occupational therapy manager communicates these to his or her staff members. The manager must screen the decisions to be made and determine which ones will benefit from involvement of team members.

A decision is required when people must choose between different courses of action. The greater the degree of uncertainty in the outcome of a decision, the greater the potential for error and the greater the challege decision making becomes. Decision making is not difficult when the choice is obvious. Decisions involve risks; one outcome may be fun and exciting, another fun and dangerous.

Identifying the decisions that can be made is a necessary first step. The need to make some decisions is apparent: Whether to hold a meeting on Monday or Wednesday is clearly a decision that needs to be made if team members are to gather. The need to make other decisions may not be apparent. At these times the chance to make a decision may be lost, and the course of events may unwind in an unintended direction. By not taking these opportunities, the person has made a decision not to choose among alternatives, but to stay on the present path. For example, assuming that a group as a whole must address all group issues is a decision; not questioning whether to handle some group issues in task groups is an unconscious decision to involve all group members equally in all tasks. This may not be the best choice if the group has a number of concrete responsibilities, such as determining where to store adaptive equipment or how to celebrate Occupational Therapy Month. On the other hand, involving all group members is a great choice if the task is to develop a mission statement. The important point is to look under the surface to identify the decisions that can and should be made.

Once it is clear which decisions to make, individuals and groups use various strategies to choose among options. Probably the least effective approach is decision making by habit. Choosing an option because something has always been done that way is sure to minimize the potential for success and to lower team morale. Treating significant decisions as opportunities to ensure excellence, to achieve the mission of the organization effectively and efficiently, can boost team cooperation and heighten the intrinsic rewards of team involvement. People are more likely to endorse a decision that they have had a part in making.

Deciding how to choose among alternatives becomes part of the overall decision-making process. Noted theorists in decision making (Raiffa, 1968; von Winterfeldt & Edwards, 1986) suggest that decision makers follow specific steps:

1. List all the possible options—think broadly. This implies that problems and their causes are clear.

2. Identify the possible consequences of each option, both positive and negative. How might the outcome of the decision be used?

3. Evaluate each outcome. How desirable is it? Would one alternative be more risky than another?

4. Determine the likelihood of each outcome.

5. Select the best option.

Successfully carrying out these steps requires a wide range of skills and attributes—for example, tolerance of ambiguity, willingness to choose, creativity in considering alternatives, problem solving, willingness to compromise, flexibility, commitment to a decision, judgment, evaluative and analytical thinking, self-efficacy, and emotional control. Also essential is the ability to evaluate how individual values and life experiences may be influencing the decision. The leader's and the manager's role is to ensure objectivity throughout the decision-making process.

Decision-Making Techniques

A number of techniques can prove beneficial in the decision-making process, as follows. Learning and practicing them until they become familiar will help leaders and managers build a solid foundation for decision making.

1. *Problem analysis:* breaking a problem down into its parts and teasing out the kinds of influences at play.

2. *Brainstorming:* freely expressing and noting all the possibilities. This is helpful in identifying the causes of problems and in generating possible solutions.

3. *Flow charting:* pinpointing the parts of a decision to be made, clarifying the effects of the decision on other elements of the problem, and tracking the different consequences of possible choices, their likelihood, and their relative significance.

4. *Prioritizing:* determining which decision must be made first, which second, and so on.

5. *Generation of alternatives:* creating a number of different ways to solve a problem; searching for a broad range of possibilities, without forming judgments about them.

6. *Determination of advantages and disadvantages:* assessing the pros and the cons of each alternative.

7. *Force-field analysis:* examining the effects of external and internal influences on attainment of the goal or solution of the problem; considering what might help (driving forces) and what might hinder (restraining forces) achievement of the desired outcomes (Lewin, 1951).

8. *Rank ordering and sorting by category:* grouping like ideas into categories and prioritizing within and between categories; comparing and contrasting the significance of influences on the decision, or aspects of the decision.

9. *SWOT analysis:* evaluating the characteristics of the decision environment; identifying the <u>s</u>trengths, the <u>w</u>eaknesses, the <u>o</u>pportunities, and the <u>t</u>hreats associated with each alternative.

10. *Role clarification:* carefully defining and setting boundaries for the decision maker; determining who is responsible for a decision on which aspects of the problem.

11. *Values clarification:* understanding which values will be supported and which undermined by each alternative. Values that might be affected include autonomy, utilitarianism, and beneficence, for example.

The skilled decision maker thoughtfully applies these levels of analysis to the problem to be solved or the decision to be made. Some decisions are weighty and require time to process and analyze; others have less far-reaching effects. Careful reflection on the type of decision and its significance to the mission of the organization guides the decision maker in when and how to use these techniques.

Causes of Faulty Decision Making

Effective decisions position an organization to achieve its goals efficiently and strategically. They are based on an ability to predict what will happen when a decision is made. A keen competence to form realistic judgments is crucial. Decision makers face a number of pitfalls, however.

Bandura (1986) suggests that decision makers may misperceive the threat that a problem represents. Those who worry excessively or distrust other people may make poor decisions. They may base a decision about the present on a bad experience in the past, or having been unsuccessful in a prior decision, they may doubt their ability to cope with a present dilemma.

An additional deterrent to sound decision making is misjudgment about the decision and its effect (Bandura, 1986). The decision maker may fail to gain a broad perspective and thus overlook information that might have an effect on the decision and its outcome. He or she may minimize significant factors. Further, the decision maker may process information poorly, not evaluate and analyze it fully, or not link it appropriately to features of the problem.

Following are some trigger questions to help decision makers identify possible misjudgments:

1. How accurate was the group's assessment of the situation?

2. Did the group define the problem too narrowly or too broadly?

3. Were the goals and the objectives targeted at accomplishing the mission?

4. How well did the group evaluate the alternatives?

5. Did the group thoroughly research the decision? Was its information base complete?

6. Was the group's analysis logical and clearly reasoned?

7. What biases and judgments did each person involved in the decision bring to the table? How might these have influenced his or her position?

8. Did the group allow sufficient time to analyze the possibilities and make sound judgments?

Some decisions are best made alone; others are more sound when made by groups. Concerns about a decision are indications that it is time to seek the opinion of others. Leaders and managers are continually building their decision-making skills by evaluating each decision before and after it is made. Using power and making decisions come into play in many situations and result in how the leader and the manager behave.

Leaders and managers play different yet interdependent roles in an organization. Because these roles are complementary, knowing how to behave and understanding the behavior of others are assets in developing a team quickly. The next section describes behaviors of managers that contribute to implementing the goals of an organization.

BEHAVIORS OF MANAGERS

There are four major functions of management essential to producing results: planning, organizing, controlling, and directing. These functions are as applicable to homemaking as they are to the federal government, and they are useful in managing both personal and career goals.

PLANNING

Managers engage their organization in strategic planning on the basis of a forecast of environmental trends, the mission of the organization, and an audit of the internal resources of the organization. Long-term objectives and strategies set the boundaries for the work of the organization and provide direction for day-to-day activities. Short-term objectives and strategies distinguish the yearly and monthly tasks that each team member undertakes to achieve the mission envisioned by the organization's leadership. Planning leads to active engagement in support of a group's goals; it is the basis of teamwork.

ORGANIZING

To clarify workers' roles and to facilitate efficiency, an organization needs a formal structure that links groups of people. The manager forms a structure to carry out long- and short-term strategies articulated in the plan.

He or she may create departments or committees. Whatever the hierarchical relationships and the span of control, the manager assigns responsibility and authority for specific duties through the structure.

Within the set of formal relationships defined by the pattern of work, informal relationships develop and flourish. Ideally these personal relationships foster the growth not only of individuals but of the organization as a whole.

CONTROLLING

Evaluating progress toward goals enables the manager to shape organizational activities within budgetary guidelines and with an eye to goal attainment. Controlling involves establishing standards, translating them into performance criteria, and correcting deviations between actual performance and goals. All this is best achieved through a reliable and frequent feedback loop among workers and managers.

DIRECTING

People are what make goals a reality. The manager, like the director of a play or the conductor of an orchestra, guides people to perform their assigned duties and evaluates their effectiveness. The manager communicates with team members, motivating them at the individual level. Unless a sense of personal satisfaction develops among team members, people are likely to look elsewhere for ways to meet their needs.

The function of directing people in an organization requires a manager to take on many of the attributes of a leader. By influencing how others perform work duties, a manager creates a vision with each employee, enables others to act, models the way, and encourages the heart. The next section explores the function of directing in supervision and mentoring.

SUPERVISION AND MENTORING

Like power, supervision has acquired negative connotations. Some people take the view that the supervisor tells them what to do. Indeed, that is the responsibility of the supervisor. To do his or her job, the supervisor takes on the directing function of management. The supervisor assigns work, consults on or defines implementation strategies, and evaluates the outcomes. Supervisors have been entrusted to help the organization realize its mission by guiding individual behaviors, evaluating performance, and shaping it to meet established standards.

Supervisors are responsible to the organization employing them. Occupational therapy practitioners, however, are also responsible to the public for maintaining standards of practice. Through AOTA's

Representative Assembly the profession has formulated policies to guide how occupational therapists and occupational therapy assistants perform their duties. The documents that define the profession take the form of policy statements, white papers, standards, and resolutions at the national level, and practice acts, such as licensure laws and certification regulations, at the state level. Each year the profession's policies appear in the archival issue of the *American Journal of Occupational Therapy*. State laws and regulations may be obtained through each state's professional association.

Supervision is so important to occupational therapy's ability to provide high-quality care that policymakers in the profession have accorded it much attention. The most recent revision of AOTA's (1995) "Guide for Supervision of Occupational Therapy Personnel" appears as appendix 9-A. That document defines *supervision* as "a process in which two or more people participate in a joint effort to promote, establish, maintain, and/or elevate a level of performance and service." Further, it is "a mutual undertaking between the supervisor and the supervisee that fosters growth and development; assures appropriate utilization of training and potential; encourages creativity and innovation; and provides guidance, support, encouragement, and respect while working toward a goal" (p. 1027). The guide summarizes supervisory relationships among occupational therapy personnel. Managers and practitioners should use it in conjunction with "Occupational Therapy Roles" (AOTA, 1993). The latter document details the kinds of job responsibilities that occupational therapy practitioners are educated to carry out independently, with direct supervision, or with indirect supervision. It also describes what a practitioner can expect from supervision, what kinds of limits a supervisor might set on evaluation and intervention approaches undertaken by the supervisee, and what lines of authority and responsibility the profession expects of occupational therapy practitioners.

Occupational therapy managers are accountable to professional practice standards and guidelines at the same time that they are responsible to their employer. Conflicts may arise when organizational structure and the patterns of direction desired by an organization are inconsistent with professional standards of practice. Certified practitioners are entrusted with upholding quality standards defined by members of the profession. Great differences between organizational parameters and professional standards can lead therapists and assistants into soul-searching analyses of career goals and job settings, and even to job changes.

Within the definition of practice set by the profession, state legislatures, and an organization's management, there is room for individuals to contribute to how they do their work. A supervisor may tell a practitioner what to do and evaluate how well he or she has done it, but the practitioner can share in determining the best approaches to accomplishing work tasks.

Working with a supervisor as a team member enhances a supervisee's opportunity to provide services that meet or exceed the expectations of the organization. Therefore, forming a strong collaborative relationship with a supervisor is a choice that a practitioner makes for positive professional development. Collaboration with a supervisor requires an attitude of give-and-take. The supervisor becomes a person to learn from, to learn with, and to teach. To collaborate truly, the collaborators must trust in the probability that they can generate a better service or product by combining their best thinking. Respect for the strengths and the skills of each person on the team, and anticipation that projects and the people working on them will develop, is essential.

Both supervisees and supervisors grow and develop; they learn as adults (Frum & Opacich, 1987). The quality of relationships that people build forms the foundation for growth. Many people seek relationships with people outside their immediate work setting. They extend the circle of influence around them by linking with others capable of inspiring and guiding them. Successful relationships may result from networking, from sponsorship, or from mentoring.

Mentoring is the development of personal and professional skills in a less experienced person, a protégé (Robertson, 1992). Both the mentor and the protégé engage in an intimate exploration of the personal characteristics and the professional skills most desirable along the career continuum. "The mentor and protégé address questions, debate issues, and refine perspectives on problems and solutions for the purpose of building communication, decision-making, problem-solving, management, and evaluation skills" (p. 1). The bonds that a mentor and a protégé form are based on interpersonal chemistry, not on a matching of names on lists.

Mentor-protégé relationships require that the two parties have time together and a commitment to a common purpose. It helps for the protégé to have an idea of the professional goals to which he or she aspires and the personal characteristics that he or she wants to develop in order to achieve those goals. If a person is willing to learn, trusting in interpersonal growth (that is, trusting in the growth of each person in the relationship so that trust in the relationship and its development grows), able to see the link between personal and professional development, and able to communicate thoughtfully, he or she may wish to seek a mentor.

For the mentor, maturity, refinement of career skills, and the desire to nurture others contribute to successful relationships. Like a leader, the mentor provides a vision, integrity, and belief in the capabilities of others.

The managerial skills of planning, clear problem solving, and understanding of organizational structures and the political nuances of organizations contribute to a responsive relationship.

Practitioners need both supervision and mentoring to shape their professional selves. As defined earlier, supervision is the assigned responsibility of ensuring that the supervisee produces delegated tasks consistent with the mission of the organization. There is a hierarchical relationship in supervision: One person oversees the work of another. Within this structure there are plenty of opportunities to motivate, guide, teach, and nurture professional growth. Mentoring more typically rests within the informal organization or in the professional life of the protégé outside work. Having the ability to take advantage of the growth opportunities in supervision and mentoring can be one of a practitioner's greatest assets. Although there are many ways to enhance relationships, mentoring is one approach that the practitioner may find useful.

CONCLUSION

This chapter has discussed the dynamic interrelationship between teamwork and leadership with a focus on how to implement team and leader behaviors successfully. Every occupational therapy practitioner can benefit from including team membership and leadership among his or her career goals. Without large numbers of people positioned to influence the design of health care, occupational therapy will lessen in influence as a responder to public need and as a creator of innovative solutions to the complex problems facing a system on the cusp of reduced resources. The system around the profession is rapidly changing.

Change is a way of life. Team membership and leadership are about change. Being a strong team member and a visionary leader fosters creative and proactive change strategies (Belasco, 1990). Leaders strive to alter how people see their environments. Managers design plans and implement strategies that modify what the organization produces, how it accomplishes its goals, and how people contribute to the achievement of its mission. Individual practitioners must change their expectations, abilities, and roles in order to create services and products responsive to the health needs of the future.

SUMMARY

A *team* is a group of equally important people collaborating, developing cooperative goals, and building trusting relationships to achieve those goals (Kouzes & Posner, 1987). The settings in which occupational therapy practitioners work and the roles that they take on in practice, education, and research involve them in many teams. *Leadership* is an observable, learnable set of practices that "enable others to act" (Kouzes & Posner, 1987, p. xvii). Leadership encompasses many facilitative behaviors that ensure team productivity.

Successful and rewarding teamwork requires an understanding of the various types of teams and the roles that members of these teams must assume. In addition, successful teamwork requires flexibility among team members. In *multidisciplinary teams*, a member's primary allegiance is to his or her discipline. *Interdisciplinary teams* are goal directed, not bound by discipline-specific roles and functions, and better able to assign the talents of individuals to achieve the group's goals. In *transdisciplinary teams*, members may support and enhance programs and activities of other disciplines in an effort to provide the most cost-effective, timely, efficient service (American Congress of Rehabilitation Medicine, 1992). Health care trends point to greater use of interdisciplinary and transdisciplinary teams.

Recent literature draws connections between teamwork and leadership. All members of a team must take on leadership roles and behaviors, and leaders must be part of the team.

Being an effective team member requires a combination of attitudes and skills. These can be broadly categorized as interpersonal characteristics (e.g., trustful and caring, constructive, and empathic), intellectual or cognitive characteristics (e.g., outcome oriented, organized, and flexible), and personality characteristics (e.g., competent, self-aware, and equality minded).

Blake, Mouton, and Allen (1981/1987) describe five patterns possible in teams: "One alone," "One to one," "One to some," "One to all," and "All to one." Teams go through identifiable stages: (1) getting started, (2) truly beginning, (3) designing the plan, and (4) doing.

Kouzes and Posner (1987) describe five leadership practices: (1) challenging the process (searching for opportunities and then experimenting); (2) inspiring a shared vision (envisioning the future and enlisting others); (3) enabling others to act (fostering collaboration and strengthening others); (4) modeling the way (setting examples and planning small wins); and (5) encouraging the heart (recognizing individual contributions and celebrating accomplishments).

Organizations need both leadership and management. Within the boundaries of the leader's vision, managers create a structure to enact that vision.

Knowing how power works is a critical skill for both leaders and followers, managers and subordinates. Some key sources of power are (1) "legitimate power," (2) "reward power," (3) "coercive power," (4) "referent power," (5) "expertise," (6) "respect," (7) "liking," (8) "charisma," (9) "possession of knowledge," (10) ability to "communicate one's knowledge," and (11) "control and dissemination of information" (Bothwell, 1983, pp. 153–61).

Decision making is a critical skill of both leaders and managers. A decision is required when people must choose between different courses of action. Noted theorists in decision making (Raiffa, 1968; von Winterfeldt & Edwards, 1986) suggest that decision makers follow specific steps: (1) list all the possible options; (2) identify the possible consequences of each option; (3) evaluate each outcome; (4) determine the likelihood of each outcome; and (5) select the best option. Successfully carrying out these options requires a wide range of skills and attributes. A number of techniques can prove beneficial in the decision-making process: (1) problem analysis; (2) brainstorming; (3) flow charting; (4) prioritizing; (5) generation of alternatives; (6) determination of advantages and disadvantages; (7) force-field analysis; (8) rank ordering and sorting by category; (9) analysis of strengths, weaknesses, opportunities, and threats; (10) role clarification; and (11) values clarification.

Decision makers face a number of potential pitfalls. For example, they may misperceive the threat that a problem represents.

There are four major functions of management essential to producing results: planning, organizing, controlling, and directing.

AOTA's "Guide for Supervision of Occupational Therapy Personnel" defines *supervision* as "a process in which two or more people participate in a joint effort to promote, establish, maintain, and/or elevate a level of performance and service." The guide summarizes supervisory relationships among occupational therapy personnel. Managers and practitioners should use it in conjunction with "Occupational Therapy Roles" (AOTA, Occupational Therapy Roles Task Force, 1993).

Mentoring is the development of personal and professional skills in a less experienced person, a protégé (Robertson, 1992). Mentor-protégé relationships require that the two parties have time together and a commitment to a common purpose. For the mentor, maturity, refinement of career skills, and the desire to nurture others contribute to successful relationships.

Practitioners need both supervision and mentoring to shape their professional selves. Having the ability to take advantage of the growth opportunities in supervision and mentoring can be one of a practitioner's greatest assets.

REFERENCES

Abelson, R. P., & Levi, A. (1985). Decision making and decision theory. In G. Lindzey & E. Aronson (Eds.), *The Handbook of Social Psychology (3rd ed.)*, vol. 4 (pp. 231–309). New York: Random House.

American Congress of Rehabilitation Medicine. (1992). *Guide to interdisciplinary practice in rehabilitation settings.* Skokie, IL: Author.

American Occupational Therapy Association. (1995). Guide for supervision of occupational therapy personnel. *American Journal of Occupational Therapy, 49,* 1027–28.

American Occupational Therapy Association, Occupational Therapy Roles Task Force. (1993). Occupational therapy roles. *American Journal of Occupational Therapy, 47,* 1087–99.

Bandura, A. (1986). *Social foundations of thought and action: A social cognitive theory.* Englewood Cliffs, NJ: Prentice-Hall.

Batten, J. D. (1989). *Tough-minded leadership.* New York: American Management Association.

Belasco, J. A. (1990). *Teaching the elephant to dance: The manager's guide to empowering change.* New York: Penguin.

Blake, R. R., Mouton, J. S., & Allen, R. L. (1987). *Spectacular teamwork: How to develop the leadership skills for team success.* New York: Wiley. (Originally published 1981)

Bothwell, L. (1983). *The art of leadership.* Englewood Cliffs, NJ: Prentice-Hall.

Cohen, W. A. (1990). *The art of the leader.* Englewood Cliffs, NJ: Prentice-Hall.

Covey, S. R. (1990). *The seven habits of highly effective people: Powerful lessons in personal change.* New York: Simon & Schuster. (Originally published 1989)

Cribben, J. J. (1981). *Leadership: Your competitive edge.* New York: AMACOM.

DePree, M. (1989). *Leadership is an art.* New York: Dell.

Feinberg, M. R., & Levenstein, A. (1985). The transforming leader. In D. Asman & A. Meyerson (Eds.), *"The Wall Street Journal" on management* (pp. 116–18). New York: New American Library.

Frum, D. C., & Opacich, K. J. (1987). *Supervision: Development of therapeutic competence.* Bethesda, MD: American Occupational Therapy Association.

Grady, A. P. (1992). Seeing, saying, doing. In TriAlliance of Health and Rehabilitation Professions, *Interdisciplinary team development* [Workshop handout IX, p. 1]. Rockville, MD: Author.

Jones, T. (1992). Stages of team development. In TriAlliance of Health and Rehabilitation Professions, *Interdisciplinary team development* [Workshop handout VI, pp. 13–17]. Rockville, MD: Author.

Kouzes, J. M., & Posner, B. Z. (1987). *The leadership challenge: How to get extraordinary things done in organizations.* San Francisco: Jossey-Bass.

Lewin, K. (1951). *Theory in social science.* New York: Harper.

Lundy, J. (1991). *Lead, follow, or get out of the way.* New York: Berkley. (Originally published 1986)

Manz, C. C., & Sims, H. P., Jr. (1989). *Superleadership: Leading others to lead themselves.* New York: Berkley.

Miller, D. (1992). Dimensions of teamwork (micro). In TriAlliance of Health and Rehabilitation Professions, *Interdisciplinary team development* [Workshop handout]. Rockville, MD: Author.

Payne, J. W. (1982). Contingent decision behavior. *Psychological Bulletin, 92,* 382–402.

Peters, T., & Austin, N. (1986). *A passion for excellence: The leadership difference.* New York: Warner. (Originally published 1985)

Raiffa, H. (1968). *Decision analysis: Introductory lectures on choices under uncertainty.* Reading, MA: Addison-Wesley.

Robertson, S. C. (1992). *Find a mentor or be one.* Rockville, MD: American Occupational Therapy Association.

Schein, E. H. (1985). *Organizational culture and leadership: A dynamic view.* San Francisco: Jossey-Bass.

Tichy, N. M., & Devanna, M. A. (1990). *The transformational leader.* New York: Wiley.

von Winterfeldt, D., & Edwards, W. (1986). *Decision analysis and behavioral research.* New York: Cambridge University Press.

Ziglar, Z. (1986). *Top performance: How to develop excellence in yourself and others.* New York: Berkley. (Originally published 1985)

ADDITIONAL RESOURCES

Ackoff, R. L. (1986). *Management in small doses.* New York: Wiley.

Ancona, D. G. (1990). Outward Bound: Strategies for team survival in an organization. *Academy of Management Journal, 33,* 334–65.

Anthony, R. (1988). *Dr. Robert Anthony's magic power of super persuasion.* New York: Berkley.

Bales, R. F. (1950). *Interaction process analysis: A method for the study of small social groups.* Cambridge, MA: Addison-Wesley.

Bennis, W. (1990). *Why leaders can't lead: The unconscious conspiracy continues.* San Francisco: Jossey-Bass.

Boyte, H. C. (1989). *Commonwealth: A return to citizen politics.* New York: Free Press.

Celente, G., & Milton, T. (1991). *Trend tracking.* New York: Warner.

Cohen, H. (1980). *You can negotiate anything.* New York: Bantam.

DeVille, J. (1984). *The psychology of leadership: Managing resources and relationships.* New York: Signet.

Doyle, R. J. (1992). *Gain management: A process for building teamwork.* New York: American Management Association.

Dutfield, M., & Eling, C. (1990). *The communicating manager: A guide to working effectively with people.* Longmead, England: Element Books, Ltd.

Dyer, W. G. (1987). *Team building: Issues and alternatives* (2nd ed.). Reading, MA: Addison-Wesley.

Gardner, J. W. (1990). *On leadership.* New York: Free Press.

Grady, A. P. (1990). Leadership is everybody's practice [Nationally Speaking]. *American Journal of Occupational Therapy, 44,* 1065–68.

Grady, A. P. (1991). Directions for the future: Opportunities for leadership [Nationally Speaking]. *American Journal of Occupational Therapy, 45,* 7–9.

Hackman, J. R. (1990). *Groups that work (and those that don't): Creating conditions for effective teamwork.* San Francisco: Jossey-Bass.

Heider, J. (1985). *The tao of leadership: Leadership strategies for a new age.* New York: Bantam.

Helgesen, S. (1990). *The female advantage: Women's ways of leadership.* New York: Doubleday.

Hersey, P., & Blanchard, K. H. (1982). *Management of organizational behavior: Utilizing human resources* (4th ed.). Englewood Cliffs, NJ: Prentice-Hall.

Huszozo, G. B. (1990, February). Training for team building. *Training and Development Journal,* 37–43.

Jessup, H. R. (1990, November). New roles in team leadership. *Training and Development Journal,* 79–83.

Kanter, R. M. (1983). *The change masters: Innovation and entrepreneurship in the American corporation.* New York: Simon & Schuster.

Loden, M., & Rosener, J. B. (1991). *Workforce America! Managing employee diversity as a vital resource.* Homewood, IL: Business One Irwin.

MacKenzie, R. A. (1990). *Teamwork through time management.* Chicago: Dartnell Group.

Martel, L. (1986). *Mastering change.* New York: Mentor.

O'Neil, E. H., Shugars, D. A., & Bader, J. D. (Eds.). (1993, November). *Health professions education for the future: Schools in service to the nation* (Report of Pew Health Professions Commission). San Francisco: Pew Health Professions Commission.

Parker, G. M. (1990). *Team players and teamwork: The new competitive business strategy.* San Francisco: Jossey-Bass.

Phillips, D. T. (1992). *Lincoln on leadership.* New York: Warner.

Phillips, N. (1995). *From vision to beyond teamwork: Ten ways to wake up and shake up your company.* Burr Ridge, IL: Irwin Professional Publishing.

Randolph, W. A., & Posner, B. Z. (1988, Summer). What every manager needs to know about project management. *Sloan Management Review,* 65–73.

Shashkin, M. (1994). *The new teamwork: Developing and using cross-function teams.* New York: AMA Membership Publications Division, American Management Association.

Von Wartburg, W. P. (1991). *How to lead with genius: Words of wisdom for the common sense manager.* New York: Markus Wiener.

Zander, A. F. (1994). *Making groups effective.* San Francisco: Jossey-Bass.

APPENDIX 9-A

Guide for Supervision of Occupational Therapy Personnel

The intent of this document is to clarify the supervisory relationships and responsibilities between registered occupational therapists, certified occupational therapy assistants, and other personnel involved in the provision of occupational therapy services. Supervision is a process in which two or more people participate in a joint effort to promote, establish, maintain, and/or elevate a level of performance and service. Supervision is a mutual undertaking between the supervisor and the supervisee that fosters growth and development; assures appropriate utilization of training and potential; encourages creativity and innovation; and provides guidance, support, encouragement, and respect while working toward a goal. As described here, supervision helps promote quality occupational therapy and fosters professional development of the individuals involved.

The American Occupational Therapy Association (AOTA) holds and maintains the principle that those persons not trained and qualified as occupational therapy practitioners (occupational therapy practitioners refers to both registered occupational therapists and certified occupational therapy assistants) are not acceptable to supervise occupational therapy practice. It is recognized that occupational therapy practitioners may be administratively supervised by others, such as principals, facility administrators, or physicians. During the supervision of occupational therapy practice, it is the supervisor who is responsible for setting, encouraging, and evaluating the standard of work performed by the supervisee. The amount of supervision required varies, depending upon the occupational therapy practitioner's clinical experience, responsibilities, and level of expertise. Supervision occurs along a continuum that includes close, routine, general, and minimal.

- *Close supervision* requires daily, direct contact at the site of work.

- *Routine supervision* requires direct contact at least every 2 weeks at the site of work, with interim supervision occurring by other methods, such as telephonic or written communication.

- *General supervision* requires at least monthly direct contact, with supervision available as needed by other methods.

- *Minimal supervision* is provided only on a need basis, and may be less than monthly. (AOTA, 1993a, p. 1088)

The amount, degree, and pattern of supervision a practitioner requires varies depending on the employment setting, method of service provision, the practitioner's competence, and the demands of service (i.e., facility standards, state laws and regulations, diagnoses served, techniques used). The method of supervision is determined by the supervising registered occupational therapist. The method should be the one most suitable to the situation. Methods of supervision should be determined before the individual enters into a supervisor–supervisee relationship and should be reevaluated regularly for effectiveness. In all cases, it is the occupational therapy practitioner's ethical responsibility to ensure that the amount, degree, and pattern of supervision are consistent with the level of role performance. As changes in the practice situation occur, the intensity of required supervision may also change to reflect new demands.

The registered occupational therapist has the ultimate responsibility for service provision. By virtue of their education and training, registered occupational therapists are able to provide services independently. Nevertheless, AOTA recommends that entry-level registered occupational therapists receive close supervision and that intermediate-level registered occupational therapists receive routine or general supervision. Certified occupational therapy assistants at all levels require at least general supervision by a registered occupational therapist. The level of supervision is related to the ability of the certified occupational therapy assistant to safely and effectively provide those interventions delegated by a registered occupational therapist. Typically, entry-level certified occupational therapy assistants and certified occupational therapy assistants new to a particular practice environment will require close supervision, intermediate level practitioners routine supervision, and advanced-level practitioners general supervision. When occupational therapy aides are delegated selected, routine tasks in specific situations, they must work under the close supervision of an occupational therapy practitioner.

These supervision guidelines are to assist occupational therapy practitioners in the provision of occupational therapy services (see Appendix).

The guidelines themselves cannot be interpreted to constitute a standard of supervision in any particular locality; rather, they indicate ideal patterns and types of supervision. All practitioners are expected to meet state and federal regulatory mandates, adhere to relevant Association policies regarding supervision standards, and participate in continuing professional developments.

Occupational Therapy Personnel	Supervision	Supervises:
Entry-level OTR*	Not required. Close supervision by an intermediate-level or an advanced-level OTR recommended.	Occupational therapy aides, technicians, care extenders, all levels of COTAs, volunteers, Level I fieldwork students.
Intermediate-level OTR*	Not required. Routine or general supervision by an advanced-level OTR recommended.	Occupational therapy aides, technicians, care extenders, all levels of COTAs, volunteers, Level I and Level II fieldwork students, entry-level OTRs.
Advanced-level OTR*	Not required. Minimal supervision by an advanced-level OTR is recommended.	Occupational therapy aides, technicians, care extenders, all levels of COTAs, volunteers, Level I and II fieldwork students, entry-level and intermediate-level OTRs.
Entry-level COTA*	Close supervision by all levels of OTRs, or an intermediate or an advanced-level COTA, who is under the supervision of an OTR.	Occupational therapy aides, technicians, care extenders, volunteers.
Intermediate-level COTA*	Routine or general supervision by all levels of OTRs, or an advanced-level COTA, who is under the supervision of an OTR.	Occupational therapy aides, technicians, care extenders, entry-level COTAs, volunteers, Level I occupational therapy (OT) fieldwork students, Level I and II occupational therapy assistant (OTA) fieldwork students.
Advanced-level COTA*, **	General supervision by all levels of OTRs, or an advanced-level COTA, who is under the supervision of an OTR.	Occupational therapy aides, technicians, care extenders, entry-level and intermediate-level COTAs, volunteers, Level I and OT fieldwork students, Level I and II OTA fieldwork students.
Personnel other than occupational therapy practitioners assisting in occupational therapy intervention***	Close supervision by all levels of occupational therapy practitioners.	No supervisory capacity.

*Refer to the Occupational Therapy Roles document for descriptions of entry-level, intermediate-level, and advanced-level OTRs and COTAs (AOTA, 1993a).

**Although specific state regulations may dictate the parameters of certified occupational therapy assistant practice, the American Occupational Therapy Association supports the autonomous practice of the advanced certified occupational therapy assistant practitioner in the independent living setting (AOTA, 1993b, p. 1079).

***Students are not addressed in this category. The student role as a supervisor is addressed in the Essentials and Guidelines of an Accredited Educational Program for the Occupational Therapist and Essentials and Guidelines of an Accredited Program for the Occupational Therapy Assistant (AOTA, 1991a, 1991b).

REFERENCES

American Occupational Therapy Association (1991a). Essentials and guidelines of an accredited educational program for the occupational therapist. *American Journal of Occupational Therapy, 45,* 1077–84.

American Occupational Therapy Association (1991b). Essentials and guidelines of an accredited educational program for the occupational therapy assistant. *American Journal of Occupational Therapy, 45,* 1085–92.

American Occupational Therapy Association (1993a). Occupational therapy roles. *American Journal of Occupational Therapy, 47,* 1087–99.

American Occupational Therapy Association (1993b). Statement: The role of occupational therapy in the independent living movement. *American Journal of Occupational Therapy, 47,* 1079–80.

Prepared by
Commission on Practice
Jim Hinojosa, PhD, OTR, FAOTA, Chairperson

Approved by the Representative Assembly March 1981, edited July 1988
Revised in 1994 and adopted by the Representative Assembly July 1994
Copyright © by the American Occupational Therapy Association, Inc., and published in the *American Journal of Occupational Therapy, 49,* 1027–28.

This replaces the 1981 document, "Guide for Supervision of Occupational Therapy Personnel" (*American Journal of Occupational Therapy, 35,* 815–16), which was rescinded by the 1994 Representative Assembly.
This document appeared previously in the *American Journal of Occupational Therapy, 48,* 1045–46.

SECTION 5

Controlling

Section 5 takes up the managerial role of controlling, which is defined in this text as influencing the accomplishment of goals through formalized means such as organizational charts, policies and procedures, and job descriptions. Chapter 10 offers a theoretical model of personnel management that places this function at the interface between the organization's resources, values, and goals, and the individual's values, goals, and skills. The chapter takes the reader step by step through all aspects of personnel management, from projecting staffing needs to terminating employees. Appended materials include sample job descriptions, sample appraisal forms, a brochure on recruitment agencies, a summary of major legislation affecting employment, and a feedback form for use in selection of new employees.

"Roles, Relationships, and Career Development," chapter 11, addresses controlling in terms of roles and relationships, stressing their function in specifying sets of responsibilities and connecting the persons performing those sets of responsibilities to one another. The chapter gives particular attention to the different roles that occupational therapy personnel may play—practitioner, educator, supervisor, administrator, consultant, researcher, and so forth—both simultaneously, as their own interests and their organizations' needs dictate, and longitudinally, as their careers develop. The chapter also addresses policies and procedures as ways of controlling what happens in an occupational therapy organization.

CHAPTER 10

Personnel Management

Barbara A. Boyt Schell, PhD, OTR, FAOTA
John W. Schell, PhD

KEY TERMS

Expectancy theory. A theory useful in explaining motivation in the workplace, namely that employees seek to maximize their satisfaction by paying attention to the aspects of work that they feel are important, constantly evaluating how those aspects are likely to affect them.

Full-time equivalent (FTE). The amount of work time of one full-time staff person in a year.

Job description. A statement of a job's purpose or a summary of the job, a list of the job's duties, an explanation of supervisory relationships, and a statement of the specifications for the job.

Performance standard. A detailed delineation of job performance expectations that are based on duties identified in a job description.

Productive days. The average number of days per year a person is actually on the job as opposed to the number of days for which the person is paid.

Productivity standard. The quantity of work that a given employee (or an FTE) can be expected to produce.

Relative value unit (RVU). An index of the level of staff expertise, sophisticated equipment, and specialized facilities required to provide service; used to quantify productivity.

Staffing plan. A manager's statement of how many and what kinds of personnel are needed for an identified work unit.

Treatment unit (TU). A given amount of treatment of patients or clients, frequently based on practitioners' time.

Visit. An occasion of service, regardless of the length of time spent.

Barbara A. Boyt Schell, PhD, OTR, FAOTA, is an associate professor and the chair of the Department of Occupational Therapy at Brenau University. She has extensive management experience in both the private and the public sector, along with over 15 years of consultation experience. She has taught management at several universities and has published articles and chapters on the subject. Her doctoral work, done at the University of Georgia, focused on staff development and professional development.

John W. Schell, PhD, is an associate professor at the University of Georgia. He has 5 years of experience teaching management courses, 15 years of experience as an administrator of educational programs, and 5 years of experience as a state supervisor for the Missouri Department of Elementary and Secondary Education. He earned his doctorate at the University of Missouri.

Management in occupational therapy involves overseeing a complex array of services provided by a range of practitioners and support personnel. This chapter highlights concepts important to efficient and effective management of these personnel resources. The initial section presents a theoretical model of personnel management that summarizes the ways in which managers integrate individual efforts into organizational performance. The balance of the chapter discusses personnel practices and techniques relevant to occupational therapy management. The emphasis is on practical strategies synthesized from the literature and the shared experiences of numerous occupational therapy managers. Included are approaches to identifying and justifying staffing needs; managing productivity; anticipating employees' expectancies; developing job descriptions; recruiting, selecting, and orienting staff; evaluating employees' performance; dealing with difficult personnel management situations; rewarding successful employees; and supporting staff development.

A THEORETICAL MODEL OF PERSONNEL MANAGEMENT

A manager serves as the interface between the individuals forming a work unit and the larger organization. The manager must design work roles, recruit individuals to perform the roles, and provide support for these individuals to improve their performance. To do this effectively, a manager must understand organizational resources, values, and goals. This knowledge provides a context for staffing, by focusing attention on the identification of individuals with skills, values, and goals consistent with the organization. Figure 10-1 illustrates this pivotal function of personnel management. It also reflects the role of personnel management in performance. Individual performance is assessed against the desired performance of the work unit and the larger organization. Performance is enhanced through staff development activities. Individual efforts are channeled into effective work groups.

In recent years the turbulence in health care has also required managers to tune in to the strategic planning process of their organization (Hernandez, Fottler, & Joiner, 1994; see chapter 2 of this book, "Strategic Planning"). Awareness of where their programs and services fit within the larger strategic plan is critical. It is important to recognize the implications of strategic planning for human resource management. For instance, to begin a new program, a manager may direct staffing efforts at the identification of highly entrepreneurial individuals who have the levels of skill needed to market the service. Alternatively, in a well-developed, well-recognized program, there may be room to recruit less experienced

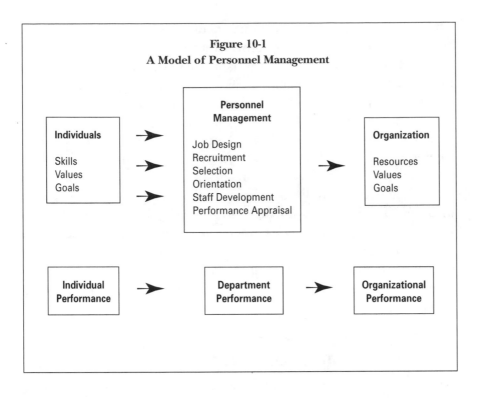

Figure 10-1
A Model of Personnel Management

personnel, assuming that a systematic plan is implemented to help them achieve desired levels of performance. Managers who are in tune with the directions of their organization and the expectations of employees are in the best position to facilitate a good fit between the staff and the goals of the organization.

QUANTIFICATION OF STAFFING NEEDS

One component of personnel management is the ability to quantify and project staffing needs accurately in order to support effective communication of productivity and budgetary information. This requires expressing human resources in quantifiable terms.

UNDERSTANDING FULL-TIME EQUIVALENTS

The concept of a full-time equivalent (FTE) is frequently used as a way to quantify personnel. An *FTE* is the amount of work time of one full-time staff person. Full-time employment in the United States usually represents an 8-hour day, a 5-day week, and a 52-week year—thus 2,080 paid hours per year, or 260 paid days. This measure is helpful for representing the amount of staffing (both full-time and part-time) in an organization.

For example, an occupational therapy department in a large regional medical center employs 12 persons: 1 full-time manager; 3 full-time therapists and 1 full-time assistant assigned to the rehabilitation unit;

1 full-time therapist for inpatient acute care; 1 full-time therapist and 1 half-time activity aide in psychiatry; and 3 half-time therapists and 1 half-time assistant for outpatient services, which include a work-hardening program and a neurorehabilitation program. The manager could express this staffing in several ways. Two are illustrated in figure 10-2. Although there are 12 persons in the department, there are only 9.5 FTEs. This is because the 5 half-time employees each represent only 0.5 FTE.

Figure 10-2
Examples of Ways to Describe Staffing in a 12-Person
Occupational Therapy Department

Staffing by Type of Personnel		Staffing by Program Allocation	
1.0 FTE	Manager	1.0 FTE	Management
6.5 FTE	Occupational therapists	4.0 FTE	Rehabilitation Program
1.5 FTE	Occupational therapy assistants	1.0 FTE	Acute Care Program
		1.5 FTE	Psychiatry Program
0.5 FTE	Activity aide	1.0 FTE	Work-Hardening Outpatient Program
9.5 FTE	Total	1.0 FTE	Neurorehabilitation Outpatient Program
		9.5 FTE	Total

DEVELOPING PRODUCTIVITY STANDARDS

A *productivity standard* is the quantity of work that a given employee (or an FTE) can be expected to produce. Inherent in the concept of productivity is the expectation that work will be of acceptable quality. A later section of this chapter, and the next chapter, address quality management in some depth. This section attends to the development and the use of measures that assess the volume of productivity.

Productivity standards vary according to setting and population served. To develop a productivity standard, a manager must determine units of productivity. There are two major approaches to this process. One is based on the amount of clinician time spent. The other is an attempt to quantify additional factors, such as staff expertise and specialized equipment, into an index known as a *relative value unit* (RVU). The examples in this chapter use the first (and simpler) approach. However, to acquaint the reader with more complex systems, the next paragraph describes the use of RVUs.

In 1979, AOTA developed a *product output reporting system* for quantifying aspects of occupational therapy services. Designed for use with computer-based billing, this system combined a standardized set of descriptors with a weighting scheme for measuring productivity. The uniform terminology that was part of this document has since been revised several times (AOTA, 1989, 1994b), although the relative value system has not. Some organizations have continued to use the original framework (see, e.g., McCarthy & Lieberman, 1992). When the product output reporting system is used as a productivity system, data are collected reflecting the number of RVUs generated by each employee or FTE. RVUs are indices of the level of staff expertise, sophisticated equipment, and specialized facilities required to provide service. These are reflected in terms of a 15-minute session. For example, an intervention at bedside to retrain a patient in self-care would be assigned a relatively low value because an inexperienced occupational therapist or occupational therapy assistant could do it without a specially equipped clinic. In contrast, an evaluation of a child's sensory integration would be assigned a relatively high value for the same amount of time spent, because only a specially trained occupational therapist could do it, using special equipment. Built into the relative values is an accounting for whether treatment is delivered in a one-to-one ratio or in groups. Thus a manager can compare staff members with differing responsibilities using the same productivity standard. Each staff member would be expected to generate a predetermined average number of RVUs in a given time frame. Readers interested in a more detailed explanation of this approach may consult the original description of the system (AOTA, 1979).

Simpler measures of productivity are treatment units and visits. *Treatment units* (TUs) represent a given amount of treatment of patients or clients and are frequently based on practitioners' time, such as 15 minutes of treatment. For instance, a practitioner who spent six hours in treatment in one day would record 24 TUs (1 hour = 4 TUs; 6 hours x 4 TUs/hour = 24 TUs). *Visits* represent occasions of service, regardless of the length of time spent. If the same practitioner saw three patients for two hours each, she would record three visits. If she saw six patients in the same amount of time, she would record six visits. TUs and visits are less sensitive than RVUs because they do not account for the skill and the experience level of the practitioners. Also, their definitions may vary from setting to setting, so it is important for managers to clarify them in the local context. Whatever unit of measure an organization uses, it should be meaningful to both staff and administration. Measures of staff members' use of time are the basis for determining the need for more staff members, for different staff composition, or for fewer staff members.

Once the methods for quantifying work have been identified, productivity standards can be developed. These standards may reflect several parameters of productivity, including the number of patients or clients, the number of RVUs, the number of treatment units, or the number of visits per day. They should reflect, indirectly, what is believed to be necessary to produce quality care. Consequently, before setting expectations for volume of care, managers must be sufficiently informed about what is needed for quality service to the populations being served. Literature reviews, consultation with expert clinicians, and case reviews of patients who have been successfully treated can all assist the manager in addressing these issues (Schell, 1992).

In using productivity standards, managers must understand that they are based on averages. In reality, on days when everything is running smoothly (or when short staffing requires treating more than one patient at a time), staff members will be able to exceed the productivity standards. On other days, perhaps because of scheduling conflicts or ill patients, they will fall below the standards. Further, many programs experience seasonal fluctuations in the number of patients or clients seen. A staff member's productivity is closely tied to availability of service recipients. All these factors suggest that productivity must be evaluated over a long period and in conjunction with other organizational factors.

DEVELOPING STAFFING PLANS

Once the manager has an idea about what the service needs of patients or clients are and what is practical for practitioners to achieve within a given setting, the manager can easily develop staffing plans. A *staffing plan* is the manager's statement about how many and what kind of personnel are needed for an identified work unit. Sometimes the term *staffing pattern* is used to reflect a more detailed plan that addresses the kinds of personnel hired (occupational therapists, occupational therapy assistants, and support personnel) and the way in which they are allocated across multiple work units, programs, or teams. A staffing plan should reflect the amount and the kind of staff necessary to provide acceptable care in the most cost-efficient way. To develop staffing plans, managers relate their expectations about productivity to the therapy needs of the population to be served. Often this requires clinical judgment. Also, to assess realistically the extent of services to be provided within a given setting, managers must be sensitive to organizational goals. Factors to consider include the ratio of staff to patients or clients and the amount of time needed for indirect care (such as billing, documentation, and transport). The consistency of demand may also affect productivity. The manager can use staff input, time studies, AOTA guidelines, and information gained from continuing education and peer professionals to assist him or her in determining staffing needs. The following example may help clarify how a manager can weave various factors together into a staffing plan.

A Scenario:
Planning a Rehabilitation Unit

A manager is responsible for determining occupational therapy staffing needs for a 10-bed inpatient rehabilitation unit that is being planned. The manager has a fairly good understanding of the diagnoses to be admitted. Based on information obtained from a variety of clinical sources, the manager estimates that each patient will require a minimum of 1 hour of individual treatment and 1 hour of group treatment daily. The maximum group size will be five patients. Top management wants this unit to be fully occupied throughout the year. In general, the staff members can expect to engage in direct treatment 6 of 8 hours daily, allowing 2 hours for indirect service. In this facility, patient-related activities, such as team conferences and family meetings, are considered part of the overhead and not billed for separately. The manager calculates the total number of hours per day that practitioners will spend in direct treatment (see figure 10-3). The analysis reveals that the unit needs 12 hours of practitioners' direct time daily.

Before a manager can convert such figures to FTE requirements, he or she must identify *productive days,* the average number of days per year that a person is actually on the job. As noted earlier, there are 260 possible working days a year, assuming a 40-hour week. This does not reflect the actual days of work per employee, however, because vacations, holidays, sick days, and other leave days have not been deducted. A manager should adjust the figure based on actual experience or on estimates that reflect his or her organization's leave policies.

Figure 10-3

Example of Calculation of Expected Treatment Volumes in Program Planning

	Per Patient	Multiplied by 10 Patients	Total Time with Patients	Total of Practitioners' Time (Direct Treatment)
Individual treatments	1 hour	× 10 =	10 hours	10
Group treatments (maximum of 5 patients/group)	1 hour	× 10 =	10 hours	2 hours (5 patients/group)
			20 hours	12 hours

At this facility, staff members are away for an average of 33 days per person per year (10 holidays, 15 vacation days, 6 sick days, and 2 days of educational leave). The manager uses this information to calculate productive days:

260 possible work days/year
−   33 days of leave/year

= 227 productive days/year

As already explained, the staff members at this facility have only 6 hours a day for direct service. The estimated number of hours per year in direct patient contact therefore would be as follows:

227 productive days
×   6 hours of direct care/day

= 1,362 hours of direct care/year

The manager's earlier computations have indicated that 12 hours of direct patient contact will be required for each working day of the year. Therefore:

260 working days
×   12 hours of direct care/day

= 3,120 hours of direct care required/year

The manager now has sufficient data to project staffing needs. By dividing the projected demand by the actual productivity per FTE, the manager determines the number of FTEs she will require:

3,120 direct hours needed
÷ 1,362 direct hours/FTE

=   2.3 FTEs

A conservative manager would probably recommend two FTEs initially, with contingency plans for allocating additional, part-time staff to the new unit.

The manager then decides to set a productivity standard for these employees by converting planning assumptions to TUs. Using 15 minutes of direct treatment as the measure of productivity, she assumes that each practitioner will see five patients a day individually for an hour, and lead one group of five patients. She calculates the TUs as follows:

1 hour = 4 TUs

5 individual treatments @ 1 hour/pt
× 4 TUs/hour

= 20 individual TUs

5 group treatments @ 1 hour/pt
× 4 TUs/hour

= 20 group TUs

20 individual TUs
+ 20 group TUs

= 40 TUs/practitioner/day

Personnel assigned to this program would now have an understanding of the average volume of treatment that would be expected of them.

QUALITATIVE ASPECTS OF STAFFING

It takes only a moment's reflection to recognize that there is a lot more to effective personnel management than figuring out the numbers. Managers need to identify the best mix of personnel to deliver quality services in a cost-efficient manner. Managers also need to recruit and retain staff members who are motivated and compatible both with the work team and with organizational demands. The remainder of this chapter deals with these qualitative concerns.

Selecting the appropriate level of staff is important. AOTA has resource information that addresses staffing levels (AOTA, 1993, 1994a, 1995a). Table 10-1 shows major terms used to reflect different kinds of staff.

All occupational therapy services require that a registered occupational therapist (OTR) be involved to assess the need for and the effect of intervention. The level of skill and experience required of OTRs will vary

---

Table 10-1

Terminology for Persons Involved in Delivery of Occupational Therapy Services

Occupational therapy personnel	Refers to OTRs, COTAs, occupational therapy students and aides, and support personnel who are involved in delivery of occupational therapy services
Occupational therapy practitioner	Refers only to person credentialed by American Occupational Therapy Certification Board to practice at professional level, OTR, or technical level, COTA
Occupational therapist, registered—OTR	Refers to person credentialed by American Occupational Therapy Certification Board to practice at professional level
Certified occupational therapy assistant—COTA	Refers to person credentialed by American Occupational Therapy Certification Board to practice at technical level
Occupational therapy student	Refers to person enrolled in program accredited by Accreditation Council for Occupational Therapy Education
Occupational therapy aide	Refers to person assigned by OTR or COTA to do delegated routine tasks under close supervision

Note. *From "Policy 1.44. Categories of Occupational Therapy Personnel," by American Occupational Therapy Association, 1994, in* American Occupational Therapy Association Policy Manual, *Rockville, MD: Author. Copyright ©1994 by the American Occupational Therapy Association, Inc.*

with the practice situation and the complexity of the problems addressed. Certified occupational therapy assistants (COTAs) may contribute to assessment, as well as to implementation of a range of services. Readers are encouraged to familiarize themselves with "Occupational Therapy Roles" (AOTA, 1993; see appendix A at the end of this book), a document that describes the range of practice expectations for both OTRs and COTAs, and the related skills and experiences needed to meet those expectations. This information can assist managers in determining reasonable expectations of entry-level staff and experienced practitioners.

Managers should also know how to use support personnel as appropriate for unit functioning. Effectively used, support personnel free occupational therapy practitioners to attend to the aspects of service provision that require their expertise. Use of support personnel is currently a subject of great debate, for there is little research to guide managerial decisions. AOTA has begun to address the issue through adoption of positions regarding the use of aides (e.g., AOTA, 1995b, 1995c). When managers use support personnel to extend occupational therapy services, a number of practical, ethical, and legal considerations arise. First, the occupational therapy manager must determine the level of skill and the nature of intervention required for effective results. Occupational therapy services can range from consultation to provision of direct service. Situations requiring evaluation of patients' or clients' status must be reserved for OTRs because they are the only level of personnel with the background for occupational therapy evaluation. When the emphasis is on skilled observation and treatment, either OTRs or COTAs may be appropriate. Occupational therapy aides may perform selected, routine tasks under close supervision. In all treatment situations, OTRs retain the overall responsibility for the appropriateness of services provided. Further, the manager is responsible for understanding both the ethical and the legal issues associated with occupational therapy services. For instance, the legal use of aides varies from state to state.

Even within the various levels of personnel, there is always the need for consideration of individual talents and preferences. Some therapists are more effective in developing new programs; others function better in already established programs. Some assistants enjoy working with several therapists; others prefer teaming with one person. Successful staffing patterns capitalize on these variances, placing people in organizational niches in which they are most likely to succeed.

MOTIVATION OF PERSONNEL

Because of the shortage of occupational therapy personnel and the complexity of occupational therapy itself, managers are often challenged to understand how to retain and motivate personnel. One scheme that is useful in thinking about these issues is the *expectancy model*, originally developed by Vroom (1965). Under expectancy theory, employees seek to maximize their satisfaction with regard to their expectations about a particular situation. Because of the complexity and the volatility of most employment situations, people attempt to maximize their satisfaction by paying attention to the aspects of work that they feel are important, constantly evaluating how those aspects are likely to affect them. In other words, when the future is not predictable, people create their own internal logic and use it to guide actions in their own self-interest.

Two parts of expectancy theory are important in explaining employee motivation (Heneman, Schwab, Fossum, & Dyer, 1980): expectancies and the perceived consequences of behaviors. *Expectancies* are a person's perceptions, or beliefs, about his or her capability to engage in an activity successfully. *Perceived consequences* are the expected results of a behavior. Most occupational therapy practitioners can readily relate these concepts to experiences that they have had with patients or clients. Similar issues operate with employees in a work setting.

Expectancies deal with the question, "How likely is it that I can successfully accomplish the task?" Having looked at that issue, a person asks, "If I am successful, what are the rewards likely to be?" This assessment of the degree to which successful performance will lead to rewards is referred to as *instrumentality*. Finally, a person considers, "How much do I value those rewards?" This positive or negative evaluation of the rewards is referred to as *valence*. A person's motivation is the result of his or her evaluation of the links between the expectation of success, the rewards of success, and the importance of those rewards. In this way the expectancies that link behaviors to rewards shape motivation. Expectancy theory addresses how people interpret, and subsequently act in, any situation that they encounter. Figure 10-4 graphically displays the elements of a specific act of behavior.

For example, an occupational therapy practitioner is very interested in working with children in a school system, but also relishes the support of colleagues offered in a hospital setting. This person likes starting new programs and enjoys having the freedom to schedule his own time flexibly. If this practitioner, who is currently working in an outpatient pediatric setting, was given the opportunity to service a school contract, he would likely be highly motivated as long as he felt capable of successfully achieving treatment goals. Of course, he would have to believe that his behavior would result in a desirable reward or lead to other attractive gains. The value of such expected rewards is individual to the employee. The plea-

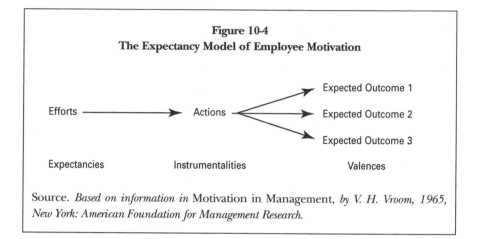

Figure 10-4
The Expectancy Model of Employee Motivation

Source. *Based on information in* Motivation in Management, *by V. H. Vroom, 1965, New York: American Foundation for Management Research.*

sure of starting a new program may be sufficient reward to one therapist. Another therapist, who is less interested in changing routine and insecure about his or her skills with school-based treatment, might resist taking on this opportunity. As the example illustrates, each person has his or her own interpretation of the work situation and its present and anticipated rewards.

The expectancy model as shown in figure 10-4 can be very misleading. What appears to be a very simple theory is in reality a complex network of interacting factors subject to constant change (Schell & Black, in press). For example, if there is insufficient time to complete a task adequately, a practitioner may reevaluate his or her willingness to invest effort in achieving the expected returns (valence). Circumstances such as shifting financial resources can affect a person's perception of the availability of the reward (instrumentality). When these shifts occur, people often reconstruct their expectancies because the previous ones no longer make sense. The result is constantly changing perceptions that can easily affect employee motivation.

Today's rapidly changing health care environment can result in high levels of ambiguity and rapid fluctuations in employee motivation. Effective managers are skilled at anticipating constantly changing expectancies among employees and the rewards desired by them. Managers who use expectancies positively to direct the motivation of practitioners and support personnel stand a better chance of being effective.

JOB DESCRIPTIONS:
FORMULAS FOR PERFORMANCE

DEVELOPING PERSONNEL JOB DESCRIPTIONS

A *job description* is a statement of a job's purpose or a summary of the job, a list of the job's duties, an explanation of supervisory relationships, and a statement of the specifications for the job. The latter section addresses the qualifications necessary for a person to do the job, including education, training, experience, skills, and physical ability. A basic tool of management, the job description is used in employee recruitment, selection, evaluation, and development. It forces the identification of critical aspects of work that are necessary to meet an organization's demands and clients' needs. Job descriptions should reflect organizational expectations and parameters.

In most employment situations, job descriptions are developed and modified in conjunction with human resource personnel and are based on a systematic job analysis (Fottler, 1994). Occupational therapy managers are usually expected to develop and regularly to review the list of duties and the delineation of specifications for jobs under their direction. AOTA has published several documents that can assist managers in developing job descriptions. One major resource is "Occupational Therapy Roles" (AOTA, 1993; see appendix A at the end of this book). This document provides examples of typical duties associated with a broad range of occupational therapy roles, as well as indications of typical expectations of entry-level and advanced personnel. Another important resource is the "Guide for Supervision of Occupational Therapy Personnel" (AOTA, 1995b). This document can help managers frame reporting relationships that they must understand in order to develop appropriate job descriptions. Appendix 10-A contains examples of job descriptions and related performance evaluation forms used in an educational setting.

DEVELOPING FUNCTIONAL JOB DESCRIPTIONS

At times a more specific description or delineation of duties is desirable to augment job descriptions—for example, when a manager is delegating a function such as student fieldwork coordination. *Functional job descriptions* describe in detail the specific duties associated with a particular delegated responsibility. Also, in organizations in which personnel job descriptions are rather general, functional job descriptions serve to provide detail. Functional job descriptions are kept in a unit's own records and are used in conjunction with relevant job descriptions approved by the human resource unit of the organization.

WRITING PERFORMANCE STANDARDS

Related to job descriptions are performance standards. *Performance standards* are detailed delineations of job performance expectations that are based on duties identified in a job description. These standards are useful in orienting new employees, and they form the basis for performance appraisal. Figure 10-5 is an example of how a performance standard might be written. Appendix 10-B is an example of how one facility combined job descriptions and their related performance standards into single forms for use during orientation and performance appraisals.

Figure 10-5

Example of Performance Standards Related to One Aspect of a COTA's Job

Responsibility
Assists with data collection and evaluation under supervision of OTR

Performance Standards
Performance is satisfactory when COTA consistently does following:

1. Accurately identifies to OTR team member own service competencies for assisting in data collection and evaluation

2. Implements standard data collection procedures according to departmental protocols; identifies to OTR team member when procedures were modified in response to patient's needs

3. Reports data and clinical observations accurately in format easily used by OTR team member

4. Reports information to OTR team member in timely manner

5. Identifies to OTR team member and other members of treatment team when patient's situation requires that OTR proceed with data collection or assessment

---

RECRUITMENT

Recruiting occupational therapy personnel is challenging in the current circumstance of shortages. Even with the cost-containment strategies being implemented by government and third-party payers, the demand for occupational therapy personnel remains high in many regions. Managers must develop strategies to predict turnover and to identify potential replacements, often in advance of actual vacancies. This section addresses approaches to forecasting vacancies and recruiting new staff.

FORECASTING VACANCIES

Forecasting vacancies requires the ability to identify the variables associated with staff turnover in a unit. Understanding individual staff members' personal and professional goals, as discussed in the earlier section Motivation of Personnel, can be helpful. A high level of trust between manager and staff facilitates open communication and aids in forecasting. In such an environment, staff members may share intentions far enough in advance for the manager to plan for turnover. Staff members who fear negative responses will not change their plans; they will just give less warning. Knowledge of the turnover history of a unit and familiarity with information obtained from exit interviews may increase a manager's accuracy in predictions. Review of the characteristics of existing staff members can also help, along with calculation of the annual percentage of turnover and identification of any recurring cycles of turnover. For instance, the manager of a particular facility may realize that she hired many new graduates in the fall; when they leave, they will go in late summer because their apartment leases will expire at that time.

All these approaches help forecast staff turnover. However, with the extreme shortages of therapists that are occurring in some areas, units will lose staff members unexpectedly because of aggressive recruitment efforts by a variety of agencies and organizations. Therefore many managers find themselves involved in recruiting as a continuing part of their jobs. This requires that they have a keen sense of their organization's strategic plan and a related awareness of the progress of their own programs in the planning cycle. Managers can more effectively plan recruitment when they can accurately predict vacancies and combine their predictions with a knowledge of positions to be added or eliminated.

RECRUITING NEW STAFF MEMBERS

Recruitment involves using a variety of communication strategies to attract qualified applicants. AOTA permits paid advertisements in *OT Week*. There are a number of other recruiting newspapers that managers may use, some of which are national or regional in scope. State and local occupational therapy associations may have mechanisms for advertising, or they may operate job-listing services. Classified advertisements in local and regional daily newspapers are a possibility, particularly in metropolitan areas. Managers can post job openings at conferences and workshops and on bulletin boards in college and university occupational therapy departments. They can also use direct mail to a segment of practitioners who meet certain requirements (such as geographic location, specialty certification, or membership in a special interest section). Mailing lists can be obtained from AOTA, state associations, and state regulatory bodies. Some occupational therapy departments or programs will provide a list of their graduates. Finally, there are recruitment and placement agencies. In some circumstances these companies can save an organization time in locating particular kinds of staff. Managers must weigh the advantages against the costs, which are charged to the hiring organization and may be as much as one-third of the employee's annual salary. Appendix 10-C contains a guide developed by the AOTA Administration and Management Special Interest Section to introduce graduating students to recruiters. Managers may find the guide helpful as a summary of key issues to consider.

The selection of one or more of these approaches depends on an assessment of which approaches are most likely to attract qualified candidates who could become effective and stable employees. Sometimes managers must experiment to identify consistently successful strategies. They can improve their recruiting by carefully tracking how candidates become aware of positions, as well as by monitoring which methods draw the most desirable candidates.

A variety of indirect approaches can be equally effective. Managers can encourage current employees to recruit occupational therapy personnel with whom they socialize or share educational experiences. Some organizations provide a bonus to employees for recruiting a candidate who is hired and stays for a specified time. Managers can also develop networks through active participation in professional groups such as local, state, and national associations, and use these networks to identify and refer candidates. Articles and chapters by staff members in professional journals, books, and newsletters, and presentations by staff members at professional meetings indirectly advertise an organization as a good place for professional growth. This strategy is effective in attracting potential job candidates. Becoming a site for students' clinical fieldwork experiences often provides organizations with an introduction to promising new graduates. It may also attract candidates interested in an opportunity to supervise students. Finally, development of reentry opportunities can assist managers in identifying occupational therapy personnel who may have stopped working for a time and want to return to the workforce gradually. Often volunteer work, part-time positions, and temporary-coverage jobs are attractive to this group and may pay off in a full-time candidate at a future date.

SELECTION

The recruitment and selection process should be tailored to identify candidates who will perform well and stay for a desirable length of time. Managers can address these considerations by developing selection criteria. Such criteria should go beyond specifying basic qualifications, such as appropriate occupational therapy credentials, to stating characteristics and skills important for successful job performance. A manager might review the characteristics of current successful employees to determine those apparently related to their success. For example, preferred treatment approaches, experience in supervising staff, engaging interpersonal style, high-quality educational background, and clear professional goals may be indicators of success. Staff members' personal preferences about the size and the nature of the patient or client population, the size of the department, and the general pace of work may all have a bearing on job success. Longevity of employment may be linked to the geographic origin of the employees or their history of job tenure. With a sufficient number of employees, the predictive value of some characteristics can be statistically determined. Human resource departments can assist managers in this process, or managers may refer to the literature on personnel for methodologies (Heneman, Schwab, Fossum, & Dyer, 1980; Landau & Abelson, 1994). Even without statistical treatment these variables can add an important dimension to the considerations already formulated in the job specifications.

Once managers have determined selection criteria, they can begin the actual process of staff selection. In organizations with human resource departments, the manager and human resource staff members collaborate in selection of employees. It is desirable for them to predetermine the division of duties, thereby avoiding confusion and unnecessary delays. The selection process usually involves five stages: screening, ranking, interviewing, checking references, and selecting the best candidate and making a job offer. Although the following sections describe these stages sequentially, in areas where there is a shortage of personnel, managers may shorten or skip some stages in order to be responsive to attractive candidates in a timely manner.

STAGE 1: SCREENING

Applicants usually submit résumés and may complete application forms standard to the organization. In the screening stage, managers and human resource department personnel should first identify applicants who lack the necessary qualifications and immediately inform them that they cannot be considered. If they might qualify for some future position, the organization can keep their applications on file. This approach allows for the development of a bank of potential candidates and should be considered for use with any unselected but possibly desirable candidates.

STAGE 2: RANKING

When there are multiple qualified candidates, they should be ranked according to how well they meet the predetermined criteria. Managers should then contact the most suitable candidates for an interview, keeping others on hold pending the results of interviews. At this stage, and throughout the rest of the selection process, managers must be sensitive to local, state, and federal employment regulations (see appendix 10-D for a summary of the latter).

STAGE 3: INTERVIEWING

The interview is a critical stage in the selection process. Not only does a manager gain impressions of the candidates, but the candidates form opinions of the job, the manager, and the organization. A manager can see expectancy theory in action! It is important for the interview to be

---

Figure 10-6
Tips for Effective Interviewing

1. Focus questions on job-related issues and characteristics.

2. Use semistructured, open-ended questions. Ask them of every candidate.

3. Use formal scoring method to evaluate each characteristic separately.

4. Use multiple interviewers whenever possible, and orient all interviewers to key questions that each should ask.

5. Train interviewers to avoid inappropriate or illegal questions.

6. Make notes as you go along, and finalize them right after interview. Avoid discussing candidate with others until you have completed your own notes.

7. Ask candidates to describe previous situations or experiences in which they dealt with issues similar to those that they will encounter on job.

Source. *Based on information in "Selection and Placement" (p. 318), by J. Landau and D. S. Fogel, 1994, in M. D. Fottler, S. R. Hernandez, and C. L. Joiner (Eds.),* Strategic Management of Human Resources in Health Services Organizations *(2nd ed.), Albany, NY: Delmar.*

---

organized in such a way as to maximize the exchange of information (see figure 10-6). The candidate should be informed in advance about the interview process, including how long it will take and who will be involved.

Adequate time should be allowed for the candidate to tour the facility, obtain an overview of the unit's functioning, and be informed about the general conditions of employment. One or more people may participate in the interviews, depending on time constraints, the setting, and the manager's leadership style. Some evidence suggests that interviews become more valid predictors of job success when multiple interviewers are used along with a semistructured interview format (Landau & Fogel, 1994). All who are involved should document their impressions on a feedback form that reflects the major selection concerns (see appendix 10-E). This is best done very soon after the interview to minimize the effects of selective memory and the influence of others. Interviewers can also use the feedback form to note specific areas for exploration during reference checks and to record preliminary impressions on whether the organization should consider the candidate further.

STAGE 4: CHECKING REFERENCES

At the time of application or during the interview process, the candidate should be asked to provide the names of references. These should include persons with enough knowledge of the candidate to discuss his or her potential success in the job. Human resource departments frequently have standard forms that they mail to references; however, this procedure may not be fast enough when several organizations are competing for the same candidate. An alternative approach is to check references by telephone, with the caller documenting the results or requesting a written confirmation. Checking references by telephone has the added advantage of yielding more information because of its interactive nature; however, the caller must be sure to pose all key questions to all references in order to have comparable information.

STAGE 5: SELECTING THE BEST CANDIDATE AND MAKING A JOB OFFER

Using the data obtained through all the sources described earlier, the manager along with other persons involved in the selection process must decide who seems to be the best candidate. When there are multiple candidates, a ranking process may be necessary. The manager or another appropriate person then makes a job offer to the highest-ranked candidate, usually by telephone. This job offer may be made conditional on successful completion of a physical examination to determine that the person has the physical capacities to perform the job (Landau & Fogel, 1994). During the telephone conversation, the caller identifies the starting date, and if necessary, the caller and the candidate negotiate salary. Other incentives that may have been offered, such as a sign-on bonus or use of a company car, should be confirmed at this time. When there is room for negotiation, the manager must know in advance what is an acceptable range of possibilities. It is advisable to maintain salary equity among employees with similar experience, skills, and responsibilities. Salaries need not be exactly the same, but if consideration is not given to existing personnel, there is a strong possibility of upsetting their expectations of fairness.

Once a manager has made a job offer and a candidate has accepted it, the manager should send a letter of confirmation. Only then should any remaining candidates be notified of the decision, and if appropriate, be informed that they might be considered for future openings. After the manager has received a verbal or written acceptance of employment, he or she can schedule the new employee for orientation.

ORIENTATION

Any new employee feels insecure during the first days and weeks on a job. An effective orientation program can minimize this feeling. Although the human resources department may handle some aspects of orientation, the manager and co-workers will need to provide much of the specific information on how to perform the job effectively. They should develop a plan for communicating this information in advance, and modify it in process to suit the learning style of the particular employee. A checklist verifying key competencies, a manual of information, and various hand-outs help ensure that all employees receive the necessary information about their jobs, and also serve as evidence of competency assurance for accrediting agencies. Introduction to key co-workers and identification of one primary resource person help to facilitate the development of positive peer relations. A tour of the facility and time to learn the location of relevant tools and materials can help the new staff member feel at home in the new work site. Chances to observe, assist, and practice are helpful in developing and reinforcing job skills. Regular opportunities to discuss progress and ask questions create a safe environment in which to learn. Every effort should be made to identify organizational values and practices to help the new employee know how to succeed.

PERFORMANCE EVALUATION

The evaluation of staff performance is probably the most threatening of the various supervisory duties. Consequently the temptation is to procrastinate or to provide only positive or very general feedback. Inexperienced supervisors are often surprised to learn that the performance appraisal can be a mutually rewarding experience when they see it as an opportunity for communication and for discussion of the staff member's goals and plans for professional development.

ESTABLISHING PERFORMANCE EXPECTATIONS

The key to effective performance evaluation is development and articulation of clear performance expectations, as described earlier in this chapter. If an employee understands how to do a job correctly and receives regular praise and guidance, the performance appraisal itself becomes merely a summary of this information and an opportunity to discuss options for continued growth.

DOCUMENTING PERFORMANCE

Just as in care of patients and clients, good documentation is necessary in supervision of employees. Documentation of positive performance is often necessary to substantiate recommendations for merit increases in salary. Lack of documentation or inadequate documentation can severely hamper the manager in dealing effectively with a problem employee. Most human resource departments require one or more performance appraisals during the probationary period of employment, with regular evaluations at least annually thereafter.

There are a variety of approaches to performance appraisal (Joiner & Hyde, 1994). One very successful approach combines a behaviorally anchored rating scale with individually negotiated performance objectives. A behaviorally anchored rating scale uses descriptors such as "Does not meet standards," "Meets standards," and "Exceeds standards" to reflect how well a person performs on identified job expectations. The sample appraisal forms found in appendixes 10-A and 10-B use such an approach. This appraisal helps a manager determine whether a staff member is performing all the basic job expectations. To facilitate growth, the manager might then identify specific objectives for the employee to work on in the coming time period. These objectives might be geared toward improving any areas that were weak in the performance appraisal, or they might reflect particular growth objectives of the employee. By looking for opportunities that are interesting to the employee and valuable to the organization, the manager can use this part of the evaluation to further both individual and organizational goals.

Because occupational therapy personnel function in a wide variety of settings, great diversity exists in performance appraisal processes. Occupational therapy managers are encouraged to augment the system used in their setting, if necessary, to maximize the effectiveness of performance appraisal. One approach is to develop an "upward" appraisal form, which employees use to provide feedback to supervisors (see appendix 10-F). Before the performance appraisal, the employee completes this form, which the employee and the manager then review orally during the appraisal meeting. Soliciting such feedback promotes more open communication and allows potential concerns to be addressed before they turn into major problems.

DISCUSSING THE APPRAISAL

Once the manager has completed the written appraisal, he or she should schedule a meeting with the employee to discuss it. A private and quiet place should be used, with sufficient time allotted to discuss the evaluation and allow the employee to provide feedback on his or her reaction to it.

During this time, the manager should encourage the employee to discuss any feedback that he or she has, and the manager should be open to this information. The session should be a two-way communication period. The manager should convey information in a relaxed and matter-of-fact manner, focusing on documented performance. When the manager must provide sensitive or negative feedback, he or she should remind the employee that the information is based on observable work-related behavior and is not a reflection of perceived capability. The manager and the employee should then make plans to assist the employee in performing more effectively, and document the plans as part of the performance appraisal. With employees whose work is satisfactory or better, development of plans or objectives for continued growth and accomplishment is an effective approach to maintaining employee motivation. This strategy allows employees to formalize their expectations with regard to their future professional directions. Whether the purpose of the objectives is to remedy problems or to promote continued growth, subsequent appraisals should include an assessment of whether the objectives were attained. In this way, performance changes can be positively channeled.

DISCIPLINARY ACTION

Special evaluations are required when an employee is demonstrating undesirable performance. For unionized employees the special evaluation procedures and related grievance procedures are spelled out in a contract. Even in nonunion situations, good personnel practice dictates that the manager provide clear information to let the employee know that his or her performance is unacceptable. This usually takes the form of written disciplinary actions or warning notices. Information provided to the employee should also refer to the organization's grievance procedures. These rules often delineate the process that employees use for administrative review of disciplinary actions. The importance of clear policies and effective orientation of employees to these policies becomes evident during difficult situations.

Managers considering disciplinary action may find the "red-hot stove" rule to be a useful guide (Strauss & Sayles, 1972). This rule states that good disciplinary action is like touching a red-hot stove:

1. There is *warning* of the consequences: Anyone can see that the stove is red-hot.

2. The consequences are *immediate:* As soon as a person touches the stove, he or she is burned.

3. The consequences are *impersonal:* Anyone who touches the stove is burned.

4. The consequences are *consistent:* Touching the stove always results in a burn.

After a series of written notices accompanied by related counseling sessions, it may be necessary to terminate an employee from employment. Although the occasion of termination is not a comfortable situation for either the employee or the manager, at times it cannot be avoided in the face of consistently poor performance. Sidestepping of the issue inevitably affects the performance of other employees and creates morale problems. Therefore, effective managers make employee performance problems a priority and deal with them until the employee either sustains a satisfactory performance, resigns, or is terminated.

REWARD SYSTEMS

Rewarding the successful employee is a much more pleasant part of supervision than taking disciplinary action. The obvious rewards for good per-

---

Figure 10-7
Ideas for Staff Rewards, Collected from Occupational Therapy Managers Across the Country

Celebrations
Flowers
Spirit awards
Dinner at nice restaurant
Office Hall of Fame
Birthday cards
Thank you notes
Food treats
Service anniversary awards
Holiday treats or costumes
Funny awards

Humor and Fun
Humorous bulletin board
Cartoons to circulate
Funny stick-on notes
Pictures of staff members with room to
    write notes under
Baby-picture guessing game
Pictures of older practitioners in first
    years of practice
Secret pals or Santas
Theme luncheon (e.g., most bizarre
    chocolate dish)
Auctions or swaps between clinics

General Recognition
Verbal praise
Lunch with boss
Nameplates for desks
Business cards
Routine job satisfaction surveys
Mentoring programs
Opportunities to be part of planning
Flexibility and trust in setting work hours

Employee Benefits
Continuing education days
On-site day care
Compensatory time
Payment of professional dues
Payment of licensure fees
Job sharing
Flexible maternity leaves
On-site library
Access to fitness equipment
Company discount cards
Exchange programs with other
    practitioners

Source. *Based on information in "Staff Rewards" (p. 3), by B. A. Schell, S. J. Rask, and M. Cohn, 1991, September,* Administration and Management Special Interest Section Newsletter, 7*(3).*

formance are salary adjustments, such as merit increases. An astute manager soon becomes aware that although money is a pleasing reward, it is not sufficient to sustain employee motivation. Oral and written praise and recognition, paid attendance at continuing education seminars, increased responsibility for program development, opportunities to supervise students, and flexible working hours can all be perceived as rewards (see figure 10-7). Opportunities for promotion can also be powerful motivators.

Each employee has his or her own perceptions of what is important, and they change over the course of personal and professional development. This is consistent with the expectancy theory model discussed earlier. Employees also form perceptions of the likelihood of being rewarded in meaningful ways. To use rewards successfully, the manager must (1) identify what is meaningful to the employee, (2) find an organizational context that allows the expression of that meaningful reward, and (3) relate the reward to desired performance. The manager must also communicate accurately the range of rewards that are available in a given situation so that employees can set realistic expectations. Careful monitoring of staff reward systems and expectations pays off in dedicated and productive personnel.

STAFF DEVELOPMENT

Orientation, performance evaluation, and reward systems are all tools critical to the basic development of staff. In addition, continual upgrading of knowledge and skills is required to support occupational therapy services in the changing health care environment. This a professional responsibility of individuals, but increasingly there is a recognition that it is an organizational responsibility as well (Senge, 1990; Watkins & Marsick, 1993). The manager plays a key role in facilitating both individual and organizational development.

To facilitate staff development effectively, the manager must first target areas of concern. He or she should develop systematic methods to assess needs and to follow up on the effectiveness of staff development activities (Bullard, 1983). Activities to monitor quality may identify areas needing improvement. The organization's strategic plan may reveal new areas of service provision for which staff need preparation. Periodic surveys and meetings involving teams or work groups can be planned to identify needs. Individual staff members can identify areas in which improved competence would enhance the care of patients or clients. A summary of weaknesses noted in performance appraisals over the last year may also reveal patterns of staff development needs. In most cases the manager will rely on multiple sources to identify important areas for staff development.

Staff development can occur in a variety of ways. Usually it involves a mix of practical experience and education (Schell, 1992, 1994). Much learning can and does go on in the course of daily practice; the manager should recognize and capitalize on this fact. For instance, vacancies or short-term leaves permit other staff members to engage in explorative practice, in which they "try on" new demands and learn new skills. Assignments to particular projects or organizational committees can also provide learning opportunities. Alternatively, allowing staff members to stay in particular practice settings for extended periods enables them to gain a depth of experience necessary for expert practice. Encouraging reflection on practice helps staff members critically evaluate their experiences and consider alternatives to their customary routines (Gambrill, 1990; Parham, 1987; Senge, 1990; Slater & Cohn, 1991).

Many staff members engage in self-directed education when they use professional resources such as journals, books, and informational interviews to gain knowledge needed for practice. In addition to learning gained from occupational therapy practice, formal educational approaches are required. Structured continuing education opportunities include inservice education, professional conferences and seminars, self-study courses, and distance education events such as teleconferences and computer on-line network conferencing. Both self-directed and continuing education approaches, when appropriately combined with experiential learning, are effective for enhancing current competencies or gaining new skills. Formal education, such as graduate study, provides staff with the opportunity to study in greater depth within a cohesively planned curriculum. These activities are designed to help staff members think more critically about a wider range of issues. Additionally, advanced education may be required for staff to assume certain roles, or to meet long-term career goals, such as becoming a faculty member.

PERSONNEL MANAGEMENT IN TODAY'S SETTINGS

A discussion of personnel management would be incomplete without an acknowledgment of the challenging staffing issues that occupational therapy practitioners have encountered as they have moved into a variety of community-based settings. Much of what has been written about personnel management in occupational therapy has presumed the existence of an occupational therapy department within a health care organization, often a hospital or a rehabilitation center. Although these traditional organizational patterns continue in many settings, it is becoming equally typical for practitioners to find themselves in different situations. Examples include program models in which occupational therapy staff members report to managers who are not occupational therapists, and solo- or distance-practice situations in which practitioners serve a number of facilities such as nursing homes, schools, or community mental health settings. In rural settings, where occupational therapy personnel shortages are most often acute, practitioners may not have supervision in the traditional sense of the word. Nonetheless, the issues discussed in this chapter must be addressed. The basic principles and strategies presented here apply in these new settings. What changes are the innovative ways that managers and practitioners find to respond. For example, in school-based practices, in which practitioners may be independent contractors, professional networks such as local and national special interest sections can play a critical role by providing peer mentoring in place of traditional supervision. In private practices that may have one occupational therapy manager for the state or the region, systems that do not solely depend on daily observation by the manager for monitoring the quality of care and the concerns of staff members become critical. In such situations the manager may develop a combination of on-site consultations, regional meetings, and regular accessibility by telephone or electronic mail to respond to the needs of staff members. In institutions where there are program teams rather than occupational therapy departments, senior occupational therapists may serve in dual capacities as both team members and occupational therapy consultants to administrators and clinicians on other teams. Finally, where occupational therapy managers themselves are responsible for multidisciplinary staffs, there are new challenges to develop appropriate expectations that both meet organizational demands and respond to the standards of the different professions represented. The many new settings for practice reflect a growing appreciation of the variety of contexts in which occupational therapy services can be effective. Managers should take advantage of these opportunities.

SUMMARY

A manager serves as the interface between the individuals forming a work unit and the larger organization. To do this effectively, a manager must understand organizational resources, values, and goals. This knowledge provides a context for staffing.

In recent years the turbulence in health care has also required managers to tune in to the strategic planning process of their organization (Hernandez, Fottler, & Joiner, 1994). Awareness of where their programs and services fit within the larger strategic plan is critical.

One component of personnel management is the ability to quantify and project staffing needs accurately. This requires understanding the concept of full-time equivalents and using it to develop productivity standards and staffing plans.

On the qualitative side, managers need to identify the best mix of personnel to deliver quality services in a cost-efficient manner. They also need to recruit and retain staff members who are motivated and compatible both with the work team and with organizational demands. Selecting the appropriate level of staff is important. So is using support personnel appropriately.

A scheme that is useful in thinking about how to retain and motivate personnel is the *expectancy model,* originally developed by Vroom (1965). Under expectancy theory, employees seek to maximize their satisfaction with regard to their expectations about a particular situation. Two parts of expectancy theory are important in explaining employee motivation (Heneman, Schwab, Fossum, & Dyer, 1980): expectancies and the perceived consequences of behaviors.

A *job description* is a statement of a job's purpose or a summary of the job, a list of the job's duties, an explanation of supervisory relationships, and a statement of the specifications for the job. A basic tool of management, the job description forces the identification of critical aspects of work that are necessary to meet an organization's demands and clients' needs. Related to job descriptions are *performance standards,* detailed delineations of job performance expectations that are based on duties identified in a job description. These standards are useful in orienting new employees, and they form the basis for performance appraisal.

Recruiting occupational therapy personnel is challenging in the current circumstance of shortages. Managers must develop strategies to predict turnover and to identify potential replacements, often in advance of actual vacancies. Forecasting vacancies requires the ability to identify the variables associated with staff turnover in a unit. It also requires that managers have a keen sense of their organization's strategic plan and a related awareness of the progress of their own programs in the planning cycle. Recruitment involves using a variety of communication strategies to attract qualified applicants. Direct approaches include placing advertisements in periodicals, posting job openings, mailing announcements to practitioners, and contracting with recruitment and placement agencies. A variety of indirect approaches can be equally effective: encouraging current employees to recruit personnel; developing networks; encouraging publications and presentations by staff members; becoming a site for students' clinical fieldwork experiences; and developing reentry opportunities.

The recruitment and selection process should be tailored to identify candidates who will perform well and stay for a desirable length of time.

Managers can address these considerations by developing selection criteria. The selection process itself usually involves five stages: screening, ranking, interviewing, checking references, and selecting the best candidate and making a job offer.

In advance of a new employee's arrival, the manager and co-workers should develop a plan for communicating specific information on how to perform the job effectively and then modify the plan to suit the learning style of the employee. Regular opportunities to discuss progress and ask questions create a safe environment in which to learn.

The key to effective performance evaluation is development and articulation of clear performance expectations. Good documentation is necessary in supervision of employees. Once the manager has completed the written appraisal, he or she should schedule a meeting with the employee, with sufficient time allotted to discuss the evaluation and allow the employee to provide feedback on his or her reaction to it. Special evaluations are required when an employee is demonstrating undesirable performance. Good personnel practice dictates that the manager provide clear information to let the employee know that his or her performance is unacceptable. Effective managers make employee performance problems a priority and deal with them until the employee either sustains a satisfactory performance, resigns, or is terminated.

Rewarding the successful employee is a much more pleasant part of supervision than taking disciplinary action. An astute manager soon becomes aware that although money is a pleasing reward, it is not sufficient to sustain employee motivation.

Continual upgrading of staff members' knowledge and skills is required to support occupational therapy services in the changing health care environment. The manager should develop systematic methods to assess needs and to follow up on the effectiveness of staff development activities (Bullard, 1983). Staff development can occur in a variety of ways: in the course of daily practice; in self-directed education; in structured continuing education opportunities; and through formal education.

Although traditional organizational patterns continue in many settings, it is becoming equally typical for practitioners to find themselves in different situations. Examples include program models in which occupational therapy staff members report to managers who are not occupational therapists, and solo- or distance-practice situations in which practitioners serve a number of facilities such as nursing homes, schools, or community mental health settings. The basic principles and strategies presented in this chapter apply in these new settings. What changes are the innovative ways that managers and practitioners find to respond.

REFERENCES

American Occupational Therapy Association. (1979). *Occupational therapy product output reporting system and uniform terminology for reporting occupational therapy services.* Rockville, MD: Author.

American Occupational Therapy Association. (1989). Uniform terminology for occupational therapy (2nd ed.). *American Journal of Occupational Therapy, 43,* 808–15.

American Occupational Therapy Association. (1994a). Policy 1.44. Categories of occupational therapy personnel. In *American Occupational Therapy Association policy manual.* Rockville, MD: Author.

American Occupational Therapy Association. (1994b). Uniform terminology for occupational therapy (3rd ed.). *American Journal of Occupational Therapy, 48,* 1047–54.

American Occupational Therapy Association. (1995a). *Developing, maintaining, and updating competency in occupational therapy: A guide to self-appraisal.* Bethesda, MD: Author.

American Occupational Therapy Association. (1995b). Guide for supervision of occupational therapy personnel. *American Journal of Occupational Therapy, 49,* 1027–28.

American Occupational Therapy Association. (1995c). Use of occupational therapy aides in occupational therapy practice [Position paper]. *American Journal of Occupational Therapy, 49,* 1023–25.

American Occupational Therapy Association Occupational Therapy Roles Task Force. (1993). Occupational therapy roles. *American Journal of Occupational Therapy, 47,* 1087–99.

Bullard, M. (1983). A needs assessment strategy for educational planning. *American Journal of Occupational Therapy, 37,* 624–29.

Fottler, M. D. (1994). Job analysis. In M. D. Fottler, S. R. Hernandez, & C. L. Joiner (Eds.), *Strategic management of human resources in health services organizations* (2nd ed., pp. 249–63). Albany, NY: Delmar.

Gambrill, E. D. (1990). *Critical thinking in clinical practice: Improving the accuracy of judgments and decisions about clients.* San Francisco: Jossey-Bass.

Heneman, H. G., III, Schwab, D. P., Fossum, J. A, & Dyer, L. D. (1980). *Personnel/human resource management.* Homewood, IL: Irwin.

Hernandez, S. R., Fottler, M. D., & Joiner, C. L. (1994). Integrating strategic management and human resources. In M. D. Fottler, S. R. Hernandez, & C. L. Joiner (Eds.), *Strategic management of human resources in health services organizations* (2nd ed., pp. 1–23). Albany, NY: Delmar.

Joiner, C. L., & Hyde, J. C. (1994). Performance appraisal. In M. D. Fottler, S. R. Hernandez, & C. L. Joiner (Eds.), *Strategic management of human resources in health services organizations* (2nd ed., pp. 365–92). Albany, NY: Delmar.

Landau, J., & Abelson, M. (1994). Recruitment and retention. In M. D. Fottler, S. R. Hernandez, & C. L. Joiner (Eds.), *Strategic management of human resources in health services organizations* (2nd ed., pp. 265–98). Albany, NY: Delmar.

Landau, J., & Fogel, D. S. (1994). Selection and placement. In M. D. Fottler, S. R. Hernandez, & C. L. Joiner (Eds.), *Strategic management of human resources in health services organizations* (2nd ed., pp. 299–333). Albany, NY: Delmar.

McCarthy, D., & Lieberman, D. (1992). National Rehabilitation Hospital. In American Occupational Therapy Association, *Managing productivity in occupational therapy* (pp. 101–12). Rockville, MD: AOTA.

Parham, D. (1987). Toward professionalism: The reflective therapist [Nationally Speaking]. *American Journal of Occupational Therapy, 41,* 555–61.

Schell, B. A. (1992). Setting realistic goals. *Occupational Therapy in Practice, 3*(3), 11–20.

Schell, B. A. (1994). *Career exploration and development: A companion guide for the occupational therapy roles document.* Bethesda, MD: American Occupational Therapy Association.

Schell, J. W., & Black, R. S. (in press). On becoming reflective scholars: An inductive case study. *Adult Education Quarterly.*

Senge, P. M. (1990). *The fifth discipline: The art and practice of the learning organization.* New York: Doubleday.

Slater, D. Y., & Cohn, E. S. (1991). Staff development through analysis of practice. *American Journal of Occupational Therapy, 45,* 1038–44.

Strauss, G., & Sayles, L. R. (1972). *Personnel: The human problems of management* (3rd ed.). Englewood Cliffs, NJ: Prentice-Hall.

Vroom, V. H. (1965). *Motivation in management.* New York: American Foundation for Management Research.

Watkins, K. E., & Marsick, V. J. (1993). *Sculpting the learning organization: Lessons in the art and science of systemic change.* San Francisco: Jossey-Bass.

ADDITIONAL RESOURCES

American Occupational Therapy Association. (1992). *Managing productivity in occupational therapy.* Rockville, MD: Author.

Bordieri, J. E. (1988). Job satisfaction of occupational therapists: Supervisors and managers versus direct service staff. *Occupational Therapy Journal of Research, 8,* 155–63.

Brollier, C. (1985). Occupational therapy management and job performance of staff. *American Journal of Occupational Therapy, 39,* 649–54.

Cervero, R. M. (1988). *Effective continuing education for professionals.* San Francisco: Jossey-Bass.

Dickerson, A. (1990). Evaluating productivity and profitability in occupational therapy contractual work. *American Journal of Occupational Therapy, 44,* 133–37.

Gilbert, J. A. (1990). *Productivity management: A step-by-step guide for health care professionals.* Chicago: American Hospital.

Lave, J., & Wenger, E. (1991). *Situated learning: Legitimate peripheral participation.* Cambridge, England: Cambridge University Press.

Metzger, N. (Ed.). (1990). *Handbook of health care human resources management* (2nd ed.). Rockville, MD: Aspen Publishers.

Mitchell, M. M. (1985). Professional development: Clinician to academician. *American Journal of Occupational Therapy, 39,* 368–73.

Nowlen, P. M. (1987). *A new approach to continuing education for business and the professions: The performance model.* New York: Macmillan.

Smith, B. C. (Ed.). (1992). Taking charge of professional growth [Entire issue]. *Occupational Therapy in Practice, 3*(3).

APPENDIX 10-A

Sample Job Descriptions and Evaluation Forms

Position Descriptions for Registered Occupational Therapist, and Occupational Therapist Assistant

Self-Appraisal Form

Professional Staff Evaluation Form

Performance Objective Form

Parents' Perception of Performance Form

HEARTLAND AEA 11   Certified Personnel

Position Title: Occupational Therapist
                      Special Education Division

Qualifications: Completed program in occupational therapy.
                      Current state license to practice occupational therapy in the state of Iowa.
                      Statement of professional recognition.
                      Experience or interest in pediatrics desired.

Accountable to: Specialty Supervisor

Primary Objective of the Position: Assist Director while under the direct supervision of the supervisor to organize and administer the occupational therapy component of the education program for children and youth with disabilities who are handicapped in obtaining an education because of an impairment in self-care, meal-time skills, and/or manipulation skills.

Major Areas of Accountability:*
1. Collaborate with LEA and AEA staff, other agencies, parents, and caregivers regarding motor-based concerns.
2. Provide self-care, meal-time skills, manipulation skills, and prevocational assessment of the student in his/her educational environment.
3. Manage time, organize materials, and communicate with AEA and LEA staff to effectively manage cases of assigned children and youth.
4. Utilize individualized occupational therapy interventions for children and youth with disabilities.
5. Participate in supervising clinical interns and in other student training.
7. Supervise certified occupational therapy assistants.
8. Develop and/or participate in professional enrichment activities to maintain a high standard of service delivery.
9. Engage in public awareness activities to assist consumers in understanding the services and outcomes of the occupational therapy profession in the educational setting.
10. Serve as an advocate for all children and youth.
11. Report any and all violations of rules and regulations to supervisor/coordinator.
12. Other duties as assigned.

Requirements: Bending, carrying, climbing, must be able to travel between job sites, lifting, pushing-pulling, reaching, sitting, standing, and walking.

Working Conditions: 1. Includes extremes of temperature and humidity.
                          2. Hazards include stairs and communicable diseases.

Length of Contract: 190 days
                          Certified Union

*All areas of accountability considered essential functions of the job.

Note. *From Heartland Area Education Agency #11, Johnston, IA. Reprinted with permission.*

HEARTLAND AEA 11   Certified Personnel

Position Title: Certified Occupational Therapist Assistant
                        Special Education Division

Qualifications: Completion of approved training program and awarding of certificate upon completion of national examination.
Current state license to practice occupational therapy under the supervision of an occupational therapist in the state of Iowa.
Experience desirable but not required.

Accountable to: Specialty Supervisor
                        Supervising Occupational Therapist

Primary Objective of the Position: Assist Director and Specialty Supervisor while under the direct supervision of occupational therapist(s) to provide occupational therapy interventions.

Major Areas of Accountability:*
1. Assist students under direction of occupational therapist to maximize their potential in areas of self-care, meal-time skills, and manipulation skills.
2. Carry out observations and assist occupational therapist in administering formal evaluations.
3. Maintain written reports and records on interventions.
4. Construct adaptive equipment, self-help devices as recommended by occupational therapist.
5. Participate in staffings, annual reviews, parent/teacher conferences, and make parent/teacher contacts as necessary; communicate with team members regarding the children's programming.
6. Engage in public awareness activities.
7. Provide clinical internship opportunities for COTA students.
8. Serve as an advocate for all children and youth.
9. Report any and all violations of rules and regulations to supervisor/coordinator.
10. Other duties as assigned.

Requirements: Bending, carrying, climbing, must be able to travel between job sites, lifting, pushing-pulling, reaching, sitting, standing, and walking.

Working Conditions: 1. Includes extremes of temperature and humidity.
                            2. Hazards include stairs and communicable diseases.

Length of Contract: 190 days
                            Classified Union

*All areas of accountability considered essential functions of the job.

Note. *From Heartland Area Education Agency #11, Johnston, IA. Reprinted with permission.*

HEARTLAND AREA EDUCATION AGENCY
Self-Appraisal
Special Education

Staff Member _____ Date _____

Rate yourself (X or O) in these areas and use the comment section to state other good things you do and concerns you have.

X = Satisfactory   O = Opportunity for Improvement

I. Interpersonal Skills

1. Students

   Shows respect for and interest in all students as individuals . . . .❏

   Can easily establish and maintain rapport with students . . . .❏

   Can adjust to individual student needs . . . .❏

2. Other Professionals

   Demonstrates willingness to share methods, materials, and ideas with co-workers . .❏

   Considers constructive criticism and guidance . . . .❏

   Is fair, impartial, and objective in dealing with others . . . .❏

   Adapts easily to unforeseen events and changing circumstances . . . .❏

   Work with others characterized by openness, respect, friendliness, and

       professional ethics . . . .❏

   Is respectful of confidences . . . .❏

   Exhibits consistent and reliable behavior . . . .❏

3. Parents

   Deals effectively with parents . . . .❏

   Keeps parents informed with involved with students . . . .❏

   Other good things I do and/or concerns I have: _____

   _____

   _____

II. Professional Qualities

1. Professional Interest and Growth

   Remains professionally current . . . .❏

   Is innovative and undertakes new projects . . . .❏

   Knows and uses appropriate resources . . . .❏

   Participates in the improvement of services . . . .❏

   Employs strategies that are ethically sound . . . .❏

   Shows evidence of self-confidence, emotional maturity, and flexibility . . . .❏

2. Cooperation

Accepts extra responsibilities ....❑

Complies with rules and regulations of the system ....❑

Follows established communication channels ....❑

3. Dependability

Submits required reports promptly and accurately ....❑

Attends required meetings ....❑

Informs appropriate individuals of work schedule ....❑

Other good things I do and/or concerns I have: _____

_____

_____

III. Job Management

1. Time Management

Maintains an acceptable attendance record ....❑

Meets the workday time requirements ....❑

Utilizes time effectively ....❑

2. Preparation

Is well organized but flexible ....❑

Has needed materials and equipment ready for use ....❑

Plans activities cooperatively ....❑

3. Communication

Communicates problems and concerns to the supervisor ....❑

Communicates with parents, teachers, and administrators regarding services ......❑

Responds promptly to telephone and written contacts ....❑

Other good things I do and/or concerns I have: _____

_____

_____

IV. Discipline Specific Section (to be completed by each discipline)

1. _____❑

2. _____❑

3. _____❑

4. _____❑

Signature _____

Date _____

Note. *From Heartland Area Education Agency #11, Johnston, IA. Reprinted with permission.*

HEARTLAND AREA EDUCATION AGENCY
Professional Staff Evaluation—Physical Therapists and Occupational Therapists
Special Education

Staff Member: _____ Zone: _____

Position: _____ Date: _____

RATING SCALE DEFINITIONS

Highly Competent (HC):   Consistently demonstrates a level of performance that exceeds
                          contemporaries.

Competent (C):   Consistently demonstrates a level of performance equal to
                          that of contemporaries.

Needs Improvement (NI):   Demonstrates a level of performance below that of most
                          contemporaries.

Unsatisfactory (U):   Does not demonstrate an acceptable level of performance.

I. Interpersonal Skills	HC	C	NI	U
1. Students				
Shows respect for and interest in all students as individuals				
Can easily establish and maintain rapport with students				
Can adjust to individual student needs				
2. Other Professionals				
Demonstrates willingness to share methods, materials, and ideas with co-workers				
Considers constructive criticism and guidance				
Is fair, impartial, and objective in dealing with others				
Adapts easily to unforeseen events and changing circumstances				
Work with others characterized by openness, respect, friendliness, and professional ethics				
Is respective of confidences				
Exhibits consistent and reliable behavior				
3. Parents				
Deals effectively with parents				
Keeps parents informed with involved with students				

Comments:

II. Professional Qualities	HC	C	NI	U
1. Professional Interest and Growth				
Remains professionally current				
Is innovative and undertakes new projects				
Knows and uses appropriate resources				
Participates in the improvement of services (committee)				
Employs strategies that are ethically sound				
Shows evidence of self-confidence, emotional maturity, and flexibility				
2. Cooperation				
Accepts extra responsibilities				
Complies with rules and regulations of the system				
Follows established communication channels				
3. Dependability				
Submits required reports promptly and accurately				
Attends required meetings				
Informs appropriate individuals of work schedule				

Comments:

III. Job Management	HC	C	NI	U
1. Time Management				
Maintains an acceptable attendance record				
Meets the workday time requirements				
Utilizes time effectively				
2. Preparation				
Is well organized but flexible				
Has needed materials and equipment ready for use				
Plans activities cooperatively				
3. Communication				
Communicates problems and concerns to the supervisor				
Communicates with parents, teachers, and administrators regarding services				
Responds promptly to telephone and written contacts				

Comments:

Note. *From Heartland Area Education Agency #11, Johnston, IA. Reprinted with permission.*

IV. Physical Therapists and Occupational Therapists	HC	C	NI	U
1. Identification and Assessment				
Selects appropriate screening and/or diagnostic tools/activities				
Demonstrates skills in conducting evaluation techniques				
2. Program Planning				
Assists in planning integrated goals and objectives				
Plans effective intervention services consistent with educational goals				
Determines appropriate model of service and amount of service				
Uses entrance and exit criteria accurately				
Facilitates integrated services				
3. Program Application				
Identifies rationale for appropriate therapeutic techniques				
Instructs and supervises others in integrated activities				
Conducts ongoing assessment and programming				
Encourages participation of child to fullest ability				
4. Communicates with team members, paraprofessionals, and others regarding the child's program				
Inservices school personnel, parents, and other team members as needed				
Attends relevant inservice training				

OVERALL SUMMARY:

Signature _____   Signature _____
               Practitioner   Supervisor

Date _____   Date _____

Note. *From Heartland Area Education Agency #11, Johnston, IA. Reprinted with permission.*

PERFORMANCE OBJECTIVE

Name: _____ Reviewed by: _____

Date: _____ Obj. No. _____ Review Date: _____

Complete sections I through IV and submit to supervisor by September 15. Complete Section V upon accomplishment of performance objective and submit to supervisor by May 15.

I. Performance Objective

II. Target Population

III. Necessary Resources

IV. Plan for Achieving Objective

V. Summary/Indicators of Success

Note. *From Heartland Area Education Agency #11, Johnston, IA. Reprinted with permission.*

Heartland Area Education Agency
Division of Special Education
Parent's Perception of Performance
PT-OT Services

Parent(s) _____

Staff Member _____

1. Were evaluation results, assessment procedures, and the time your child will be in the program discussed with you?

   _____
   _____
   _____

2. Were the annual goals discussed and agreed upon by both you and the therapist?

   _____
   _____
   _____

3. How has this therapist involved you in the process?

   _____
   _____
   _____

4. What do you like most about how this therapist works with you and your child?

   _____
   _____
   _____

5. What do you think this therapist needs to do to be more effective in providing services?

   _____
   _____
   _____

6. Did you receive a copy of the annual goals from the therapist? _____

7. Does this therapist keep scheduled appointments or notify you of any changes? _____

   _____

Your Signature _____

Date _____

Note. *From Heartland Area Education Agency #11, Johnston, IA. Reprinted with permission.*

APPENDIX 10-B

Sample Job Descriptions/Performance Reviews for Occupational Therapist, Registered, and Certified Occupational Therapy Assistant

HARMARVILLE REHABILITATION CENTER, INC.
JOB DESCRIPTION/PERFORMANCE REVIEW

Job Title: Occupational Therapist, Registered   Employee: _____

Department: Occupational Therapy   Performance Review Date: _____

Approved by: Reports to: Occupational Therapy Supervisor

Date of Original Approval: July 1, 1991   Review Type: _____ Annual

   _____ Special

Date of Revision: September 15, 1994   Salary Level: _____

Position Requirements:

Graduate of an AOTA-accredited occupational therapy program, current certification with the AOTA as a registered occupational therapist, licensed and/or eligible for licensure as an occupational therapist in the state of Pennsylvania. Related experience in occupational therapy with disabled adults preferred, Level II fieldwork experience in rehabilitation strongly preferred for newly graduated candidates.

Job Purpose:

To plan, develop, and administer occupational therapy services with a goal of facilitating the resumption of the patient's former life roles in a full or altered capacity.

Physical Demands:

Must be able to ambulate freely about the unit; must be able to see and hear normally or to normal range with assistive devices; must be able to perform occasional heavy lifting tasks; must be able to stoop, bend, stretch, and kneel; must be able to work safely with persons of infectious disease; must be cognitively and emotionally able to care for patients, observe their condition, perform treatments, and record results.

The above requires excellent general health and normal immune status; functional gait/ambulatory status adequate to perform job duties; normal vision and hearing abilities; acuity of 20/40 each eye and in both eyes alone or with corrective lenses, as measured by the Snellen Chart. Hearing grossly measured by whisper testing. Normal strength in extremity muscles as measured by manual muscle testing. Ability to display fair to excellent strength in back and abdominal muscles as measured by Krasu-Weber testing. No abnormalities inconsistent with job requirements found in x-rays. Normal cognitive ability and emotional state as observed during the process of taking the history and performing the physical examination, and during orientation process. Must be able to demonstrate safe and appropriate transfer activities.

Demonstrates manual dexterity to perform tasks required (i.e., splinting, patient evaluation, self-care, wheelchair positioning). Cognitively and emotionally able to communicate with patients and families, observe patient's performance, and adjust treatment accordingly.

Supervisory Responsibilities:

Note. *From Harmarville Rehabilitation Center, Inc., Pittsburgh, PA. Reprinted by permission.*

Job Description/Performance Review   Job Title: Occupational Therapist, Registered

Job Responsibilities & Performance Standards	Expectation		
	Below (−)	Meets (+)	Above (++)
1. Responds to referral by performing initial evaluation to establish baseline information from which to plan treatment, as observed by supervisor and through chart review.			
1.1 Administers occupational therapy initial evaluation per departmental procedure 90% of the time. EXCEEDS: When documentation highlights those areas that directly impact on occupational performance 90% of the time.			
1.2 Establishes goals and treatment plan that reflect patient's life roles and patient's family's concerns and valued goals 100% of the time. EXCEEDS: When 90% of patient goals are measurable and functionally based or outcome oriented.			
1.3 Identifies need for and performs or recommends special evaluations to supplement initial assessment as indicated.			
1.4 Monitors response to intervention on an outgoing basis and modifies treatment as necessary to attain goals.			
Total:			
Comments:			
2. Provides quality occupational therapy treatment to ensure optimum patient recovery/adaptation as observed by supervisor or senior clinician, and/or through chart review.			
2.1 Provides appropriate therapeutic interventions based upon the patient's specific needs including, but not limited to, cognitive status, behavior, physical limitations, and age, clearly addressing the age appropriateness of evaluation batteries, treatment strategies, and expected outcomes in all age groups from adolescent through geriatric populations.			
2.2 Treatment modalities reflect consideration of patient's life roles, valued goals, and interests 100% of the time.			
2.3 As scheduled, pre-plans and implements goal-directed, age-relevant, functionally oriented group sessions. EXCEEDS: By recognizing patients who will not benefit from planned group activities, making recommendations for, and ensuring provision of more customized treatment approaches.			

Note. *From Harmarville Rehabilitation Center, Inc., Pittsburgh, PA. Reprinted by permission.*

Job Responsibilities & Performance Standards	Expectation		
	Below (−)	Meets (+)	Above (++)
2.4 Implements treatment plan in accordance with departmental, team, and patient goals 100% of the time. EXCEEDS: When treatment and documentation routinely link occupational therapy intervention with activities of the multi-disciplinary team.			
2.5 Coverage is provided in therapist's absence 100% of the time. EXCEEDS: When coverage plans are detailed, goal directed, and outcome oriented.			
2.6 Complies with departmental productivity standards 100% of the time while maintaining acceptable level of quality care. EXCEEDS: When statistics reflect productivity 20% above expectations on an annual basis (10% for OTR/COTA team).			
2.7 Identifies need for and provides family/caregiver education relevant to patient status 100% of the time. EXCEEDS: When family performance abilities, concerns, and reactions to the patient's program (or lack of participation) are routinely documented 100% of the time.			
2.8 Promotes carryover of occupational therapy interventions upon discharge by providing appropriate home and/or community programming recommendations 100% of the time. EXCEEDS: When customized home programs are developed and provided to patient and/or family.			
2.9 Accurately assesses priorities for patient treatment and implements accordingly 100% of the time. EXCEEDS: When customized home programs are developed and provided to patient and/or family.			
2.10 Documents instances of and rationale for treatment occurring less than five (5) days/week for inpatients 100% of the time.			
2.11 Demonstrates knowledge of roles/functions of other members of the department 100% of the time. Elicits appropriate assistance and supervises/coordinates services for each patient. EXCEEDS: Interactions are directive, timely, and respectful of others' areas of expertise.			
Total:			
Comments:			

Note. *From Harmarville Rehabilitation Center, Inc., Pittsburgh, PA. Reprinted by permission.*

Job Responsibilities & Performance Standards	Expectation		
	Below (−)	Meets (+)	Above (++)
3. Communicates information relevant to patient care to ensure quality service delivery and maximum reimbursement as observed by supervisor or senior clinician and/or through chart review.			
3.1 Complies with departmental documentation protocols as evidenced by complete records and justified medical record deficiencies of less than 10 per year. EXCEEDS: When justified medical record delinquency notifications do not exceed five (5) per year.			
3.2 Ensures that all charges are entered within 24 hours of service delivery 85% of the time. EXCEEDS: When accomplished 95% of the time.			
3.3 Provides information necessary for ongoing program evaluation and quality assurance studies as requested. EXCEEDS: By identifying potential quality problems or areas for study and reporting those to supervisor.			
3.4 Provides relevant information regarding functional performance and goal attainment at scheduled staffing conferences or provides for informed representative 100% of the time. EXCEEDS: When presentation is professional and efficient and reflects consideration of program evaluation and utilization review requirements.			
3.5 Informs patient and/or significant others of evaluation findings and treatment rationale at their level of understanding 100% of the time. EXCEEDS: When presented in a manner that is conducive to integration and interaction.			
3.6 Communicates with other health care personnel regarding patient care as necessary. EXCEEDS: When routinely initiating discussions.			
Total:			
Comments:			

Note. *From Harmarville Rehabilitation Center, Inc., Pittsburgh, PA. Reprinted by permission.*

Job Responsibilities & Performance Standards	Expectation		
	Below (−)	**Meets** (+)	**Above** (++)
4. Guest/Employee Relations: Demonstrates regard for the dignity of and respect for all patients, their families, guests, and representatives of other organizations as well as fellow employees, volunteers, and medical staff in support of the corporation's mission to provide consistent quality health care services in a professional, caring, and responsive environment.			
4.1 Maintains confidentiality of patient and/or patient and departmental information with no infractions as noted by supervision.			
4.2 Consistently displays a caring and responsive attitude and represents the corporation in a positive manner and conducts all activities respecting patient/customer rights and expectations. EXCEEDS: By consistently making extra efforts to achieve patient/customer expectations while discharging job responsibilities.			
4.3 Regularly maintains a neat appearance and adheres to departmental/corporation dress, including the wearing of appropriate identification. EXCEEDS: By consistently meeting corporation and departmental dress standards and being recognized as a role model by peers and supervisors.			
4.4 Interpersonal relations with other health care workers are regularly fostered in a courteous and friendly manner as evidenced by supervisor observation and peer input. EXCEEDS: When the employee continuously exhibits self-initiated behaviors as outlined above.			
4.5 Resolves conflicts with staff members by following established communication norms with limited involvement by supervisor to initiate resolution. EXCEEDS: By expressing feelings and venting frustrations in an appropriate place and at an appropriate time as observed by peers and supervisors, and admitting personal error and taking corrective measures.			
4.6 Consistently receives and gives suggestions and constructive criticism in a professional manner.			
Total:			
Comments:			

Note. *From Harmarville Rehabilitation Center, Inc., Pittsburgh, PA. Reprinted by permission.*

Job Responsibilities & Performance Standards	Expectation		
	Below (−)	Meets (+)	Above (++)
5. Safety: Employee follows established safety precautions and procedures in the performance of all duties in order to ensure a safe environment.			
5.1 Regularly performs job tasks in accordance with hospital and departmental policy and procedures, including appropriate use of equipment and machines, appropriate use in wearing of physical barriers and safety equipment. EXCEEDS: By continuously meeting all safety procedures, being recognized as a role model by peers and supervisor, self-identifying nonroutine, potentially unsafe conditions and responding appropriately.			
5.2 Demonstrates a complete knowledge of body mechanics by consistent use in the work setting, as evidenced by no injuries sustained as a result of improper body mechanics in the evaluation period. EXCEEDS: By continuously using proper body mechanics, being recognized as a role model by peers and supervisor.			
5.3 Demonstrates a concern for cleanliness of self and work area, and practices proper infection control and universal precautions techniques. EXCEEDS: When there are no observable variances during the review period.			
5.4 Responds in accordance with emergency procedures to codes.			
5.5 Regularly maintains work area and equipment in a neat and orderly manner; assists in cleaning of the department, and corrects any malfunctioning equipment or environmental conditions, as observed by supervisor. EXCEEDS: By self-identifying additional tasks or activities and actively working toward completion.			
Total:			
Comments:			
6. Team Work/Responsibility: Demonstrates responsibility for individual performance and efficient utilization of products, supplies, equipment, and time to ensure the timely completion of duties and to promote financial viability through provision of services at a reasonable cost.			

Note. *From Harmarville Rehabilitation Center, Inc., Pittsburgh, PA. Reprinted by permission.*

Job Responsibilities & Performance Standards	Expectation		
	Below **(−)**	**Meets** **(+)**	**Above** **(++)**
6.1 Completes assigned duties and follows through with appropriate direction as determined by supervisor. EXCEEDS: By actively participating as an effective member of the department team by accepting additional assignments, including the training of new staff as assigned, seeking additional education or information regarding related skills.			
6.2 Provides proper notification for all absences or tardiness of scheduled shift and scheduled time off in accordance with corporate and departmental policies. EXCEEDS: By volunteering to assist the department in maintaining proper shift coverage.			
6.3 Consistently uses products, supplies, and equipment in an efficient manner, keeping waste within departmental limits as observed by peers and supervision. EXCEEDS: By regularly exceeding departmental standard and regularly suggesting more efficient ways to complete tasks.			
Total:			
Comments:			
7. Professional Growth and Development: Critically self-evaluates and improves proficiency in service delivery as observed by supervisor.			
7.1 Initiates request for clinical direction/assistance when situation is beyond scope of knowledge. EXCEEDS: When request reflects an analysis of the problem, patient performance, and possible alternatives.			
7.2 Identifies, on an annual basis, areas for growth and attends 2 continuing education opportunities that enhance patient care skills and job performance. EXCEEDS: When skills and job performance reflect understanding and integration of information and/or when information is formally shared at pod or departmental level.			

Note. *From Harmarville Rehabilitation Center, Inc., Pittsburgh, PA. Reprinted by permission.*

Job Responsibilities & Performance Standards

	Expectation		
	Below (−)	Meets (+)	Above (++)
7.3 Maintains ongoing record of attendance at continuing education opportunities and submits to Coordinator of Recruitment and Staff Development at the end of the fiscal year. EXCEEDS: When inservice records are maintained independently and submitted to Coordinator by July 15 on an annual basis.			
Total:			
Comments:			

Note. *From Harmarville Rehabilitation Center, Inc., Pittsburgh, PA. Reprinted by permission.*

Job Description/Performance Review   Job Title: Occupational Therapist, Registered

PERFORMANCE REVIEW SUMMARY

Overall assessment of performance: _____

_____

_____

Recommendation for salary increase (if any): _____

_____

Developmental Plan: Identify goals and timetables if appropriate: _____

_____

_____

Employee Comments: _____

_____

_____

_____

Reviewer's Comments: Discuss strengths and areas to be improved: _____

_____

_____

_____

ADMINISTRATIVE REVIEW

Reviewer's Signature	Title	Date
Employee's Signature	Title	Date

OTHER REQUIRED SIGNATURES (WITH DATES)

Signature	Title	Date
Signature	Title	Date

Note. This form is also used with the certified occupational therapy assistant.

Note. *From Harmarville Rehabilitation Center, Inc., Pittsburgh, PA. Reprinted by permission.*

HARMARVILLE REHABILITATION CENTER, INC.
OCCUPATIONAL THERAPY DEPARTMENT

Performance Review

Employee: _____

Performance Review Date: _____

STRENGTHS

AREAS FOR GROWTH

AREAS SHOWING IMPROVEMENT

GOALS TO BE ACCOMPLISHED BY   _____

Note. This form is also used with the certified occupational therapy assistant.

Note. *From Harmarville Rehabilitation Center, Inc., Pittsburgh, PA. Reprinted by permission.*

PERFORMANCE APPRAISAL SUPPLEMENT

In the past year, this employee has been able to demonstrate the knowledge and skills necessary to provide care appropriate to the age of the patients served in his/her area of responsibility. This individual has demonstrated and possesses the ability to assess data reflective of the patient's status and interpret the appropriate information needed to identify each patient's requirements relative to his/her age-specific needs, and to provide the care needed as described in the unit's/area's/department's policies and procedures.

FOR PATIENT CARE/TREATMENT POSITIONS—
CHECK AGES OF PATIENTS SERVED

❏ Pediatric

❏ Adolescent

❏ Young Adult

❏ Adult

❏ Geriatric

Reviewer's Signature	Title	Date
Employee's Signature	Title	Date

Distribution: Employee's personnel file with current year's performance appraisal.

Note. This form is also used with the certified occupational therapist assistant.

Note. *From Harmarville Rehabilitation Center, Inc., Pittsburgh, PA. Reprinted by permission.*

HAMARVILLE REHABILITATION CENTER, INC.
JOB DESCRIPTION/PERFORMANCE REVIEW

Job Title: Certified Occupational Therapy Assistant

Department: Occupational Therapy

Approved by:

Date of Original Approval: July 1, 1991

Date of Revision: September 15, 1994

Employee: _____

Performance Review Date: _____

Reports to: Occupational Therapy Supervisor

Review Type: _____ Annual
_____ Special

Salary Level: _____

Position Requirements:

Graduate of an AOTA-accredited occupational therapy assistant program, current certification with the AOTA as a certified occupational therapy assistant in the state of Pennsylvania. Related experience in occupational therapy with disabled adults preferred, Level II fieldwork experience in rehabilitation strongly preferred for newly graduated candidates.

Job Purpose:

To assist with goal setting, treatment planning, and implementation of occupational therapy services with a goal of facilitating the resumption of the patient's former life roles in a full or altered capacity.

Physical Demands:

Must be able to ambulate freely about the unit; must be able to see and hear normally or to normal range with assistive devices; must be able to perform occasional heavy lifting tasks; must be able to stoop, bend, stretch, and kneel; must be able to work safely with persons of infectious disease; must be cognitively and emotionally able to care for patients, observe their condition, perform treatments, and record results.

The above requires excellent general health and normal immune status; functional gait/ambulatory status adequate to perform job duties; normal vision and hearing abilities; acuity of 20/40 each eye and in both eyes alone or with corrective lenses, as measured by the Snellen Chart. Hearing grossly measured by whisper testing. Normal strength in extremity muscles as measured by manual muscle testing. Ability to display fair to excellent strength in back and abdominal muscles as measured by Krasu-Weber testing. No abnormalities inconsistent with job requirements found in x-rays. Normal cognitive ability and emotional state as observed during the process of taking the history and performing the physical examination, and during orientation process. Must be able to demonstrate safe and appropriate transfer activities.

Demonstrates manual dexterity to perform tasks required (i.e., splinting, patient evaluation, self-care, wheelchair positioning). Cognitively and emotionally able to communicate with patients and families, observe patient's performance, and adjust treatment accordingly.

Supervisory Responsibilities:

Note. *From Harmarville Rehabilitation Center, Inc., Pittsburgh, PA. Reprinted by permission.*

Job Description/Performance Review   Job Title: Certified Occupational Therapy Assistant

Job Responsibilities & Performance Standards	Expectation		
	Below (−)	Meets (+)	Above (++)
1. Contributes to evaluation process by obtaining pertinent information so that thorough and appropriate treatment may be planned and implemented as indicated by chart audit, OTR, or supervisor observation.			
1.1 Reviews physical medicine evaluation and history to obtain relevant information before COTA's initial session with patient 100% of the time and upon request, records in appropriate areas of evaluation. EXCEEDS: Before COTA's initial session with patient, by identifying potential problem areas and performance deficits based on medical record review and initiating discussion with managing OTR.			

1.2 As requested, accurately provides assessment information to managing OTR from structured evaluation and observations before patient's next scheduled occupational therapy session 100% of the time in the areas of:
a. Intake interview.
b. Physical daily living skills.
c. Sensorimotor skills.
    1) Gross/fine motor.
    2) General strength and endurance.
    3) Functional range of motion.
    4) Functional transfers.
d. Orientation and cognition.
 	
EXCEEDS: By recognizing need for modified or additional evaluations and/or suggesting realistic long-term goals.			

1.3 Initiates communication with managing OTR before patient's next occupational therapy session 100% of the time when changes in patient status are recognized. EXCEEDS: By offering alternatives/options for change in goals and/or treatment plan.			
Total:			
Comments:			

Note. *From Harmarville Rehabilitation Center, Inc., Pittsburgh, PA. Reprinted by permission.*

Job Responsibilities & Performance Standards	Expectation		
	Below (−)	Meets (+)	Above (++)
2. Provides quality occupational therapy treatment to ensure optimum patient recovery/adaptation as observed by managing OTR, unit supervisor, or senior clinician, and/or through chart review.			
2.1 Implements treatment plan in accordance with departmental, team, and patient goals with the use of creative, life-role activities 100% of the time. EXCEEDS: By consistently enhancing patient's level of motivation and by routinely incorporating inter-disciplinary team information into treatment.			
2.2 Coverage is provided in assistant's absence 100% of the time. EXCEEDS: When coverage plans are detailed, goal directed, and outcome oriented.			
2.3 Complies with departmental productivity expectations 100% of the time. EXCEEDS: When statistics reflect productivity 10% above expectations on an annual basis.			
2.4 Identifies need for and in conjunction with OTR, provides family/caregiver education relevant to patient status 100% of the time. EXCEEDS: When family performance abilities, concerns, and reactions to the patient's program (or lack of participation) are documented 100% of the time.			
2.5 Demonstrated knowledge of roles/functions of other members of the Occupational Therapy Department 100% of the time, eliciting appropriate assistance and supervising/coordinating services for each patient as requested. EXCEEDS: When interactions are directive, timely, and respectful of others' areas of expertise.			
2.6 Promotes carryover of occupational therapy inter-ventions upon discharge by providing appropriate home and/or community programming recom-mendations as requested. EXCEEDS: When customized home programs are developed and presented to managing OTR before providing to patient and/or family.			

Note. *From Harmarville Rehabilitation Center, Inc., Pittsburgh, PA. Reprinted by permission.*

Job Responsibilities & Performance Standards	Expectation		
	Below (−)	Meets (+)	Above (++)
2.7 Assists managing OTR with assessing priorities for patient treatment and implements accordingly 100% of the time. EXCEEDS: By initiating alternatives/options for managing priorities for patient treatment.			
2.8 As scheduled, pre-plans and implements goal-directed, age-relevant, functionally oriented group sessions. EXCEEDS: By recognizing patients who will not benefit from planned group activities, make recommendations for, and ensuring provision of more customized treatment approaches.			
Total:			
Comments:			
3. Communicates information relevant to patient care to ensure quality service delivery and maximum reimbursement as observed by managing OTR or unit supervisor, or through chart review.			
3.1 Completes assigned documentation according to departmental protocols, including but not limited to: initial evaluations, progress notes, discharge summaries, prescriptions, PDLS cards, and nonroutine instructions in the nonmedical section of the chart, 100% of the time.			
3.2 Communicates information relevant to patient status/ performance to managing OTR within 24 hours of observation 100% of the time. EXCEEDS: When information is provided in an efficient and professional manner and reflects consideration of potential programmatic/approach modifications.			
3.3 Ensures that all treatment and equipment charges are entered within 24 hours of service delivery 85% of the time. EXCEEDS: When accomplished 95% of the time.			
3.4 Provides information necessary for ongoing program evaluation and quality assurance studies as requested. EXCEEDS: By identifying potential quality problems or areas for study and reporting those to supervisor.			

Note. *From Harmarville Rehabilitation Center, Inc., Pittsburgh, PA. Reprinted by permission.*

Job Responsibilities & Performance Standards	Expectation		
	Below (−)	Meets (+)	Above (++)
3.5 Provides relevant information regarding patient's functional skills and performance at scheduled staffing conferences or informs assigned representative as requested. EXCEEDS: When completed in an efficient and professional manner.			
3.6 Informs patient/and or significant others of evaluation findings and treatment rationale at their level of understanding 100% of the time. EXCEEDS: When presented in a manner that is conducive to integration and interaction.			
3.7 Communicates with other health care personnel regarding patient care as necessary. EXCEEDS: When routinely initiates discussions.			
Total:			
Comments:			
4. Guest/Employee Relations: Demonstrates regard for the dignity of and respect for all patients, their families, guests, and representatives of other organizations as well as fellow employees, volunteers, and medical staff in support of the corporation's mission to provide consistent quality health care services in a professional, caring, and responsive environment.			
4.1 Maintains confidentiality of patient and of patient and departmental information with no infractions as noted by supervision.			
4.2 Consistently displays a caring and responsive attitude and represents the corporation in a positive manner and conducts all activities respecting patient/customer rights and expectations. EXCEEDS: By consistently making extra efforts to achieve patient/customer expectations while discharging job responsibilities.			
4.3 Regularly maintains a neat appearance and adheres to departmental/corporation dress, including the wearing of appropriate identification. EXCEEDS: By consistently meeting corporation and departmental dress standards and being recognized as a role model by peers and supervisors.			

Note. *From Harmarville Rehabilitation Center, Inc., Pittsburgh, PA. Reprinted by permission.*

Job Responsibilities & Performance Standards	Expectation		
	Below (−)	**Meets** (+)	**Above** (++)
4.4 Interpersonal relations with other health care workers are regularly fostered in a courteous and friendly manner as evidenced by supervisor observation and peer input. EXCEEDS: When the employee continuously exhibits self-initiated behaviors as outlined above.			
4.5 Resolves conflicts with staff members by following established communication norms with limited involvement by supervisor to initiate resolution. EXCEEDS: By expressing feelings and venting frustrations in an appropriate place and at an appropriate time as observed by peers and supervisors, and admits personal error and taking corrective measures.			
4.6 Consistently receives and gives suggestions and constructive criticism in a professional manner.			
Total:			
Comments:			
5. Safety: Employee follows established safety precautions and procedures in the performance of all duties in order to ensure a safe environment.			
5.1 Regularly performs job tasks in accordance with hospital and departmental policy and procedures, including appropriate use of equipment and machines, appropriate use in wearing of physical barriers and safety equipment. EXCEEDS: By continuously meeting all safety procedures, being recognized as a role model by peers and supervisor, self-identifying nonroutine, potentially unsafe conditions and responding appropriately.			
5.2 Demonstrates a complete knowledge of body mechanics by consistent use in the work setting, as evidenced by no injuries sustained as a result of improper body mechanics in the evaluation period. EXCEEDS: By continuously using proper body mechanics, being recognized as role model by peers and supervisor.			
5.3 Demonstrates a concern for cleanliness of self and work area, and practices proper infection control and universal precautions techniques. EXCEEDS: When there are no observable variances during the review period.			

Note. *From Harmarville Rehabilitation Center, Inc., Pittsburgh, PA. Reprinted by permission.*

Job Responsibilities & Performance Standards	Expectation		
	Below (–)	**Meets** (+)	**Above** (++)
5.4 Responds in accordance with emergency procedures to codes.			
5.5 Regularly maintains work area and equipment in a neat and orderly manner; assists in cleaning of the department, and corrects any malfunctioning equipment or environmental conditions, as observed by supervisor. EXCEEDS: By self-identifying additional tasks or activities and actively working toward completion.			
Total:			
Comments:			
6. Teamwork/Responsibility: Demonstrates responsibility for individual performance and efficient utilization of products, supplies, equipment, and time to ensure the timely completion of duties and to promote financial viability through provision of services at a reasonable cost.			
6.1 Completes assigned duties and follows through with appropriate direction as determined by supervisor. EXCEEDS: By actively participating as an effective member of the department team by accepting additional assignments, including the training of new staff as assigned, seeking additional education or information regarding related skills.			
6.2 Provides proper notification for all absences or tardiness of scheduled shift and scheduled time off in accordance with corporate and departmental policies. EXCEEDS: By volunteering to assist the department in maintaining proper shift coverage.			
6.3 Consistently uses products, supplies, and equipment in an efficient manner, keeping waste within departmental limits as observed by peers and supervision. EXCEEDS: By regularly exceeding departmental standard and regularly suggesting more efficient ways to complete tasks.			
Total:			
Comments:			

Job Responsibilities & Performance Standards	Expectation		
	Below (−)	Meets (+)	Above (++)
7. Professional Growth and Development: Critically self-evaluates and improves proficiency in service delivery as observed by supervisor.			
7.1 Initiates request for clinical direction/assistance when situation is beyond scope of knowledge. EXCEEDS: When request reflects an analysis of the problem, patient performance, and possible alternatives.			
7.2 Identifies, on an annual basis, areas for growth and attends 2 continuing education opportunities that enhance patient care skills and job performance. EXCEEDS: When skills and job performance reflect understanding and integration of information and/or when information is formally shared at pod or departmental level.			
7.3 Maintains ongoing record of attendance at continuing education opportunities and submits to Coordinator of Recruitment and Staff Development at the end of the fiscal year. EXCEEDS: When inservice records are maintained independently and submitted to Coordinator by July 15 on an annual basis.			
Total:			
Comments:			

Note. From Harmarville Rehabilitation Center, Inc., Pittsburgh, PA. Reprinted by permission.

APPENDIX 10-C

Recruiters: A Student Guide

As a graduating student, a newcomer to the field of occupational therapy, you surely will come into contact with a group of individuals called RECRUITERS, who will want to assist you in finding the job of your choice.

Recruiters, or placement specialists, are companies or individuals who work for both sides of the industry: the employer and the employee. The employers may be hospitals, school systems, nursing homes, private companies, or any facility that employs therapists. The occupational therapy practitioner, or potential employee (possibly you), uses the recruiter to find a suitable job placement. The goal of the recruiter is to make matches between the potential employee and employer.

HOW RECRUITERS WORK

A recruiter generally secures resumes of potential OTRs and COTAs by a variety of means—for example, by contacting attendees at conferences, calling from licensure lists or graduating class rosters, or calling other health care facilities.

Once the recruiter has talked to the applicant and received his or her resume, the recruiter works to find a placement that suits the applicant's career wants and needs. This may involve contacting facilities with known vacancies, or, if the applicant has specific preferences, calling several facilities in a particular region or specialty. This does not prevent the therapist from seeking employment on his or her own, or from using other recruiters from other companies.

The recruiter usually receives a facility request to routinely fill vacancies with their recruits or will call facilities to offer placement of actual or anticipated recruits.

Once the request is received, the recruiter will send the facility a confirmation of the request and a copy of the fees charged. There is no cost to the therapist for the recruiter's services: the potential employer bears the cost. The cost to an employer can be up to 30% of the therapist's first-year's salary. For example, if XYZ Hospital in Somewhere, USA, hires Sally OT for $30,000 from a recruitment company, that recruiter receives up to 30% of $30,000, or $9,000, payable immediately upon Sally's employment.

CONSIDER THE PROS & CONS OF USING A RECRUITER

ADVANTAGES:

- They may assist in resume preparation.
- They can expedite a match between therapists with specific location or specialty requirements.
- They can save time in looking for positions.
- They can help with confidential searches.

DISADVANTAGES:

- Some recruiters are persistent and use aggressive business tactics, e.g., representation without written permission of the OT practitioner.

OTHER OPTIONS:

There are many other options and avenues to follow when seeking employment, such as:

1. Word of mouth,
2. Local newspaper advertising,
3. Professional journals/newspapers,
4. State association job placement listings,
5. State association newsletters,
6. University placement services,
7. University career days,
8. Annual and state conferences,
9. Referrals from friends already in the field,
10. AOTA's *OT Week*

QUESTIONS TO ASK RECRUITERS

Seeking a job can be an exciting opportunity, but it is important to be adequately prepared and aware of all that is required of you before you begin to work. Do not be afraid to ask questions to ensure that you have a clear understanding of the job description, benefit package, and stability of the company. Similarly you may wish to seek legal advice with respect to the terms of a proposed employment agreement prior to signing on. All recruiters are not the same. Increase your opportunity for success by exploring answers to the following questions.

WORKING CONDITIONS

- What is the type and amount of clinical support that will be received? Who will provide it?

- What is the staff/patient ratio at the facility? How many and what types of clients are expected on caseload? What happens when patient numbers drop?

- Will there be a team or accessible network of OTs to consult with?

- Is there a requirement to supervise support personnel and students?

- Does the state require licensure in addition to certification?

THE EMPLOYMENT AGREEMENT

- What is the employment term (length of time, start/end date)? Is employment guaranteed by the recruitment facility for this length of time? What occurs if work cannot be found?

- Are there provisions for you to select your employment setting? Will the company find work that meets your approval? What occurs if you do not approve of or refuse the placement setting?

- What are the process and the terms for repayment if you/the facility/the recruitment company does not honor the contract?

RECRUITING COMPANY CREDENTIALS

- What are the terms of the contract between the recruitment company and the employment facility? Is it more than just one placement?

- What is the company's success rate of placement?

- Is the company willing to provide references or contact numbers of therapists or facilities that have used its services?

FINANCIAL

- What wages and benefits will you receive and how will they be calculated (salary, bonus, medical, dental, holidays, vacation)? How often and with what method will you be paid?

- What provisions are available for professional growth (e.g., education/conference allowance)?

- Will the recruitment company pay for travel costs (mileage, car, accommodation), if you are hired as a traveling therapist? Relocation costs?

- If you fly in for an interview and do not get offered a job, or you do not accept a position, will the company fully reimburse you for your travel expenses?

IF RECRUITERS CALL . . .

- Interview them regarding their success rate of placements, request references, and explore with them what they plan to do with your resume and what the entire process is.

- This will help you determine if the recruiter has your best interests in mind.

- Each recruiter is different, and methods of recruiting and placement differ.

- Think before you act, and ask lots of questions before deciding to have a recruiter represent you.

- Be wise in your dealings with recruiters and realize the first point of contact is a business arrangement.

THE CHOICE IS YOURS

As one of the newest occupational therapy practitioners joining our profession, there are many choices to think about. The choice is yours to use a recruiter or not. Be sure you fully understand exactly what the recruiter is going to do for you, and weigh your options before sending a recruiter your resume.

Developed by the Administration and Management SIS Standing Committee 1991, revised 1996 with assistance of the Canadian Association of Occupational Therapy.

For detailed information on preemployment agreements, please refer to "Strategies for Negotiating Preemployment Agreements," by R. Perry & P. Crist, 1994, *American Journal of Occupational Therapy, 48*(9).

APPENDIX 10-D

Significant Federal Legislation on Employment

AMERICANS WITH DISABILITIES ACT OF 1990 (29 U.S.C. § 706)

Prohibits discrimination against qualified persons with disabilities in employment, public services, transportation, accommodations, and telecommunication services.

An individual with a disability is defined as a person with a physical or mental impairment that substantially limits one or more major life activities; a person having a record of such an impairment; or a person regarded as having such an impairment.

Title I: Employment Discrimination

- Employers may not discriminate against an individual with a disability in hiring or promotion if the person is otherwise qualified for the job.

- Employers can ask about one's ability to perform a job but cannot inquire if someone has a disability nor can employers subject a person to tests that tend to screen out people with disabilities.

- Employers must provide "reasonable accommodation" to individuals with disabilities unless such accommodations would impose an "undue hardship" on business operations.

- Employers must make and document efforts to eliminate barriers that would prevent successful employment of an individual with disabilities. Reasonable accommodation may include making existing facilities readily accessible, job restructuring, modification of work schedules, acquisition or modification of equipment, devices, materials or policies, provision of qualified readers or interpreters and other similar accommodations.

- An "undue hardship" on business operations means an action requiring significant difficulty or expense in relation to the overall financial resources of the covered employer.

- Employers may reject applicants or fire employees who pose a direct threat (a significant risk which cannot be eliminated by reasonable accommodation) to the health or safety of others in the workplace.

- Applicants and employees who are current users of drugs have no rights to claim discrimination on the basis of their illegal drug use under the ADA. Drug testing is not prohibited by the ADA.

- Employers may not discriminate against a qualified applicant or employee because of the known disability of an individual with whom the applicant or employee is known to have a relationship or association.

- Religious organizations may give preference in employment to their own members and may require applicants and employees to conform to their religious tenets.

Title II: Public Services of State and Local Governments

- State or local government, and departments, agencies or other components of government, may not discriminate against, exclude, or deny individuals with disabilities with regard to participation in or benefiting from the services, programs or activities of a public entity.

Title III: Public Accommodations and Services Operated by Private Entities

Places of public accommodation, including hospitals, professional offices of health care providers, day care centers, schools and other places of accommodation, shall not discriminate against individuals with disabilities in participation in or benefiting from a good, service, facility or other accommodation.

Auxiliary aids and services must be provided to individuals with vision or hearing impairments or other individuals with disabilities, unless an undue burden would result.

Physical barriers in existing facilities must be removed if removal is readily achievable, meaning easily accomplished and able to be carried out without much difficulty or expense.

All new construction for public accommodations must be accessible.

AGE DISCRIMINATION IN EMPLOYMENT ACT OF 1967
(29 U.S.C. § 621)

Prohibits discriminatory employment practices that unfairly affect workers 40 years old and older. Also prohibits employers from requiring older workers to retire at a given age.

TITLE VII OF THE CIVIL RIGHTS ACT OF 1964
(42 U.S.C. § 2000E)

Prohibits discrimination in employment based on sex, race, color, religion, or national origin.

CIVIL SERVICE REFORM ACT OF 1978
(U.S.C. § 7116)

Prohibits unfair labor practices by labor organizations representing federal employees. Prohibits discrimination on the basis of handicapping condition with regard to membership in the labor organization.

REHABILITATION ACT OF 1973, SEC. 504
(29 U.S.C. § 791–794)

Requires each federal agency to develop action plans for hiring, placement, and advancement of handicapped persons. Further, for federal contracts over $2,500, requires contractors to take affirmative action to employ handicapped persons. Discrimination on the basis of disability is prohibited in any program or activity receiving federal assistance.

JOB TRAINING PARTNERSHIP ACT (JTPA)
(29 U.S.C. § 1577)

Prohibits exclusion from participation, denial of benefits, and employment and other discrimination on the basis of handicap in programs receiving funds under JTPA.

OMNIBUS BUDGET RECONCILIATION ACT OF 1981
(42 U.S.C. § 300, 708, 5309, 9849, 9906)

Affirms application of Section 504 of the Rehabilitation Act of 1973 (prohibiting discrimination in federally funded programs) to the following:

- Preventive health and health services block grants

- Alcohol and drug abuse and mental health services block grants

- Primary care block grants

- Maternal and child health services block grants

- Community development programs

- Head Start programs

- Community services block grants

DEVELOPMENTAL DISABILITIES ASSISTANCE ACT
AND BILL OF RIGHTS ACT
(42 U.S.C. § 6005)

Requires entities receiving funds through this program to take affirmative action to employ and advance persons with disabilities.

APPENDIX 10-E — APPLICANT INTERVIEW ANALYSIS

APPLICANT INTERVIEW ANALYSIS   *Harmarville Rehabilitation Centers*

Name of Applicant: _____ Date of Interview: _____

Time if Interview: _____

Candidate for: _____ _____ Interview: _____

Please report your interview impressions by checking the one most appropriate box in each area

1. APPEARANCE
❑ Untidy
❑ Somewhat careless about personal appearance.
❑ Satisfactory personal appearance.
❑ Better than average appearance.

2. PERSONALITY
❑ Appears very distant and aloof.
❑ Approachable; fairly friendly.
❑ Warm; friendly; sociable.
❑ Very sociable and outgoing.

3. POISE-STABILITY
❑ Ill at ease; is "jumpy" and appears nervous.
❑ Somewhat tense; is easily irritated.
❑ About as poised as the average person.
❑ Sure of self; well composed.

4. COMMUNICATION ABILITY
❑ Expresses self poorly.
❑ Does less than average job at expressing self.
❑ Average fluency and expression.
❑ Communicates well.

5. ALERTNESS
❑ Appears slow to "catch on".
❑ Appears rather slow; requires more than average explanation.
❑ Appears to grasp ideas with average ability.
❑ Appears quick to understand; perceives very well.

6. KNOWLEDGE OF FIELD
❑ Appears to have poor knowledge of field.
❑ Appears to have some knowledge of field.
❑ An average amount of knowledge is demonstrated.
❑ Appears to have excellent knowledge of field.

7. EXPERIENCE IN FIELD
❑ No relationship between applicant's background and job requirements.
❑ Fair relationship between applicant's background and job requirements.
❑ Average amount of meaningful background and experience.
❑ Excellent background considerable experience in field.

8. DRIVE
❑ Appears to have poorly defined goals.
❑ Appears to set goals too low.
❑ Appears to have average goals.
❑ Appears to have high desire to achieve.

9. OVERALL
❑ Definitely unsatisfactory candidate.
❑ Substandard candidate.
❑ Average candidate.
❑ Definitely above average candidate.
❑ Outstanding candidate.

Notes: _____
_____
_____

This applicant should be considered further ❑ Yes   ❑ No   If no, state reason: _____
_____

If YES — Request reference check ❑ Yes   ❑ No _____
_____

If NO, would you recommend consideration at future date for this or any other position? _____

❑ Yes   ❑ No   Remarks: _____
_____

Additional comments: _____
_____

Salary Quote: _____ Start date: _____ Status: _____

RETURN COMPLETED FORM TO HUMAN RESOURCES

Note. *From Harmarville Rehabilitation Center, Inc., Pittsburgh, PA. Reprinted with permission.*

APPENDIX 10-F — FORM FOR "UPWARD" APPRAISAL

Staff Feedback

Date: _____

Name: _____ **Supervisor's Name:** _____

Self-Assessment

What do you see as your strengths?

What do you need to improve?

What accomplishments this year are you most proud of?

What do you want to work on in the coming year?

Assessment of Supervisor

What do you see as your supervisor's strengths?

How would you like to see your supervisor change or improve?

Are there any additional actions that your supervisor should take to improve your performance?

Assessment of Organization

What do you like best about working here?

What do you like least about working here?

What should the organization do to improve the care of patients?

What should the organization do to improve employees' satisfaction?

What would you be willing to do to help improve the organization's functioning?

CHAPTER 11

Roles, Relationships, and Career Development

Patricia Crist, PhD, OTR, FAOTA

KEY TERMS

Career. The sequence of positions that a person occupies in the course of his or her work history.

Career development. Progressive growth in a career.

Departmentalization. The division of labor among specialists who need coordination and leadership.

Empowerment. The ability to exercise influence and have authority within a system.

Organizational chart. A graphic representation of chains of command and position-designated authority.

Organizational structure. An organization's framework (Robbins, 1994), specifying the relationship between roles and role responsibility.

Policy. A guide that establishes a parameter for making decisions (Robbins, 1994).

Procedure. A series of interrelated sequential steps that can be used to respond to a structured problem (Robbins, 1994).

Role. "A set of behavior patterns expected of someone occupying a given position in a social unit" (Robbins, 1994, p. 445).

Role responsibility. The obligation to perform assigned job tasks.

Patricia Crist, PhD, OTR, FAOTA, is a professor and the chair of the Department of Occupational Therapy at Duquesne University. A manager herself, she chaired the AOTA task force that developed "Occupational Therapy Roles" and has taught and written on the topics of roles, systems, and fieldwork. Her doctorate is from the University of Northern Colorado.

Organizations provide a structure in which employees can per- form work efficiently and effectively. Structure in an organiza- tion produces stability and predictability. Stability and pre- dictability provide a foundation for consistently accomplishing routine or regular work tasks, as planning, organizing, and negotiating cease to be necessary. Stability and predictability also decrease the amount of super- vision needed for routine tasks. The structure of an organization engen- ders understanding among its component parts and conveys knowledge and expectations regarding the contribution of the component parts to the work of the organization.

Organizations provide this valuable structure through roles and rela- tionships. Thus it is important for occupational therapy managers to understand these organizational components. Roles specify positions or sets of prescribed occupational responsibilities. Relationships connect the various roles to one another, creating working organizations. In combina- tion, roles and relationships explain interactions and define expectations. They also facilitate change and enhance growth. When new ideas or inno- vations are under consideration in a work environment, changes in roles and relationships are also necessary.

An understanding of roles and relationships can also help managers plan and guide career development—their own and that of their staff members. Roles in organizations are defined in terms of jobs. Roles in pro- fessions are defined in terms of common sets of tasks. A given employment role may consist of several professional roles. Current career development is the result of previous choices about roles and relationships in organiza- tions. Future career development is based on an understanding of the options and the skills required to perform other roles in organizations. Thus roles, relationships, and career development are interdependent.

ROLES AND RELATIONSHIPS

A *role* is "a set of behavior patterns expected of someone occupying a given position in a social unit" (Robbins, 1994, p. 445). All persons in a social unit or an organization have a role. In fact, most persons play multiple roles. Roles in social units typically relate to behaviors used during group interaction. Roles in organizations typically reflect the primary purpose of the role. For example, the role of fieldwork educator on a rehabilitation team reflects the responsibility of training students. Any given role fits within a specific organization, and within this framework there are statements of relationships, influence, and control related to a role. Thus a role reflects expectations for job performance and gives direction regarding supervision, authority, and even power. Roles are important in organizations because each role has a specific set of responsibilities and expectations relative to outcomes. Any system depends on the outcomes of specific role performance.

PERSPECTIVES ON ROLES

In an open system or organization, roles are interactive. They are the structural component that specifies relationships among members of an organization. These relationships, not roles themselves, are the energy and the motivation for systems to be responsive, creative, and productive. As Wheatley (1992) states, "Roles and structure are created from need and interest; relationships, exchanges, and connections among employees are nurtured as the primary source of organizational creativity and success" (p. 117).

In traditional organizations, roles are the outcome of formal structures created to delineate the internal flow of power and authority. Expertise in performing a particular task or function in an organization accompanies a particular role and is frequently reflected in the role's title. For example, a *staff* occupational therapist staffs—that is, provides direct services to patients; an occupational therapy *supervisor* supervises staff members; and so on. In traditional organizations, roles specify relationships to the roles immediately above (supervisor) and immediately below (supervisee) an employee as information flows up and down the hierarchy. This provides employees with stability and makes performance predictable.

In the new type of organization, the learning organization (Senge, 1990; see chapter 7, "Organizational Effectiveness"), roles are viewed slightly differently. They are not boundaries or limitations, but the energy to create new solutions in order to perform work better (Wheatley, 1992). The focus is not on what position takes care of a problem, but on what energy, skill, or influence and wisdom are available to contribute to the solution (Pacanowski, 1988). As the systems approach to organizational effectiveness spreads, inter- and intra-organizational relationships become more important than roles that are perceived as rigid and inflexible, if not incapable of responding to environmental demands. For example, in this time of rapid reform in health care, the key to survival is not to cling to specified roles but to form new roles and relationships in the emerging system. Attention to roles alone focuses on the parts of an organization, not on the related processes. Relationships facilitate the flow of information throughout layers of organizational hierarchy. In learning organizations, specifying roles is a hindrance to inter- and intra-organizational exchanges (Wheatley, 1992).

This shift in perspective on roles and relationships permeates business. Attention to how effective organizations work is essential in health care too, as reform goes forward. For example, private practices and contract organizations in occupational therapy are scurrying to establish relationships as part of managed care systems. Institutions that provide occupational therapy as a specific service are seeking alliances with larger health care systems to be part of the seamless system of the future. In addition, rehabilitation professionals are forming new interdisciplinary alliances, which are redefining work relationships and in some cases even roles. In the years ahead, roles will be important only in establishing expertise to perform a specific service. Roles that specify rigid order, reduce ability to perform for the greater good of the organization, or limit a system's response to new demands from the environment will not be evident in dynamic systems.

PROFESSIONAL RESPONSIBILITIES

Professions, as a special kind of group providing resources for systems, have their own role definitions to facilitate communication regarding mastery or competency. These professional role functions reflect values and needs in relation to current social and cultural demands. For example, with health care decreasing the length of stay in hospitals, dependence on good caregiving from family members has markedly increased. Thus the role of consumer educator in occupational therapy is increasing in prevalence. There is no longer the luxury of training patients until they learn skills. Instead, occupational therapy practitioners instruct family caregivers in techniques to use after discharge.

Regardless of the specific roles that occupational therapy practitioners perform, the individual practitioner must understand that he or she typically occupies more than one role within a system and should strategically use the related responsibilities to empower himself or herself to influence the system positively. *Empowerment,* or the ability to exercise influence and have authority within a system, depends on (1) organization of work, (2) definition of roles, (3) determination of supervisees' behavior, and (4) establishment of boundaries and goals for performance. The key to using roles effectively is to be able to form relationships and alliances with important persons within a system and to ensure that requisite information is available to support role functions and organizational processes.

The word *roles* takes on various meanings today depending on need and experience. Just as roles are important to a client's reengagement in society, professional roles specify an occupational therapy practitioner's contribution to the delivery of health care. Each role carries specific performance expectations and responsibilities. In the past the role of occupational therapy practitioner on a health care team was central to role definition in the profession. However, roles have been influenced not only by the changing health care system but by the types of systems in which occupational therapy practitioners practice. Providing services in schools and industry, in addition to hospitals, has required the profession to broaden its perspective on roles and functions. Likewise, there are differences between occupational therapy roles in academic and clinical environments. The system within which a practitioner provides occupational therapy services requires a clarification of role regarding professional responsibility to maintain flexible relationships.

ORGANIZATIONAL STRUCTURE AND DESIGN

Organizational structure describes an organization's framework (Robbins, 1994). Formal rules and procedures direct the behaviors of employees in organizations. Organizational structure specifies the relationship between roles and role responsibility. *Role responsibility* is the obligation to perform assigned job tasks. In *organizational design,* managers construct or change organizational structure to respond to a system's needs. Over 60 years old, the concepts of organizational structure and design are salient today for managers as means of planning and controlling effective and efficient organizations. Managers create and use organizational charts to identify unity of command, to stipulate authority and power, and to specify chain of command. Robbins (1994) provides definitions for each of these key terms related to organizational structure: *Unity of command* is the principle that a worker should have only one direct supervisor; having multiple bosses can present conflicting expectations. *Authority* is the rights accorded to a person in a managerial role who gives orders and expects them to be obeyed. Authority is inherent in a position, not a person; that is, when a person leaves a position that has authority, the authority remains with the position. *Power* is a person's capacity to influence decisions. Authority relates to a person's position in an organization, whereas power is the method a person uses to direct human performance. *Chain of command* reflects the flow of authority from top management to the bottom of the organization.

An *organizational chart* is a graphic representation of chains of command and position-designated authority. Major roles within an organization are included in an organizational chart so that individual employees understand where they are in the organization, who their supervisor is, and when appropriate, whom they direct or command. The chain of command and administrative authority is represented by vertical relationships among roles. Persons or roles with similar levels of authority within the organization are represented in a horizontal arrangement. In figure 11-1 the chief executive officer has authority over the executive vice-president. The executive vice-president has authority over the four vice-presidents. The vice-presidents manage specific operations within the organization, but their fundamental administrative responsibilities are at the same level; they do not supervise one another.

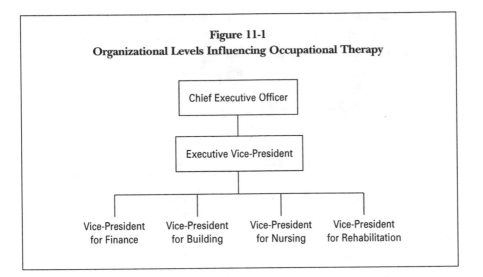

Figure 11-1
Organizational Levels Influencing Occupational Therapy

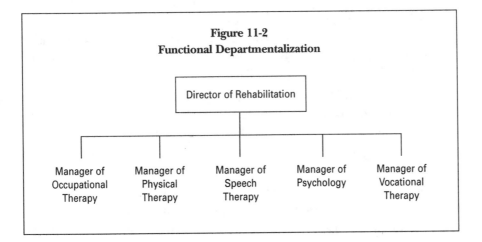

Figure 11-2
Functional Departmentalization

An organizational chart depicts *departmentalization,* or the division of labor among specialists who need coordination and leadership. Departmentalization is based on roles or work tasks.

Managers can use a variety of organizational charting methods to depict departmentalization, depending on the objectives and the goals of the organization. Robbins (1994) identifies five approaches: (1) functional, (2) product, (3) customer, (4) geographic, and (5) process. The explanations of each approach that follow identify an example in occupational therapy practice and review it in terms of general strengths and weaknesses.

Functional departmentalization is the grouping of an organization's activities by function. For example, a department of rehabilitation might be organized around the different service delivery professions, as in figure 11-2. Organizing by function or professional discipline is a traditional approach in many hospitals and rehabilitation centers. The strength of this model is intradisciplinary communication and support. The weakness is potential for interdisciplinary turf wars or conflict.

Product departmentalization is the grouping of organizational components by product line, or service. As figure 11-3 shows, the manager has considerable control over the overall program. Functions or professions are replicated under each major product. This approach to designing rehabilitation services is rapidly growing in popularity. The strength of the model is that the team in each service can become highly specialized in its particular area and very efficient in delivering services. The weakness is that practitioners do not receive supervision or daily support from someone in their own discipline.

Customer departmentalization is the grouping of an organization into component activities on the basis of common consumers. Figure 11-4 illustrates customer departmentalization of an occupational therapy department. The strength of this organizational structure is that practitioners become highly specialized in a comprehensive program for a particular group of patients or referrals. The weakness is that staff members lose flexibility to treat in other areas and may lose perspective on shared departmental goals.

Geographic departmentalization, an emerging organizational structure, is based on geography or location. It has applications in two kinds of organizations: large contract organizations and managed care systems. Because of their size and their geographic comprehensiveness, large contract organizations use this approach to oversee services on a regional basis. This

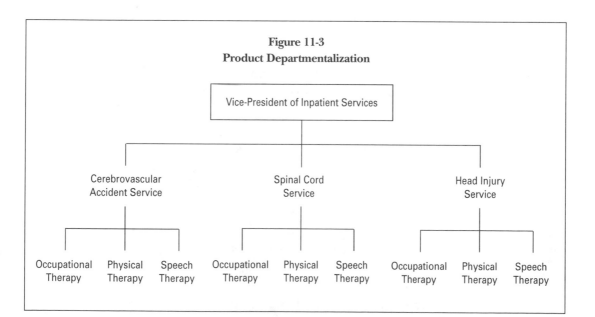

Figure 11-3
Product Departmentalization

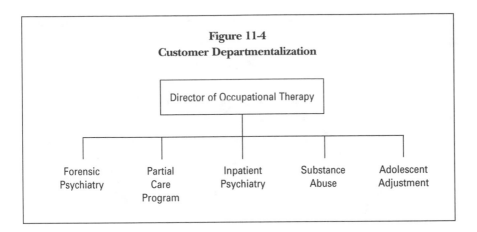

Figure 11-4
Customer Departmentalization

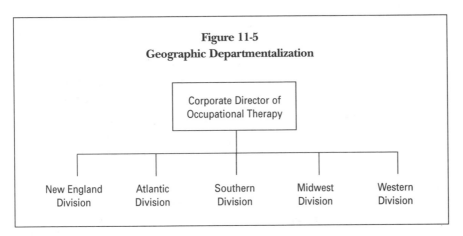

Figure 11-5
Geographic Departmentalization

model is presented in figure 11-5. A second application is emerging in managed care. For example, a health maintenance organization may have numerous satellites in a city, with replication of essential services at each site or provision of specialty services at single locations. The first approach offers easy access to consumers; the second creates efficiency in operation. The strength of this kind of organizational structure is that resources are located where services are needed or provided. The negative side is that staff members may experience professional isolation and limited role definition. Further, the quality of management across locations may vary considerably, thus creating variation in the quality of service based on location.

Process departmentalization is the grouping of activities by flow of product or consumer. In figure 11-6, occupational therapy services are organized around the major components of the service delivery continuum. This approach is compartmentalized. It is successful when a high degree of cooperation and coordination occurs among the units, decreasing consumers' perception of duplication of services and ultimately increasing efficiency. The challenge with this approach is to deliver

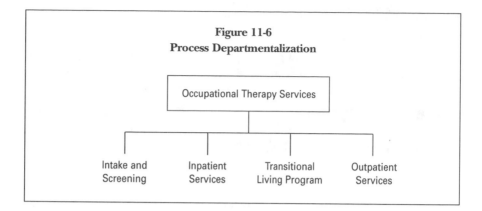

Figure 11-6
Process Departmentalization

services so that transitions between departments are effortless for the consumer and information is shared openly and easily at each step. For example, evaluations completed during intake and screening should be meaningfully related throughout treatment and be used by later services. Critical pathways can be organized within managed care systems using the process model.

ROLES AND CAREER DEVELOPMENT

Role, or the ability to provide a set of expected behaviors, varies on the basis of educational preparation, professional boundaries and responsibilities, and previous experience in the role. Participation in various roles develops into careers. A *career* is the sequence of positions that a person occupies in the course of his or her work history. Professional philosophy and responsibilities within systems permeate careers, helping determine role options. For example, the background of occupational therapy practitioners makes the role of case manager a viable one for them, but contributes little to their ability to be fiscal managers. Likewise, advancement in roles can contribute to career development that engages new skills. For example, an occupational therapy practitioner who plans to become a middle or top manager may earn a master's degree in business administration to perform better an administrative role that requires management of fiscal resources.

Career development is progressive growth in a career. Career development can also be an organization's mission for its personnel. Development in a career can occur randomly, or purposefully through personal choices guided by on-the-job-training, continuing education, and involvement in structured programs such as advanced education and specialty certification. Effective organizations include career development in their personnel practices because it ensures the presence of requisite skills in the workforce, helps provide equal opportunities for persons with diverse backgrounds, and aids in both recruitment and retention of competent personnel.

With the reengineering of health care in the 1990s, career development in many organizations is more likely to occur through lateral moves than through vertical advancement. Most health care organizations are flattening their management hierarchies, leaving few options for ascent on the career ladder within one organization. Whereas lateral career shifts were previously seen primarily as options for mediocre workers, they are now viewed as viable career options because (1) they provide a wider range of experiences to develop skill mastery and competency in a role within an organization, (2) they can enhance long-term mobility across organizations, and (3) the novelty of a new environment can energize work.

Careers and career development can occur through two types of roles: specific roles in an organization and roles that are recognized by a profession. Thus in reality, careers, career development, and roles can be situation specific, as in an organization, or reflect professional boundaries.

ORGANIZATIONS AND ROLE OPTIONS

Human resources in an organization consist of workers performing specific job responsibilities to meet organizational goals. In organizations, roles are frequently encapsulated in job titles that describe the major job function. These job titles are linked together in functional organizational charts. Figures 11-7 and -8 are examples of typical organizational structures for occupational therapy—an academic department in a university (figure 11-7) and a clinical department in a hospital (figure 11-8). In the organizational chart for the hospital, the supervisor of the mental health program is responsible to the chief of occupational therapy. As part of the position, this supervisor must oversee the performance of three staff therapists. The chief, a middle manager, negotiates programming issues with two directors in order to manage the occupational therapy services for both Physical Medicine and Rehabilitation, and Psychiatry.

Good organizational charts meet a specific purpose and are as simple as possible to support organizational effectiveness. For example, figures 11-7 and -8 present overall organizational structures. Within these structures the occupational therapy department itself may have an organizational chart to describe internal relationships. Figure 11-9 is a department-level chart in the hospital presented in figure 11-8, which is used for fieldwork education. This chart more specifically delineates the responsibilities of the supervisor of mental health, who also has the role of overseeing the fieldwork program. This involves supervision of staff members as fieldwork educators in both physical medicine and mental health. A different chart may be in place to depict clinical service relationships.

Figure 11-7

An Organization-wide Chart for an Occupational Therapy Department in a University

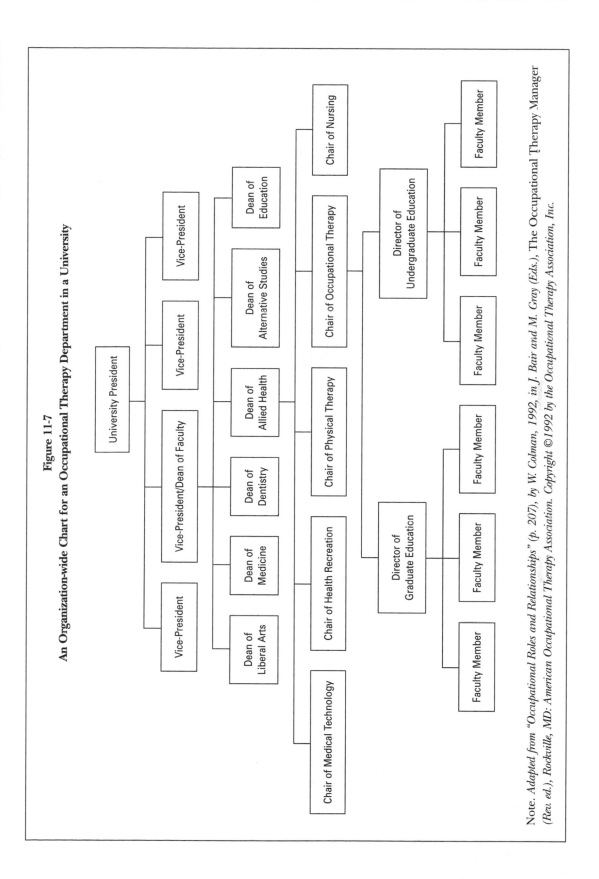

Note. Adapted from "Occupational Roles and Relationships" (p. 207), by W. Colman, 1992, in J. Bair and M. Gray (Eds.), The Occupational Therapy Manager (Rev. ed.), Rockville, MD: American Occupational Therapy Association. Copyright ©1992 by the Occupational Therapy Association, Inc.

Figure 11-8

An Organization-wide Chart for an Occupational Therapy Department in a Hospital

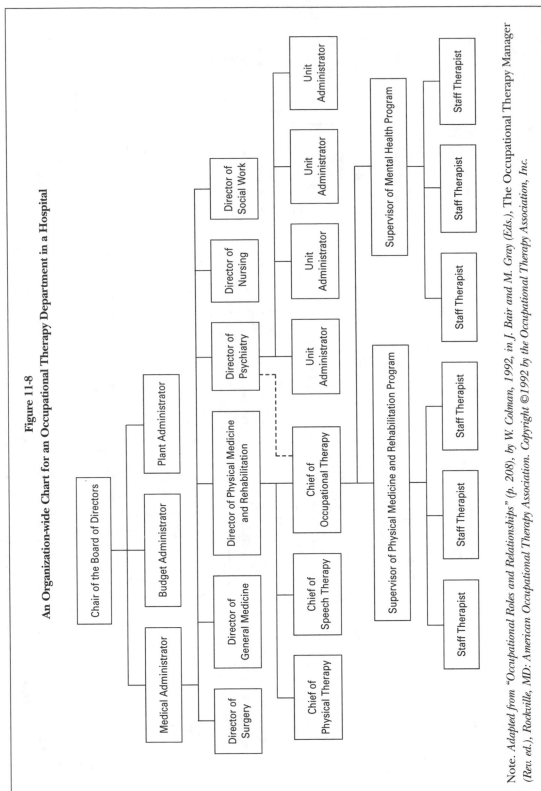

Note. Adapted from "Occupational Roles and Relationships" (p. 208), by W. Colman, 1992, in J. Bair and M. Gray (Eds.), The Occupational Therapy Manager (Rev. ed.), Rockville, MD: American Occupational Therapy Association. Copyright ©1992 by the Occupational Therapy Association, Inc.

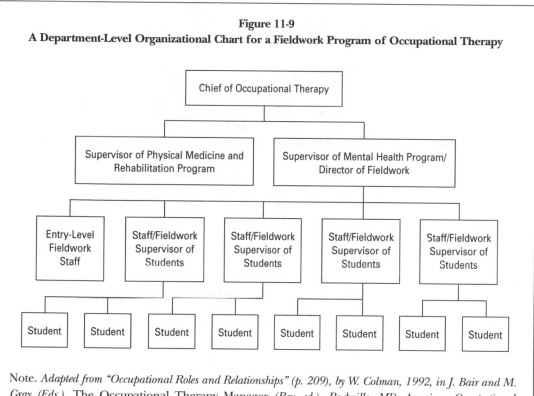

Figure 11-9
A Department-Level Organizational Chart for a Fieldwork Program of Occupational Therapy

Note. *Adapted from "Occupational Roles and Relationships" (p. 209), by W. Colman, 1992, in J. Bair and M. Gray (Eds.),* The Occupational Therapy Manager *(Rev. ed.), Rockville, MD: American Occupational Therapy Association. Copyright ©1992 by the Occupational Therapy Association, Inc.*

PROFESSIONAL ROLE OPTIONS

The growing prevalence of occupational therapy in different service delivery systems has resulted in an increase over the past decade in the number and the complexity of roles that occupational therapy practitioners perform. Multiple roles are now more the norm than before because practitioners frequently address multiple purposes within an organization. Thus roles are combined to describe jobs or positions in particular environments.

In recognition of its growth and diversification, the profession has identified 12 occupational therapy roles that are salient in today's health care system. These roles are listed in table 11-1 along with their function or primary purpose in the profession.

Table 11-1
Major Professional Roles and Functions in Occupational Therapy

Role	Major Function
Practitioner—OTR	Provides quality occupational therapy services, including assessment, intervention, program planning and implementation, discharge planning–related documentation, and communication.
Practitioner—COTA	Provides quality occupational therapy services to assigned individuals under the supervision of an OTR.
Educator (Consumer, Peer)	Develops and provides educational offerings or training related to occupational therapy to consumer, peer, and community individuals or groups.
Fieldwork Educator (Practice Setting)	Manages Level I or II fieldwork in a practice setting. Provides occupational therapy or occupational therapy assistant students with opportunities to practice and carry out practitioner competencies.
Supervisor	Manages the overall daily operation of occupational therapy services in a defined practice area(s).
Administrator (Practice Setting)	Manages department, program, services, or agency providing occupational therapy services.
Consultant	Provides occupational therapy consultation to individuals, groups, or organizations.
Fieldwork Coordinator (Academic Setting)	Manages student fieldwork program within the academic setting.
Faculty	Provides formal academic education for occupational therapy or occupational therapy assistant students.
Program Director (Academic Setting)	Manages the occupational therapy educational program.
Researcher/Scholar	Performs scholarly work of the profession including examining, developing, refining, and evaluating the profession's body of knowledge, theoretical base, and philosophical foundations.
Entrepreneur	Entrepreneurs are partially or fully self-employed individuals who provide occupational therapy services.

Note. *From "Occupational Therapy Roles" (pp. 1088–97), by American Occupational Therapy Association, Occupational Therapy Roles Task Force, 1993,* American Journal of Occupational Therapy, 47. *Copyright ©1992 by the Occupational Therapy Association, Inc.*

The 12 roles are described in greater detail in "Occupational Therapy Roles" (AOTA, 1993), summarized in Appendix 11–A. Each role description in this document consists of the following components:

Major function: Describes the primary purpose(s) of the role.

Scope of role: Delineates the range of responsibility and complexity that typically occurs within the role.

Key performance areas: Specifies common activities and expectations associated with role function . . .

Supervision: Describes the typical oversight required or recommended for individuals at the various levels of role performance . . .

Qualifications: Lists the critical credentials, education, and work experience necessary as a prerequisite to adequate role performance.

(pp. 1087–88)

Two issues under each role require close scrutiny during career development planning. First, the key performance areas are organized in levels to indicate degree of expertise within a role: entry level, intermediate level, and high-proficiency level. "Progression within a role through the three levels of professional development is based on accumulation of higher-level skills through experience, education, guided self-development, and professional socialization" (p. 5). Time spent in a role does not necessarily equate with progression in a role. Second, if a job consists of several roles, a practitioner may perform each one at a different level of expertise. For example, a therapist may be an intermediate-level practitioner in a direct care setting, but be performing at the entry level as a new fieldwork educator. Reviewing the complete document will increase the reader's understanding; the present discussion offers only highlights of this important career development resource.

To use "Occupational Therapy Roles" correctly, the reader should understand that roles are not job titles but that jobs in occupational therapy consist of blends of occupational therapy roles. For example, the supervisor of the mental health program in figures 11-8 and -9 would have the following simultaneous professional roles in occupational therapy: practitioner–OTR, supervisor, and fieldwork educator.

CAREER CHOICES

Career development in occupational therapy occurs in three ways. First, practitioners may move up the organizational chart to progressively higher positions. Second, they may move horizontally within an organization or between organizations to increase their breadth of experience with or without a significant change in role. Third, they may mature within their given role by becoming able to perform at more advanced levels of expertise. A companion guide to "Occupational Therapy Roles," titled "Career Exploration and Development" (Schell, 1994), in Appendix B provides descriptions of career decision-making processes.

Vertical Movement Within a Setting

"Occupational Therapy Roles" does not assume that all 12 roles can be hierarchically organized. In fact, some are independent, such as the two practitioner roles, and some occur in very distinct environments, like faculty in the university, fieldwork educator in the clinic, and entrepreneur in private practice. However, a few roles may be linked vertically within particular settings. For example:

Practice Setting

Practitioner —> Fieldwork educator —> Supervisor —> Administrator

Academic Setting

Fieldwork coordinator —> Faculty —> Scholar —> Program director

To make transitions in roles that can be linked, practitioners must focus their career development activities on the *key performance areas* and the *qualifications* for the new role. An example of this professional transition process is contained in case 3 of the companion guide to "Occupational Therapy Roles": an occupational therapist considers advancing on the career ladder within his setting.

Lateral Movement Across Settings

To support movement across organizations, which might or might not involve a role change, practitioners would concentrate their attention on the key performance expectations for the new role. In case 6 of the companion guide, a master clinician aspires to perform an academic educator role not linked to her current clinical one, in a totally different environment. She couples self-assessment of skills with relevant professional activities to make the transition to an assistant professorship.

Maturation Within a Role

A third way to facilitate professional role development is to study the *levels of performance* for a specific role. Each role has key performance descriptions at the entry, intermediate, and advanced levels. Practitioners can use these to plan appropriate career development activities. Mentoring and supervision by role specialists and carefully coordinated education activities can facilitate this process. For example, in case 3, the occupational therapist explores becoming a clinical specialist by observing and interviewing advanced-level practitioners in his place of employment.

Regardless of the path that practitioners select for career development, it is important that they realize the expectations for any role advancement or change. By matching their abilities and talents with role demands and organizational expectations, practitioners can minimize pitfalls and disappointments. Avoiding jumping into performance expectations that are beyond professional abilities can prevent failure, job dismissal, and even professional liability crises. Professionals are expected to know their limits and not to accept job responsibilities beyond their abilities, regardless of encouragement or enticement from employers. For example, in case 1 of the companion guide, a graduating senior assesses her performance abilities in relation to two job offers, and opts for the one that is more compatible with her level of education, experience, and skill.

Successful career development is planned, even though opportunities to engage in roles arise almost serendipitously in the occupational therapy profession. Careful self-assessment of readiness for a role is essential. Occupational therapy managers can be excellent resources for their staff members, encouraging and modeling appropriate preparation for role enhancement or change in annual negotiations of job goals or during supervisory sessions.

Managers themselves should engage in career development activities for their own professional growth in a current or future role. Excellent role development means excellent job performance, quality service, and even career mobility. In this decade of rapid change, having occupational therapy practitioners in top organizational roles increases the likelihood that the profession will be represented in health care reform policies and organizational leadership.

ORGANIZATIONAL RELATIONSHIPS

Organizational effectiveness is directly related to identified relationships. Relationships help organizations meet goals, they guide development of competencies in the workforce, and they provide continuity between internal operations and external demands. Although the formal structure of relationships can be described in organizational charts and roles, managers realize that the energy to do work behind these structures is really based on relationships. Managers facilitate relationships through their use of communication skills, flow of information, and policies and procedures.

COMMUNICATION SKILLS

Effective communication skills are essential for a manager because communication is the primary function of this role. (See also chapter 14, "Principles of Communication.") Occupational therapy managers can draw on their background in group dynamics and therapeutic communication as a basis. However, beyond the basics, management communication is different. The function of communication in organizations is to transmit information so that work objectives are understood and given meaning. The typical organizational methods used for communication are oral interaction, written information, nonverbal behaviors, and electronic communication.

Oral Interaction

Oral interaction is the most frequently used form of organizational communication. Speeches, inservice programs, group discussions, supervisory sessions, rounds, and even the grapevine are some of the types of oral interaction in occupational therapy organizations. Oral communication is quick and allows for rapid feedback. However, it is easily distorted or interpreted differently by the receiver.

Written Information

Written information includes reports, periodicals such as in-house newspapers, memos, bulletin boards, and now Post-its. It is permanent, tangible, and verifiable. It takes more time than oral communication, however, and eliciting feedback from the receiver is more difficult. Further, seldom is there verification that the written information was received.

Nonverbal Behaviors

Communication without words, or nonverbal communication, is meaningful. The most common types of nonverbal behaviors are body language and voice intonation, both of which communicate the emotional content behind a message. The advantage of using nonverbal behaviors is that the sender can quickly and easily give cues validating performance or signaling the need for a change in behavior. The disadvantage is that the receiver can readily misinterpret or devalue the cues.

Electronic Communication

Electronic media used in communication include personal computers, facsimile (fax) machines, modems, fax modems, and more. Among their applications are electronic mail (E-mail) and networking on the information superhighway (the Internet). Modern technologies increase the amount of information available to managers, but they require effective time-management strategies for processing. For example, avoiding addiction to "surfing the Internet" and making good use of the information obtained are significant challenges. Also, managers and practitioners must be careful to use electronic communication ethically and professionally. A staff member should not, for instance, notify a supervisor by E-mail that he or she is resigning.

FLOW OF INFORMATION

Effective relationships are based on the flow of information between people in an organization. The *downward* flow of communication from the manager is used to inform subordinates, to coordinate their work, and to evaluate their performance. Downward communication in an organization includes describing jobs, establishing annual job performance goals, pointing out performance problems, and requesting actions. The *upward* flow of communication keeps managers aware of employee-related issues, such as satisfaction, relationships with co-workers, and the general health of the organization, and it supports continuous quality improvement activities. Upward communication includes performance summaries, annual reports, job satisfaction surveys, and focus groups. Managers rely on upward communication to document and improve organizational operations. *Lateral* communication takes place among horizontally equivalent managers within an organization. This type of communication can provide consistency in operations, save time, and facilitate coordination while limiting input from upper-level managers. An experienced middle manager can easily communicate laterally about the implementation of procedures to a middle manager new to the role or to management activity.

Managers always have information from all three sources. An effective manager uses this information judiciously, fairly, and equitably to support beneficial work relationships. Deciding what, when, where, how, and with whom information is shared is the basis of control. Frequently it is also the basis on which upper-level managers as well as supervisees differentiate effective managers from ineffective managers.

The flow of information in any organization reflects the style of the manager and the culture of the organization. In participatory cultures, upward communication is encouraged so that employees provide input for decisions. Upward communication is best in organizations that create cultures based on trust and respect. In authoritarian cultures, by contrast, the communication is primarily downward except that top managers expect lower-level managers to communicate upward when they need control information.

POLICIES AND PROCEDURES

One major influence on managerial relationships is an organization's rules and regulations, known as *policies and procedures*. Policies and procedures, which are established by top management, communicate the values of the system and provide the basis for effective and efficient decision making in organizations. Typically an organization publishes its policies and procedures and makes the document readily available to all employees by placing copies in strategic places such as offices throughout the organization. Both managers and staff members are expected to be familiar with the document because it sets forth the *standard operating procedures* (SOPs) of the organization. SOPs communicate expectations regarding commonly occurring organizational issues, provide consistency in expectations for all employees, and most important, program decisions regarding routine tasks, allowing managers to focus on unique, nonrecurring events that influence work performance.

A *policy* is a guide that establishes a parameter for making decisions (Robbins, 1994). For example, an organization may have policies regarding vacation, promotion, or documentation. Given that policies are guides, the role of the manager is to judge and interpret the policy in relation to the current situation. When a new employee requests support to attend a continuing education event, for example, the manager and the employee may find a policy stating whether or not the employee may receive financial support for this activity during the probation period, and if not, whether the employee may take leave without pay to attend. A manager is given authority to make decisions interpreting policy in light of a given situation. If a manager renders a decision different from the stated policy, he or she must frequently follow the organization's guidelines for documenting this exception, which may include approval by the manager's administrator. In the example just given, the organization may have hired the new employee as a supervisor, and the manager may have agreed to provide immediate professional development activities in supervisory competencies. In this case the manager might waive a policy requiring a new employee to complete a six-month probation period before receiving financial support for continuing education.

Some policies are "cast in stone"; no managerial discretion is permitted regarding them. These policies are frequently referred to as *rules and regulations*. For example, an organization establishes rules and regulations for which days are considered annual holidays and how vacation time is accrued and used. These issues are invariant.

A *procedure* is a series of interrelated sequential steps that can be used to respond to a structured problem (Robbins, 1994). Procedures offer ready answers to common problems in organizations and provide consistent, efficient operations. These usually are so common that a form is created to ensure that all required conditions for each step are met. In the previous example the new employee might complete a form to request continuing education support, stating when he or she would be gone and how this event would improve his or her job performance. Decision making and communication of expectations by the manager are thereby simplified and directed. For example, most organizations have very specific procedures to follow when purchasing equipment, which include not only identifying the product but also securing required approvals from other key managers. Procedures support organizational efficiency.

In organizations, one of the main responsibilities of first-line and middle managers is to know the organization's policies and procedures and to communicate these expectations to their supervisees. Also, if a policy requires frequent interpretation or decisions, or seems contrary to new organizational procedures, managers are expected to alert top managers so that policies can be reviewed. As SOPs, all policies are reviewed annually by a group of specified individuals within an organization who are expected to oversee these processes.

SUMMARY

A *role* is "a set of behavior patterns expected of someone occupying a given position in a social unit" (Robbins, 1994, p. 445). All persons in a social unit or an organization have a role. In fact, most persons play multiple roles. In traditional organizations, roles are the outcome of formal structures created to delineate the internal flow of power and authority. In the learning organization, roles are not boundaries or limitations, but the energy to create new solutions in order to perform work better (Wheatley, 1992). As the systems approach to organizational effectiveness spreads, inter- and intra-organizational relationships become more important than roles that are perceived as rigid and inflexible. This shift in perspective on roles and relationships permeates business. Attention to how effective organizations work is essential in health care too.

Professions have their own role definitions. The individual practitioner must understand that he or she typically occupies more than one role within a system and should strategically use the related responsibilities to empower himself or herself to influence the system positively. The key to using roles effectively is to be able to form relationships and alliances with important persons within a system and to ensure that requisite information is available to support role functions and organizational processes.

Organizational structure describes an organization's framework (Robbins, 1994). It specifies the relationship between roles and *role responsibility,* the obligation to perform assigned job tasks. An *organizational chart* is a graphic representation of chains of command and position-designated authority. It depicts *departmentalization,* or the division of labor among specialists who need coordination and leadership. Robbins (1994) identifies five approaches to departmentalization: by function, by product, by customer, by geographic region, and by process.

Participation in various roles develops into careers. A *career* is the sequence of positions that a person occupies in the course of his or her work history. *Career development* is progressive growth in a career. Development in a career can occur randomly or purposefully. In the 1990s, career development in many organizations is more likely to occur through lateral moves than through vertical advancement.

Careers and career development can occur through two types of roles: specific roles in an organization and roles that are recognized by a profession. In organizations, roles are frequently encapsulated in job titles that describe the major job function. The profession of occupational therapy has identified 12 roles that are salient in today's health care system. Jobs in occupational therapy consist of blends of these roles.

Career development in occupational therapy occurs in three ways: by moving up the organizational chart; by moving horizontally within an organization or between organizations; or by maturing within a given role. Successful career development is planned.

Organizational effectiveness is directly related to identified relationships. Managers facilitate relationships through their use of communication skills, the upward and downward flow of information, and policies and procedures. A *policy* is a guide that establishes a parameter for making decisions (Robbins, 1994). A *procedure* is a series of interrelated sequential steps that can be used to respond to a structured problem (Robbins, 1994).

REFERENCES

American Occupational Therapy Association, Occupational Therapy Roles Task Force. (1993). Occupational therapy roles. *American Journal of Occupational Therapy, 47,* 1087–99.

Pacanowski, M. (1988). Communication in the empowering organization. In J. A. Anderson (Ed.), *International Communications Association Yearbook II* (pp. 356–79). Beverly Hills, CA: Sage.

Robbins, S. P. (1994). *Management* (4th ed.). Englewood Cliffs, NJ: Prentice-Hall.

Schell, B. A. B., for American Occupational Therapy Association, Use Document Task Force. (1994). Career exploration and development: A companion guide to the "Occupational therapy roles" document. *American Journal of Occupational Therapy, 48,* 844–51.

Senge, P. M. (1990) *The fifth discipline: The art and practice of the learning organization.* New York: Doubleday.

Wheatley, M. J. (1992). *Leadership and the new science: Learning about organizations from an orderly universe.* San Francisco: Berrett-Koehler.

APPENDIX 11-A

Occupational Therapy Roles

This document is a guide to major roles common in the profession of occupational therapy. It is intended to assist the practitioner in identifying career options and developing career paths. *Practitioner* refers to anyone who is certified by the National Board for Certification in Occupational Therapy (NBCOT) as an occupational therapist (OTR) or an occupational therapy assistant (COTA). Practitioners work in a variety of systems including health care, educational, academic, governmental, social, corporate, and industrial settings. This document can be a resource for planning career ladders, developing job descriptions, and suggesting educational content for formal and continuing education programs.

Roles listed in this document are those frequently held by certified practitioners and are not all inclusive. The nature of the experience as an occupational therapy practitioner prepares individuals for other specialized roles (e.g., activity director, case manager, rehabilitation coordinator, dean). Roles described in this document are valued equally. Although different roles may vary in their scope and in the experience required to perform them, each role fulfills a specific function within the profession and contributes to the profession's growth, development and strength.

An individual's employment setting, method of service delivery, performance competence, and career goals are all interdependent and result in an individualized composite of roles during actual job performance. In this document, roles are not exclusive because jobs performed by practitioners may include aspects of more than one role. For example, an occupational therapist may have a job that includes practitioner and fieldwork educator roles. Another individual may function as a faculty member, researcher, and consultant.

Career progression involves advancement within roles as well as transition to different roles. When transitioning occurs, practitioners need to have demonstrated performance potential and appropriate educational preparation for the new role. Individuals entering into a new role typically require closer supervision and will begin at a relatively lower level of expertise than in their other roles. Preparation for new roles often involves self-reflection, continuing or advanced education, and acquisition of experience and skills required for the new role. The development of a mentoring relationship assists in understanding the context in which role performance will occur. For example, an individual who is an advanced-level administrator in a practice setting may move into an entry-level faculty role in an academic setting. Preparation for this transition may include acquiring appropriate academic degrees; understanding the educational environment; and demonstrating potential for teaching, scholarly activity, and professional service.

ROLE DESCRIPTIONS

Each role in this document consists of the following components: major function, scope of role, performance areas, qualifications, and supervision. These components are described as follows:

- **Major Function:** Describes the primary purpose(s) of the role.

- **Scope of Role:** Delineates the range of responsibility and complexity that typically occurs within the role.

- **Key Performance Areas:** Specifies common activities and expectations associated with role function. Performance that occurs within each area is built upon the unique philosophy and perspective of occupational therapy. Practitioners are expected to take personal responsibility for functioning within the ethical code and standards of the profession. Specific knowledge, skills, and attitudes fundamental for performance are beyond the scope of this document.

Individuals develop varying degrees of expertise in role performance. Levels of expertise are those skills that are fundamental to the entry level (noted by ♦), those skills that are intermediate (noted by ♦♦), or those skills that require a high degree of proficiency (noted by ♦♦♦). These three levels describe the professional development process for each role and are described in Figure 1. Progression within a role through the three levels of professional development is based on accumulation of higher level skills through experience, education, guided self-development, and professional socialization. Progression is not simply the amount of time in a role. Each person progresses along this continuum at an individualized pace. Some individuals may remain at one level for the duration of their career and not everyone progresses to the advanced level. An individual may function in more than one role simultaneously. When this occurs, it is possible to function at different levels within each role. For example, a new faculty member may be at an entry level in teaching, though at an advanced level in clinical practice. All roles described in this document build on the performance expectations of the Practitioner-OTR and Practitioner-COTA, as this is the entry point into the profession. Consequently, the entry-level performance areas are considered to be an inherent part of all other roles described in this document.

- **Supervision:** Describes the typical oversight required or recommended for individuals at the various levels of role performance. The amount of supervision required is closely linked to both the role and the level of expertise in a role. The supervision recommended is intended to be a collaborative relationship that serves to promote quality service and the professional development of the individuals involved.

All COTAs will require more than a minimal level of supervision by an OTR when providing services. Formal supervision occurs along a continuum including close, routine, general, and minimal. Refer to Figure 2 for descriptions of these levels.

Figure 1
Levels of Role Performance

Level	Major Foci	Supervision
Entry	• The development of skills. • Socialization in the expectations related to the organization, peers, and the profession. Acceptance of responsibilities and accountability in role-relevant professional activities is expected.	Close
Intermediate	• Increased independence. • Mastery of basic role functions. • Ability to respond to situations based on previous experience. • Participation in the education of personnel. Specialization is frequently initiated, along with increased responsibility for collaboration with other disciplines and related organizations. Participation in role-relevant professional activities is increased.	Routine or General
Advanced	• Refinement of specialized skills. • Understanding of complex issues affecting role functions. Contribution to the knowledge base and growth of the profession results in being seen as an expert, resource person, or consultant within a role. This expertise is recognized by others within and outside the profession through leadership, mentoring, research, education and volunteerism.	Minimal

---

Figure 2
Types of Formal Supervision

Type	Description
Close	Daily, direct contact at the site of work.
Routine	Direct contact at least every 2 weeks at the site of work, with interim supervision occurring by other methods such as telephone or written communication.
General	At least monthly direct contact, with supervision available as needed by other methods.
Minimal	Provided only on a need basis, and may be less than monthly.

In addition to formal supervision, individuals may provide or receive functional supervision. Functional supervision implies the provision of information and feedback to coworkers. Individuals who provide functional supervision have specialized knowledge as a result of their own experience and expertise. Based on this specialized knowledge or skill, the individual supervises peers relative to this expertise in a particular function. For example, a fieldwork educator may provide functional supervision to coworkers who are supervising students, although he or she is not responsible for evaluating the overall performance of the other therapists.

- **Qualifications:** Lists the critical credentials, education, and work experience necessary as a prerequisite to adequate role performance. Qualifications are listed in a range to reflect changing expectations associated with higher levels of role functioning. As all roles are within the profession, professional certification as a practitioner is a consistent requirement. Additionally, all practitioners are expected to meet state and federal regulatory mandates, and adhere to relevant Association policies, and participate in continuing professional development.

PRACTITIONER—OTR

Major Function: Provide quality occupational therapy services, including assessment, intervention, program planning and implementation, discharge planning related documentation, and communication. Service provision may include direct, monitored, and consultative approaches.

Scope of Role: OTR practitioners advance along a continuum from entry to advanced level based on experience, education, and practice skills. The OTR has the ultimate responsibility for service provision (AOTA, 1990, p.1093).

Key Performance Areas (♦ entry-level skills, ♦♦ intermediate skills, ♦♦♦ high-proficiency skills):

♦ Responds to requests for service and initiates referrals when appropriate.

♦ Screens individuals to determine the need for intervention.

♦ Evaluates individuals to obtain and interpret data necessary for planning intervention and for intervention.

♦ Interprets evaluation findings to appropriate individuals.

♦ Develops and coordinates intervention plans, including goals and methods to achieve stated goals.

♦ Implements the intervention plan directly or in collaboration with others.

♦ Adapts environment, tools, materials, and activities according to the needs of the individual and his or her social cultural context.

♦ Monitors the individual's response to intervention and modifies plan as needed.

♦ Communicates and collaborates with other team members, individuals, family members, or caregivers.

♦ Follows policies and procedures required in the setting.

♦ Develops appropriate home and community programming to support performance in natural environment.

♦ Terminates services when maximum benefit is received and formulates discontinuation and follow-up plans.

♦ Documents services as required.

♦ Maintains records required by practice setting, third party payors, and regulatory agencies.

♦ Performs continuous quality improvement activities and program evaluation using predetermined criteria.

♦ Provides inservice education to team members and the community.

♦ Maintains treatment area, equipment, and supply inventory.

♦ Identifies and pursues own professional growth and development.

♦ Schedules and prioritizes own workload.

♦ Participates in professional and community activities.

♦ Monitors own performance and identifies supervisory needs.

♦ Functions according to the AOTA *Code of Ethics* (AOTA, 1988) and *Standards of Practice* (AOTA, 1992) of the profession.

♦ Supervises/teaches occupational therapy practitioners, students, and other staff performing supportive services and/or other aspects of service provision.

♦♦ Assists other practitioners in the development of professional skills.

♦♦ Participates in committees and activities of larger systems in the development of service operations, policies, and procedures.

♦♦ Participates in the fieldwork education process.

♦♦ Critically examines own practice and integrates new knowledge.

♦♦♦ Performs advanced, specialized evaluations or interventions.

♦♦♦ Develops protocols and procedures for intervention programs based on current occupational therapy theory and practice.

♦♦♦ Provides expert consultation to practitioners and outside groups about area of expertise.

QUALIFICATIONS

• Certified by the National Board for Certification in Occupational Therapy (NBCOT) as an OTR.

• Meets state regulatory requirements.

• Progressive levels of expertise will require one or more of the following: work experience, self-study, continuing education, special certification, or post- professional education.

Supervision: Practice supervision must be performed by an experienced OTR. Administrative supervision is determined by individual settings and may or may not be performed by an OTR.

• Entry-Level Practitioners-OTRs in a particular practice area will require closesupervision for service delivery aspects and routine supervision for administrative aspects (AOTA, 1981).

• Intermediate Practitioners-OTRs require routine to general supervision from advanced practitioners.

• Advanced Practitioners-OTRs require minimal supervision within area of expertise and general supervision for administrative aspects.

PRACTITIONER—COTA

Major Function: Provides quality occupational therapy services to assigned individuals under the supervision of an OTR.

Scope of Role: COTA practitioners advance along a continuum from entry to advanced level, based on experience, education, and practice skills. Development along this continuum is dependent on the development of service competency. The OTR has ultimate overall responsibility for service provision (AOTA, 1990, p.1093).

Key Performance Areas (♦ entry-level skills, ♦♦ intermediate skills, ♦♦♦ high-proficiency skills):

♦ Responds to request for services in accordance with service agency's policies and procedures.

♦ Assists with data collection and evaluation under the supervision of an OTR.

♦ Develops treatment goals under the supervision of an OTR.

♦ Implements and coordinates intervention plan under the supervision of an OTR.

♦ Provides direct service that follows a documented routine and accepted procedure under the supervision of an OTR.

♦ Adapts intervention environment, tools, materials, and activities according to the needs of the individual and his or her sociocultural context under the supervision of an OTR.

♦ Communicates and interacts with other team members and the individual's family or caregivers in collaboration with an OTR.

♦ Monitors own performance and identifies supervisory needs.

♦ Follows policies and procedures required in a setting.

♦ Performs continuous quality improvement activities or program evaluation in collaboration with an OTR.

♦ Maintains treatment area, equipment, and supply inventory as required.

♦ Identifies and pursues own professional growth and development.

♦ Maintains records and documentation required by work settings under the supervision of an OTR.

♦ Participates in professional and community activities.

♦ Functions according to the AOTA *Code of Ethics* (AOTA, 1988) and *Standards of Practice* (AOTA, 1992) of the profession.

♦♦ Schedules and prioritizes own workload.

♦♦ Supervises volunteers, COTAs, OTA students, and personnel other than OT practitioners under the direction of an OTR.

♦♦ Participates in development of policies and procedures in collaboration with an OTR.

♦♦ Participates in the fieldwork education process under the direction of an OTR.

♦♦ Selects, adapts, and implements intervention under the supervision of an OTR.

♦♦ Administers standardized tests under the supervision of an OTR after service competency has been established.

♦♦ Modifies treatment approaches to reflect changing needs under the supervision of an OTR.

♦♦ Formulates discontinuation and follow-up plans under the supervision of an OTR.

♦♦ Participates in organizational activities and committees.

♦♦♦ Serves as a resource person to the agency in areas of specific expertise.

♦♦♦ Educates others in the area of established service competency under the supervision of an OTR.

♦♦♦ Contributes to program planning and development in collaboration with an OTR.

QUALIFICATIONS

• Certification by the NBCOT as a COTA.

• Meets state regulatory requirements.

• Progressive levels of expertise will require one or more of the following: work experience, self-study, continuing education, and formal education including advanced degrees.

Supervision: COTAs at all levels require at least general supervision by an OTR. The level of supervision is related to the ability of the COTA to safely and effectively provide those interventions delegated by an OTR. Typically, entry-level COTAs and COTAs new to a particular practice environment will require close supervision, intermediate-level practitioners routine supervision, and advanced-level practitioners general supervision. COTAs will require closer supervision for interventions that are more complex or evaluative in nature and for areas in which service competencies have not been developed. Service competency is the ability to use the identified intervention in a safe and effective manner.

EDUCATOR (CONSUMER, PEER)

Major Function: Develops and provides educational offerings or training related to occupational therapy to consumer, peer, and community individuals or groups.

Scope of Role: Practitioners advance along a continuum of providing informal education to individuals and small groups in the course of service provision, to developing and providing comprehensive educational programs targeted to consumers and peers. At entry level of role, education typically occurs with peers and consumers within the individual's own service system (e.g., patient education, department, or school district inservice). At higher levels of expertise, provision of educational offerings may involve individuals or groups from multiple systems (e.g., provision of injury-prevention programs to industry, caregiver education programs to community, and continuing education seminars).

Key Performance Areas (♦ entry-level skills, ♦♦ intermediate skills, ♦♦♦ high-proficiency skills):

♦ Implements strategies to assist individual learner to identify own learning needs.

♦ Develops or collaborates with individual learner in developing learning objectives.

♦ Implements educational methods designed to support learner's objectives.

♦ Responds to feedback about the teaching-learning process, and modifies own educational strategies to support learning.

♦ Supports the evaluation of educational effectiveness.

♦ Monitors own performance and identifies own development needs.

♦ Functions according to the AOTA Code of Ethics (AOTA, 1988) and Standards of Practice (AOTA, 1992) of the profession.

♦♦ Selects or designs strategies to identify individual learner needs.

♦♦ Develops program plans and materials for formal program offerings (e.g., conference presentations, workshops, seminars).

♦♦ Uses a variety of teaching-learning methods appropriate to the learning objectives and learner needs.

♦♦♦ Evaluates strategies to identify learning needs of individuals and groups.

♦♦♦ Develops program plans and educational methods for extended or multiple program offerings.

◆◆◆ Designs evaluation strategies to assess impact of educational programs.

QUALIFICATIONS

- Certification by NBCOT as an OTR or a COTA.

- Progressive levels of expertise will require combinations of the following: self-study, continuing education, experience, and post-entry-level formal education.

- Appropriate level of practice or service expertise is necessary as it relates to provision of these education services.

Supervision: Supervision depends on the nature of the project and the skills of the educator. COTAs at all levels usually will require OTR supervision for educational activities that occur related to occupational therapy consumers.

FIELDWORK EDUCATOR (PRACTICE SETTING)

Major Function: Manages Level I or II fieldwork in a practice setting. Provides occupational therapy or occupational therapy assistant students with opportunities to practice and carry out practitioner competencies.

Scope of Role: The fieldwork educator role may range from supervision of an individual student to full responsibility for an entire fieldwork program.

Key Performance Areas (◆ entry-level skills, ◆◆ intermediate skills, ◆◆◆ high-proficiency skills):

- ◆ Establishes, mediates, and supports relationships between practice-based and academic personnel.

- ◆ Initiates and maintains communication and correspondence between the practice and academic settings.

- ◆ Schedules students in collaboration with the academic fieldwork coordinator.

- ◆ Provides orientation for student to fieldwork site including policies, procedures, and student responsibilities.

- ◆ Facilitates student learning activities to achieve desired student competence.

- ◆ Facilitates student's clinical reasoning and reflective practice.

- ◆ Evaluates student performance throughout fieldwork.

- ◆ Provides the student with both formative and cumulative feedback and supervision.

♦ Ensures student's integration of professional standards and ethics into practice.

♦ Ensures students' compliance with agencies' standards, goals, and objectives.

♦ Attends meetings, programs, or continuing education related to fieldwork education.

♦ Develops learning objectives for fieldwork in collaboration with academic institution(s) and consistent with current student fieldwork evaluation(s).

♦ Functions according to the AOTA *Code of Ethics* (AOTA, 1988) and *Standards of Practice* (AOTA, 1992) of the profession.

♦♦ Provides functional supervision to OTRs and COTAs specific to their roles as student fieldwork supervisors.

♦♦ Facilitates assignment of students to appropriate practitioners for supervision.

♦♦ Counsels or arbitrates students' concerns.

♦♦ Oversees the administrative aspects of the fieldwork program, including the formal agreement with academic programs.

♦♦ Conducts ongoing fieldwork program evaluations and monitors changes in program.

♦♦ Organizes or participates in appropriate fieldwork education support groups (e.g., local fieldwork councils, Commission on Education).

♦♦ Coordinates continuing education and inservice opportunities to develop staff fieldwork education skills.

♦♦♦ Participates at leadership level in appropriate fieldwork groups.

♦♦♦ Facilitates the development of clinical fieldwork programs and related student supervision skills.

♦♦♦ Contributes to student learning by modeling leadership in professional organizations and facilitating student involvement.

QUALIFICATIONS

- Certified by NBCOT as an OTR or a COTA.
- Meets appropriate state regulatory requirements.
- Continuing education regarding fieldwork education and supervision.
- Entry-level OTRs and COTAs may supervise Level I fieldwork students.

- OTRs with 1 year of practice-based experience may supervise OT and OTA Level II fieldwork students.

- COTAs with 1 year of practice-based experience may supervise OTA Level II fieldwork students.

- Three years of experience are recommended for individuals overseeing programs involving multiple student supervisors and multiple students.

Supervision: Supervision provided by an administrator or specifically designated individual. Level of supervision varies with skills of educator, complexity of setting, and nature of student's learning needs.

SUPERVISOR

Major Function(s): Manages the overall daily operation of occupational therapy services in a defined practice area(s).

Scope of Role: The supervisor is involved in managing other occupational therapy practitioners, personnel, and volunteers in a defined practice setting or program.

Key Performance Areas (♦ entry-level skills, ♦♦ intermediate skills, ♦♦♦ high-proficiency skills):

- ♦ Assists in selection, orientation, and training of staff, students, and volunteers.

- ♦ Promotes professional growth through staff development.

- ♦ Coordinates scheduling of work assignments.

- ♦ Evaluates, monitors, and provides feedback regarding job performance of assigned staff.

- ♦ Assists in establishment, implementation, and evaluation of agency goals and objectives.

- ♦ Monitors and facilitates staff compliance with established standards and guidelines.

- ♦ Provides for acquisition, care, and maintenance of physical facilities, supplies, and equipment.

- ♦ Oversees implementation of continuous quality improvement activities.

- ♦ Represents personnel, fiscal, professional, and program needs to occupational therapy administrator.

- ♦ Functions according to the AOTA *Code of Ethics* (AOTA, 1988) and *Standards of Practice* (AOTA, 1992) of the profession.

◆◆ Develops, implements, and monitors department policies and procedures in collaboration with occupational therapy administrator.

◆◆ Coordinates specific activities for department or service unit.

◆◆ Facilitates collaboration among occupational therapy and non-occupational therapy personnel and administrators.

◆◆◆ Serves as liaison to specialty program coordinators and administrators.

QUALIFICATIONS

- Certified by NBCOT as an OTR or COTA.

- Meets appropriate state regulatory requirements.

- Two to 3 years of practice experience in service area prior to supervising others is recommended.

- One year of experience is recommended prior to supervising a COTA. Experienced COTAs may supervise other COTAs administratively, as long as service protocols and documentation are supervised by an OTR.

- Continuing or postprofessional education relevant to supervisory function.

Supervision: Routine to minimal supervision provided by the occupational therapy administrator. Supervision ranges from routine to minimal, depending on the experience and expertise of the supervisor. Consultation from more advanced practitioners should be available as needed.

ADMINISTRATOR (PRACTICE SETTING)

Major Function: Manages department, program, services, or agency providing occupational therapy services.

Scope of Role: This role encompasses those individuals who organize and manage occupational therapy service units.

Key Performance Areas (◆ entry-level skills, ◆◆ intermediate skills, ◆◆◆ high-proficiency skills):

◆ Plans, develops, and monitors occupational therapy services to ensure quality service.

◆ Achieves service unit goals and objectives through allocation of resources.

◆ Recruits and hires employees.

♦ Conducts performance evaluation and staff development activities.

♦ Establishes policies and standard operating procedures.

♦ Formulates and manages budget.

♦ Maintains effective information management systems.

♦ Assures safe work environments, procedures, and methods.

♦ Develops and monitors reimbursement processes to support services.

♦ Monitors the acquisition and maintenance of supplies, equipment, and facilities.

♦ Develops and supervises a continuous quality improvement program.

♦ Ensures compliance with accreditation, certification, and government standards.

♦ Advocates for appropriate use of occupational therapy services.

♦ Oversees fieldwork education process.

♦ Functions according to the AOTA Code of Ethics (AOTA, 1988) and Standards of Practice (AOTA, 1992) of the profession.

♦♦ Establishes a long-range plan for staff recruitment, development, and retention.

♦♦ Collaborates with other administrators within the organization to develop and manage organizational systems.

♦♦ Collaborates with others outside of the organization regarding pertinent administrative management issues.

♦♦ Participates at a leadership level in professional, community organizations.

♦♦♦ Participates in organizational strategic planning and establishes strategic plan for assigned areas.

♦♦♦ Develops and implements marketing strategies for assigned areas.

♦♦♦ Facilitates development of systems supporting clinical research.

♦♦♦ Assumes leadership role within the organization and in interorganizational projects.

QUALIFICATIONS

• Certification by NBCOT as an OTR.

• Meets appropriate state regulatory requirements.

- Graduate degree or continuing education relevant to management.

- Recommended experience varies with size and scope of department; a minimum of 3 years experience is preferred for small programs and 5 or more years for larger programs.

Supervision: General supervision by administrative personnel within the organization is required. Individuals with fewer than 3 years experience should have access to an occupational therapy management consultant. Consultation from more advanced practitioners should be available as needed.

CONSULTANT

Major Function: Provides occupational therapy consultation to individuals, groups, or organizations.

Scope of Role: Consultative services may take place within the case, colleague, or systems model. Consultation may relate to practice, education, administration, or research.

Key Performance Areas (♦ entry-level skills, ♦♦ intermediate skills, ♦♦♦ high-proficiency skills):

- ♦ Communicates scope of professional expertise.

- ♦ Assists consumers in identifying problems to be addressed in the consultative process.

- ♦ Collaborates with consumers in developing appropriate consultation outcomes.

- ♦ Develops recommendations that are relevant within the cultural context of the consumers' environment.

- ♦ Assists consumers in developing and implementing interventions, or identifying alternate resources necessary to obtain consumer objectives.

- ♦ Complies with applicable local, state, and federal laws and regulations.

- ♦ Functions according to the AOTA *Code of Ethics* (AOTA, 1988) and *Standards of Practice* (AOTA, 1992) of the profession.

- ♦♦ Assesses quality of own consultative efforts, and identifies own continuing professional development needs.

- ♦♦♦ Participates at a leadership level in professional, community organizations.

QUALIFICATIONS

- Certified by NBCOT as an OTR or COTA.
- Meets appropriate state regulatory requirements.
- Intermediate or advanced practice level.
- Recommend minimum of 6 months experience for case consultation, 1 year for colleague consultation, and 3 to 5 years for systems consultation.

Supervision: Practitioners are expected to function as consultants within the scope of practice appropriate to their level of competence. The OTR functioning as a consultant is responsible for obtaining supervision when needed to meet regulatory and professional standards. The COTA functioning as a consultant is expected to seek the appropriate level of OTR supervision to meet regulatory and professional standards.

FIELDWORK COORDINATOR (ACADEMIC SETTING)

Major Function: Manages student fieldwork program within the academic setting.

Scope of Role: The fieldwork coordinator role may be decentralized among the faculty or may be managed entirely by one individual. This encompasses all fieldwork experiences required by a curriculum.

Key Performance Areas (♦ entry-level skills, ♦♦ intermediate skills, ♦♦♦ high-proficiency skills):

- ♦ Identifies and secures sites for fieldwork education.
- ♦ Reviews the quality and appropriateness of fieldwork sites in collaboration with other academic faculty.
- ♦ Develops fieldwork objectives in collaboration with the fieldwork sites.
- ♦ Initiates and maintains communication and correspondence between the academic and fieldwork sites.
- ♦ Communicates with fieldwork educators regarding the curriculum model, course content, and fieldwork expectations.
- ♦ Oversees the administrative aspects of the fieldwork program including agreements with fieldwork sites.
- ♦ Assigns students to fieldwork settings.
- ♦ Orients students to responsibilities and protocol for fieldwork.
- ♦ Maintains communication with fieldwork educators and students during fieldwork.

- ◆ Monitors the facilitation of clinical reasoning and reflective practice in Level II fieldwork settings.

- ◆ Counsels and arbitrates with students and fieldwork educators on matters of concern.

- ◆ Collaborates with the fieldwork educator in assigning the final appraisal (grading) of the student.

- ◆ Supports research.

- ◆ Functions according to the AOTA *Code of Ethics* (AOTA, 1988) and *Standards of Practice* (AOTA, 1992) of the profession.

- ◆ Participates in appropriate fieldwork educational support groups (e.g., local fieldwork councils, Commission on Education).

- ◆◆ Provides educational opportunities to prepare and enhance fieldwork educators' knowledge and skills.

- ◆◆ Coordinates contlŒuing education pertaining to fieldwork education processes for clinical fieldwork educators.

- ◆◆ Participates actively in professional, volunteer organizations.

- ◆◆ Supervises support personnel carrying out administrative aspects of fieldwork.

- ◆◆◆ Participates at leadership level in appropriate fieldwork group.

- ◆◆◆ Facilitates the development of fieldwork programs and related student supervision skills.

QUALIFICATIONS

- • Certified by NBCOT as an OTR or COTA.

- • Three years of practice experience and experience in supervising and advising fieldwork students are recommended.

Supervision: General supervision by academic administrator who is usually the program director. Close to routine supervision for new faculty.

FACULTY

Major Function: Provides formal academic education for occupational therapy or occupational therapy assistant students.

Scope of Role: This role varies among institutions and the subsequent balance expected between teaching, service, and scholarly activities. Progression within this role typically advances from lecturer and instructor to the professorial ranks, including assistant, associate, full, and emeritus professorships. Included in the faculty role may be adjunct, clinical, or academic appointments.

Key Performance Areas (♦ entry-level skills, ♦♦ intermediate skills,
♦♦♦ high-proficiency skills):

- ♦ Develops educational course objectives and sequences the content to promote optimal learning.

- ♦ Designs and structures effective educational experiences, including methods, media, content areas, and types of student interactions.

- ♦ Facilitates students' learning through lectures, discussions, practical and laboratory exercises, or practice-related experiences.

- ♦ Evaluates and addresses student learning needs within their social and cultural environmental context.

- ♦ Reviews educational media and published resources and selects class readings or supplemental materials.

- ♦ Plans and prepares course materials to include course syllabi, lectures, case studies, teaching/learning handouts, and questions for group discussion.

- ♦ Prepares evaluation materials and measures student attainment of stated course objectives.

- ♦ Develops and maintains proficiency in teaching areas through investigation, formal education, continuing education, or practice.

- ♦ Participates in curriculum development.

- ♦ Participates in teaching evaluation and uses outcome data to modify teaching.

- ♦ Advises students and student groups.

- ♦ Serves on department, school, college, or university committees.

- ♦ Assists with designated departmental administrative tasks such as student admissions, recruitment, and course scheduling.

- ♦ Maintains students' records according to regulations and procedures.

- ♦ Functions according to AOTA *Code of Ethics* (AOTA, 1988) and *Standards of Practice* (AOTA, 1992) of the profession.

- ♦ Engages in service to the university or community.

- ♦♦ Prepares innovative curriculum or instructional methods.

- ♦♦ Evaluates and incorporates emerging research findings and technology into teaching and research.

- ♦♦ Participates in research and scholarly activities.

♦♦ Collaborates in the preparation of academic reports and accreditation self-studies.

♦♦ Participates actively in professional organizations.

♦♦♦ Provides expert consultation to practitioners, educators, and outside groups about area of expertise.

♦♦♦ Chairs or leads groups or organizations outside the department.

♦♦♦ Mentors students through scholarly investigation process to develop student skills in research.

♦♦♦ Mentors other faculty in the development of their teaching, research, and practice skills.

QUALIFICATIONS

- Certified by NBCOT as an OTR or COTA.

- For OTR, in professional programs, a doctoral degree is preferred (a master's degree is recommended).

- In technical programs, a master's degree is preferred (a bachelor's degree is recommended).

- Intermediate to advanced skills in primary area of teaching.

- Skills as a classroom instructor and understanding of the educational system.

Supervision: General supervision by academic program director and other appropriate academic administrators. Close to routine supervision by academic program directors for new, adjunct, and part-time faculty.

PROGRAM DIRECTOR (ACADEMIC SETTING)

Major Function: Manages the occupational therapy educational program.

Scope of Role: The program director's role varies depending on the level of the program (e.g., technical, professional, or postprofessional level) and the demands of the academic setting (e.g., technical school, community college, college, university, or health sciences center). The academic program director facilitates the education of competent graduates through faculty development and supervision and effective program management. Dependent on their academic environment, program directors may oversee both academic and practice-related activities, externally funded projects, and continuing education programs.

Key Performance Areas (♦ entry-level skills, ♦♦ intermediate skills, ♦♦♦ high-proficiency skills):

♦ Oversees student recruitment, selection, evaluation, advisement, retention, and professional development.

♦ Oversees institutional and professional accreditation activities and reports.

♦ Manages faculty recruitment, development, evaluation, and retention.

♦ Assigns and monitors faculty and staff responsibilities.

♦ Ensures the quality of the program.

♦ Formulates and implements a fiscal plan.

♦ Represents the program to university administrators and negotiates for the needs of the program.

♦ Fosters an academic climate that facilitates faculty, student, and staff learning and professional growth.

♦ Promotes effective instructional techniques for faculty.

♦ Oversees student and faculty rights and responsibilities.

♦ Produces narrative and data-based reports for internal and external communication.

♦ Facilitates library acquisitions of resources for teaching and research.

♦ Fosters beneficial relationships among faculty and practitioners.

♦ Functions according to the AOTA *Code of Ethics* (AOTA, 1988) and *Standards of Practice* (AOTA, 1992) of the profession.

♦♦ Develops and implements long-range or strategic plans.

♦♦ Produces scholarly work.

♦♦ Facilitates the development of useful information management systems.

♦♦ Participates at the leadership level in professional and community organizations.

♦♦♦ Leads in the acquisition of externally funded projects.

♦♦♦ Designs and implements marketing for program enhancement.

♦♦♦ Promotes central theme within the occupational therapy programs that contributes to the knowledge base of the profession.

QUALIFICATIONS

Technical-Level Program Director:

• An OTR with a bachelor's degree (a master's degree is preferred) who is certified by NBCOT.

• Recommend 3 years professional practice with experience supervising COTAs.

- Recommend 3 years experience as a faculty member.

- Experience or continuing education in academic management.

Professional-Level Program Director:

- An OTR with a master's degree (a doctoral degree is preferred) who is certified by NBCOT.

- Recommend 5 years experience in practice.

- Recommend 5 years experience as a faculty member.

- Experience or continuing education in academic management.

Post-Professional-Level Program Director:

- An OTR with a doctoral degree who is certified by NBCOT.

- Recommend 5 years experience in practice.

- Recommend 5 years experience as a faculty member.

- Experience or continuing education in academic management.

- Intermediate to advanced competence as a researcher/scholar.

Supervision: General to minimal administrative supervision from designated administrative officer. Individuals with fewer than 3 years experience should have access to occupational therapy education and accreditation consultants.

RESEARCHER/SCHOLAR

Major Function: Performs scholarly work of the profession including examining, developing, refining, and evaluating the profession's body of knowledge, theoretical base, and philosophical foundations.

Scope of Role: The role of the researcher ranges from the individual who critically examines and interprets empirical studies to independent investigator. The scholar is an individual who has in-depth knowledge and who engages in examination, development, or refinement of the profession's body of knowledge.

Key Performance Areas (♦ entry-level skills, ♦♦ intermediate skills, ♦♦♦ high-proficiency skills):

- ♦ Promotes and engages in research/scholarly activities.

- ♦ Reads, interprets, and applies scholarly information relative to occupational therapy.

- ♦ Collects research data.

- ♦ Assumes responsibility for the ethical concerns in research and complies with institutional bio-ethics committee protocols.

♦ Functions according to the AOTA *Code of Ethics* (AOTA, 1988) and the *Standards of Practice* (AOTA, 1992) of the profession.

♦♦ Directs the completion of studies, including data analysis, interpretation, and dissemination of results.

♦♦ Collaborates with others to facilitate studies of concern to the profession.

♦♦ Monitors resources which facilitate research and scholarly activities.

♦♦♦ Probes methods of science, theoretical information, or research designs to answer questions important to the profession.

♦♦♦ Conceptualizes the body of knowledge in the profession to develop new theories, frames of reference, or models of practice.

♦♦♦ Mentors novice researchers.

♦♦♦ Participates at the leadership level in professional, volunteer organizations.

QUALIFICATIONS

- Certified by NBCOT as an OTR or COTA.

- Progressive levels of expertise will require combinations of the following: self-study, continuing education, experience, and formal education for independent research or scholarly activities.

- COTAs can contribute to the research process. COTAs need additional academic qualifications to be a principal investigator.

Supervision: Supervision ranges from close to minimal, depending on the nature of the project and the skills of the researcher/scholar.

ENTREPRENEUR

Major Function: Entrepreneurs are partially or fully self-employed individuals who provide occupational therapy services.

Scope of Role: Entrepreneurs may function in a variety of roles, including independent contractor and private practice owner or operator. The form of organization may be sole proprietorship, partnership, corporation, group practice, or joint venture.

Key Performance Areas (♦ entry-level skills, ♦♦ intermediate skills, ♦♦♦ high-proficiency skills):

♦ Delivers quality occupational therapy services within scope of endeavor.

♦ Develops and implements business plan designed to ensure viability using financial and legal consultation.

- ◆ Establishes a business organization appropriate to nature and scope of activities.

- ◆ Negotiates contractual relationships that take into account the setting, services, and reimbursement.

- ◆ Uses legal, financial, and practice consultation as needed to support business operations.

- ◆ Establishes and collects fees for service, complying with reimbursement requirements.

- ◆ Manages business support services.

- ◆ Complies with local, state, and federal laws and regulations related to business and practice.

- ◆ Complies with standards and guidelines of accrediting or regulating organizations.

- ◆ Develops and maintains personnel policies and records.

- ◆ Develops and implements marketing strategies, as appropriate.

- ◆ Evaluates consumer satisfaction and business operations.

- ◆ Develops and implements risk management plan that includes business property, liability, and employee or employer benefits.

- ◆ Functions according to the AOTA *Code of Ethics* (AOTA, 1988), *Standards of Practice* (AOTA, 1992) of the profession, as well as business ethics.

- ◆◆ Participates in, supervises, or oversees fieldwork program.

- ◆◆ Participates at a leadership level in professional, community organizations.

QUALIFICATIONS

- • Certified by NBCOT as an OTR or COTA.

- • Meets appropriate state regulatory requirements.

- • A minimum of 3 years of practice experience.

Supervision: In cases in which a COTA provides direct service, it is the COTA's responsibility to obtain the appropriate level of supervision from an OTR. Expert consultation or mentorship is obtained as needed to support the business, legal, financial, regulatory, and practice aspects of role performance.

REFERENCES

American Occupational Therapy Association. (1981). Guide to supervision of occupational therapy personnel. *American Journal of Occupational Therapy, 35,* 815-816.

American Occupational Therapy Association. (1988). Occupational therapy code of ethics. *American Journal of Occupational Therapy, 42,* 795-796.

American Occupational Therapy Association. (1990). Entry-level role delineation for registered occupational therapists (OTRs) and certified occupational therapy assistants (COTAs). *American Journal of Occupational Therapy, 44,* 1091-1102.

American Occupational Therapy Association. (1992). Standards of practice. *American Journal Journal of Occupational Therapy, 46,* 1082-1085.

RELATED BACKGROUND MATERIALS

American Occupational Therapy Association. (1991). Essentials and guidelines for an accredited educational program for the occupational therapist. *American Journal of Occupational Therapy, 45,* 1077-1084.

American Occupational Therapy Association. (1991). Essentials and guidelines for an accredited education program for the occupational therapy assistant. *American Journal of Occupational Therapy, 45,* 1085-1092.

American Occupational Therapy Association. Guide to supervision of occupational therapy personnel. (1988). In *Reference manual of official documents of The American Occupational Therapy Association, Inc.* Bethesda, MD: Author. (Original work published 1981, *American Journal of Occupational Therapy, 35,* 815-816.)

Beeler, J. L., Young, P. A. & Dull, S. M. (1990). Professional development framework: Pathway to the future. *Journal of Nursing Staff Development, 6,* 296-301.

Mitchell, M. M. (1985). Professional development: Clinician to academician. *American Journal of Occupational Therapy, 39,* 368-373.

APPENDIX A

BACKGROUND

The need for a broader description of career options for occupational therapy was identified as part of the Entry-Level Study Report (AOTA, 1987) presented to the Representative Assembly (RA). The RA charged the Executive Board to study the recommendation of the Entry-Level Report and develop an action plan. The Executive Board formed a Directions for the Future (DFF) Coordinating Committee and charged that committee to develop an overall action plan. Part of the action plan was the implementation of a DFF Symposium to examine the future needs of practice and education.

Following the symposium, the DFF Coordinating Committee directed the Commission on Education (COE) and Commission on Practice (COP) to form a combined task force of members to develop a document describing a hierarchy of occupational therapy roles. The chairpersons of both commissions selected representatives from a wide variety of arenas in both practice and education. The task force included individuals directly involved in both professional and technical levels of education and practice. Special Interest Section Steering Committee (SISSC) representation was added to the task force to further broaden the scope of the task force. Reference to current professional literature provided a foundation for committee work. The most important references are listed at the end of this section.

Throughout the entire document development process, the document was reviewed by the members of the full COE, COP, COTA Task Force, and SISSC, as well as program directors for professional and technical curricula, thus ensuring both OTR and COTA perspectives. One preliminary review of this document was followed by two formal reviews of drafts. The commission chairpersons recommended that the task force report be sent to the Intercommission Council (ICC) to further ensure that all facets of the Association were represented in the document development process.

As a result of the task force and review processes, an integrated education and practice taxonomy was recommended by the task force rather than a hierarchy. The taxonomy was preferred because it would provide practical information for a variety of uses within the profession. Since this taxonomy is a classification of categories of professional roles, it was decided to entitle the document *Occupational Therapy Roles*.

An ad hoc task force representing the Commission on Education Steering Committee (COESC), the Commission on Practice (COP), and the Special Interest Sections Steering Committee (SISSC) met in 1991 to 1992 and developed this draft entitled, *Occupational Therapy Roles.* This document is expected to replace and expand on the *Guide to Classification of Occupational Therapy Personnel* (AOTA, 1987).

REFERENCE

American Occupational Therapy Association. (1987). Guide to classification of occupational therapy personnel. *American Journal of Occupational Therapy, 39,* 803-810.

AUTHORS

Occupational Therapy Roles Task Force

Patricia A. Crist, PhD, OTR, FAOTA, Chairperson

Julie A. Halom, OTR

Jim Hinojosa, PhD, OTR, FAOTA

Scott McPhee, DrPH, OTR/L, FAOTA

Marlys M. Mitchell, PhD, OTR/L, FAOTA

Barbara A. Boyt Schell, MS, OTR/L, FAOTA

Mary Jane Youngstrom, MS, OTR

Carolyn Harsh, ScD, OTR/L, Staff Liaison

Sarah D. Hertfelder, MEd, MOT, OTR , Staff Liaison

for

Intercommission Council

Catherine Nielson, MPH, OTR/L, Chairperson

Approved by the Representative Assembly June 1993

This document replaces the following documents rescinded by the Representative Assembly in June 1993:

• American Occupational Therapy Association. Guide to classification of occupational therapy personnel. (1987). In *Reference manual of official documents of The American Occupational Therapy Association, Inc.* Bethesda, MD: Author. (Original work published 1985, *American Journal of Occupational Therapy, 39,* 803-810).

• American Occupational Therapy Association. (1990). Supervision guidelines for certified occupational therapy assistants. *American Journal of Occupational Therapy, 44,* 1089-1090.

APPENDIX 11-B

Career Exploration and Development

A Companion Guide to the
Occupational Therapy Roles Document

INTRODUCTION

Practitioner, educator, consultant, researcher . . . these are some of the many roles that occupational therapists fulfill in their careers. In order to understand the scope of these and other roles, the American Occupational Therapy Association (AOTA) developed the *Occupational Therapy Roles* document (*OT Roles*) (AOTA, 1993). *OT Roles* identifies major roles common in the field of occupational therapy and describes for each role the major functions and scope of the role. Key performance areas, relevant qualifications, and supervision required for different levels of expertise are also included. This companion guide illustrates some of the applications of the *OT Roles* document. This companion guide is intended to be used with *OT Roles* and was developed to facilitate an understanding of how roles within the profession interface to permit a variety of career opportunities. The ideas in this guide have been summarized from many sources and reflect related AOTA documents. Readers are referred to the bibliography at the end for selected literature providing more in-depth information about the issues addressed in this document.

OT Roles describes 12 roles (Figure 1). Although not all-inclusive, these roles serve to illustrate the breadth of the profession. The basis for these roles is the OTR or COTA practitioner, as these are the entry paths into the profession. Many employment situations require the individual to perform several roles simultaneously. For example, an occupational therapy department manager at a medium-sized acute care hospital may be called upon to be a supervisor, fieldwork educator, and practitioner in the course of his or her daily duties. Similarly, a member of an occupational therapy curriculum may function as a faculty member, consultant, and researcher.

Figure 1
Occupational Therapy Roles*

Role	Major Function
Practitioner-OTR	Provides quality occupational therapy services, including assessment, intervention, program planning and implementation, discharge-planning-related documentation, and communication. Service provision may include direct, monitored, and consultative approaches.
Practitioner-COTA	Provides quality occupational therapy services to assigned individuals under the supervision of an OTR.
Educator (Consumer, Peer)	Develops and provides educational offerings or training related to occupational therapy to consumer, peer, and community individuals or groups.
Fieldwork Educator (Practice Setting)	Manages Level I or II fieldwork in a practice setting. Provides occupational therapy or occupational therapy assistant students with opportunities to practice and carry out practitioner competencies.
Supervisor	Manages the overall daily operation of occupational therapy services in a defined practice area(s).
Administrator (Practice Setting)	Manages department, program, services, or agency providing occupational therapy services.
Consultant	Provides occupational therapy consultation to individuals, groups, or organizations.
Fieldwork Coordinator (Academic Setting)	Manages student fieldwork program within the academic setting.
Faculty	Provides formal academic education for occupational therapy or occupational therapy assistant students.
Program Director (Academic Setting)	Manages the occupational therapy educational program.
Researcher/Scholar	Performs scholarly work of the profession, including examining, developing, refining, and evaluating the profession's body of knowledge, theoretical base, philosophical foundations.
Entrepreneur	Entrepreneurs are partially or full self-employed individuals who provide occupational therapy services.

*Note: *Many jobs involve more than one role, and job titles vary by setting.*

Individuals can also perform in similar roles, but at differing levels of expertise. For instance, a practitioner supervising his or her first student would be attempting to perform in key areas appropriate for an entry-level fieldwork educator. In contrast, an advanced-level fieldwork educator might coordinate all fieldwork education experiences at a facility and mentor other staff in their fieldwork educator roles.

This companion guide has been designed to help readers use *OT Roles* to meet their specific needs. The first section addresses issues of role development and transition that are applicable to individual uses of the document. These include uses for guiding personal growth and supporting the

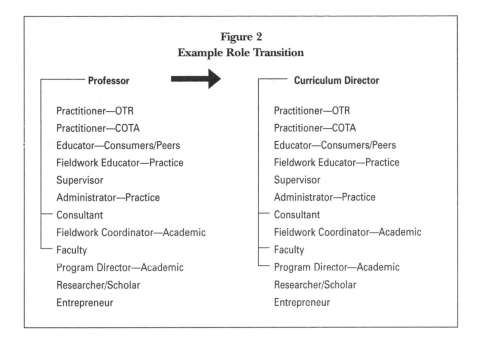

Figure 2
Example Role Transition

Professor	Curriculum Director
Practitioner—OTR	Practitioner—OTR
Practitioner—COTA	Practitioner—COTA
Educator—Consumers/Peers	Educator—Consumers/Peers
Fieldwork Educator—Practice	Fieldwork Educator—Practice
Supervisor	Supervisor
Administrator—Practice	Administrator—Practice
Consultant	Consultant
Fieldwork Coordinator—Academic	Fieldwork Coordinator—Academic
Faculty	Faculty
Program Director—Academic	Program Director—Academic
Researcher/Scholar	Researcher/Scholar
Entrepreneur	Entrepreneur

development of others. Consideration is also given to the document's potential use by administrators, educators, and researchers. In the second section, case studies have been developed to illustrate specific applications for the document. Some cases were developed to highlight common situations. Others were selected because they represent demanding role adjustments.

SECTION I:
USING *OCCUPATIONAL THERAPY ROLES*

DEVELOPMENT AND TRANSITION

Effective career development involves thoughtful transition from one pattern of roles to another. *OT Roles* can be useful in several ways during transition. Individuals can identify qualifications and key performance expectations for relevant roles. They can also identify what levels of expertise may be required for successful role functioning in different environments. For example, a professor at an OT educational program might decide to accept a promotion to direct the program (Figure 2).

In this new job, the curriculum director would add the role of program director to the existing roles of faculty and consultant. This new role would require the development of new abilities, such as curriculum management, faculty development, and skilled negotiation, all necessary for obtaining resources in the politically charged education environment. Similarly, a master clinician might decide to become an entrepreneur and

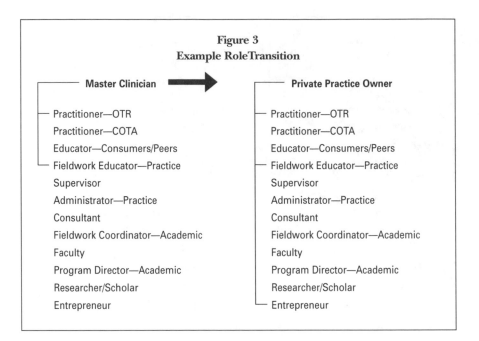

Figure 3
Example Role Transition

Master Clinician ➡ Private Practice Owner

Master Clinician	Private Practice Owner
Practitioner—OTR	Practitioner—OTR
Practitioner—COTA	Practitioner—COTA
Educator—Consumers/Peers	Educator—Consumers/Peers
Fieldwork Educator—Practice Supervisor	Fieldwork Educator—Practice Supervisor
Administrator—Practice	Administrator—Practice
Consultant	Consultant
Fieldwork Coordinator—Academic	Fieldwork Coordinator—Academic
Faculty	Faculty
Program Director—Academic	Program Director—Academic
Researcher/Scholar	Researcher/Scholar
Entrepreneur	Entrepreneur

develop a private practice (Figure 3), while continuing to provide fieldwork educator supervision.

Although the individual would continue as an advanced practitioner and fieldwork educator, a variety of entry-level skills related to the business aspects of practice would be needed in order to succeed as an entrepreneur. Through this process, individuals may realize that they have already gained some of the needed skills important to the new roles under consideration. Additionally, gaps in preparation and ability will become evident, highlighting areas for new skill development.

In addition to role transition, individuals often demonstrate changes in the levels of expertise in each of the roles performed (see Figure 4). Although individuals may stay in the same role, such as practitioner, they advance through development of intermediate or advanced abilities in key performance areas of that role. For instance, a certified occupational therapy assistant was interested in becoming an expert practitioner in the area of pediatrics. Based on this, the individual asked to rotate from the current assignment, which involved treating both children and adults, to working only with children. In the new assignment, the practitioner would continue to work with an OTR in daily treatment of outpatient children, but would have more responsibility for fitting children with and training them in the use of assistive technology devices. These new responsibilities would require planned continuing education, supervised practice, and peer support by other advanced practitioners to further individual practice skills.

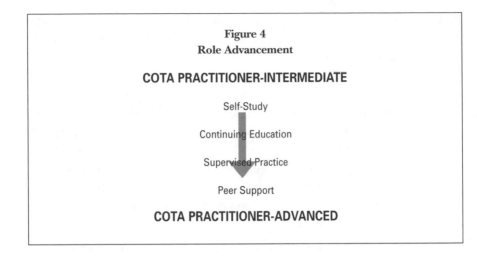

Figure 4
Role Advancement

COTA PRACTITIONER-INTERMEDIATE

Self-Study

Continuing Education

Supervised Practice

Peer Support

COTA PRACTITIONER-ADVANCED

Another person might wish to move from managing a small department to managing a large department. This would require the development of greater knowledge and expertise in the administrative key performance areas, thus prompting the manager to obtain management education. Once the manager assumed the new administrative responsibilities, this same manager might experience a loss of expertise in the practitioner role, if direct patient care is no longer a component of the new job. Active role engagement and ongoing development of skills are necessary to maintain expertise in role functioning.

MAKING CAREERS HAPPEN

Career development is an ongoing process in which systematic planning combines with circumstances, opportunities, individual interests, and ethical considerations. It involves assessment and goal development, environmental scanning, and preparation through education and experience. Each of these processes is described here, with illustrations of how they can be supported with use of *OT Roles.*

Assessment and goal planning. Assessment involves both self-assessment and assessment by others. Self-assessment involves reflection on personal and professional abilities, weaknesses, goals, and growth needs. It also involves examining how work fits into larger life circumstances, such as family obligations, living preferences, and financial resources. At different stages of personal and family development, employment assumes varying levels of importance. Effective career planning and implementation evolve from an assessment process that considers individuals within their unique social contexts.

In conjunction with self-assessment, feedback from others can be crucial in making successful career decisions. Supervisors, peers, and mentors all may have information that can be useful. This information may relate to how they perceive a person's skills and talents relative to various job demands. Additionally, these individuals may have knowledge of the different cultures associated with roles in different settings. The key performance areas emphasized in one situation or work culture may vary dramatically from those emphasized in another. For instance, a professor at a large research institution may be expected to very actively generate original research and supervise student research, while teaching only one course at a time. A professor at a small private college may be expected to spend most of his or her time in teaching and the rest in student advisement. Although these individuals are both professors, the culture in which they work is very different.

Similarly, the practice demands on a therapist in a small, private, for-profit agency may differ from those in a large, nonprofit, public institution. The private agency may place a premium on a high volume of patient service, whereas the other institution may be more supportive of program development and student training. By gaining feedback from individuals who are knowledgeable about both the potential work culture and the particular skills and abilities of the individual, the chances for a better fit are optimized.

Performance areas addressed in *OT Roles* were developed with the recognition that successful function is much broader than mastery of techniques. Communicating with others, understanding systems in which the individual performs, and evaluating both the positive and negative results of one's efforts are all important to career success. Both self-assessment and feedback from others should address these broad issues.

OT Roles can be an important adjunct to the assessment process. Individuals can review the scope and key performance areas within roles and compare these to their own skills. They are also encouraged to review their skills against the demands of new roles, in order to adequately prepare for them. Such comparisons can help to reveal areas in which improvement is needed in order to perform a role satisfactorily or to improve expertise. Supervisors and mentors can use key performance areas within roles as resources in advising others. Suggested qualifications can be reviewed and the level of supervision required can be anticipated.

Environmental scanning. Careers don't happen in a vacuum . . . rather, they reflect the possibilities available in the social environment. Consequently, environmental scanning is important in order to recognize and take advantage of opportunity, as well as to guard against unwelcome career disruptions. Environmental scanning means staying aware of the changes that are happening that may affect job opportunities and responsibilities. This can include becoming aware of policy changes affecting health and education at national and state levels, shifting management philosophies and organizational structures, or learning about changes in populations that require service. *OT Roles* can be a stimulus for considering new options with which to capitalize on change.

Preparing through experience. Whether advancing within a role or transitioning among roles, preparation is usually required for success. There are many forms of preparation, as reflected in the qualification descriptions found in *OT Roles*. Specific experiential approaches to consider are explorative practice, sustained performance, and reflective practice.

- Explorative practice is a temporary or short-term assumption of duties that allows one to experience the demands in a particular situation.

- Sustained performance is the ongoing development of expertise through experience in a role.

- Reflective practice involves the active review of experiences, followed by critical analysis leading to possible improvements.

Each of these experiential approaches can be enhanced by discussions with other knowledgeable individuals, such as supervisors and respected colleagues, allowing for understandings to emerge that otherwise might have not been considered.

Preparing through education. In addition to experience, education can also support career development. Education can take the form of self-directed inquiry, continuing education, or formal education. Self-directed inquiry includes reading, seeking consultation, observing, and initiating informational interviews in order to gain knowledge and develop skills. Continuing education may include participation in self-study programs, seminars, teleconferences, and professional meetings. Such programs tend to focus on very specific topics and are often designed to advance the knowledge and skills obtained through performance. Both self-directed and continuing education can be most effective if they are carefully selected for their potential to enhance current competencies or gain new skills required for transitions.

Formal education is critical for entry into certain roles, such as the education required to become a COTA or an OTR. In other roles, education may be highly desirable. For example, although a doctoral degree is not required to gain employment in some faculty positions, it may be necessary in order for individuals to function effectively or retain their job in an academic environment. *OT Roles* provides information about necessary and desirable educational preparation to qualify for particular roles and helps individuals recognize the relative merits of continuing education versus formal education for given roles.

APPLICATIONS FOR ADMINISTRATION, EDUCATION, AND RESEARCH

In addition to using the document for individual career development and counseling, *OT Roles* has other potential uses for those both within and outside the profession. Administrators will find it useful for developing job descriptions, performance standards, and career ladders. Recognition of the variety of roles to fulfill can assist administrators in enriching existing jobs and creating clusters of roles within jobs to meet organizational needs. Once this is done, staff can be evaluated by matching individual performance abilities against the key performance areas. A review of key qualifications and supervisory requirements can help administrators to match the level of personnel to job demands.

OT Roles can also be used to study group performance. By looking at patterns of performance abilities and gaps across individuals, administrators can recognize strengths and weaknesses of a given department or faculty group. This team assessment can be the basis for staff development programs or strategic recruitment of individuals needed to support team functioning. In this way, groups may be able to more effectively support the mission of their particular setting.

Educators can incorporate *OT Roles* into course work that is designed to orient students to career opportunities and to help students recognize the contributions of various kinds of personnel to the profession. *OT Roles* can stimulate consideration of educational experiences critical for advanced performance, which can be incorporated into graduate programs. For instance, postprofessional academic programs that wish to prepare advanced practitioners and consultants can use the performance areas within these roles as the basis for thinking about important educational course work and experiences. In this way, *OT Roles* serves as the basis for development of hierarchical systems of knowledge, skills, and attitudes useful for curriculum planning.

Researchers and scholars may choose to validate the understandings of professional practice that are inherent in the *OT Roles* or suggest alternative understandings of professional activity. The descriptions of roles could serve as the basis for empirical studies that examine the frequency and quality of role functioning within the field, the nature of supervisory relationships, common career paths, and the importance of various performance areas. In this way, *OT Roles* can serve as a starting point for further knowledge development.

SECTION II: CASE EXAMPLES

In this section, case examples have been used to illustrate how *OT Roles* might be helpful. Case topics have been selected representing career dilemmas that are either common, or carry with them potentially high-stress situations. In each case, there is a brief introduction to the dilemma, followed by a summary of relevant information about the situation. A possible use of *OT Roles,* along with other resources, is described next, followed by the action taken by the individuals in the situation.

Case 1: Student to Practitioner-OTR

In many areas of the country, new graduates are faced with a variety of tempting job offers. This first case shows how students might use OT Roles *as a resource in deciding about a first job.*

During her senior year, Beth Woods had attended both her state and the AOTA Annual Conference, as she had successfully submitted papers for student presentations. While there, she met a number of recruiters. The recruiters were impressed with her academic record, outgoing personality, and experience as a technician in a sheltered workshop prior to enrolling in an academic program. Since then, she had been bombarded by both telephone and mail recruitment offers. Two offers looked particularly promising, especially in light of the heavy school loans that Beth had to pay back. One company offered her a salary of $60,000. This job would require her to perform work capacity evaluations, consult to several work-hardening programs in three different sites, and supervise COTAs. Additionally, she would be expected to develop the OT policies for her facilities and help administration market injury prevention programs to local industries. The money sounded very good, but the responsibilities seemed overwhelming, as she had no previous experience with work capacity programming. A second company was offering $40,000, with a very generous continuing education and tuition reimbursement package. This company provided outpatient rehabilitation services to neurologically and orthopedically involved adults. There was a more experienced therapist to provide her with supervision while she developed her skills. She would, however, be expected to give regular inservice presentations to community groups and participate in support groups for patients and their family members.

Beth referred to *OT Roles* to help her analyze what both jobs would entail, and whether she was qualified to meet them. She realized that the higher paying job had elements from several roles, including practitioner, consultant, and administrator. The other job was a combination of practitioner and educator. Given her experience, Beth decided that realistically she did not have the skills or experience to succeed in the higher paying job, particularly since there would be little supervision available. Based on conversations with more experienced therapists, she anticipated high stress due to ethical concerns and the pressure to perform beyond her current skills. The other job still offered an excellent salary and allowed her to develop her practitioner skills, and capitalize on her early experiences in giving educational presentations. She decided to accept that position.

Case 2: Entry-Level COTA . . . In Search of Supervision

COTAs must analyze the supervisory resources available to support their practice when considering employment. This case shows how an entry-level COTA used OT Roles *to help his employer understand his needs.*

Harry Johnson lived in a rural area of a state in the midwest, not far from where his family had farmed when he was a child. The farm had since been sold, but like many in his family, Harry had found work locally, preferring to stay in the area. He had been a nursing assistant at the county-run nursing home. This facility had difficulty attracting rehabilitation staff and usually relied on contract services. Harry had talked to the administrator who indicated that if Harry were willing to go to the COTA program located across the state, the county would pay for his tuition and expenses. In return, Harry agreed to work a year for every semester of tuition reimbursement. Harry leaped at the opportunity to have a college education paid for, and was now returning home, having completed and passed his certification examination.

On meeting with the administrator, he was dismayed to learn that the contract OTR came in only once a month for 3 hours. Harry felt he was in a bind, because by now he had obligated himself to work at the facility for 6 years. He called the AOTA Practice Department and the state licensure board for guidance. The licensure board advised him that a minimum of 3 hours a week of supervision was required by an OTR, if he was working full-time. Harry did not feel that was enough, since he was an entry-level practitioner. AOTA sent him OT Roles, which supported his belief that he needed close supervision as an entry-level practitioner.

Harry showed *OT Roles* to the nursing home administrator. After hearing Harry's concerns, and reviewing *OT Roles*, the administrator called a number of rehabilitation agencies to find OTR support. He was able to negotiate a contract in which Harry's time would be split between the county nursing home and a long-term- care facility in a nearby community. An OTR (who had no COTA to work with) would be able to float between the two facilities, with Harry as her partner. In this way, both facilities would be covered, Harry would have adequate supervision, and Harry's contract could be honored with his employer. Harry felt comfortable that this situation would be stable enough until he developed sufficient skills to function with less OTR supervision.

Case 3: Supervisor or Clinical Specialist

When practitioners have several years of experience, they often desire to move up career ladders that are now available through many employers. For instance, the supervisor and clinical specialist roles are potential options. The question becomes, what career development activities are needed to explore and prepare for these new roles? This case shows strategies one therapist used to explore two different career options.

Jaime Gonzalez was an occupational therapist who had been working at a rehabilitation center for 2 years. Prior to that position, he worked at an acute care facility. At that facility he found he enjoyed helping individuals with neurological problems regain their independence. After spending a year working with acute care patients, he made the transition to rehabilitation because he felt he could provide more in-depth services to patients in this setting. He believed that he had developed good intermediate skills as a practitioner and was now interested in exploring promotional opportunities within his setting. Because he worked in such a large facility with a well-developed career ladder, he felt he had several possibilities for advancement within his setting. He talked to several of his colleagues in the department about what they thought he should consider. He also raised the issue at his annual performance appraisal. He and his supervisor used the *OT Roles* as a resource to consider some options. After reviewing several roles, Jaime expressed the most interest in the supervisor, advanced-level practitioner, and consultant roles. Based on this, his supervisor arranged several explorative practice opportunities for Jaime. One was to cover for the supervisor of the neurology service when she was on maternity leave. In this way, he could experience first hand some of what was involved in supervision. The other was to spend time observing and talking with each of the other clinical specialists in the department to better understand the mix of consulting and practitioner expectations that made up their jobs. Jaime and his supervisor agreed to meet again after he had done these things so they could make future plans.

After several months, Jaime followed up with his supervisor. She had obtained information from the staff that Jaime had supervised. Jaime was well-liked by the staff, but it was evident that he had some time management problems when placed in the supervisory role, as little of the paperwork required of supervisors was completed on time. He was very good at balancing caseloads and encouraging new staff. Jaime had also been able to complete all of his informational interviews with the clinical specialists. Based on his interviews with clinical specialists, Jaime had decided he did not want to specialize in a practice area at this time. He wished to pursue a supervisory role. Jaime and his supervisor planned to enroll him in continuing education courses on time and project management. He also increased his student and volunteer supervision responsibilities and planned to meet regularly with both his supervisor and the department manager to reflect on his supervision experiences. As he gained skills in supervision, he would be considered for future supervisory openings as they occurred.

Case 4: Practice Administrator to Curriculum Director

Changing jobs requires careful analysis of current skills, and anticipated demands. The expectations of the new work culture must also be understood.

Susan Chen was considering accepting a position as director of a developing occupational therapy assistant program at the local community college. She had been in occupational therapy practice for 15 years, most recently as a regional manager for a large health care corporation where she was responsible for a staff of 60 OTRs and COTAs who served 12 facilities in 7 states.Susan had consulted with other health care corporations, presented adult education workshops, and been active in her state OT association. She had extensive continuing professional education, but no graduate education. Susan was considering accepting this position because she enjoyed her experiences in teaching workshops and wanted to decrease her travel time away from home.

Using the AOTA *OT Roles* document, Susan realized she did not have all the suggested qualifications for faculty and academic program director. While her management experience was quite extensive, she realized she needed to adapt her administrative skills to fit a new setting. Additionally, in reviewing performance expectations, she saw some gaps in her skills. Although she had taught seminars, she had never done the student selection, advising, or curriculum planning inherent in this job. Before accepting the job, she decided to obtain some mentoring to help her make a wise decision. She contacted the AOTA Departments of Accreditation and Education for initial information, and requested the names of people she might contact. She scheduled a meeting with the director of the professional OT academic program at the state university in the next town, and had several telephone consultations with other OTA program directors in different states. Based on this information, she decided to accept the job, after negotiating several additions to her employment contract. These included release time to begin her master's degree studies, a budget that included money for curriculum consultation and networking at professional leadership meetings, and a revision of the proposed start-up time, so that adequate preparations could be made prior to admitting students.

Case 5: Experienced COTA to Adult Day-Care Coordinator

Experienced practitioners may have opportunities to build on their occupational therapy experiences while moving to jobs that are outside the profession. This case shows how OT Roles *can be used to recognize skills that can be used in other settings, as well as how to determine when continued supervision within occupational therapy service provision is required.*

Mary Schmidt was a COTA who had 15 years of experience in a variety of settings, including inpatient and outpatient rehabilitation, home care, and skilled nursing facilities. Over the years, the staff at her facility had begun to rely on her extensive knowledge of a variety of individual and group activities suitable for physically and cognitively impaired adults. She often supervised volunteers and COTA students, and provided functional supervision to OTR students and staff who were learning a new activity procedure. In addition, she routinely handled all the inventory systems and billing summaries. She constantly read about new activity ideas and took every opportunity she had to evaluate new resources on the market.

Although she enjoyed her work, Mary felt ready for a new challenge. Because she was married to a local businessman and had teenage children, moving was not an option for her. However, she became aware of a position for a director with the local adult daycare program. She met with the administrator and found that the job would entail supervising attendant staff, coordinating all activity programming, and facilitating routine care planning meetings of treatment staff. She would be responsible for budgeting and marketing as well. Some of the participants received therapy at the daycare center, but most required only supervision and activity programming to maintain their performance skills.

Mary was excited about the possibility of functioning in a more autonomous role, but wanted to be sure that she had the skills and qualifications to do this new job. She referred to *OT Roles*, which confirmed her belief that she had been functioning as an advanced COTA practitioner. After reviewing the various roles, she realized that her new job would be a blend of administrator, supervisor, and family educator. She would actually not be functioning as a COTA, although it was possible that she might be involved in delivering OT services to those participants who required them. In those circumstances, she would still require practice supervision by an OTR. Otherwise, she would be performing in a job that built on her OT skills, but in fact was outside of the profession. She realized that she had developed many of the skills required in that new job, particularly related to supervision and programming. She was less confident about her administrative skills, especially budgeting and marketing. She decided to take the new position and negotiated for monies to allow her to attend some seminars and courses that would help her develop her administrative skills. She arranged with her prior employer to provide OTR services when required, so that she could continue to provide occupational therapy to those participants who required it.

Case 6: Master Clinician to Assistant Professor

Moving between different work cultures, such as from community practice to an educational institution, can involve many challenges for practitioners. OT Roles, along with the support of mentors, can be an important resource for identifying skills needed to succeed in new roles.

Karen Knotts, MA, OTR/L, was admired locally as a master clinician with an innovative community practice in mental health. Because of her reputation for handling fieldwork students, as well as her clinical expertise, she was asked to consider applying for a faculty position at a large research university to teach in the professional baccalaureate program. The tenure track position would involve teaching courses in activity analysis and mental health, along with engaging in research activities. Karen negotiated and signed the final contract in July.

As the full impact of the career move began to dawn on Karen, she sought *OT Roles* to help her estimate what tasks the new position would entail. Her skills were those of an expert practitioner and fieldwork supervisor. Her new job description was a combination of the roles of faculty and researcher. As Karen scanned the key performance areas for these roles, she identified skills she had and those she would need to develop. She was confident of her course content knowledge and her ability to relate to students, but the faculty role required additional knowledge, such as developing course materials that would integrate her course into the total undergraduate curriculum design. She decided to use her available time before the quarter started to review materials developed by other faculty members as possible models for her courses. She enrolled in a continuing education course on educational methods. She set up a meeting with the program director to become fully oriented to the curriculum philosophy and university mission.

The research role also required some thought. Karen had an interest in depression and had completed one research project as a part of her master's degree program. She still felt she needed guidance and assistance in initiating and executing independent research, especially in the areas of research design and statistical methods. She knew that obtaining a doctoral degree was a necessary condition of tenure at this university and felt that the right doctoral program would help her develop her research skills. Her problem was how to get all of this done! To help her develop a plan to balance her teaching, research, and new doctoral studies responsibilities, Karen sought mentoring from her program director and a tenured faculty member. Karen and her mentors collectively established a time frame and plan for scholarship, as well as for enrolling in a doctoral program during her 1st year. Knowing that tenure decisions would be made after 6 years, her mentors helped her develop activities to be completed on an annual basis that would prepare her to meet the institution's and program's expectations for successful tenure review.

Case 7: A Department Personnel System

OT Roles *can be used to develop career ladders, including job descriptions and performance expectations. This case shows how this might be done.*

Monique LaFleur was hired to manage an occupational therapy department that had recently expanded from 5 to 15 therapists, due to the addition of several new programs within the organization. Prior to the expansion, there had been only an occupational therapy manager and several staff positions. Monique was interested in developing a personnel system in her department that would support orientation, performance appraisal, and the opportunity for therapists to advance as they gained education and experience. She consulted *OT Roles* in order to identify major roles that were relevant to her facility. These were identified as OTR and COTA practitioner (entry-level through (peers, consumers, and fieldwork), supervisor, and consultant. Based on this, she had a committee of staff members reflect on typical daily demands and how these might be met by job descriptions that entailed one or more of these advanced), educator (peers, consumers, and fieldwork), supervisor, and consultant. Based on this, she had a committee of staff members reflect on typical daily demands and how these might be met by job descriptions that entailed one or more of these roles. By combining key performance areas from several roles and defining job functions that included major areas of concern, Monique was able to construct a performance management and career laddering system within the department. She referenced the *OT Roles* in her report to administration and the human resources department, demonstrating that her suggested system was based on an official document from the AOTA. This, combined with supportive information gained from her staff and other OT administrators whom she had contacted, gave her report more credibility.

SUMMARY

The AOTA has developed OT Roles for practitioners, administrators, educators, researchers and others to help them appreciate the broad range of opportunities in occupational therapy. This document also helps individuals and groups understand important qualifications for successful performance of key role components. Continuums of typical progression from entrylevel to expert are suggested.

This companion document demonstrates how *OT Roles* can be used as a resource for career planning, administration curriculum planning, and the basis for research in the field. Case studies have been presented to show some of the many applications of *OT Roles*. It is anticipated that through the use of both *OT Roles* and this companion document, individuals and groups will be able to support continued growth and diversification of the many opportunities within the field of occupational therapy.

REFERENCE

American Occupational Therapy Association. (1993). Occupational therapy roles. *American Journal of Occupational Therapy, 47,* 1087–1098.

BIBLIOGRAPHY

Beeler, J., Young, P., & Dull, S. (1990). Professional development framework: Pathway to the future. *Journal of Nursing Staff Development, 6,* 296–301.

Benner, P. (1984). *From novice to expert.* Menlo Park, CA: Addison-Wesley.

Cervero, R. (1988). *Effective continuing education for professionals.* San Francisco: Jossey-Bass.

Cervero, R., & Dimmock, K. (1987). A factor analytic test of Houle's typology of professionals' modes of learning. *Adult Education Quarterly, 37,* 125–139.

Daloz, L. (1986). *Effective teaching and mentoring.* San Francisco: Jossey-Bass.

Fidler, G. (1966)). Learning as a growth process: A conceptual framework for professional education. *American Journal of Occupational Therapy, 20,* 1–8.

Hall, D. (1976). *Careers in organizations.* In L. W. Porter (Ed.), *Scott, Foresman series in management and organizations.* Glenview, Il: Scott, Foresman.

Houle, C. (1990). *Continuing learning in the professions.* San Francisco: Jossey-Bass.

Mitchell, M. (1985). Professional development: Clinician to academician. *American Journal of Occupational Therapy, 39,* 368–373.

Schell, B. (1992). Setting realistic goals. *Occupational Therapy in Practice, 3,* 3, 11–20.

Schell, B., & Kieshauer, M. (l987). Beyond the job description: Managing for performance. *American Journal of Occupational Therapy, 4l,* 305–309.

Schon, D. (1983). *The reflective practitioner: How professionals think in action.* New York: Basic Books.

Schon, D. (1987). *Educating the reflective practitioner.* San Francisco: Jossey-Bass.

Slater, D., & Cohn, E. (1991). Staff development through analysis of practice. *American Journal of Occupational Therapy, 45,* 1038–1044.

Super, D. (1980). A life-span, life-space approach to career development. *Journal of Vocational Behavior, 16,* 282–298.

AUTHOR

Barbara A. Boyt Schell, MS, OTR, FAOTA

for

The Use Document Task Force:

Patricia Crist, PhD, OTR, FAOTA, Chairperson

Louise C. Fawcett, PhD, OTR

Jim Hinojosa, PhD, OTR, FAOTA

Scott McPhee, DrPH, OTR/L, FAOTA

Marlys M. Mitchell, PhD, OTR/L, FAOTA

Annette M. Port, COTA

Mary Jane Youngstrom, MS, OTR

Carolyn Harsh, ScD, OTR/L, Staff Liaison

Sarah D. Hertfelder, MEd, MOT, OTR/L, Staff Liaison

for

The Intercommission Council 1994

Catherine Nielson, MPh, OTR/L, Chairperson

Previously copyrighted and published by the American Occupational Therapy Association, Inc., in the *American Journal of Occupational Therapy, 48,* 844–51.

SECTION 6

Evaluating

Section 6 treats the important managerial role of evaluating, that is, determining the extent to which programs are achieving the goals and the objectives established for them and using that information as necessary to modify activities. Two chapters constitute the section, "Evaluation of Program" and "Voluntary Accrediting Agencies." The first of these, chapter 12, addresses internal evaluation of program, explaining the origins and the features of program evaluation and quality improvement, two widely used outcome-oriented systems that an organization might adopt to assess its effectiveness and efficiency. The chapter also explains documentation, a basic and necessary process in any kind of evaluation of program.

Chapter 13 turns to external evaluation, as represented in voluntary accreditation, a mechanism for establishing standards and assessing organizations' compliance with them. The chapter highlights the three voluntary accrediting agencies with which occupational therapy managers and practitioners have the most experience: the Joint Commission on Accreditation of Healthcare Organizations; CARF, The Rehabilitation Accreditation Commission; and the Accreditation Council on Services for People with Disabilities.

CHAPTER 12

Evaluation of Programs

KEY TERMS

Criterion measure. In program evaluation, a measure that identifies in absolute terms the specific objective that a program aims to achieve. Compare *improvement measure*.

Documentation. The written record of evaluation and treatment provided.

Effectiveness. (1) In program evaluation, the achievement of benefits by the patient; (2) in quality improvement, a key indicator of a quality program, referring to the results obtained from care. Compare *efficiency*.

Efficiency. (1) In program evaluation, the containment of costs in providing services; (2) in quality improvement, a key indicator of a quality program, referring to the resources employed in achieving a certain outcome. Compare *effectiveness*.

Improvement measure. In program evaluation, a measure that assesses relative change, often through the use of a gain scale. Compare *criterion measure*.

Long-term goal. In documentation, a description of the functional status that a practitioner expects a patient to have reached by the end of treatment in a given facility or program; the goal must be functional, measurable, and objective.

Outcomes management. "A technology of patient experience designed to help patients, payers, and providers make rational medical care–related choices based on better insight into the effect of these choices on the patient's life" (Ellwood, 1988, p. 1551).

Program evaluation system. A system that provides information an organization can use to improve performance to an agreed-on level that meets desired outcomes.

Quality assurance (QA). A set of activities designed to monitor the performance of an organization against specified quantitative thresholds of quality.

Quality improvement (QI). A system through which better and more efficient processes in an organization continuously raise the levels of performance and the outcomes of all functions, eliminate errors, and reduce cost.

Short-term goal. In documentation, a specification of the steps to be taken to reach a long-term goal; the short-term goal (and the long-term goal) must be functional, measurable, and objective.

Total quality management (TQM). A paradigm for business management, emphasizing three themes: continuous quality improvement, doing things right the first time, and empowerment of workers at all levels of an organization to make improvements and take pride in the organization's success.

Value. In quality improvement, the ratio of quality to price.

Christine M. MacDonell, BSOT, is the national director of the Medical Rehabilitation Division of CARF, The Rehabilitation Accreditation Commission. Before joining CARF in 1991, she served as the executive director of the California Alliance of Rehabilitation Industries, and earlier, as education and training coordinator of the California Association of Rehabilitation Facilities. She received her training in occupational therapy at the University of Southern California.

Deborah L. Wilkerson, MA, is now director of research and quality improvement at CARF, The Rehabilitation Accreditation Commission. At the time she contributed to this book, she was the director of program evaluation and outcome studies, and co-director of quality improvement, at the National Rehabilitation Hospital. She was also an adjunct instructor in the Department of Family Medicine at Georgetown University. Her master's degree is from Wake Forest University.

Jane D. Acquaviva, OTR, is a self-employed consultant based in Washington, D.C.'s northern Maryland suburbs. From 1986 to 1992, she was director of continuing education at AOTA, during which time she directed development of AOTA's Documentation Workshop Series. Earlier, as a member of AOTA's Government Relations staff, she was responsible for the reimbursement program. She earned her undergraduate degree in occupational therapy at Columbia University.

Occupational therapy practitioners are living and working in a world of high-velocity change. Consumers of occupational therapy expect accountability and a higher quality of service than ever before, and the workload never seems to become smaller or less demanding. Competition among individual practitioners, among care delivery systems (hospitals, merged organizations, etc.), and between individual practitioners and care delivery systems is at an all-time high, and it continues to stiffen. Messages to managers are sometimes at odds: Cost cutting, cost containment, and efficiency are paramount; yet quality care and effective services are imperative.

Efforts at massive reform of the health care system in the United States have called many prior assumptions into question. Although Congress did not pass major legislation proposed in 1993 to reform health care, the system continues to evolve, with state-level legislation altering payment structures, access to care, and types of care available.

To meet these challenges and gain a competitive edge, occupational therapy managers must make their organization's services effective and efficient. As costs are ratcheted downward, providers who are able to maintain high-quality services may be the survivors of radical changes in the American system of health care delivery. An outcome-focused system of service provision can do more and become better with fewer resources than a system that is not outcome focused. This chapter discusses program evaluation and quality improvement, two systems in widespread use that support an organization in setting goals and objectives, planning and implementing programs to achieve them, monitoring progress toward outcomes, and modifying programs based on outcome data. The chapter also describes documentation, that is, individual practitioners' record keeping on patients. Good and efficient documentation is a necessary element of systems to monitor performance and improve quality.

PART 1

Program Evaluation

Christine M. MacDonell, BSOT

One of the ways to lead an organization to a new level of effectiveness is to develop, implement, and use a program evaluation system. A *program evaluation system* provides information that an organization can use to improve performance to an agreed-on level that meets desired outcomes. Such a system can give managers information that will help them act to affect how staff members provide treatment. A program evaluation system demands that organizations identify what they do and measure how effectively and efficiently they do it. It allows organizations to measure the outcomes of occupational therapy after patients have left the service. In today's marketplace this information is vital for success.

HISTORICAL PERSPECTIVES

Program evaluation grew out of the rapid growth of social programs in the late 1960s. In the early 1970s, rehabilitation providers began to realize that they had focused on process (number of clinical staff, qualifications of staff, etc.) and had no way to measure outcomes that the patient achieved or maintained. In March 1973, CARF, The Rehabilitation Accreditation Commission[1] sponsored an invitational conference to discuss and establish systems for providers to use in measuring the outcomes of their services. This work became the basis of program evaluation standards in CARF.

Throughout the rest of the 1970s, the field of rehabilitation studied and refined outcome measurement systems. In 1982, CARF revised its program evaluation standards with input from the field. There was an increased emphasis on the actual use of outcome information to make decisions about programming for the persons served (Johnston, Wilkerson, & Maney, 1993). In 1995 the CARF Board of Trustees approved a three-year project to facilitate quality improvement through measurement and management of outcomes. Project activities chiefly involve (1) information gathering and networking on tools and techniques, the latest developments

---

1. *CARF is an acronym for Commission on Accreditation of Rehabilitation Facilities. Formed in 1966, the organization changed its name in August 1994 to CARF, The Rehabilitation Accreditation Commission, retaining the acronym as a well-recognized short form of the old designation.*

in research, and best practices, and (2) dissemination of the resulting knowledge to consumers, providers, purchasers, and accreditation personnel (CARF, Board of Trustees, 1995).

STEPS IN PROGRAM EVALUATION

There are 10 major steps in developing, implementing, and using a program evaluation system: (1) gaining awareness, (2) obtaining involvement, (3) justifying use, (4) developing a design, (5) making decisions about data gathering, (6) training staff, (7) processing the data, (8) developing report forms, (9) using the data, and (10) reviewing the system.

GAINING AWARENESS

First, managers must identify an impetus for change. They must recognize that their organization is providing services in a different environment and that this environment demands responsiveness and accountability. They must then ask themselves, Do I want to have a competitive advantage among occupational therapy providers? Do I want to have new patients who are satisfied, referring others to our services, and paying for our services? Do I want to make my job easier and more secure?

Managers who answer yes to these questions are ready to lead their organization through an analysis of the environments in which it operates. This analysis must take into account the emerging forces that are affecting occupational therapy—managed care, product line development, reengineering of organizations, flattening of organizations, and so forth—and the related threats to and opportunities for the organization.

OBTAINING INVOLVEMENT

Managers should lead their environmental analysis with the active participation of all levels of staff members. Identification of challenges and impending changes in the provision of occupational therapy services will elicit cooperation and innovation from staff members and provide a business focus for the organization.

There must be a commitment from all levels of the organization to develop and use this system of accountability. Management must visibly and verbally demonstrate its intentions to use the program evaluation approach to improve services. Staff members should have this verification so that the quality of the information gathered and the use of the information for decision making are not impaired.

JUSTIFYING USE

Once staff members understand management's commitment to a program evaluation system, it is important to have clear statements of why the organization will use the system. The subjects that the statements should clarify are as follows:

1. *Purposes of the system.* These might include improving outcomes for patients, providing information about efficiency to purchasers of services, providing information about satisfaction to referral sources, and so forth.

2. *Services that will be subject to evaluation.* If the occupational therapy organization is large, the manager might choose to begin evaluation in one area, such as inpatient rehabilitation, home health, or outpatient day treatment, or to begin with one product line, such as hands, orthopedic services, neurological services, sports medicine, or occupational rehabilitation.

3. *Major elements of the system.* The elements that an organization includes in its system will depend on the model that it uses. CARF has had program evaluation standards since 1973. Over 11,000 rehabilitation programs in the United States and Canada currently use CARF's model (Commission on Accreditation of Rehabilitation Facilities, 1991c). Small organizations can use it as well. The model has 13 elements. They are identified and discussed later in the chapter.

4. *Development process.* Questions to address in this area include who will be responsible, what resources are needed, what resources will be available, what are the general time frames, how will staff members participate, and so forth.

5. *Use.* Decisions to make in this area are who will receive the information, how frequently will the information be reported, how will the organization use the data, and what will the budget for the operation be.

The manager and key staff members of the occupational therapy organization should specify these elements in a *written* document that provides readers with a broad understanding of the program evaluation system. The organization can then use the document as a tool to orient new employees and to communicate to staff members about the nature of the system and the ways in which the organization intends to use it. This is not a secret document, but one that is shared with and distributed to those who are concerned about the provision of services and organizational policies.

DEVELOPING A DESIGN

When the manager and key staff members have completed the specifications for the system, it is time to develop the evaluation design. This process will vary greatly from organization to organization, depending on staff members' talents in program evaluation. If some staff members have expertise in this area, they might organize themselves as a task force to develop and obtain reactions to the program evaluation elements. This approach can be time-consuming, but it has the advantage of soliciting input from staff members throughout the process. Having the opportunity to provide input appears to decrease resistance as the system moves through development, implementation, and use. It also facilitates staff members' understanding of the entire system.

Some small organizations may not have staff members who are interested in program evaluation. If they do not, the manager must take on the responsibility of design or seek assistance outside the organization. Many consultants and companies provide this type of technical assistance. The CARF standards (published annually) and two CARF monographs on program evaluation (Commission on Accreditation of Rehabilitation Facilities, 1991c, 1992) are also sources for the manager. Decisions about responsibility for development of the design depend on the financial resources of the organization and its overall commitment to the program evaluation system.

MAKING DECISIONS ABOUT DATA GATHERING

The next step is to decide how to gather data for program evaluation and how to measure change. Methods might include formal or informal measurement instruments, interview protocols, and follow-up forms and procedures. The organization will need to gather the same kinds of information on patients at admission, discharge, and follow-up.

The importance of the data-gathering and measurement tools is evident from the number available and the number of companies and individuals that are working on development and revision of them. It is impossible to list all the possibilities. AOTA's Practice Division can assist organizations when they reach this stage of development.

There are many ways to conduct follow-up: The organization can do the work itself by telephone, by mail, or through face-to-face reevaluation; or it can contract with a company to do the work. The important elements in follow-up are the efficiency of the system and its capacity for gathering the information that the organization needs.

TRAINING STAFF

Staff training occurs next. The success of the system depends on how much staff members concur on the importance of the data that they need to collect. Staff members also need to understand how management will use the information to develop, modify, revise, and eliminate what they do as clinicians. Staff members should see the system as a valuable resource for gaining new equipment, positions, and resources, and as a tool to assist them in doing more with less.

Most organizations that have developed a program evaluation system have found it helpful to develop a manual that can be used to train and orient staff members and administration, as well as to explain the system. This will ensure uniformity and consistency in use of the forms. Staff members must learn how and when to record information on individual patients. Procedures should be in place that address the feeding of information into the program evaluation system at appropriate times.

PROCESSING THE DATA

Once the program evaluation system is operational, the organization must decide whether to process the data manually or use an automated system. The decision is usually based on the volume of data, the number and the complexity of the reports needed, and the costs involved in automating. Regardless of the decision, the occupational therapy organization must go through the same steps of designing the system, developing measurement instruments, and establishing reporting and follow-up procedures to obtain data for processing. Also, it must still analyze and interpret the data for use in decision making and planning.

DEVELOPING REPORT FORMS

Concurrently with system design and staff training, the organization should develop forms to report and interpret the data obtained through the program evaluation system. The occupational therapy manager will most likely be responsible for the program evaluation management report, so if the manager has sought technical assistance from an outside consultant, he or she should work with the consultant in developing the forms.

USING THE DATA

The crucial component of use of the information now comes into play. The occupational therapy manager should use the information in making all decisions on modification, revision, addition, or elimination of services. The information will assist the manager in making appropriate and usually difficult decisions about staffing, allocation of resources, lengths of stay, and so forth. If the manager does not use the program evaluation system in this way, it will only consume organization dollars and be viewed as one more "thing" that should never have been done.

REVIEWING THE SYSTEM

A program evaluation system is a guide. It cannot be a static system, however, because of the environment in which practitioners provide services today. Priorities change. Staff members change. Patients, purchasers, and referral sources change. So organizations must periodically review their program evaluation system to determine if it is still accurate and appropriate, or needs modification.

Occupational therapy managers should regularly ask themselves these questions:

1. Is the system achieving the purpose for which the organization created it?

2. Is the system comprehensive in scope? Is it complete in terms of the value of the information it is producing?

3. Is the cost of maintaining the system reasonable in terms of the value of the information it is producing?

4. Is the system producing accurate information?

5. Is the system providing the information in a timely manner?

The answers will help occupational therapy managers determine the changes necessary to make their organization's program evaluation system a vital management tool in today's health care environment.

ELEMENTS OF THE CARF PROGRAM EVALUATION MODEL

A program evaluation system can be as simple or as difficult as an organization makes it. It may be a very expensive, computerized system, or it may be a small, manually operated system. Regardless of its size and complexity, it must have 13 key elements if it is to help an organization measure and manage outcomes: (1) a purpose statement, (2) a program structure, (3) program goal statements, (4) admission criteria, (5) a list of types of patients served, (6) a list of services provided, (7) a statement of objectives, (8) measures, (9) a specification of the time of application of measures, (10) a specification of the patients to whom measures will be applied, (11) patient descriptors, (12) an expression of performance expectancies, and (13) a statement of the relative importance of objectives. For many people, development of the 13 elements of the program evaluation system is the most complex and technically difficult portion. This section discusses the rationale for each element and gives examples of how to deal with the element.

A PURPOSE STATEMENT

A statement of purpose is necessary for persons outside the organization to gain a general understanding of the organization's mission and the needs that it is meeting for the general community or a specific population. This statement becomes a foundation for the other components of the program evaluation system. The statement should be in sufficient detail that the reader can see the relationship between the organization's purpose and its specific goals and objectives. For example:

> The mission of the XYZ Occupational Therapy Department is to assist adults with physical disabilities in achieving maximum independence and returning to their communities through a coordinated program of physical restoration, training in activities of daily living, cognitive retraining, and community-integration activities.

A PROGRAM STRUCTURE

An occupational therapy organization has an administrative structure that is usually displayed in an organizational chart. A program structure describes the organization in terms of function. A program structure should facilitate management of resources and be comprehensive enough to measure outcomes for all patients receiving services. For example:

> One or more liaisons from each program or service offered (return-to-work program, inpatient program, home care program, etc.) are responsible for coordination of the outcome system. Ultimately the occupational therapy manager is responsible for the efficiency of their plan for measurement of outcomes across programs and services.

PROGRAM GOAL STATEMENTS

The program goal statements provide a specific description of a major characteristic of each service. They help clarify the specific intent of a program, indicating whom it serves, what services it offers, and what outcomes its managers expect. For example:

> The Occupational Rehabilitation Program of the XYZ Occupational Therapy Department provides functional capacity evaluations, and physical restoration activities that will return an injured worker to work.

ADMISSION CRITERIA

The admission criteria detail characteristics, behaviors, capabilities, disabilities, or other qualifications that a person must possess to be admitted to the occupational therapy program. These criteria ensure that the persons for whom the program is intended are admitted. They also give objective reasons to persons who are not admitted to the program. Further, criteria assist referral sources and purchasers of services in directing people appropriately to the services they need. It is important that the occupational therapy manager distinguish specific criteria for admission to an occupational therapy program from the larger organization's criteria. For example:

The patient must be medically stable.

The patient must be able to respond to verbal or physical stimuli.

The patient must have a referral from a physician.

The patient must have a job to which he or she can return.

PATIENTS SERVED

The list of types of patients served is a simple list of the types of characteristics and needs apparent in the patients whom the occupational therapy organization serves. This list clarifies and justifies the nature of the persons whom the organization expects to benefit from occupational therapy services. There should be a logical relationship between patients served and the description of the program (in the program goal statements) and between patients served and the admission criteria. Examples of some characteristics and needs of patients are as follows:

Dependence in some area of activities of daily living

An upper-extremity injury with loss of function

Psychosocial impairments related to physical disability

Neurological disorders

Psychological disorders

SERVICES PROVIDED

The list of services provided is a list of the services that the occupational therapy organization offers, the services that will assist the organization in reaching its program goals. The list describes the resources that are available for a patient to achieve his or her goals. There should be a logical relationship between services provided, patients served, and program goal statements. Examples are as follows:

Functional capacity evaluations

Training in stress management

Driver education and training

Splinting

Assistance in community integration

Training in activities of daily living

OBJECTIVES

The objectives element is a series of statements of the results that the occupational therapy services are intended to achieve. There are two types of objectives: One type is related to *effectiveness,* the achievement of benefits by the patient; the other type is related to *efficiency,* the containment of costs in providing services. Each occupational therapy organization will have numerous objectives. Not all patients can be expected to achieve all the objectives. The program evaluation system should be able to summarize the results that patients have achieved and the cost of achieving the results. The objectives should express desired changes following the provision of service rather than desired changes during the provision of service. They should be specific enough to be measured—for example, "Reduce patient's dependency on others in the home" rather than "Improve patient's home life." Other examples of objectives are as follows:

Maintain patient's health status

Contain program costs

Prevent institutionalization of patient

MEASURES

Measures are the methods that an organization uses to determine whether it has achieved its objectives. One should always start with objectives; measures follow logically. There are two kinds of measures: improvement measures and criterion measures. An *improvement measure* assesses relative change, often through the use of a gain scale. For example, if the objective is to maximize independence in dressing, an improvement measure is the percentage of patients who improve one level on a dressing scale. Patients' gains on a scale may be quite significant or very insignificant, depending on how the scale is constructed. Also, interpreting gain results can be difficult, especially for people outside the organization who may be unfamiliar with the scale.

A *criterion measure* identifies in absolute terms the specific objective that a program aims to achieve. In the preceding example, a criterion measure is the percentage of patients who become independent in dressing. This kind of information has more meaning and a greater effect on the parties that need to understand what an occupational therapy organization does and how well the organization does it—for example, referral sources, administrators, and purchasers (insurance companies, managed care corporations, employers, etc.).

Measures should gauge improvement from time of admission to discharge to a point after discharge. To lessen the possibility that the practitioner who treated a patient will interpret statements in a more favorable light, he or she should not do the follow-up measurement on that patient.

In establishing measures the occupational therapy manager must be sure that the organization is measuring outcomes, not process. If all the qualified staff members left and were replaced by inexperienced practitioners with little skill level in the area that the organization is measuring, there should be a definite decrease in effectiveness.

Efficiency measures should facilitate an understanding of the relationship between the amount of resources that the organization has expended and the level of benefit that patients have achieved. Examples of resources are level of staff (registered occupational therapists versus certified occupational therapy assistants), dollars, and days required to reach objectives.

Examples of objectives and measures are as follows:

Objective	Measure
Maximize patient's independent living	Percentage of patients residing in an independent-living situation
Help patients obtain employment	Percentage of patients returning to work
Maintain patient's health status	Percentage of patients who remain free of health problems related to their disability

TIME OF APPLICATION OF MEASURES

Time of application of measures refers to the time when measurement takes place. It should be appropriate to the objective being measured. If staff members apply a measure too soon after the provision of occupational therapy services, the benefit of the services may not yet have occurred. If staff members apply the measure too long after the provision of services, there may be changes that are not the result of the services. Examples of time of application are as follows:

At discharge

One week after discharge

Ninety days after discharge

PATIENTS TO WHOM MEASURES WILL BE APPLIED

The program evaluation system should identify the patients whom the organization will assess with each measure. In most evaluation systems, all measures are not applied to all patients. It is important for the organization to specify clearly to whom it will apply measures so that it will be able to gather appropriate and reliable data. This determination should be an official act, not a chance occurrence. Examples:

Measure	To Whom Applied
Percentage of patients achieving independence in dressing	All patients receiving dressing training
Percentage of patients returning to work or school	All patients over 16 years of age and under 65 years of age
Percentage of patients obtaining transfer to more independent living situation	All patients in dependent-living situation at admission

PATIENT DESCRIPTORS

Patient descriptors define the persons whom occupational therapy is serving. They should express severity of problems or barriers to success. They should also facilitate judging the adequacy of program results. Patient descriptors can be helpful in marketing the program. For example, by tracking the number of patients with arthritis, an organization might be able to receive additional funds from the local arthritis foundation. Examples of patient descriptors are as follows:

Percentage of patients admitted from an extended-care facility

Percentage of patients recently disabled (within the past six months)

Percentage of patients dependent on pain-relieving medications

Percentage of patients requiring driver training

PERFORMANCE EXPECTANCIES

Performance expectancies reflect the degree to which an organization expects to achieve an objective. When an organization gathers data about the objectives that it has established, comparing the data against an expectancy is helpful. This adds an evaluative element to the data that are gathered. For example:

Measure	Expectancy	Actual Result
Patients who achieve independent living	85%	78%
Cost per patient	$15,000	$12,500

A comparison of expectancies and actual results reveals that the program is below its expectancy of benefit on the independence measure, but well within its expectancy of cost.

Setting a *range* of expectancies helps to put the actual results in perspective if they are below or above the goal. The *minimal level* is a level of performance that the occupational therapy organization would judge to be unacceptable. It would indicate a need for a substantial corrective action. The *optimal level* is a level of performance that the occupational therapy organization thinks it could achieve under ideal situations. Following is the preceding example recast in this format:

Measure	Expectancy			Actual Result
	Minimal	Goal	Optimal	
Patients who achieve independent living	70%	85%	95%	78%
Cost per patient	$22,000	$15,000	$10,000	$12,500

The comparison of expectancies and actual results in this framework reveals that the program is above its minimal expectancy of benefit, though below its goal and its ideal. On the cost measure, it is well below the unacceptable figure and comfortably below its goal, though not within its ideal.

RELATIVE IMPORTANCE OF OBJECTIVES

The occupational therapy organization will not view all objectives as equally important. The program evaluation system must weight or prioritize the objectives. The occupational therapy manager needs to ask the question, If all 10 of our objectives fell below an acceptable level of performance, into which one would we put our resources first, second, and so forth? If the organization chooses to use a weighted system, it should give greater weight to objectives that contribute to achieving the overall program goals than it gives to objectives that do not.

A program evaluation system gives occupational therapy managers a valuable tool that will move them from a reactive role to a proactive one. When market forces alone drive the provision of health care, everyone becomes reactive. Occupational therapy practitioners, not people external to the occupational therapy profession, can and should initiate all changes in the delivery of occupational therapy services. Occupational therapy practitioners should not underestimate their capability to become effective and efficient. An internal evolution in each occupational therapy manager's practice will collectively create the health care revolution required to address the challenges of cost-effectiveness and continuing recognition of occupational therapy as a valuable service.

SUMMARY OF PART 1

One of the ways to lead an organization to a new level of effectiveness is to develop, implement, and use a *program evaluation system,* a type of system that provides information an organization can use to improve performance to an agreed-on level that meets desired outcomes.

There are 10 major steps in developing, implementing, and using a program evaluation system: (1) gaining awareness, (2) obtaining involvement, (3) justifying use (clarifying purposes, services subject to evaluation, major elements, the development process, and use), (4) developing a design, (5) making decisions about data gathering, (6) training staff, (7) processing the data, (8) developing report forms, (9) using the data, and (10) reviewing the system.

Regardless of its size and complexity, a program evaluation system must have 13 key elements: (1) a purpose statement, (2) a program structure, (3) program goal statements, (4) admission criteria, (5) a list of types of patients served, (6) a list of services provided, (7) a statement of two types of objectives (one type related to *effectiveness*, the achievement of benefits by the patient; the other type related to *efficiency*, the containment of costs in providing services), (8) two kinds of measures (*improvement measures*, which assess relative change, often through the use of a gain scale; and *criterion measures*, which identify in absolute terms the specific objectives that a program aims to achieve), (9) a specification of the time of application of measures, (10) a specification of the patients to whom measures will be applied, (11) patient descriptors (definitions of the persons who are served), (12) an expression of performance expectancies, and (13) a statement of the relative importance of objectives.

PART 2

Quality Improvement

Deborah L. Wilkerson, MA

Quality improvement systems, transmutations of quality assurance systems, provide a mechanism for monitoring the quality of care, reviewing the appropriateness and the effectiveness of care, assessing the use of health care resources, and modifying programs and services as a result. As noted in part 1 of this chapter, it is not sufficient for occupational therapy organizations to assess and monitor outcomes of care. They must apply the knowledge gained to making changes in the system of service delivery. Neither is it sufficient to document that a practitioner has provided quality services to the persons whom he or she serves. As quality improvement systems have evolved, the mandate has become to *improve* the quality of care continually through changes in the processes and the outcomes. What is of importance is the relationship between the processes of care—treatments and interventions, ways of doing things in the organization—and their results—clinical outcomes, consumer satisfaction, and efficiency of operations.

The earlier notion of quality assurance has undergone a transformation during the 1980s and 1990s, based in large part on the spillover of quality improvement concepts from manufacturing industries. The transformation has brought the concept of quality improvement more in line with the long-standing emphasis on program evaluation promoted by CARF for rehabilitation organizations. This part of chapter 12 discusses quality improvement because of its widespread use in many types of American organizations.[2] Occupational therapy managers would do well to consider merging the concepts of program evaluation and quality improvement into one effort at providing the highest-quality service possible.

A DEFINITION OF QUALITY IMPROVEMENT

Quality in occupational therapy and rehabilitation services can and has been described in many ways. At a minimum the highest quality demands that the right things be done, that things be done right, that what is done

---

2. *The sections of this part titled Early Lessons in the Importance of Quality Review, Emergence of Quality Assurance in Health Care, and Relationship of Quality Improvement to Research and Program Evaluation, are based in part on "Quality Assurance," by B. E. Joe, 1992, in J. Bair and M. Gray (Eds.),* The Occupational Therapy Manager *(Rev. ed., pp. 251–58), Rockville, MD: American Occupational Therapy Association.*

be done efficiently, that desirable outcomes be achieved, that errors not be made, that decisions be appropriate, and that people be treated well (Crosby, 1979; Deming, 1982). Beyond these basics are many angles on quality specific to occupational therapy and rehabilitation: positive outcomes for recipients of care, individualized care, well-trained staff members, involvement of patients and clients and their families in care decisions, and lack of complications and rehospitalizations (England, Glass, & Patterson, 1989; Johnston & Wilkerson, 1992; National Rehabilitation Hospital, 1992).

Quality improvement (QI) is a system through which better and more efficient processes in an organization continuously raise the levels of performance and the outcomes of all functions, eliminate errors, and reduce cost.[3] All persons in the organization, in all departments, have a responsibility to assess and improve quality. Conceptually very similar to the notion in formative program evaluation of using information to improve the program, QI tends to focus more sharply on the processes of care, using outcomes and other information as pointers to areas needing improvement. In addition, as an emerging field, QI has developed well-honed tools for separating processes into their component parts, analyzing where problems exist, and reformatting the processes to improve them. Data on outcomes, cost, and consumers' satisfaction are then used as evidence that the process changes actually created a quality improvement.

HISTORICAL PERSPECTIVES

EARLY LESSONS IN THE IMPORTANCE OF QUALITY REVIEW

The examination of whether medical treatments really work has evolved through history, but even early observations in quality aimed at reducing error and variation. In the 1860s, nurse Florence Nightingale observed and reported on the deficiencies of health care services provided to those wounded in the war (Huxley, 1975). As the first person to collect and compare mortality statistics from different hospitals, she documented a plunge in the death rate in military hospitals during the Crimean War, from 42 percent to 2.2 percent.

Florence Nightingale's efforts were continued by a physician, Abraham Flexner. His 1910 report on the poor quality of medical education in the United States and Canada was instrumental in closing 60 of 155 United States medical schools then in existence.

---

3. *Quality improvement (QI) is sometimes referred to as continuous quality improvement (CQI). The term quality improvement and its abbreviation QI imply continuous improvement of performance, as compared with the notion of improvement of performance to a threshold that need not be altered once it has been reached.*

In 1912 a revolutionary and prophetic resolution from the Third Clinical Congress of Surgeons of North America began to change health care. The resolution stated,

> Some system of standardization of hospital equipment and hospital work should be developed, to the end that those institutions having the highest ideals may have proper recognition before the profession, and that those of inferior equipment and standards should be stimulated to raise the quality of their work. (as quoted in Davis, 1960, p. 476)

Five years later the American College of Surgeons initiated the process of hospital accreditation, formulating *Minimum Standards for Hospitals.*

EMERGENCE OF QUALITY ASSURANCE IN HEALTH CARE

In 1951 the American College of Surgeons, in concert with other professional medical groups, established the Joint Commission on Accreditation of Hospitals, now the Joint Commission on Accreditation of Healthcare Organizations (JCAHO). The Joint Commission's quality assurance program evolved over the next several decades. In 1955 the Joint Commission began to stress the importance of medical audits. By 1974 its standards required hospitals to audit medical records and make quarterly reports. In 1981, judging that the audit system was producing good medical records but not necessarily better care, the Joint Commission began urging the introduction of additional *monitors,* or measures of important outcomes of care, and a focus on problem resolution.

As late as 1990, key literature still used the term *quality assurance* (QA), meaning a set of activities designed to monitor the performance of an organization against specified quantitative thresholds of quality. QA had as its hallmark (1) the sampling of case records for review, (2) peer study of case records, and (3) identification of thresholds of performance. Once performance reached those thresholds, an organization could claim to have met quality screens. Nonetheless, QA was rooted in discovering the relationship between process and outcome.

FROM QUALITY ASSURANCE TO QUALITY IMPROVEMENT

The concepts and the activities surrounding the review and the enhancement of quality health and rehabilitation services have undergone a gradual but major transformation during the 1980s and the 1990s. In the 1980s a quality revolution occurred in American business and manufacturing and began to spread into health care. The concept of *total quality management* (TQM) influenced several key shifts in the paradigm of QA (McLaughlin & Kaluzny, 1990). First, the notion of a quality threshold gave way to the ideas of continuous improvement and zero defects.

Second, the notion that quality could be assured gave way to the idea that quality is a matter of perception of the consumer of a service; although quality must be quantified and measured, satisfaction of the consumer is the ultimate demonstration of quality products. Today these ideas are being refined in health care in ways that affect the occupational therapy manager.

KEY CONCEPTS

Several concepts are key to the evolution and the consideration of QI and the design and the implementation of QI systems. Each concept has contributed to modern QI activities.

DONABEDIAN'S FRAMEWORK: STRUCTURE, PROCESS, AND OUTCOME

In 1966, Donabedian proposed a framework for assessing the quality of medical care, and in 1983 and 1988 he elaborated on his now-classic scheme. The framework includes three dimensions: *structure,* or the "attributes of the settings in which care occurs"; *process,* "what is actually done in giving and receiving care"; and *outcome,* "the effects of care on the health status of patients and populations" (1988, p. 1745). These concepts parallel a systems analysis framework (input, process, and output). For a long while, the focus of QA in rehabilitation and occupational therapy was on the structure and the processes of care. The heightened attention to outcomes in health care during the 1980s and the 1990s has brought this third dimension more actively into the QI equation.

The practical implication of the Donabedian framework for QI activities is to focus attention on the relationship between structure, process, and outcome. Causal relationships are difficult to establish, and they must be determined not by QI efforts, but by careful prior research (Donabedian, 1988). Yet the assessment of each component of the triad is essential to a thorough review of quality. Organizations are led, then, to include in a quality review all their departments and functions, from clinical program operations (structure and process) and effectiveness (outcome), to support systems—referrals and admissions, finance, housekeeping, food service, and other administrative structures and processes.

TOTAL QUALITY MANAGEMENT

TQM is a paradigm for business management that was first developed in the United States by American W. Edwards Deming (1982). Initially ignored in this country, the innovation was adopted by the Japanese manufacturing industry, which subsequently soared to success in the global economy (McLaughlin & Kaluzny, 1990). Central to TQM are 14 points, which emphasize the three TQM themes:

1. Quality, and processes that produce quality products, can always be improved.

2. It is possible for things to be done right the first time, and this should become the standard.

3. Workers at all levels of an organization should be empowered to make improvements and be provided with avenues to take pride in the organization's success.

Health care as an industry has been slower to adopt TQM concepts than business has because of the challenges of translating a paradigm originating in manufacturing into the language of service organizations. However, with JCAHO refocusing its standards on the concepts of TQM (JCAHO, 1995a; McLaughlin & Kaluzny, 1990), health care organizations of all kinds are now implementing TQM strategies and tools to help improve quality.

FOCUS ON THE CONSUMER

Consumer Satisfaction

An important element of TQM is its focus on the consumer's satisfaction with a product. The QI paradigm recognizes that processes of care are successful only to the extent that they result in a high-quality product or service for the consumer and minimize costs to the consumer and the payer. Consequently, consumer satisfaction has become a key new outcomes measure in the tool kit of program evaluation and QI. The implications of this new element for occupational therapy managers are that they must establish systems for tapping the satisfaction of patients, families, other advocates, and payers, and for incorporating their findings into action plans for quality improvements.

Consumer Service

Consistent with the focus on the consumer's satisfaction, QI programs often include specific activities teaching that it is every employee's responsibility to serve the consumer, whether the consumer is internal (other staff members and colleagues) or external (patients, families, referral sources, and payer representatives) to the organization. Occupational therapy managers may find themselves engaged in full-fledged training programs designed to orient staff members to entirely new ways of thinking for a health care organization. Based in the TQM philosophy, a heightened focus on service to consumers is founded on the premise that higher-quality care means meeting the needs of the users of the service. This is in fact a fairly radical shift in medical and health services; traditionally the professional has presumed to know best what is right for the patient, and fee-for-service arrangements have put providers, rather than payers, in charge of what services are rendered. The practice is now changing to place explicit value on including the consumer in decisions about care.

OUTCOMES MANAGEMENT

Paul Ellwood, a leader in outcomes and health policy research, first proposed *outcomes management* in 1988. He defines it as "a technology of patient experience designed to help patients, payers, and providers make rational medical care–related choices based on better insight into the effect of these choices on the patient's life" (p. 1551). It employs four key techniques:

1. Use of standards and guidelines to help physicians choose appropriate treatments

2. Routine and systematic measurement of patients' functioning and well-being, and of disease-specific outcomes

3. Pooling of outcome data and information on the clinical process to form large databases for study

4. Analysis and dissemination of results in appropriate form for the use of various decision makers in health care

Outcomes management forms a link between the traditional arena of program evaluation and the newer notion of QI. At the core is the notion of studying and identifying the relationship between the outcomes of care and the processes that influence those outcomes. Variation in care not attributable to patients' needs should be minimized, and the cost of care should retreat (Berwick, 1989, 1990). The concepts inherent in outcomes management resonate particularly well in the already outcome-oriented field of rehabilitation, to such a degree that CARF adopted the phrase *outcome measurement and management* beginning with its 1995 standards (see part 1 of this chapter).

An implication of outcomes management for occupational therapy managers is that quality review mechanisms will increasingly include the building of an ongoing database on patients—perhaps in addition to sample case review methods—from which to examine trends in the outcomes of programs. Ongoing data systems are likely to encompass outcomes measures and to be used as a source of evidence that QI efforts are working. Top management will expect occupational therapy managers both to contribute to, and to be able to understand and use information from, an outcomes management system as part of an overall QI initiative.

EFFECTIVENESS, EFFICIENCY, AND VALUE

Many program evaluation and QI systems refer to the twin concepts of effectiveness and efficiency as key indicators of a quality program. *Effectiveness* refers to the outcome dimension: What results are obtained from care? For example, what gains did patients make in functional status? What proportion of clients were able to return to the living arrangements that they enjoyed before incurring a disability? What proportion of consumers received and were able to make use of recommended assistive devices? *Efficiency* considers the resources employed in achieving a certain outcome: What did it cost to obtain certain results of care? How much gain was achieved for a given expenditure of resources? For example, what measurable change in functional status occurred for every thousand dollars of charges?

Value is the principal concept that brings together effectiveness (outcome), cost and price, and efficiency. *Value* is the ratio of quality to price: Although high-quality programs can certainly be provided at high cost, the highest quality for the lowest price is the highest value. A premise of TQM is that quality can be maximized while cost from doing things wrong (error) and doing the wrong things (misfocus) is reduced. The long-range goals of QI and program evaluation are to encourage and communicate value in an organization.

CURRENT PLAYERS AND DRIVING FORCES

In addition to serving as an organization's means of reviewing and enhancing the value of its services, QI systems are required by external reviewers of quality. As consumers, payers, and the public call on accrediting bodies and peer review organizations to certify the quality of health care providers, those bodies and organizations in turn want assurance that mechanisms are in place to identify problems, find opportunities and implement strategies for improvement in processes and outcomes, and continually maximize the quality of care provided.

ACCREDITING BODIES

CARF, The Rehabilitation Accreditation Commission

For more than two decades CARF has required that rehabilitation programs use an ongoing, outcome-based program evaluation system to assess effectiveness and efficiency of services. CARF further requires that organizations apply the resulting knowledge to planning and management of clinical programs. Although the CARF standards use terms different from TQM and QI jargon—for example, *program evaluation* and *outcome management*—they describe QI efforts. Three sections of the 1995 CARF standards are especially relevant: "Promoting Organizational Quality," "Promoting Program Quality," and "Promoting Outcome Measurement and Management." Chapter 13 describes CARF and its standards in greater detail.

Joint Commission on Accreditation of Healthcare Organizations

JCAHO heavily influences the QI activities of many provider organizations, and with its 1995 standards it has made a major philosophical shift consistent with TQM concepts. Instead of focusing on identifying errors and measuring whether or not a quantitative threshold for quality has been met (as in traditional QA), the agency is now concentrating on improving processes to eliminate errors, and on *continuously* improving quality (eliminating the threshold) (McLaughlin & Kaluzny, 1990).

Particularly relevant to QI are two sections of the JCAHO (1995a) standards: "Improving Organizational Performance," which requires that the organization "continuously measure, assess and improve all important patient care and organizational functions" (p. 222); and "Information Management," which requires that the organization "obtain, manage and use information to enhance and improve individual and organizational performance in patient care, governance, management and support processes" (p. 377). Information from individual case records, aggregate data, external knowledge-based information (e.g., scientific literature and practice guidelines), and comparative data are all components. Chapter 13 contains more information about JCAHO and its standards.

PEER REVIEW ORGANIZATIONS

Peer review, as the name implies, is a system by which professionals review the quality of work of their peers. Berwick (1990) has defined it as "inspection and evaluation of health care structures, practices, or results, conducted or guided by medical professionals" (p. 247). In a peer review model, individual clinicians (physicians, therapists, nurses, etc.) are assigned to review sample records of the patients of other professionals in their organization and typically to report to a committee that oversees the enterprise (e.g., during a regular morbidity and mortality review).

The Peer Review Improvement Act of 1982 requires each state to designate a single agency as responsible for monitoring the quality of care for Medicare beneficiaries. As a result, provider organizations must review their own work and respond to the inquiries of peer review organizations about the quality of care.

The underlying philosophy of traditional peer review (inspection and sanction by individuals) is in many ways fundamentally at odds with the QI mentality (statistical examination of outcomes, focus on process, and empowerment of individuals). Berwick (1990) suggests, however, that peer review and QI efforts can coexist and complement each other, with peer review professionals playing a role in measurement and information analysis. It is likely that samples of individual case records for peer review will be augmented—and in some organizations replaced—by ongoing clinical information systems and computer databases in which key elements are routinely recorded for statistical analysis.

Occupational therapy managers can expect to be involved at some level in a peer review activity. Another use of peer review is the monitoring and the improvement of individual clinicians' skills. *Developing, Maintaining, and Updating Competency in Occupational Therapy: A Guide to Self-Appraisal* (AOTA, Commission on Practice, 1995) identifies peer review as one of the methods by which practitioners can achieve competency. The document is the product of a task force established in 1991 by AOTA's Commission on Practice to examine competency issues at all levels and in all practice settings. Establishing, maintaining, and measuring competency is essential for the survival of the occupational therapy profession in today's health care and education systems.

ELEMENTS AND STEPS IN QUALITY IMPROVEMENT

A number of tools for information management, outcome measurement and monitoring, process analysis, and applied organizational change are available and frequently used in conducting QI programs. Many are drawn from the TQM movement and applied to a health care environment. Occupational therapy managers may well become involved in or be asked to lead QI activities as part of an organizational effort, and therefore should educate themselves on the use of these tools and surrounding structures.

ORGANIZATIONAL INFRASTRUCTURE: QUALITY COUNCILS

A focal point for the activities associated with QI may be an organization's quality council and supporting subgroups responsible for compiling and reviewing plans and data on outcomes and processes of care. Although the specific organizational layout for such councils, committees, and task forces will vary widely (Berwick, 1990), those that are most effective will be guided from the highest levels of the organization (e.g., executive and medical management) and will commit significant time to analyzing findings from the QI reviews and translating findings into actions for improving processes. Occupational therapy managers may well be called on to participate in or report to such groups and should build these activities into their regular work expectations.

DATA COLLECTION

At the core of modern QI efforts is the need to gather data on outcomes, conformance to prescribed standards, and the proportion of persons meeting quality-indicator conditions (Ellwood, 1988; Johnston & Wilkerson, 1992). Methods of data collection may range from retrospective reviews of randomly sampled patients' records to highly automated computer technologies supporting ongoing clinical information systems. Combinations of these methods are likely, depending on the size and the sophistication of the organization. However, even the smallest organizations may have personal computer–based software designed to record and to help analyze outcome and other quality-indicator data.

With the influence of TQM and outcomes management paradigms, QI efforts are placing increased emphasis on the statistical analysis of aggregate data, requiring large databases on the populations served by the organization. Relying solely on a small peer-reviewed sample of records is inadequate. Thus occupational therapy managers will benefit from at least a general understanding of what databases and information systems have to offer and the ways in which information must be recorded to accommodate these systems (Lieberman, 1991).

TOOLS AND TECHNIQUES

A variety of tools can be employed to structure an organization's improvement activities, including some described in detail by JCAHO (1992a, 1992b, 1994a, 1994b, 1995b), others stemming from the TQM movement (Plsek, 1993), and program evaluation techniques such as those endorsed by CARF (Commission on Accreditation of Rehabilitation Facilities, 1991a, 1991b, 1991c, 1992; see also part 1 of this chapter). At the core of each is a cycle of planning, implementing, gathering and analyzing data, developing plans for improvement, implementing changes, and reassessing the status of the system in comparison with its status before the change or with the goals for improvement (see figure 12-1).

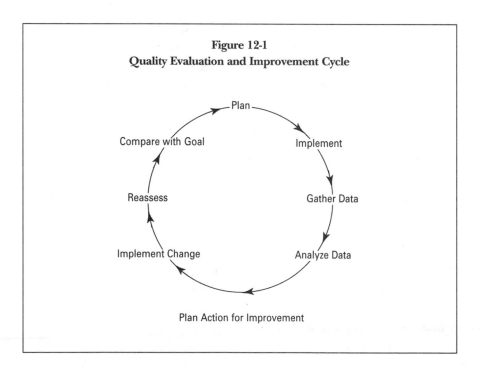

Figure 12-1
Quality Evaluation and Improvement Cycle

Plan

Compare with Goal

Implement

Reassess

Gather Data

Implement Change

Analyze Data

Plan Action for Improvement

JCAHO refers to and diagrams this learning-and-change cycle as plan-do-study-act, or PDSA. The templates for CARF program evaluation suggest slightly different labels: objective-measurement-performance-action. Occupational therapy managers should understand that whatever the labels and the organizational placement of QI activity, the goal is a change of processes in order to improve outcomes and consumer satisfaction.

Common tools used in QI efforts include charts and graphs for display of data in formats that facilitate understanding of patterns and trends, and comparisons with external data sources; flow charts that clarify processes and sequences of events; and diagrams that display potential causes of variation and error in processes (Carefoote, 1994; Plsek, 1993). AOTA's (1994) *QI Resource Guide* is a valuable publication that will assist occupational therapy managers and practitioners with QI activities. The guide contains an extensive bibliography, a list of resources, and sample forms.

QI teams are also a hallmark of many QI efforts. A task force is convened whose work is temporary but focused on improving a single major process. Based on the premise that persons who do the work know the processes best, QI teams typically involve employees at all levels of the organization and across departments—all those who participate in or use the products of an organization's process. For example, occupational therapy managers or their staff members may be involved with admission personnel, medical records employees, physicians, and administrative representatives on a team to improve the flow of documentation on the care of patients. The potential team member must learn the use of specific tools, as well as understand the overall goals of improving an outcome (in this example, complete and timely documentation of care).

RELATIONSHIP OF QUALITY IMPROVEMENT TO RESEARCH AND PROGRAM EVALUATION

Distinctions have been drawn in the past between quality assurance and research, and skepticism has arisen regarding the validity of decisions based on the relatively unsophisticated early QA activities. The shift from QA to QI and the inherent shift from reviews of small samples of case records to use of population databases move QI toward health services research. Demands on modern systems include valid and reliable outcomes measures, secure and properly used databases, and sound sampling and statistical analysis techniques (Fuhrer, 1987; Johnston, Keith, & Hinderer, 1992). Organization-specific and pooled databases [e.g., the Uniform Data System for Medical Rehabilitation (Hamilton, Granger, Sherwin, Zielzny, & Tashman, 1987)] are the most efficiently designed to meet the needs of QI efforts as well as to provide a foundation for epidemiological and health services research.

Although randomized clinical trials are outside the usual practice of QI projects, *de facto* controls from pre- and post-intervention designs are possible. Analysis of patterns of variation, effectiveness, and efficiency from program evaluation and QI efforts can point to and set the groundwork for more focused and controlled outcomes research. In turn, treatment efficacy suggested by clinical research should be tested in the real-world laboratory of clinical practice. In fact, real-world effectiveness of treatment can often be verified only through outcomes management-type analyses. Research efforts can also lead to changes in practice, clinical guidelines, and evaluation goals. Practice guidelines, which include clinical processes that may be among the targets for improvement, are based in part on efficacy findings from controlled clinical research.

OVERCOMING OF OBSTACLES TO QUALITY IMPROVEMENT

Resistance to QI efforts can come from several angles. The culture and the behavior of an organization are being challenged and changed through QI, and people resist change. The flattening of an organizational structure and the empowerment of line staff members that often take place with a TQM philosophy can be very threatening, especially to mid-level managers (Gillem, 1988; McLaughlin & Kaluzny, 1990). Constant change is indeed at the core of continuous improvement. Preparing an organization for change, conveying excitement for better care and service from the top of the organization, and understanding new roles of managers and staff members are critical to a successful QI program (McLaughlin & Kaluzny, 1990).

Managers and staff must also become accustomed to new demands for data collection, which if not implemented carefully can place undue burdens on clinical operations. Involving staff in the design and the use of information systems, as well as on specific teams for quality or process improvement, will help make the information collected and changes recommended meaningful and successful.

SUMMARY OF PART 2

Quality improvement (QI) is a system through which better and more efficient processes in an organization continuously raise the levels of performance and the outcomes of all functions, eliminate errors, and reduce cost. Several concepts are key to QI:

1. Donabedian's (1988) framework for assessing the quality of medical care, which includes three dimensions: *structure,* or the "attributes of the settings in which care occurs"; *process,* "what is actually done in giving and receiving care"; and *outcome,* "the

effects of care on the health status of patients and populations"
(p. 1745)

2. *Total quality management* (TQM), which emphasizes three
    themes: continuous quality improvement; doing things right
    the first time; and empowering workers at all levels to make
    improvements

3. Focus on the consumer, which includes two elements: consumer
    satisfaction and consumer service

4. Outcomes management, which employs four key techniques: use
    of standards and guidelines to help physicians choose appropri-
    ate treatments; routine and systematic measurement of function-
    ing, well-being, and disease-specific outcomes; pooling of out-
    come data and information on the clinical process; and analysis
    and dissemination of results to decision makers

Effectiveness refers to the outcome dimension. *Efficiency* considers the
resources employed in achieving a certain outcome. Value is the principal
concept that brings together effectiveness (outcome), cost and price, and
efficiency. *Value* is the ratio of quality to price: The highest quality for the
lowest price is the highest value. The long-range goals of QI and program
evaluation are to encourage and communicate value in an organization.

QI systems are required by accrediting bodies and peer review organizations. A focal point for QI activities may be an organization's quality
council and supporting subgroups. At the core of modern QI efforts is the
need to gather data on outcomes, conformance to prescribed standards,
and the proportion of persons meeting quality-indicator conditions
(Ellwood, 1988; Johnston & Wilkerson, 1992). A variety of tools can be
employed to structure an organization's QI activities. At the core of each
is a cycle of planning, implementing, gathering and analyzing data, developing plans for improvement, implementing changes, and reassessing the
status of the system in comparison with its status before the change or with
the goals for improvement. QI teams, also a hallmark of many QI efforts,
typically involve employees at all levels of the organization and across
departments.

PART 3

Documentation of Occupational Therapy Services

Jane Davy Acquaviva, BS, OTR

Documentation is the written record of evaluation and treatment provided. This part of chapter 12 identifies the critical elements of good and efficient occupational therapy documentation that meets the needs of all interested parties. It emphasizes evaluation, treatment planning, and functional goal setting because success with these elements helps guarantee the practitioner success in the overall documentation process. Learning to document is somewhat like learning a second language. If the practitioner initially learns the correct grammar and pronunciation, mastery will come faster and more easily.

HISTORICAL PERSPECTIVES

Good documentation is an important responsibility of all professionals because it is an indication that they are accountable for their actions and that they recognize their obligation to share the product of their efforts with others. Occupational therapy practitioners have been documenting their services in some fashion for decades. Practitioners' notes frequently consisted of long narrative descriptions of evaluation results, treatment methods, and patients' response to treatment. In the late 1960s and early 1970s, as the profession sought to assess the quality of the treatment provided, it looked for a way to document such that the response to treatment could be measured. Practitioners learned to write goals in the RUMBA format: real, understandable, measurable, behavioral, and achievable. Although this approach is no longer emphasized, it started practitioners thinking about how to document progress so that they could measure it by retrospective or continuing chart review. Government programs like Medicare and Medicaid that began to pay for more health care provided additional incentive. As health care became more expensive, all payers started to require documentation to determine the necessity for and the appropriateness of care.

The medical record has always been the legal documentation of medical care provided. As workers' compensation, personal injury, and malpractice litigation have increased, court scrutiny of the record has become common. This is yet another reason for practitioners to pay close attention to the quality and the clarity of documentation.

The medical record serves many purposes, and the documenting practitioner is writing for many audiences: the legal system; third-party payers; accrediting agencies; quality improvement and research personnel; other treatment team members; and patients and their families. Serving all these audiences is not as difficult as it may seem, however, because each wants essentially the same information:

1. How did the patient function at the beginning of treatment?
2. How did the patient function at the end of treatment?
3. Briefly, what procedures did the practitioner follow, and what treatments did he or she provide?
4. How long did treatment take?

To serve the variety of potential readers of occupational therapy notes, practitioners must use clear and consistent language. Before the mid-1970s there was no universal description of occupational therapy accepted by both the profession and third-party payers. When Medicare published the *Medicare Intermediary Manual,* it included a description of occupational therapy developed with input from AOTA. Medical reviewers used this description to determine whether the occupational therapy services provided were appropriate under the Medicare program. Although there were problems with this description, reviewers used it extensively because it was the best available at the time.

In 1979, AOTA adopted uniform terminology for reporting occupational therapy services, which provided the profession with its first comprehensive lexicon of consistent treatment terminology. AOTA has revised its uniform terminology twice since 1979, publishing the most recent edition in 1994 (see appendix 12-A for an outline).

In 1990 the Health Care Financing Administration (HCFA), the federal agency responsible for Medicare, published a new description of occupational therapy called "Medical Review (MR) Guidelines for Outpatient OT Services" (see appendix 12-B). Occupational therapy practitioners had considerable input to this document, a vast improvement over the description of occupational therapy published earlier.

Because "Uniform Terminology for Occupational Therapy" and "Medical Review (MR) Guidelines" have national approval and use, especially among third-party payers, they often form the basis for documenting occupational therapy services. Practitioners should be conversant with both of these documents.

EVALUATION AND TREATMENT PLANNING

Documentation begins when a person is referred to occupational therapy for evaluation. A practitioner interviews a patient and his or her family members or caregivers to determine the patient's prior level of functioning and the activities that the patient is unable to perform. The practitioner observes the patient performing selected functional activities to determine what might be causing the disability. Then through further assessment, the practitioner identifies the underlying factors (performance components) that are causing the functional problems. Keeping in mind the many contextual factors, such as the patient's environment, age, support systems, and cultural traditions, the practitioner discusses the treatment options with the patient and the family. Together they plan the treatment and set goals and priorities. These evaluation data form the baseline necessary for discussing treatment options, writing functional goals, and assessing progress.

The following checklist provides guidance for documenting evaluation and treatment planning. Some items are general and administrative, such as the date of the evaluation; others are specific to the patient.

❏ The facility or the agency at which the service is being performed (usually printed on forms or notes)

❏ The physician referring the patient, and the date of the referral

❏ The date of the occupational therapy evaluation

❏ The date of onset of the condition for which occupational therapy is required

❏ Relevant medical history and previous occupational therapy treatment for the condition

❏ The patient's abilities and deficits in functional performance areas (see appendix 12-A)

❏ Deficits in underlying factors or performance components causing functional deficits

❏ A description of the patient's and the family's motivation

❏ If treatment is indicated, a statement that there is a reasonable expectation that the patient will benefit from occupational therapy services

❏ The estimated frequency and duration of treatment

❏ A statement indicating that the practitioner has discussed the treatment options with the patient and the family, and that the patient and the family have agreed on the goals

❏ Measurable, functional occupational therapy goals

FORMULATION OF FUNCTIONAL GOALS

The manner in which practitioners write functional goals tends to set the direction for their documenting of the remainder of a patient's record. All occupational therapy is directed toward a patient's performing functional activities; therefore the goals and the subsequent notes should reflect those activities. Although some treatment is specifically directed at changing the underlying factors or components of function, such as strength or coordination, the goals still need to tie into functional activity. For example, a practitioner might use a program of graded activities to improve a patient's coordination in one or more performance areas. The goals for that patient might therefore read as follows:

1. Within two weeks, patient will be able to dress with minimal assistance.

2. Within one week, patient will be able to bathe using adapted equipment with moderate assistance.

The program of coordination activities will assist the patient in achieving these goals, but changes in coordination must be expressed in terms of the desired functional activities. Sometimes patients change so slowly that the practitioner may observe changes in underlying factors but not see a higher level of functioning. When this occurs, the practitioner should document it in the progress notes, indicating that the patient is, in fact, improving in an area that is prerequisite to a change in function. For example:

Patient can now maintain sitting balance for one minute without support, in preparation for transfers.

SETTING OF LONG- AND SHORT-TERM GOALS

Long-term goals describe the functional status that the practitioner expects the patient to reach by the end of treatment in a given facility or program. Short-term goals specify the steps to reach the long-term goals. All goals must be functional, measurable, and objective.

Long-term goals might read as follows:

1. Within two months, patient will be ADL independent with assistive devices.

2. Within three months, patient will be ADL independent and safe living alone at home with assistance for shopping and some meal preparation.

The practitioner should be mindful that goals are an indication of what the patient needs to accomplish, not what the practitioner intends to do. For example, "Refer for driving evaluation" is not a goal, but a practitioner's plan; therefore it should not be listed among the patient's goals.

Following is a long-term goal and some initial short-term goals for a patient with a recent hip fracture who must remain non-weight-bearing for three months:

History

Patient is overweight, her endurance poor, and her strength only fair+. She has history of cognitive problems (memory, problem solving) as well as depression. She lives with her son and daughter. Patient and family are hoping to reach long-term goal in two months. She is being treated in her home.

Long-Term Goal

1. Within two months, patient will be ADL independent with minimum assistance at home.

Short-Term Goals

1. Within two days, patient will roll and come to sitting position independently.

2. Within one week, patient will bathe upper body with setup.

3. Within one week, patient will dress upper body.

Following completion of the first set of short-term goals, the second set might be these:

1. Within one week, patient will transfer to wheelchair using sliding board with maximum assistance.

2. Within one week, patient's son will learn techniques and assist patient in transferring safely using sliding board.

3. Within two weeks, patient will bathe and dress upper body independently.

4. Within one week, patient will demonstrate compliance with home exercise program to prevent pressure ulcers and strengthen upper extremities for more independent transfers.

TREATMENT

The orderly flow of evaluation information, goal development, and outcome reporting will reflect the practitioner's thinking in combination with the patient's goals. If the goals and the outcomes show a logical progression of the patient becoming more independent, the caregiver becoming more capable, and the patient needing less assistance, any reader will understand the purpose of the occupational therapy treatment as well as the outcomes.

Documentation of the type of treatment provided or emphasized on a particular visit or in the course of a week is necessary, but a summary of methods and procedures is sufficient. For example:

> Treatment emphasized transfer training, compensatory dressing techniques, and activities to improve movement in right upper extremity.

> Treatment sessions this week consisted of activities to improve attention to left side, wheelchair mobility, transfers, and upper-extremity dressing.

> Treatment emphasized activities to improve group work skills, appropriate social interaction with peers, and grooming and dressing for work environment.

PROGRESS NOTES AND WEEKLY OR MONTHLY SUMMARIES

The practitioner should periodically review a patient's progress to determine whether the long-term goal continues to be realistic, whether the short-term goals reflect what is happening in treatment, and whether treatment has been modified without a corresponding change in the goals. The timing of the review will depend on the intensity of the treatment and in some cases a facility's reporting requirements. For example, an inpatient rehabilitation facility may require weekly summaries of progress, whereas a home health practitioner treating patients only eight to twelve times a month may review progress monthly. Whichever interval applies, the following format may be useful for documenting progress:

Summary

Goal	Outcome
[List short-term goals.]	[Specify whether goal has been met, modified, or not achieved, and why; or why goal is no longer applicable.]

[List any new goals.]

[Follow with information about patient's continued rehabilitation potential, frequency and duration of future occupational therapy treatment, and any referrals that will be made or additional resources that will be needed for patient.]

Following is an example of a monthly summary using the format just presented:

Monthly Summary

Short-Term Goal	Outcome
1. Patient will independently dress upper body.	Achieved.
2. Patient will transfer from bed to chair with minimum assistance.	Achieved.
3. Patient's family will have grab bars installed in bathroom.	Not achieved. Family unable to schedule workman this week.
4. Patient will use affected right upper extremity as gross assist in self-care.	Not achieved. Patient's gross grasp was insufficient.

Modify goal 4: Patient will use affected right upper extremity as stabilizer.

The Medicare Part B guidelines provide uniform descriptions of levels of assistance, which are helpful in reporting changes in a person's level of functioning. Using these levels, the practitioner can measure small amounts of improvement even with patients who still need much assistance. For example:

Patient transfers with total assistance using Hoyer lift.

Patient transfers with total assistance of one person using sliding board.

Patient does sliding board transfer with moderate assistance of one.

Each time a practitioner treats a patient, he or she must make a notation in the patient's medical chart. In some cases a practitioner may need only to note the date of the treatment and the procedures that he or she followed, then initial or sign the notation. A practitioner can effectively document this type of information using a checklist or an attendance record. Such a system reduces the time that the practitioner must devote to daily progress notes, focusing attention on the weekly or monthly summaries in which he or she addresses progress toward goals.

DISCHARGE SUMMARY

The discharge summary follows a format similar to that of weekly or monthly summaries, but succinctly recapitulates the entire treatment process. It states the patient's functional level at the beginning of treatment, restates all the general functional goals for the patient, and indicates the outcome; if the patient did not meet the goals, it gives the reason. Following is an example:

History

Patient was referred for home care four weeks post stroke. Patient was dependent in all self-care activities with exception of grooming and eating. Patient was seen two times a week for six weeks, followed by one time a week for two weeks.

Long-Term Goals

1. Within six weeks, patient will dress independently.

2. Within five weeks, patient will bathe with supervision.

3. Within six weeks, patient will prepare breakfast and lunch independently.

4. Within six weeks, patient will toilet independently.

Outcomes

1. By 9/1/95 (five weeks), patient dressed independently using adapted shoe closures.

2. By 9/1/95 (five weeks), patient bathed using tub seat and wall grab bar, with supervision from his son for safety.

3. By 8/30/95 (four weeks), patient prepared breakfast independently. He preferred meals-on-wheels for lunch. Lunch leftovers were sufficient for evening snack.

4. By 9/15/95 (seven weeks), patient toileted independently with use of two grab bars.

Family did not arrange for installment of necessary equipment until last week; therefore, complete goal attainment was delayed approximately one week.

Patient was discharged on 9/19/95. He will receive assistance with shopping from his son and supervision in bathing as needed from his son.

CONCLUSION

The reader of documentation is interested in the outcome of treatment, not the practitioner's methods for achieving the outcome. However, if the patient is not reaching the expected outcome, the practitioner should take a careful look at the treatment plan and make a change.

One of the best ways for a practitioner to improve his or her documentation is to read the documentation of others and think about the following:

1. Do the evaluation data present a vivid picture of the patient's level of functioning?

2. Is there evidence that the patient is improving in functional activities, or is improvement apparent only in underlying factors such as strength, coordination, and attention span?

3. Is there evidence that the patient and his or her family were involved in the treatment planning?

4. Are the reasons for any changes in treatment clear?

5. Are the treatment methods mentioned consistent with the occupational therapy goals?

Again, documenting is like learning a new language. When the practitioner learns the rules correctly in the beginning, the task is easier and more efficient. Documenting requires clear logical thinking, involvement of the patient, and an orientation to results.

SUMMARY OF PART 3

Documentation is the written record of evaluation and treatment provided. The documenting practitioner is writing for many audiences. Each, however, wants essentially the same information: (1) how the patient functioned at the beginning of treatment; (2) how the patient functioned at the end of treatment; (3) what procedures the practitioner followed and what treatments he or she provided; and (4) how long treatment took.

To serve a variety of potential readers, practitioners must use clear and consistent language. AOTA's "Uniform Terminology for Occupational Therapy" and the Health Care Financing Administration's "Medical Review (MR) Guidelines for Outpatient OT Services" often form the basis for documenting occupational therapy services.

Documentation begins when a person is referred for evaluation. The following list provides guidance for documenting evaluation and treatment planning: agency; referral source and date; date of evaluation; date of onset; relevant medical history and previous treatment for condition; abilities and deficits in functional performance areas; deficits in underlying factors or performance components; motivation; reasonable expectation of benefit; estimated frequency and duration of treatment; discussion of treatment options with patient and family, and agreement on goals; and measurable, functional goals.

The manner in which practitioners write functional goals tends to set the direction for documenting. Long-term goals describe the functional status that the practitioner expects the patient to reach by the end of treatment in a given facility or program. Short-term goals specify the steps to reach the long-term goals.

Documentation of the type of treatment provided or emphasized on a particular visit or in the course of a week is necessary, but a summary of methods and procedures is sufficient. The practitioner should review a patient's progress weekly or monthly. A suggested format for reporting data displays short-term goals in one column and specifies outcomes in another. The discharge summary follows a format similar to that of weekly or monthly summaries, but succinctly recapitulates the entire treatment process.

REFERENCES

American Occupational Therapy Association. (1994). *QI resource guide.* Bethesda, MD: Author.

American Occupational Therapy Association. (1994). Uniform terminology for occupational therapy (3rd ed.). *American Journal of Occupational Therapy, 48,* 1047–54.

American Occupational Therapy Association, Commission on Practice, Competency Task Force. (1995). *Developing, maintaining, and updating competency in occupational therapy: A guide to self-appraisal.* Bethesda, MD: Author.

Berwick, D. M. (1989). Continuous improvement as an ideal in health care. *New England Journal of Medicine, 320,* 53–56.

Berwick, D. M. (1990). Peer review and quality management: Are they compatible? *Quality Review Bulletin, 16,* 246–51.

Carefoote, R. (1994). Implementing TQM/CQI at rehabilitation hospitals: A survey. *Journal of Healthcare Quality, 16*(3), 34–38.

CARF, The Rehabilitation Accreditation Commission. (1995). *1995 standards manual and interpretive guidelines for medical rehabilitation.* Tucson, AZ: Author.

CARF, The Rehabilitation Accreditation Commission. (published annually). *Standards manual and interpretive guidelines for behavioral health.* Tucson, AZ: Author.

CARF, The Rehabilitation Accreditation Commission. (published annually). *Standards manual and interpretive guidelines for employment and community support services.* Tucson, AZ: Author.

CARF, The Rehabilitation Accreditation Commission. (published annually). *Standards manual and interpretive guidelines for medical rehabilitation.* Tucson, AZ: Author.

CARF, The Rehabilitation Accreditation Commission, Board of Trustees. (1995). *Quality improvement through measurement and management of rehabilitation outcomes: Tools for application of knowledge of rehabilitation outcomes management* [Proposal]. Tucson, AZ: Author.

Commission on Accreditation of Rehabilitation Facilities. (1991a). *Program evaluation: A first step.* Tucson, AZ: Author.

Commission on Accreditation of Rehabilitation Facilities. (1991b). *Program evaluation: A guide to utilization.* Tucson, AZ: Author.

Commission on Accreditation of Rehabilitation Facilities. (1991c). *Program evaluation: For inpatient medical rehabilitation programs* (1991 ed.). Tucson, AZ: Author.

Commission on Accreditation of Rehabilitation Facilities. (1992). *Program evaluation: Utilization and assessment principles* (1992 ed.). Tucson, AZ: Author.

Crosby, P. B. (1979). *Quality is free.* New York: Mentor/New American Library.

Davis, L. (1960). *Fellowship of surgeons: A history of the American College of Surgeons.* Springfield, IL: Charles C Thomas.

Deming, W. E. (1982). *Out of the crisis.* Cambridge, MA: Massachusetts Institute of Technology, Center for Advanced Engineering Study.

Donabedian, A. (1966). Evaluating the quality of medical care. *Milbank Quarterly, 44,* 166–203.

Donabedian, A. (1983). Quality, cost and clinical decisions. *Annals of the American Academy of Political and Social Science, 468,* 196–204.

Donabedian, A. (1988). The quality of care: How can it be assessed? *Journal of the American Medical Association, 260,* 1743–48.

Ellwood, P. (1988). Outcomes management: A technology of patient experience [Shattuck Lecture]. *New England Journal of Medicine, 318,* 1549–56.

England, B., Glass, R. M., & Patterson, C. H. (Eds.). (1989). *Quality rehabilitation: Results-oriented care.* Chicago: American Hospital.

Flexner, A. (1910). *Medical education in the United States and Canada.* New York: Carnegie Foundation, Merrymount Press.

Fuhrer, M. J. (Ed.). (1987). *Rehabilitation outcomes: Analysis and measurement.* Baltimore: Brookes.

Gillem, T. R. (1988). Deming's 14 points and hospital quality: Responding to the consumer's demand for the best value health care. *Journal of Nursing Quality Assurance, 2,* 70–78.

Hamilton, B. B., Granger, C. V., Sherwin, F. S., Zielzny, M., & Tashman, J. S. (1987). A uniform national data system for medical rehabilitation. In M. J. Fuhrer (Ed.), *Rehabilitation outcomes: Analysis and measurement* (pp. 137–50). Baltimore: Brookes.

Health Care Financing Administration. (1990, September). Medical review (MR) guidelines for OT outpatient services (DHHS Transmittal No. 1489). In *Medicare intermediary manual* (sec. 3906ff, pp. 23–43). Baltimore, MD: Author.

Huxley, E. (1975). *Florence Nightingale.* New York: Putnam.

Joint Commission on Accreditation of Healthcare Organizations. (1992a). *Examples of quality improvement in a hospital setting.* Oakbrook Terrace, IL: Author.

Joint Commission on Accreditation of Healthcare Organizations. (1992b). *Using quality improvement tools in a healthcare setting.* Oakbrook Terrace, IL: Author.

Joint Commission on Accreditation of Healthcare Organizations. (1994a). *Forms, charts, and other tools for performance improvement.* Oakbrook Terrace, IL: Author.

Joint Commission on Accreditation of Healthcare Organizations. (1994b). *Framework for improving performance: From principles to practice.* Oakbrook Terrace, IL: Author.

Joint Commission on Accreditation of Healthcare Organizations. (1995a). *Accreditation manual for hospitals.* Oakbrook Terrace, IL: Author.

Joint Commission on Accreditation of Healthcare Organizations. (1995b). *Leadership skills for performance improvement: Planning for quality.* Oakbrook Terrace, IL: Author.

Johnston, M. V., Keith, R. A., & Hinderer, S. R. (1992). Measurement standards for medical rehabilitation (Work of the American Congress of Rehabilitation Medicine's Task Force on Measurement and Evaluation) [Special supplement]. *Archives of Physical Medicine and Rehabilitation, 73*(supp. no. 12-5).

Johnston, M. V., & Wilkerson, D. L. (1992). Program evaluation and quality improvement systems in brain injury rehabilitation. *Journal of Head Trauma Rehabilitation, 7,* 68–82.

Johnston, M. V., Wilkerson, D. L., & Maney, M. (1993). Evaluation of the quality and outcomes of medical rehabilitation programs. In J. A. DeLisa & B. Gans (Eds.), *Rehabilitation medicine: Principles and practice* (2nd ed., pp. 240–68). Philadelphia: Lippincott.

Lieberman, D. (1991). Foreword. *Occupational Therapy Practice, 2*(2), v–vi.

McLaughlin, C. P., & Kaluzny, A. D. (1990). Total quality management in health: Making it work. *Health Care Management Review, 15*(3), 7–14.

National Rehabilitation Hospital. (1992). *Quality in medical rehabilitation: Definitions and dimensions.* Washington, DC: Author.

Peer Review Improvement Act of 1982, Pub. L. No. 97–248, 96 stat. 324, § 141.

Plsek, P. E. (1993). Tutorial: Management and planning tools of TQM. *Quality Management in Health Care, 1*(3), 59–72.

ADDITIONAL RESOURCES

Boon, B. (1995, February 15). *Creating an effective results-oriented organization.* A Best Practice Presentation at the 1995 CARF Medical Rehabilitation Conference on Standards and Best Practices, Tucson, AZ.

Johnston, M. V., Stineman, M., & Maney, M. (1993, June 17). *Improving the reliability and integrity of functional measures in medicine and rehabilitation* [Abstract]. West Orange, NJ: Kessler Institute for Rehabilitation.

MacDonell, C. M. (1993, February/March). A tool for the future. *Rehab Management* (Marina del Ray, CA: CurAnt Communications), *6,* 112–13.

McNally, D. (1990). *Even eagles need a push.* New York: Delacorte Press.

Wiley, G. (1993, June/July). A scramble for facts. *Rehab Management* (Marina del Ray, CA: CurAnt Communications), *6,* 165–67.

Wilkerson, D. L. (1991). Program and outcome evaluation: Opportunity for the 1990's. *Occupational Therapy Practice, 2*(2), 1–15.

Wilkerson, D. L. (1995, October-November). Implementing outcomes. *Rehab management* (Marina del Ray, CA: CurAnt Communications), *8,* 97–99.

Wilkerson, D. L. (1995, December-January). Developing outcomes management tools. *Rehab Management* (Marina del Ray, CA: CurAnt Communications), *8,* 114–15.

Wilkerson, D. L. & Johnston, M. V. (in press). Outcomes research and clinical program monitoring systems: Current capability and future directions. In M. J. Fuhrer (Ed.), *Medical rehabilitation research.* Baltimore: Brookes.

APPENDIX 12-A

Uniform Terminology for Occupational Therapy
Third Edition Outline

I. Performance Areas

A. Activities of Daily Living
   1. Grooming
   2. Oral Hygiene
   3. Bathing/Showering
   4. Toilet Hygiene
   5. Personal Device Care
   6. Dressing
   7. Feeding and Eating
   8. Medication Routine
   9. Health Maintenance
   10. Socialization
   11. Functional Communication
   12. Functional Mobility
   13. Community Mobility
   14. Emergency Response
   15. Sexual Expression
B. Work and Productive Activities
   1. Home Management
     a. Clothing Care
     b. Cleaning
     c. Meal Preparation/Cleanup
     d. Shopping
     e. Money Management
     f. Household Maintenance
     g. Safety Procedures
   2. Care of Others
   3. Educational Activities
   4. Vocational Activities
     a. Vocational Exploration
     b. Job Acquisition
     c. Work or Job Performance
     d. Retirement Planning
     e. Volunteer Participation
C. Play or Leisure Activities
   1. Play/Leisure Exploration
   2. Play/Leisure Performance

II. Performance Components

A. Sensorimotor Component
   1. Sensory
     a. Sensory Awareness
     b. Sensory Processing
       (1) Tactile
       (2) Proprioceptive
       (3) Vestibular
       (4) Visual
       (5) Auditory
       (6) Gustatory
       (7) Olfactory
     c. Perceptual Processing
       (1) Stereognosis
       (2) Kinesthesia
       (3) Pain Response
       (4) Body Scheme
       (5) Right-Left Discrimination
       (6) Form Constancy
       (7) Position in Space
       (8) Visual-Closure
       (9) Figure Ground
       (10) Depth Perception
       (11) Spatial Relations
       (12) Topographical Orientation
   2. Neuromusculoskeletal
     a. Reflex
     b. Range of Motion
     c. Muscle Tone
     d. Strength
     e. Endurance
     f. Postural Control
     g. Postural Alignment
     h. Soft Tissue Integrity
   3. Motor
     a. Gross Coordination
     b. Crossing the Midline
     c. Laterality
     d. Bilateral Integration
     e. Motor Control
     f. Praxis
     g. Fine Coordination/Dexterity
     h. Visual-Motor Integration
     i. Oral-Motor Control
B. Cognitive Integration and Cognitive Components
   1. Level of Arousal
   2. Orientation
   3. Recognition
   4. Attention Span
   5. Initiation of Activity
   6. Termination of Activity
   7. Memory
   8. Sequencing
   9. Categorization
   10. Concept Formation
   11. Spatial Operations
   12. Problem Solving 13. Learning
   14. Generalization
C. Psychosocial Skills and Psychological Components
   1. Psychological
     a. Values
     b. Interests
     c. Self-Concept
   2. Social
     a. Role Performance
     b. Social Conduct
     c. Interpersonal Skills
     d. Self-Expression
   3. Self-Management
     a. Coping Skills
     b. Time Management
     c. Self-Control

III. Performance Contexts

A. Temporal Aspects
   1. Chronological
   2. Developmental
   3. Life Cycle
   4. Disability Status
B. Environmental Aspects
   1. Physical
   2. Social
   3. Cultural

APPENDIX 12-B

Medical Review (MR) Guidelines for Outpatient OT Services

Refer to: Medicare Intermediary Manual (sec. 3906ff)

Occupational Therapy Review These guidelines assist the reviewer in understanding the field of OT as well as facilitate the MR process. They are flexible and neither guarantee a minimum amount of coverage nor establish a maximum coverage amount. They do not cover all situations.

The following is criteria for MR of OT services. Use the edits in Exhibit I to assist you in conducting focused MR within your budgeted levels. Conduct focused review using other selection criteria which you determine to be effective. If you choose to use any of the diagnostic edits listed in Exhibit I, do not change the visits and/or duration parameters without approval from CO [*HCFA central office*]. Conform to the MR requirements for all outpatient claims from rehabilitation agencies, SNFs, hospitals, and HHAs that provide OT in addition to home health services (bill types: hospital-12 and 13, SNF-22 and 23, rehabilitation agency, public health agency or clinic-74 and CORF-75). These criteria do not apply to OT services provided under a home health plan of care.

The criteria for MR case selection are based on ICD-9-CM diagnoses, elapsed time from stat of care (at the billing provider) and number of visits. (See Exhibit I.)

<u>Denial of a bill solely on the basis that it exceeds the criteria in the edits is prohibited.</u>

The edits are <u>only</u> for assisting you to select bills to review or for paying bills if they meet Level I criteria. Do not provide automatic coverage up to these criteria. They neither guarantee minimum nor set maximum coverage limits.

<u>Use of OT Edits (Exhibit I) Level I Review.</u> OT edits have been developed for a number of diagnoses. The diagnoses were selected on the basis that, when linked with a recent date of onset, there is a high probability that

Medicare patients with these diagnoses will require skilled OT. The edits do not specify every diagnosis which may require OT, and the fact that a given diagnosis does not appear in the edits does not create a presumption that OT services are not necessary or are inappropriate. Do not approve or deny claims at Level I for medical necessity. Pay claims that span or pass the edits in Exhibit I without being subjected to Level II MR. However, refer all claims which meet your focused MR criteria to Level II MR.

For patients receiving OT services only (V57.2) during an encounter/visit, list the appropriate V code for the service first, and, if documented, list the diagnosis or problem for which the services are performed second. Program your system to read the diagnosis or problem listed second to determine if it meets the Level I OT edits.

EXAMPLE: Outpatient rehabilitation services, V57.2, for a patient with multiple sclerosis, 340. The V code will be listed first, followed by the code for multiple sclerosis (V57.2, 340). Edit for multiple sclerosis not the V code. Use this same procedure for V57.81 (orthotic training), V57.89 (other), and V57.9 (unspecified rehabilitation procedure).

Evaluate bills at Level I based upon:

1. Facility and Patient Identification. (Facility name, patient name, provider number, HICN, age)

2. Diagnosis. List the primary diagnosis for which OT services were furnished by ICD-9-CM code first. List other DX(s) applicable to the patient or that influence care second.

3. Duration. The total length of time OT services have been furnished (in days) from the date treatment was initiated for the diagnosis being treated at the billing provider (including the last day in the current billing period).

4. Number of Visits. The total number of patient visits completed since OT services were initiated for the diagnosis being treated by the billing provider. The total visits to date (including the last visit in the billing period) must be given rather than for each separate bill (value code 51).

5. Date Treatment Started (Occurrence Code 44). The date OT services were initiated by the billing provider for the primary medical DX for which OT services are furnished.

6. Billing Period. When OT services began and ended in the billing period (from/through dates).

Level II Review Process. If a bill is selected for focused or intensified review, refer it to the Level II health professional MR stall. If possible, have occupational therapists review OT bills.

Once the bill is selected for focused MR, review it in conjunction with the medical information submitted by the provider.

1. Reimbursable OT Services. Reimburse OT services only if they meet all requirements established by the Medicare guidelines and regulations. Each bill for OT services that is subjected to Level II MR must be supported with adequate medical documentation for you to make a determination.

2. MR and Documentation. When a claim is referred to Level II review, use the following pertinent data elements in addition to those used for Level I review:

a. Medical History. Obtain only the medical history which is pertinent to, or influences the OT treatment rendered, including a brief description of the functional status of the patient prior to the onset of the condition requiring OT, ;and any pertinent prior OT treatment.

b. Date of Onset (Occurrence code 11). The date of onset or exacerbation of the primary medical diagnosis for which OT services are being rendered by the billing provider.

c. Physician Referral and Date.

d. OT Initial Evaluation and Date.

e. Plan of Treatment and Date Established.

f. Date of Last Certification. Obtain the date on which the plan of treatment was last certified by the physician.

g. Progress Notes. Obtain updated patient status reports concerning the patient's current functional abilities/limitation.

The following explains specific Level II documentation principles:

Medical History. *[3906.1]*

If a history of previous OT treatment is not available, the provider supplies a general summary regarding the patient's past relevant medical history recorded during the initial evaluation with the patient/family or through contact with the referring physician. Information regarding prior OT treatment for the current condition, progress made, and treatment by the referring physician is provided when available. The level of function prior to the current exacerbation or onset is described.

The patient's medical history as it relates to OT, includes the date of onset and/or exacerbation of the illness of injury. If the patient has had prior therapy for the same condition, use that history in conjunction with the patient's current assessment to establish whether additional treatment is reasonable.

The history of treatments from a previous provider is necessary for patients who have transferred to a new provider. For example, if surgery has been performed, obtain the type and date. The date of onset and type of surgical procedure should be specific for diagnoses such as fractures. For other diagnoses, such as arthritis, the date of onset may be general. Establish it from the date the patient first required medical treatment. For other types of chronic diagnoses, the history gives the date of the change or deterioration in the patient's condition and a description of the changes that necessitate skilled OT.

Evaluation *[3906.2]*

Approve an OT initial evaluation, (excluding routine screening) when it is reasonable and necessary for the therapist to determine if there is an expectation that either restorative or maintenance services are appropriate. Approve reevaluations when the patient exhibits a demonstrable change in physical functional ability, to reestablish appropriate treatment goals, or when required for ongoing assessment of the patient's rehabilitation needs. Approve initial evaluations or reevaluations that are reasonable and necessary based on the patient's condition, even though the expectations are not realized, or when the evaluation determines that skilled rehabilitation is not needed.

The OT evaluation established the physical and cognitive baseline data necessary for assessing expected rehabilitation potential, setting realistic goals, and measuring progress. The evaluation of the patient's functional deficits and level of assistance needed forms the basis for the OT treatment goals. Objective tests and measurements are used (when possible) to establish base-line data.

The provider documents the patient's functional loss and the level of assistance requiring skilled OT intervention resulting from conditions such as:

Activities of Daily Living (ADL) Dependence—The individual is dependent upon skilled intervention for performance of activities of daily living. These include, but are not limited to, significant physical and/or cognitive functional loss, or loss of previous functional gains in the ability to eat and drink, bathe, dress, perform personal hygiene, groom, or perform toileting. This could include management and care of orthoses and/or other adaptive equipment, or other customized therapeutic adaptations.

Functional Limitation—The individual is dependent upon skilled OT intervention in functional training, observation, assessment, and environmental adaptation due to, but not limited to:

- Lack of awareness of sensory cues, or safety hazard;
- Impaired attention span;
- Impaired strength;
- Incoordination;
- Abnormal muscle tone;
- Range of motion limitations;
- Impaired body schema;
- Perceptual deficits;
- Impaired balance/head control; and
- Environmental barriers.

Safety Dependence/Secondary Complications—A safety problem exists when a patient, without skilled OT intervention, cannot handle him/herself in a manner that is physically and/or cognitively safe. This may extend to daily living or to acquired secondary complications which could potentially intensify medical sequelae such as fracture nonunion or skin breakdown. Safety dependence may be demonstrated by high probability of falling, lack of environmental safety awareness, swallowing difficulties, abnormal aggressive/destructive behavior, severe pain, loss of skin sensation, progressive joint contracture, and joint protection/preservation requiring skilled OT intervention to protect the patient from further medical complication.

If the goal for the patient is to increase functional abilities and decrease the level of assistance needed, the initial evaluation must measure the patient's starting functional abilities and level of assistance required.

Plan of Treatment *[3906.3]*

The OT plan of treatment must include specific functional goals and a reasonable estimate of when they will be reached (e.g., 6 weeks). It is not adequate to estimate "1 to 2 months on an ongoing basis." The plan must include specific OT procedures, frequency, and duration of treatment. The provider submits changes in the plan with the progress notes.

The plan of treatment contains:

- *Type of OT Procedures*—Describes the specific nature of the therapy to be provided.

- *Frequency of Visits*—An estimate of the frequency of treatment to be rendered (e.g., 3x week). The provider's medical documentation should justify the intensity of the services rendered. This is crucial when the treatments are given more frequently than 3 times a week.

- *Estimated Duration*—Identifies the length of time over which the services are to be rendered. It may be expressed in days, weeks, or months.

- *Diagnoses*—Includes the OT diagnosis if different from the medical diagnosis. The OT diagnosis should be based on objective tests, whenever possible.

- *Functional OT Goals (short or long-term)*—Reflects the occupational therapist's and/or physician's description of what functional physical/cognitive abilities the patient is expected to achieve. Assume that certain factors may change or influence the level of achievement. If this occurs, the occupational therapist explains the factors which led to the change in functional goal(s).

- *Rehabilitation Potential*—The occupational therapist's and/or physician's expectation concerning the patient's ability to meet the established goals.

Progress Reports [3906.4]

The provider documents and reports:

- The initial functional status of the patient;

- The patient's functional status and progress (or lack of progress) specific for this reporting period; including clinical findings (amount of physical and/or cognitive assistance needed, range of motion, muscle strength, unaffected limb measurements, etc.); and

- The patient's expected rehabilitation potential.

Where a valid expectation of improvement exists at the time OT services are initiated, or thereafter, the services are covered even though the expectation may not be realized. However, in such instances, the OT services are covered only to the time that no further significant practical improvement can be expected. Progress reports or status summaries must document a continued expectation that the patient's condition will continue to improve significantly in a reasonable and generally predictable period of time.

"Significant," means a generally measurable and substantial increase in the patient's present level of functional independence and competence, compared to that when treatment was initiated. Do not interpret the term "significant" so stringently that you deny a claim simply because of a temporary set back in the patient's progress. For example, a patient may experience an intervening medical complication or a brief period when lack of progress occurs. The medical reviewer may approve the claim if there is still a reasonable expectation that significant improvement in the patient's overall safety or functional ability will occur. However, the provider should document such lack of progress and briefly explain the need for continued skilled OT intervention.

The provider must provide treatment information regarding the status of the patient during the billing period. The provider's progress notes and any needed reevaluation(s) must update the baseline information provided at the initial evaluation. If there is a change in the plan of treatment, it must be documented. Additionally, when a patient is continued from one billing period to another, the progress report(s) must reflect the comparisons between the patient's current functional status and that during the previous billing and/or initial evaluation.

Conduct MR of claims with an understanding that skilled intervention may be needed, and improvement in a patient's condition may occur, even where a patient's full or partial recovery is not possible. For example, a terminally ill patient may begin to exhibit ADL, mobility and/or safety dependence requiring OT services. The fact that full or partial recovery is not possible or rehabilitation potential is not present, does not affect MR coverage decisions. The deciding factor is whether the services are considered reasonable, effective, treatment for the patient's condition and they require the skills of an occupational therapist, or whether they can be safely and effectively carried out by nonskilled personnel, without the occupational therapist's supervision. The reasons for OT must be clear to you as well as their goals, prior to a favorable coverage determination. They often require review at Level III.

It is essential that the provider documents the updated status in a clear, concise, and objective manner. Objective tests and measurements are stressed when these are practical. The occupational therapist selects the appropriate method to demonstrate current patient status. However, the method chosen, as well as the measures used, should be consistent during the treatment duration. If the method used to demonstrate progress is changed, the reasons for the change should be documented, including how the new method relates to the old. You must have an overview of the purpose of treatment goals in order to compare the patient's currently functional status to that in previous reporting periods.

Documentation of the patient's current functional status and level of assistance required compared to previous reporting period(s) is of paramount importance. The deficits in functional ability should be clear. Occupational therapists must document functional improvements (or lack thereof) as a result of their treatments. Documentation of functional progress must be stated whenever possible in objective, measurable terms. The following illustrates these principles and demonstrates that significant changes may occur in one or more of these assistance levels:

a. *Change in Level of Assistance*—Occupational therapists document assistance levels by describing the relationship between functional activities and the need for assistance. Within the assistance levels of minimum, moderate, and maximum, there are intermediate gradations of improvement based on changes in behavior and response to assistance. *Improvements at each level must be documented.* Documentation should compare the current cognitive and physical level achieved to that achieved previously. While the need for cognitive assistance often is the more severe and persistent disability, the requirement of physical assistance often is the major obstacle to successful outcomes and subsequent discharge. Interpret the levels as follows:

- *Total Assistance* is the need for 100% assistance by one or more persons to perform all physical activities and/or cognitive assistance to elicit a functional response to an external stimulation.

  A patient requires total assistance if the documentation indicates the patient is only able to initiate minimal voluntary motor actions and requires the skill of an occupational therapist to develop a therapeutic program or implement a maintenance program to prevent or minimize deterioration.

  A cognitively impaired patient requires total assistance when documentation shows external stimuli are required to elicit automatic actions such as swallowing or responding to auditory stimuli. Skills of an occupational therapist are needed to identify and apply strategies for eliciting appropriate, consistent automatic responses to external stimuli.

- *Maximum Assistance* is the need for 75% assistance by one person to physically perform any part of a functional activity and/or cognitive assistance to perform gross motor actions in response to direction.

  A patient requires maximum assistance if maximum OT physical support and proprioceptive stimulation is needed for performance of each step of a functional activity every time it is performed.

A cognitively impaired patient, at this level, may need propriocep-tive stimulation and/or one-to-one demonstration by the occupa-tional therapist due to the patient's lack of cognitive awareness of other people or objects in the environment.

- *Moderate Assistance* is the need for 50% assistance by one person to perform physical activities or constant cognitive assistance to sustain/complete simple, repetitive activities safely.

A physically impaired patient requires moderate assistance if documentation indicates that moderate OT physical support and proprioceptive stimulation is needed for the patient to perform a functional activity, every time it is performed.

The records submitted should state how a cognitively impaired patient, at this level, requires intermittent one-to-one demonstra-tion or intermittent cuing (physical or verbal) throughout perfor-mance of the activity. Moderate assistance is needed when the occupational therapist/caregiver needs to be in the immediate environment to progress the patient through a sequence to com-plete a functional activity. This level of assistance is required to halt continued repetition of a task and to prevent unsafe, erratic or unpredictable actions that interfere with appropriate sequencing.

- *Minimum Assistance* is the need for 25% assistance by one person for physical activities and/or periodic, cognitive assistance to per-form functional activities safely.

A physically impaired patient requires minimum assistance if doc-umentation indicates that activities can only be performed after physical set-up by the occupational therapist or caregiver, and if physical help is needed to initiate, or sustain an activity. A review of alternate procedures, sequences, and methods may be required.

A cognitively impaired patient requires minimal assistance if doc-umentation indicates help is needed in performing known activi-ties to correct repeated mistakes, to check for compliance with established safety procedures, or to solve problems posed by unexpected hazards.

- *Standby Assistance* is the need for supervision by one person for the patient to perform new activity procedures which were adapt-ed by the therapist for safe and effective performance. A patient requires standby assistance when errors and the need for safety precautions are not always anticipated by the patient.

- *Independent Status* means that no physical or cognitive assistance is required to perform functional activities. Patients at this level are able to implement the selected courses of action, consider potential errors, and anticipate safety hazards in familiar and new situations.

b. *Change in Response to Treatment Within Each Level of Assistance*—Significant improvement must be indicated by documenting a change in one or more of the following categories of patient responses within any level of assistance:

- *Decreased Refusals.* The patient may respond by refusing to attempt performance of an activity because of fear or pain. The documentation should indicate what activity and performance is refused, the reasons, and how the OT plan addresses them.

  These responses are often secondary to a change in medical status or medications. If the refusals continue over several days, the therapy program should be put on "hold" until the documentation indicates the refusal response has changed and the patient is willing to attempt performance of functional activities.

  For the cognitively impaired patient, refusal to perform can escalate into aggressive, destructive or verbally abusive behavior if pressed by the therapist or caregiver to perform. In these cases, a reduction in these behaviors is significant and must be clearly documented, including the skilled OT provided to reduce the abnormal behavior.

  For the psychiatrically impaired patient, refusals to participate in an activity frequently are symptoms of the diagnosis. This patient should not be put on a "hold" status due to refusal. If the documentation indicates the patient is receiving OT, contacted regularly, and actively encouraged to participate, medically review the claim to determine if reasonable and necessary skilled care has been rendered.

- *Increased Consistency.* The patient may respond by inconsistently performing functional tasks from day-to-day or within a treatment session. approve the claim when the documentation indicates a significant progression in consistency of performance of functional tasks within the same level of assistance.

- *Increased Generalization.* The patient may respond by applying previously learned concepts and performance of one activity to another, similar activity. The records submitted should document a significant increase in scope of activities that the patient can perform, the type of activities, and the skilled OT services rendered.

c. *A New Skilled Functional Activity is Initiated.*—Two examples of skilled care are:

— Adding teaching of lower body dressing to a current program of upper body dressing;

— Increasing the ability to perform personal hygiene activities for health and social acceptance.

d. *A New Skilled Compensatory Technique is Added.*—(With or without adapted equipment.) Two examples are:

— Teaching a patient techniques such as one-handed shoe tying;

— Teaching the use of a button hook for buttoning shirt buttons.

e. *Length of Time in Treatment.*—The acceptable length of time in treatment for various disorders is determined by the patient's functional abilities and progress as reflected in the documentation.

Level of Complexity of Treatment *[3906.5]*

Base decisions on the level of complexity of the services rendered by the occupational therapist and not what the patient is asked to do. Examples of complexity of treatment are:

a. **Skilled OT**—The documentation must indicate that the severity of the physical/emotional/perceptual/cognitive disability requires complex and sophisticated knowledge to identify current and potential capabilities. In addition, consider instructions required by the patient and/or the patient's caregivers. Instructions may be required for activities that most healthy people take for granted. The special knowledge of an occupational therapist is required to decrease or eliminate limitations in functional activity performance imposed by illness or disability. Occupational therapists must often address underlying factors which interfere with the performance of specific activities. Some of these factors could be cognitive, sensory, or perceptual deficits.

The occupational therapist modifies the specific activity by using adapted equipment, making changes in the environment and surrounding objects, altering procedures for accomplishing the task, and providing specialized assistance to meet the patient's current and potential abilities. Skilled services include, but are not limited to reasonable and necessary:

— Evaluations of the patient;

— Determinations of effective goals and services with the patient and patient's caregivers and other medical professionals;

— Analyzing and modifying functional tasks;

— Determining that the modified task obtains optimum performance through tests and measurements;

— Providing instructions of the task(s) to the patient/family/caregivers; and

— Periodically reevaluating the patient's status with corresponding readjustment of the OT program.

A period of practice may be approved for the patient and/or patient's caregivers to learn the steps of the task, to verify the task's effectiveness in improving function, and to check for safe and consistent activity performance.

b. **Nonskilled OT**—When the documentation indicates a patient has attained the therapy goals or has reached the point where no further significant improvement can be expected, the skills of an occupational therapist are not required to **maintain function** at the level to which it has been restored. Examples of maintenance procedures are:

— Daily feeding programs after the adapted procedures are in place;

— Routine exercise and strengthening programs;

— The practice of coordination and self-care skills on a daily basis; and

— Presenting information on energy conservation or pacing, but not having the patient perform the activity.

You may approve a claim because the patient requires the judgement and skills of the occupational therapist to design a safe and effective maintenance program and make **periodic** checks of its effectiveness. The services of an occupational therapist in **carrying out** the established maintenance program are not considered reasonable and necessary for the treatment of illness or injury and may not be approved.

Reporting on New Episode or Condition *[3906.6]*

Occasionally, a patient who is receiving or who has received OT services, experiences a new illness. The provider must document the significance of any change to the patient's functional capabilities. This may be through pre and post episodic nursing notes or physician reports. If the patient is receiving treatment, it might be lengthened. If the patient has completed treatment for the functional deficit; a significant change in the patient's functional status must be documented that warrants a new treatment plan.

Other MR Considerations *[3906.7]*

A. **Pain**—Documentation describing the presence or absence of pain and its effect on the patient's functional abilities must be considered in MR decisions. A description of its intensity, type, changing pattern, and location at specific joint ranges of motion materially aids correct MR decisions. Documentation should describe the limitations placed upon the patient's ADL, mobility and/or safety, as well as the subjective progress made in the reduction of pain through treatment.

B. **Therapeutic Programs**—The objective documentation should support the skilled nature of the program, and/or the need for the design and establishment of a maintenance OT program. The goals should generally be to increase functional abilities in ADL, mobility or patient safety. Documentation should indicate the goals and type of program provided.

Approve claims when the therapeutic program, because of documented medical complications, the condition of the patient, or complexity of the OT employed, must be rendered by, or under, the supervision of an occupational therapist. For example, while functional ADL may often be performed safely and effectively by nonskilled personnel, the presence of fracture nonunion, severe joint pain, or other medical or safety complications may warrant skilled occupational therapist intervention to render the service and/or to establish a safe maintenance program. In these cases, the complications and the skilled services, they require, must be documented by physician orders and/or occupational therapist notes. To make correct MR decisions, the patient's losses and/or dependencies in ADL, mobility and safety must be documented. The possibility of adverse effects from the improper performance of an otherwise unskilled service does not make it a skilled service unless there is documentation to support why skilled OT is needed for the patient's medical condition and/or safety.

Approved establishment and design of a maintenance exercise program to fit the patient's level of ADL, function, and any instructions supportive personnel and/or family members need to safely and effectively carry it out. Reevaluation may be approved when reasonable and necessary to readjust the maintenance program to meet the changing needs of the patient. There must be adequate justification for readjusting a maintenance program, e.g., loss of previous functional gains.

C. **Cardiac Rehabilitation Exercise**—Occupational therapy is not covered when furnished in connection with cardiac rehabilitation exercise program services (see Coverage Issues Manual 35-25) unless there is also a diagnosed noncardiac condition requiring it e.g., where a patient who is recuperating from an acute phase of heart disease may have had a stroke which requires OT. (While the cardiac rehabilitation exercise program may be considered by some a form of OT, it is a specialized program conducted and/or supervised by specially trained personnel whose services are performed under the direct supervision of a physician.)

D. **Transfer Training**—The documentation should describe the patient's functional limitations in transfer ability that warrant skilled OT intervention. Documentation should include the special transfer training needed to perform functional daily living skills and any training needed by supportive personnel and/or family members to safely and effectively carry it out. Approve transfer training when the documentation supports a skilled need for evaluation, design and effective monitoring and instruction of the special transfer technique for safety and completion of the functional activities of daily living or mobility task.

Documentation that supports only repetitious carrying out of the transfer method, once established, and monitored for safety and completion is noncovered care.

E. **Fabrication of and Training in Use of Orthoses Prostheses and Adaptive Equipment**—Approve reasonable and necessary fabrication of orthoses, protheses, adaptive equipment, and any reasonable and necessary skilled training needed in their safe and effective use. The documentation must indicate the need for the device and training required.

F. **OT Forms**—Documentation may be submitted on a specific form you [the carrier] require or may be copies of the provider's record. However, your form must capture the needed MR information. If you choose to require a particular form, show the OMB clearance number. The information you require to review the bill is that which is required by an occupational therapist to properly treat a patient.

G. **Certification and Recertification**—OT services must be certified and recertified by a physician and must be furnished while the patient is under the care of a physician. OT services must be furnished under a written plan of treatment established by the physician or a qualified occupational therapist. If the plan is established by an occupational therapist, it must be reviewed periodically by the physician.

The plan of treatment must be established (reduced to writing by either professional or the provider when it makes a written record of oral orders) before treatment is begun. When outpatient OT services are continued under the same plan of treatment for a period of time, the physician must certify at least at 30-day intervals that there is a continuing need for them. Obtain the recertification when reviewing the plan of treatment since the same interval of a least 30 days is required for review of the plans. A recertification must be signed by the physician, who reviewed the plan of treatment. Any changes to the treatment plan established by the occupational therapist must be in writing and signed by the therapist or by the attending physician. The physician may change a plan of treatment established by the occupational therapist. However, the occupational therapist may not alter a plan of treatment established by a physician.

Occupational Therapy availability—Two or more disciplines may provide therapy services to the same patient. There may also be occasions where these services are duplicative. In many instances, the description of the services appears duplicative, but the documentation proves that they are not. Some examples where there is <u>not</u> a duplication include:

A. <u>Transfers</u>—PT instructs the patient in transfers to achieve the level of safety with the techniques. OT utilizes transfers as they relate to the performance of daily living skills (e.g., transfer from wheelchair to bathtub.).

B. <u>Pulmonary</u>—PT instructs the patient in an adapted breathing technique. OT carries the breathing retraining into activities of daily living.

C. <u>Hip Fractures/Arthroplasties</u>—PT instructs the patient in hip precautions and gait training. OT reinforces the training with precautions for activities of daily living, e.g., lower extremity dressing, toileting, and bathing.

D. <u>CVA</u>—PT utilizes upper extremity neurodevelopmental (NDT) techniques to assist the patient in positioning the upper extremities on a walker and in gait training. OT utilizes NDT techniques to increase the functional use of the upper extremity for dressing, bathing, grooming, etc.

Focused MR Analysis—The HCFA edits may assist you in identifying OT claims for focused MR. Perform regular evaluations of provider claims which pass or fail the edits. Change your focused review claims selection based on the results of the evaluation. For example, a provider billing at an aberrantly consistent rate just below the edit parameters is subject to intensified review.

Develop procedures for focused MR based on each of the following trends or characteristics:

- Edits with high charges per aggregate bill charges;

- Providers billing a higher than average utilization of specific diagnostic codes that fall just below the edit parameters; and

- Specific principal DX codes, such as those with longer visits and duration; those representing the most frequent denials in prepay MR; special codes, e.g., 585, Chronic Renal Failure; 733.1, Senile Osteoporosis; and 290.0-290.9, Senile and Presenile Organic Psychotic Conditions; and/or certain edit groups such as 17, 19, and 29 in one quarter and others in the next quarter.

Medical and Medicaid Guide Utilization and Medical Review
Special Instructions for Dysphagia Claims

For your MR of dysphagia claims for speech-language pathology (SLP), occupational therapy (OT), and physical therapy (PT) services follow these procedures:

A. Medical Workup—Documentation by the physician must establish a preliminary diagnosis and form the basis of estimates of progress. Patients must be selected for therapy after a proper medical diagnostic evaluation by a physician. The medical workups must document whether the difficulty involves the oral, pharyngeal, or esophageal phase of swallowing. This may involve collaboration with therapists or speech-language pathologists.

B. Dysphagia Criteria—Oral, Pharyngeal, or Esophageal (upper one third) Phase of Swallowing—Documentation must indicate the patient's level of alertness, motivation, cognition, and deglutition. In addition, at least one of the following conditions must be present:

- History of aspiration problems or aspiration pneumonia, or definite risk for aspiration, reverse aspiration, chronic aspiration, nocturnal aspiration, or aspiration pneumonia. Nasal regurgitation, choking, frequent coughing up food during swallowing, wet or gurgling voice quality after swallowing liquids or delayed or slow swallow reflex.

- Presence of oral motor disorders such as drooling, oral food retention, leakage of food or liquids placed into the mouth.

- Impaired salivary gland performance and/or presence of local structural lesions in the pharynx resulting in marked oropharyngeal swallowing difficulties.

- Incoordination, sensation loss, (postural difficulties) or other neuromotor disturbances affecting oropharyngeal abilities necessary to close the buccal cavity and/or bite, chew, suck, shape and squeeze the food bolus into the upper esophagus while protecting the airway.

- Post-surgical reaction affecting ability to adequately use oropharyngeal structures used in swallowing.

- Significant weight loss directly related to non-oral nutritional intake (g-tube feeding) and reaction to textures and consistencies.

- Existence of other conditions such as presence of tracheostomy tube, reduced or inadequate laryngeal elevation, labial closure, velopharyngeal closure, laryngeal closure, or pharyngeal peristalsis, and cricopharyngeal dysfunction.

C. Esophageal (lower two thirds) Phase of Swallow.—Esophageal dysphagia (lower two thirds of the esophagus) is difficulty in passing food from the esophagus to the stomach. If peristalsis is inefficient, patients may complain of food getting stuck or of having more difficulty swallowing solids than liquids. Sometimes patients experience esophageal reflux or regurgitation if they lie down too soon after meals.

Inefficient functioning of the esophagus during the esophageal phase of swallowing is a common problem in the geriatric patient. Swallowing disorders occurring only in the lower two thirds of the esophageal stage of the swallow have not generally been shown to be amenable to swallowing therapy techniques and may not be approved. An exception might be when discomfort from reflux results in food refusal. A therapeutic feeding program in conjunction with medical management may be indicated and constitute reasonable and necessary care. A reasonable and necessary assessment of function, prior to a conclusion that difficulties exist in the lower two thirds of the esophageal phase, may be approved, even when the assessment determines that skilled intervention is not appropriate.

D. <u>Assessment</u>—Medical workup and professional assessments must document history, current eating status, and clinical observations such as:

- Presence of a feeding tube;

- Paralysis;

- Coughing or choking;

- Oral motor structure and function;

- Oral sensitivity;

- Muscle tone;

- Cognition;

- Positioning;

- Laryngeal function;

- Oropharyngeal reflexes; and

- Swallowing function.

This information is used to determine necessity for further medical testing, e.g. videofluoroscopy, upper GI series, endoscopy. If videofluoroscopic assessment is conducted (modified barium swallow), documentation must establish that the exact diagnosis of the swallowing disorder cannot be substantiated through oral exam and there is a question as to whether aspiration is occurring. The videofluoroscopy assessment is conducted and interpreted by a radiologist with assistance and input from the physician and/or individual disciplines. The assessment and final analysis and interpretation should include a definitive diagnosis, identification of the swallowing phase(s) affected, and a recommended treatment plan. An analysis by an individual discipline may be submitted as a separate line item charge.

E. <u>Care Planning</u>—Documentation must delineate goals and type of care planned which specifically addresses each problem identified in the assessment, such as:

- Patient caregiver training in feeding and swallowing techniques;

- Proper head and body positioning;

- Amount of intake per swallow;

- Appropriate diet;

- Means of facilitating the swallow;

- Feeding techniques and need for self help eating/feeding devices;

- Food consistencies (texture and size);

- Facilitation of more normal tone or oral facilitation techniques;

- Oromotor motor and neuromuscular facilitation exercises to improve oromotor control;

- Training in laryngeal and vocal cord adduction exercises;

- Conpensatory swallowing techniques; and

- Oral sensitivity training.

As with all other rehabilitation services, there must be a reasonable expectation that the patient will make material improvement within a reasonable period of time.

F.   Professional Services.—Services are sometimes performed by speech-language pathologists, occupational therapists and physical therapists in concert with other health professionals. Services are often performed as a team with each member performing unique roles which do not duplicate services of others. Services may include, but are not limited to, the following example:

EXAMPLE: One professional assisting with positioning, adaptive self help devices, inhibiting abnormal oromotor and/or postural reflexes while another professional is addressing specific exercises to improve oromotor control, determining appropriate food consistency form, assisting the patient in difficulty with muscular movements necessary to close the buccal cavity or shape food in the mouth in preparation for swallowing. Another professional might address a different role, such as increasing muscle strength, sitting balance and head control.

G.   Chronic Progressive Diseases.—Patients with progressive disorders, such as Parkinson's disease, Huntington's disease, Wilson's disease, multiple sclerosis, or Alzheimer's disease and related dementias, do not typically show improvement in swallowing function, but will often be helped through short-term assistance/instruction in positioning, diet, feeding modifications, and in the use of self help devices. Medically review documentation in support of short-term assistance/teaching and establishment of a safe and effective maintenance dysphagia program.

Chronic diseases such as cerebral palsy, status post-head trauma or stroke (old) may require monitoring of swallowing function with short-term intervention for safety and/or swallowing effectiveness. Documentation should relate to either loss of function, or potential for change.

As with other conditions/disorders, the reasonableness and necessity of services must be documented. Documentation should include:

- Changes in condition or functional status;

- History and outcome of previous treatment for the same conditions; and

- Other information which would justify the start of care.

H. <u>Nasogastric Tube or Gastrostomy Tube.</u>—The presence of a nasogastric or gastrostomy tube may be an appropriate treatment goal.

I. <u>Safety.</u>—Although the documentation must indicate appropriate treatment goals to improve a patient's swallowing function, it must also indicate that the treatment is designed to ensure that it is safe for the patient to swallow during oral feedings. Improving the patient's safety and quality of life by reduction or elimination of alternative nutritional support systems and advancement of dietary level, with improved nutritional intake should be the primary emphasis and treatment goal. The documentation must be consistent with these goals and indicate the reasonableness and need for skilled intervention.

J. <u>Skilled Level of Care.</u>—Documentation of ongoing dysphagia treatment should support the need for skilled services such as observation, treatment, and diet modification. Documentation which is reflective of routine, repetitive observation or cuing may not qualify as skilled rehabilitation.

For example, repeated visits in which the caregiver appears only to be observing the patient eating a meal, reporting on the amount of food consumed, providing verbal reminders (e. g., slow down or cough) in the absence of other skilled assistance or observation suggests a nonskilled or maintenance level of care. Maintenance programs are covered for a brief period and are usually included during the final visits of the professional.

K. <u>Professional Qualification.</u>—Swallowing rehabilitation is a highly specialized service. Assume that the professionals rendering care have the necessary specialized training and experience. Refer to the RO any suspected patterns of poor quality.

L. <u>Consultation.</u>—You are encouraged to seek consultation/advice from the American Speech-Language-Hearing Association, American Occupational Therapy Association, and American Physical Therapy Association.

CHAPTER 13

Voluntary Accrediting Agencies

KEY TERMS

Accreditation. A process by which an institution or an educational organization seeks to demonstrate to an accrediting agency that it complies with generally accepted standards set forth by appropriate professional organizations; also, a kind of status awarded to an organization that demonstrates compliance with standards.

Formative evaluation. AC: Continuous assessment of the ability to strive for and achieve improvement in quality.

Function. JCAHO: A goal-directed, interrelated series of processes (see *process*), such as patient assessment or human resource management.

Independent quality review. AC: An on-site visit during which a review team applies 30 outcome measures to a representative sample of persons with disabilities whom it has chosen, through observations and interviews. The team also conducts interviews with staff members, family members, and other persons receiving services and supports.

National consensus standards. Standards based on consensus among providers, consumers, and purchasers of services, as compared with standards derived from a research base.

Outcome-based performance measures (outcome measures). AC: Measures of the presence of outcomes that persons with disabilities want from their support or service programs (e.g., "People choose their daily routine," "People choose to participate in the life of the community," and "People are safe").

Outcomes. AC: Core benefits that persons with disabilities want from their support or service programs (e.g., choice, rights, and social inclusion).

Process. JCAHO: A goal-directed, interrelated series of actions, events, mechanisms, or steps, such as coordination of care among practitioners.

Quality. AC: An attribute determined or measured by an organization's responsiveness to the individual rather than by its compliance with traditional standards.

Review, survey. An on-site visit to an organization seeking accreditation, during which an individual or a team may review documents; conduct interviews with the persons served, staff, purchasers, and other consumers; make observations to assess an organization's compliance with standards; and conduct public hearings.

Reviewer, surveyor. A person conducting a review or a survey, or participating on a team conducting one, typically a peer in an accredited program who has experience in the type of program seeking accreditation.

Self-study, self-assessment. A self-examination conducted by an organization preparing for a review or a survey.

AC = Accreditation Council on Services for Persons with Disabilities; JCAHO = Joint Commission on Accreditation of Healthcare Organizations

Richard W. Scalenghe, BM, RMT, is an associate director of the Department of Standards at the Joint Commission on Accreditation of Healthcare Organizations, responsible for interpreting the standards related to rehabilitation, mental health, and chemical dependency. He is also the Joint Commission's Liaison Network Organization representative for AOTA.

Christine M. MacDonell, BSOT, is the national director of the Medical Rehabilitation Division of CARF, The Rehabilitation Accreditation Commission. Before joining CARF in 1991, she served as the executive director of the California Alliance of Rehabilitation Industries, and earlier, as education and training coordinator of the California Association of Rehabilitation Facilities. She received her training in occupational therapy at the University of Southern California.

Nancy MacRae, MS, OTR/L, FAOTA, is an associate professor in the Department of Occupational Therapy at the University of New England. Formerly she managed the Occupational Therapy Department at Pineland Center, an institution for persons with developmental disabilities. She represented AOTA on the Accreditation Council on Services for Persons with Disabilities for over eight years, in her last years serving as secretary, then vice-president, then president. Her master's degree is from the University of South Maine.

I n health care as in other fields, mechanisms exist for setting standards and applying them to individuals and organizations providing professional services.[1] The mechanisms serve both the public and the health care professions. For the public they ensure qualified professionals and adequately equipped, competently staffed organizations. For the professions they publicly affirm the competence of individual practitioners and the quality of individual organizations. Chapter 17 addresses the mechanisms for setting and applying standards to individuals—state regulation and specialty certification. This chapter addresses the mechanism for setting and applying standards to organizations—accreditation.

Accreditation is a process by which an institution or an educational organization seeks to demonstrate to an accrediting agency that it complies with generally accepted standards set forth by appropriate professional organizations (Wilson & Neuhauser, 1985); also, accreditation is a kind of status awarded to an organization that demonstrates compliance with standards. The chapter focuses on accreditation at the national level. Technically, accreditation at this level is voluntary, whereas accreditation at the state level, in the form of obtaining a license to operate, is often mandatory. The voluntary nature of national accreditation is questionable, however. Many third-party payers condition reimbursement on accreditation, and the federal government relies on accreditation to establish an organization's eligibility for grants and contracts. Moreover, the federal government's Health Care Financing Administration "deems" health care organizations that are accredited by certain national agencies to have met requirements for participation in the Medicare program; therefore those organizations need not undergo a separate annual review by the federal government. Similar arrangements exist in many states, organizations accredited by certain national agencies being deemed to have met state requirements for a license to operate or for participation in the Medicaid program. These factors make national accreditation virtually mandatory.

The chapter describes in detail the three national accrediting agencies with which occupational therapy managers and practitioners have the most contact: the Joint Commission on Accreditation of Healthcare Organizations (the Joint Commission or JCAHO); CARF, The Rehabilitation Accreditation Commission;[2] and the Accreditation Council on Services for People with Disabilities (the Accreditation Council). Table 13-1 identifies the domain of each agency, its sponsoring organizations, the

1. *This section is based in part on "Regulation and Standard Setting" (pp. 333–41), by S. B. Fine, J. Bair, S. P. Hoover, and J. D. Acquaviva, 1992, in J. Bair and M. Gray (Eds.), The* Occupational Therapy Manager *(Rev. ed.), Rockville, MD: American Occupational Therapy Association.*

2. *CARF is an acronym for Commission on Accreditation of Rehabilitation Facilities, the organization's original name. The commission changed its name in August 1994 to CARF, the Rehabilitation Accreditation Commission, retaining the acronym as a well-recognized short form of the old designation.*

Table 13-1

Domains, Sponsorship, and Practices of Voluntary Accrediting Agencies in Health Care and Rehabilitation

Agency	Domain	Sponsors	Responsibility for Development of Standards	Responsibility for Accreditation Decisions
Joint Commission on Accreditation of Healthcare Organizations (JCAHO)	General, behavioral health, children's, and physical rehabilitation hospitals; health care networks, including health maintenance organizations, preferred provider organizations, physicians' networks, and comprehensive delivery systems for defined populations; home care agencies and organizations, including those that provide home health, personal care and support, home infusion therapy, hospice care, or durable medical equipment services; nursing homes (including their subacute care units) and other long-term-care facilities; behavioral health care, including mental health, chemical dependency, and mental retardation/developmental disabilities services for persons of all ages in all organized service settings; ambulatory health care providers, including outpatient surgery facilities, physical rehabilitation centers, infusion centers, group practices, and others; and clinical and pathology laboratories	American College of Physicians, American College of Surgeons, American Dental Association, American Hospital Association, American Medical Association	JCAHO staff with input from task forces on particular chapters, professional and technical advisory committees, field reviews; final approval by JCAHO Board of Commissioners	Accreditation Committee of JCAHO Board of Commissioners

Agency	Domain	Sponsors	Responsibility for Development of Standards	Responsibility for Accreditation Decisions
CARF, The Rehabilitation Accreditation Commission	Free-standing rehabilitation organizations or rehabilitation programs operated as units of larger institutions; private not-for-profit, proprietary, public agency–operated, and privately owned programs; in the areas of behavioral health, employment and community support services, and medical rehabilitation	American Academy of Neurology, American Academy of Orthopedic Surgeons, American Academy of Orthotists and Prosthetists, American Academy of Pain Medicine, American Academy of Physical Medicine and Rehabilitation, American Network of Community Options and Resources, American Hospital Association, American Occupational Therapy Association, American Pain Society, American Physical Therapy Association, American Psychological Association, American Rehabilitation Association, American Speech-Language-Hearing Association, American Spinal Injury Association, American Therapeutic Recreation Association, Association of Rehabilitation Nurses, Federation of American Health Systems, Goodwill Industries International, International Association of Jewish Vocational Services, International Association of Psychosocial Rehabilitation Services, National Head Injury Foundation, Paralyzed Veterans of America, United Cerebral Palsy Association;[a] and members at large[b]	Ad hoc national advisory committees reaching consensus regarding practice in field, field reviews; final approval by CARF Board of Trustees	CARF Board of Trustees

continued

Table 13-1, continued

Agency	Domain	Sponsors	Responsibility for Development of Standards	Responsibility for Accreditation Decisions
Accreditation Council on Services for People with Disabilities	Programs or agencies serving persons with disabilities	American Association on Mental Retardation; American Network of Community Options and Resources; American Occupational Therapy Association; American Psychological Association; Association for Behavior Analysis; Association for Retarded Children; Autism Society of America; Epilepsy Foundation of America; United Cerebral Palsy Association	Select committee of advisers, service providers, and consumers; final approval by Accreditation Council Board of Directors	Accreditation Subcommittee, on behalf of Accreditation Council Board of Directors

Note. *Adapted from "Regulation and Standard Setting" (pp. 336–37), by S. B. Fine, J. Bair, S. P. Hoover, and J. D. Acquaviva, 1992, in J. Bair and M. Gray (Eds.),* The Occupational Therapy Manager *(Rev. ed.), Rockville, MD: American Occupational Therapy Association. Copyright ©1992 by the American Occupational Therapy Association, Inc.*

a. CARF also has associate members, as follows: American Association for Partial Hospitalization, American Association on Mental Retardation, American Congress of Rehabilitation Medicine, American Horticultural Therapy Association, American Osteopathic College of Rehabilitation Medicine, Association of Mental Health Administrators, National Association for the Dually Diagnosed, National Association of Addiction Treatment Providers, National Association of Alcoholism and Drug Abuse Counselors, National Association of Social Workers, National Association of State Mental Health Program Directors, National Coalition of Arts Therapy Associations, National Community Mental Healthcare Council, National Easter Seal Society, National Rehabilitation Association, National Spinal Cord Injury Association, and National Therapeutic Recreation Society.

b. These are persons from a variety of sources who represent consumers, purchasers, and professionals with an interest in rehabilitation issues.

locus of responsibility for development of standards, and the locus of responsibility for accreditation decisions. The chapter also describes in brief two national accrediting agencies with which occupational therapy managers and practitioners should be familiar: the Community Health Accreditation Program (CHAP) and the Accreditation Council for Occupational Therapy Education (ACOTE).

THE ORIGINS OF VOLUNTARY ACCREDITATION OF HEALTH CARE ORGANIZATIONS

Voluntary accreditation of health care organizations originated in 1917. Prompted by the revelations of the landmark Flexner (1910) report on the poor quality of medical education and by related apprehension about government regulation of hospital practice (Starr, 1982), the American College of Surgeons formulated *Minimum Standards for Hospitals* and began on-site inspections. The success of this voluntary effort to improve the quality of health care is obvious in the change from a 13-percent rate of accreditation the first year to a 94-percent rate by 1945 (Somers, 1969). The marked growth of the regulatory process over the years is tangibly illustrated by the increase in the length of the standards for hospitals, from 1 page in 1917 to 332 pages in 1996.

ACCREDITING AGENCIES TODAY

Today health care accrediting agencies are often collaborative in nature, their governing bodies consisting of representatives from various constituencies interested in ensuring quality in the institutions or the programs being accredited (Wilson & Neuhauser, 1985). Among these constituencies may be individual and institutional health care providers, administrators, educators, consumers, insurance companies, and the public. As table 13-1 indicates, JCAHO has 5 sponsors, CARF 43, and the Accreditation Council 9. The diversity among the sponsors is evident. Within the agencies there may be additional bodies with responsibility for certain aspects of accreditation (accreditation committees, advisory committees, standards committees, boards of review, etc.), and these too may be broadly representative of constituencies.

Accrediting agencies typically have several sources of income. The institutions that seek accreditation usually pay a substantial fee to participate in the process. Other revenue may come from sale of publications, sponsorship of training events (seminars, workshops, etc.), and grants (e.g., to develop and validate outcome measures). Also, sponsoring organizations may provide direct support.

Across accrediting agencies, some variation exists in the process for developing and revising the standards used to accredit organizations (see table 13-1). In the last two decades the standards themselves have been changing in emphasis as health care costs have escalated, concerns about accountability have mounted, and business practices have influenced health care management. Once focused almost exclusively on structure and process, standards increasingly address outcomes as well.

THE ACCREDITATION PROCESS

Typically an organization seeking accreditation initiates the accreditation process by submitting an application for a *review,* called a *survey* by some agencies. The accrediting agency then usually requires the organization to conduct a *self-study* (or *self-assessment*), a self-examination on the basis of the agency's standards. The next step is an on-site review, in which an individual *reviewer* (or *surveyor*), or a team, visits the organization. These persons are experienced, competent peers from an accredited organization, in some cases the type of organization seeking review. They typically receive orientation and continuing education to perform their role effectively. The agency usually notifies the organization in advance of the date of the visit. Depending on an organization's size and the scope of its services, the visit may last from one to four days, and one to four professionals from various fields of health care may conduct the review. The organization seeking accreditation typically bears the cost of the review. Once an organization is accredited, it must undergo periodic review to maintain its accreditation, normally every three years.

Across the agencies, different bodies may make the final decision regarding accreditation (see table 13-1). If the agency denies accreditation or renewal of accreditation, there is normally an appeals process for challenging the decision. A common practice of accrediting agencies is to publish a list of the organizations that they have accredited.

THE ROLE OF THE OCCUPATIONAL THERAPY MANAGER IN ACCREDITATION

How occupational therapy managers and practitioners view the standards, the self-assessment, and the actual review will likely influence their experience. Those who view the standards as busywork and the review as intrusive will probably gain little. Those who approach the standards and the review as a way to streamline, validate, and improve the unit, however, will gain much.

An occupational therapy manager whose organization is being reviewed should expect to participate through advanced planning with other members of the organization's administration, submission of policies and procedures manuals and other documents representing compliance with the standards, hosting of an inspection of the physical plant, and interviews with the survey team. The interviews frequently involve discussion of personnel (their formal preparation, credentials, qualifications, and experience, and provisions for continuing assessment of their competence), staff continuing education and supervision, methods of documentation, referrals, and quality improvement activities. If the occupational therapy manager handles the interviews skillfully, he or she will be able not only to demonstrate compliance but to educate reviewers about the purpose and the value of occupational therapy services.

THE IMPORTANCE OF ACCREDITATION TO OCCUPATIONAL THERAPY

Despite the shortcomings of some standards, the difficulties that frequently plague the on-site review, and the variability in reviewers' knowledge and understanding of the many aspects of an organization's services, the accreditation process provides important opportunities for occupational therapy managers to clarify program goals for their staff, themselves, and the organization's administrators, and to develop effective strategies for implementation of clinical practice, research, and education, as appropriate. Managers and practitioners should learn how to make the accreditation process—and accredited status, once it is achieved—work for them and their programs on a continuing basis:

1. The accreditation process provides organization personnel with an objective assessment of their organization's performance. It can provide a systems or holistic perspective that few if any within the organization possess.

2. The accreditation process promotes communication on all levels. The occupational therapy manager who does not communicate with his or her staff members will have a difficult time preparing for the review. During the review itself, staff members will be uncomfortable answering questions if they have not been part of the preparation and the development of policies and procedures that affect practice.

3. The accreditation process provides practitioners with an occasion to define and document their work. The occupational therapy profession can ill afford to ignore this opportunity.

4. The accreditation process offers expertise in the form of knowledgeable and responsive accrediting agency staff members and reviewers who can provide resources and training to assist occupational therapy managers and practitioners in dealing with issues related to individual or organizational outcomes. Reviewers and agency staff members can help lay the groundwork for active problem solving that both involves and addresses the individual

and the organization. Organizations are encouraged to use the accreditation process as an educational and consultative opportunity by drawing on the reviewers' and staff members' experience. Among other contributions, they can share best practices as examples.

5. The accreditation process can support managers in promoting the needs of their unit with the administration. The fact that the senior leaders and the governance groups of the organization have requested a review, and that they expect to meet the standards, should ensure that there are sufficient staff members, space, and other resources to fulfill their expectations. One role of the reviewers is to assess the adequacy of resources and make recommendations for additional resources to comply with standards if necessary.

6. The accreditation process can foster effectiveness in outcomes and efficiency in operations by helping managers monitor and improve the use and the quality of occupational therapy services and heighten the visibility and the credibility of occupational therapy within their organization.

7. The accreditation process can promote the use of outcome information to make decisions about the programs and the services offered. The information gathered from an outcome system can assist the occupational therapy manager in planning additional or new services and in modifying or eliminating certain existing services. The occupational therapy manager who learns from the overall outcome system and implements a like system in the occupational therapy unit will be a great asset to the organization. The knowledge that an outcome system can bring to the improvement of performance is also an excellent management tool.

8. Accredited status can promote increased referrals for services. The rapid changes in health care have left many purchasers and referral sources leery of programs. They are interested in a baseline of quality, financial information, and consumer satisfaction. Accreditation gives them the information that they need to make decisions about where to provide care.

9. Accredited status reassures practitioners that an organization in which they seek or obtain employment is committed to continuous improvement in the quality of the supports and the services that it offers to the people whom it serves. The organization's values are likely to be highly compatible with those expressed by occupational therapy practitioners.

Understanding and interpreting standards skillfully, logically, and sensitively, in keeping with patients' or clients' needs and the organization's objectives and resources, is the responsibility of the occupational therapy manager. Resource materials prepared by accrediting agencies are helpful in developing a fuller understanding of the intent and the potential of their standards. Information about these resources may be obtained directly from the agencies (see Additional Resources for their addresses and telephone numbers).

PART 1

Joint Commission on Accreditation of Healthcare Organizations

Richard W. Scalenghe, BM, RMT

HISTORY, MISSION, AND DOMAIN

The Joint Commission is the largest and oldest private agency involved in voluntary accreditation in health care. It dates back to the American College of Surgeons' formulation of *Minimum Standards for Hospitals* in 1917 and that group's initiation of on-site inspection of hospitals in 1918. In 1951 the American College of Physicians, the American Hospital Association, the American Medical Association, and the Canadian Medical Association joined with the American College of Surgeons to create the Joint Commission on Accreditation of Hospitals as an independent, not-for-profit organization to provide voluntary accreditation for hospitals. The Canadian Medical Association withdrew in 1959 to start its own accrediting agency. Starting in the 1960s, the Joint Commission expanded to include long-term care, mental health, and other areas. The American Dental Association became a member of the Joint Commission in 1979.

Today the Joint Commission's mission is "to improve the quality of healthcare provided to the public through the provision of healthcare accreditation and related services that support performance improvement in healthcare." It strives to achieve this mission in the following ways:

1. Developing state-of-the-art performance standards

2. Providing accreditation services for the full range of mainstream health care organizations

3. Ensuring the availability of educational and consultative support for organizations seeking accreditation

4. Incorporating outcomes and other performance measures into the accreditation process

5. Publicly disclosing organization-specific performance information to interested parties

In fulfilling its mission, the Joint Commission relies on and collaborates with multiple professional and health care organizations and individuals, including AOTA and occupational therapy practitioners.

The Joint Commission evaluates and accredits more than 5,200 hospitals and more than 6,000 other health care organizations. Joint Commission accreditation is available for the following *fields,* or types of organizations:

1. General, behavioral health, children's, and physical rehabilitation hospitals

2. Health care networks, including health maintenance organizations (HMOs), preferred provider organizations (PPOs), physicians' networks, and comprehensive delivery systems for defined populations

3. Home care agencies and organizations, including those that provide home health, personal care and support, home infusion therapy, hospice care, or durable medical equipment services

4. Nursing homes (including their subacute care units) and other long-term-care facilities

5. Behavioral health care, including mental health, chemical dependency, and mental retardation/developmental disabilities services for persons of all ages in all organized service settings

6. Ambulatory health care providers, including outpatient surgery facilities, physical rehabilitation centers, infusion centers, group practices, and others

7. Clinical and pathology laboratories

The Joint Commission has established a professional and technical advisory committee (PTAC) for each field except clinical and pathology laboratories. PTACs consist of representatives from professional and health care organizations and public representatives relevant to each field. Each PTAC includes a representative from the Coalition of Rehabilitation Organizations. Created by the Joint Commission for purposes of PTAC representation, the coalition comprises AOTA, the American Physical Therapy Association, the American Speech-Language-Hearing Association, the American Therapeutic Recreation Association, the National Therapeutic Recreation Society, and the National Coalition of Arts Therapy Associations. There are advisory committees for safety fields (fire safety, occupational health, hazardous waste, health care engineering, etc.).

For each of the health care fields just listed, the Joint Commission publishes a corresponding manual containing standards (volume 1) and a set of scoring guidelines (volume 2). Table 13-2 lists the fields, their Joint Commission accreditation programs, and the related manuals.

Table 13-2
Scope, Organizational Locus, and Related Standards Manual
of JCAHO Responsibility for Accreditation

Health Care Field	Accreditation Program	Standards Manual	Latest Edition/ Frequency of Revision[a]
Hospitals	Hospital Accreditation Services	*Accreditation Manual for Hospitals* (AMH)	1996/annually
Health care networks	Network Accreditation Services	*Accreditation Manual for HealthCare Networks* (AMHCN)	1996/biennially
Home care[b]	Home Care Accreditation Services	*Accreditation Manual for Home Care* (AMHC)	1995/biennially
Nursing homes and other long-term-care organizations[c]	Long Term Care Accreditation Services	*Accreditation Manual for Long Term Care* (AMLTC)	1996/biennially
Behavioral health, including mental health, substance abuse, and mental retardation and developmental disabilities	Behavioral Health Accreditation Services	*Mental Health Manual* (MHM) (next and subsequent editions to be called *Accreditation Manual for Behavioral Health Care* (AMBHC))	1995/biennially
Ambulatory health care	Office of Ambulatory Care	*Accreditation Manual for Ambulatory HealthCare* (AHCSM)	1996/biennially
Laboratories	No official program as yet	*Accreditation Manual for Pathology and Clinical Laboratory Services* (CAMPCLS)	1996/frequency not yet determined

a. This information is current as of April 1996.

b. This field encompasses hospice.

c. This field encompasses subacute care.

The Joint Commission also publishes *Perspectives,* a bimonthly newsletter that reports changes in standards, policies, and procedures, as well as printing a range of features to improve understanding of accreditation. At the time of survey, practitioners are held accountable not only for what is in the current manual and scoring guidelines, but also for the changes, the additions, and the corrections noted in *Perspectives.* Every accredited organization receives a complimentary *Perspectives* subscription.

The format and the content of Joint Commission standards have varied over the years. The publication of the 1995 and 1996 versions of the standards manuals as well as changes in the survey process represent the achievement of a significant milestone in the Joint Commission's Agenda for Change. An effort to make accreditation a more effective stimulus for demonstrated and continuous improvement in the performance of health care organizations, the Agenda for Change includes three major initiatives:

1. Revision of the standards to focus on the processes and the functions (both clinical and organizational) that most significantly influence care; to emphasize doing the right things and doing them well; and to give more attention to what, less to how and who

   Process—a goal-directed, interrelated series of actions, events, mechanisms, or steps, such as coordination of care among practitioners

   Function—a goal-directed, interrelated series of processes, such as patient assessment or human resource management

2. Redesign of the survey process to focus on assessment of actual performance of the processes and the functions that most significantly influence care and to give more attention to what has been/is done, less to structures or documentation

3. Use of outcomes and other performance measures to capture the results of implemented processes and functions in the survey and to provide comparative information to practitioners, organizations, the Joint Commission, and the public

In the following sections each of these initiatives is discussed, and suggestions for survey preparation are offered. AOTA and occupational therapy practitioners, along with other professions and professionals, have been important participants in the development of the initiatives.

REVISION OF THE JOINT COMMISSION STANDARDS

The first initiative of the Agenda for Change, revision of the standards, is based on the premise that health care organizations exist to maximize the health of the people whom they serve and to use resources efficiently. Therefore, existing standards have been revised and new standards developed to emphasize evaluation of organizational performance aimed at continuously improving the outcomes of care. This emphasis on performance has led to identification of the processes and the functions likely to have the most significant influence on the outcomes of care. Because carrying out these processes and functions often requires interdisciplinary teamwork involving many departments and services, the Joint Commission has reorganized standards in a functional framework that envisions the organization as an integrated system rather than a collection of discrete independent units.

Because the aim of the standards revision has been to improve outcomes, less emphasis has been placed on *how to* and *who should* achieve the objectives of a given standard. Instead, the intention has been to establish a set of consistent performance expectations and to challenge organizations to achieve them creatively. Therefore the standards that appear in the manuals are not meant to be prescriptive; rather, they are designed to encourage innovation and flexibility. Practitioners are free to develop strategies and approaches to performance improvement that best meet their organization's unique needs and the needs of the persons whom their organization serves.

The 1995 and 1996 editions of the various manuals reflect a move toward performance and functions, with standards organized into two main sections:

1. "Patient-Focused Functions," including chapters titled "Patient Rights and Organization Ethics," "Assessment of Patients," "Care of Patients," "Education," and "Continuum of Care"

2. "Organizational Functions," including chapters titled "Improving Organizational Performance," "Leadership," "Management of Information," "Management of Human Resources," "Management of the Environment of Care," and "Surveillance, Prevention and Control of Infections"

The *Accreditation Manual for Hospitals* contains a third section, "Structures with Important Functions," including chapters titled "Governance" and "Medical Staff" and standards related to the role of the chief executive officer and the nurse executive.

The scoring guidelines (volume 2 of each manual) related to the standards include additional explanatory information: preambles, intent statements, examples of implementation, examples of evidence, requirements for 1–5 scoring, suggested readings, and other resources. The Joint Commission holds organizations accountable to the standards, their intent statements, and the requirements for 1–5 scoring. The examples are for information only.

To understand how to comply with the standards, managers and practitioners should review the appropriate standards manual (along with the scoring guidelines) in its entirety, rather than review selected department-specific chapters, as in the past. For example, standards relating to involving patients and families in decisions about care are addressed in "Patient Rights and Organization Ethics"; standards relating to planning care, in "Care"; standards relating to documenting care in the clinical record, in "Management of Information"; and standards relating to defining staff qualifications and competencies, in "Management of Human Resources."

In 1995 there is a version of the *Accreditation Manual for Hospitals* (AMH) called the *Comprehensive Accreditation Manual for Hospitals* (CAMH). In addition to containing information from volumes 1 and 2 of the AMH, the CAMH includes the aggregation and decision rules used to make accreditation decisions. Comprehensive versions of the other manuals will be available in the near future.

Work has begun on collapsing all the manuals into a core set of standards. The core standards will most likely require supplemental standards for additional settings (e.g., ambulatory care), programs (e.g., rehabilitation), and populations (e.g., geriatric).

REDESIGN OF THE JOINT COMMISSION SURVEY PROCESS

The second initiative of the Agenda for Change, redesign of the survey process, was a direct response to a request from accredited organizations for a survey that was more individualized, more consistent, and more helpful than the existing one in improving performance. The transition from standards organized around departments and services, or structures, to standards focused on performance and organized around important functions has called for corresponding changes in the survey process. The revised hospital survey process focuses more on the quality of care and the performance of functions across the organization, and less on structures. The surveyors will survey the performance of important functions across the organization.

One or more surveyors may survey an organization. The number, the discipline, and the background of the surveyors are based on the manual under which an organization is accredited, the population that the organization serves, and the organization's size and complexity.

Several key changes have been made in the survey process:

1. Introduction of new protocols to help standardize the process and make it more consistent than before

2. Tailoring of the process to an organization's specific characteristics

3. Surveyors spending substantial time on care units interviewing staff, patients, and families

4. Surveyors achieving a better understanding of an organization through review of information and on-site documents before the survey

5. Greater emphasis on interactive interviews with an organization's staff and less on document review

6. Greater emphasis on actual performance and less on the structures that support care (e.g., policies and procedures)

7. When there is more than one surveyor, a team-based and interactive approach to conducting the overall survey

8. Establishment of an Organization Liaison Unit at the Joint Commission's central office to provide organizations with a personal contact to assist them through their survey

SURVEY HIGHLIGHTS FOR HOSPITALS

There are differences in the survey process for each field accredited by the Joint Commission. Most occupational therapy managers and practitioners working in JCAHO–accredited organizations work in hospitals, so this chapter describes the hospital survey process. It is similar in many respects to the process in nonhospital settings.

Preparation for a Survey

Occupational therapy managers and practitioners should begin preparing for a survey 16 months before the anticipated survey date in order to be able to demonstrate a 12-month track record of compliance with standards. A 12-month track record is required to receive a score of 1, or *substantial compliance.* It is important that managers and practitioners have access to the standards, the scoring guidelines, and the periodical *Perspectives.* The standards facilitate an interdisciplinary and systems approach to program design, execution, and improvement. To meet them, managers and practitioners must collaborate with patients and families, other consumers, their organization's leaders, and personnel in other departments and disciplines, as well as with their peers.

Survey Planning

To facilitate survey planning, a representative from the Joint Commission, an *organization liaison,* works with each hospital before the survey to develop a detailed survey agenda that tells hospital staff in advance when they will meet with surveyors. Approximately six months before the survey, the Joint Commission sends the Application for Survey/Annual Update Form to the hospital to be completed and returned. This survey/form asks for a general description of what services are provided, in which settings. Approximately four months before the survey, the Joint Commission sends the Survey Planning Package to the organization to be completed and returned. This package includes the Survey Planning Questionnaire, which asks for a detailed description of what services are provided, by whom, in which settings. Using the information provided in the questionnaire, the Joint Commission's organization liaison assists the hospital being surveyed in customizing the survey agenda to the hospital's unique structure and characteristics. The liaison attempts to make the most efficient use of hospital staff's and surveyors' time during the survey.

Surveyor Complement

Each hospital survey team includes, at minimum, a physician, a nurse, and an administrator. In psychiatric hospitals the physician will be a psychiatrist; in rehabilitation hospitals, a rehabilitation specialist. Organizations with comprehensive rehabilitation programs may choose to add a physician who is a rehabilitation specialist to the team (such a choice would result in an additional fee). Other surveyors are added to the team according to the additional services provided by the hospital (e.g., home care, long-term care, chemical dependency, and ambulatory care).

Survey Activities

The activities currently used in on-site hospital surveys are document review, interviews with the organization's leaders, visits to settings for care of patients, function interviews, review of the organization's processes for competence assessment, feedback sessions, and public information interviews. These are described in the following sections.

Document Review

After the opening conference and a performance improvement overview presentation by the organization, the survey team reviews documents that orient it to how the organization addresses the important functions covered by the AMH standards. The documents that are requested generally describe how the organization has planned for these functions and how it has designed processes to support them.[3]

Interviews with the Organization's Leaders

An interview with the organization's leaders addresses the collaboration of senior leaders in planning, designing, implementing, and improving patient care services. It is usually limited to senior staff such as the chief executive officer, the medical director, and the nurse executive. The surveyors interview other leaders (i.e., department and service directors) later in the survey.

Visits to Settings for Care of Patients

Much of the survey consists of visits to inpatient units, to other settings where patients receive rehabilitation (identified as *rehabilitative services*— e.g., an occupational therapy clinic), and to ambulatory care/outpatient sites. These visits address how the organization's important functions come together in the care of patients. Elements of such visits include a discussion with the director, a tour of the setting, a review of open clinical records, and a conversation with and/or observation of patients and their significant others in inpatient units and in other settings. Surveyors may visit only a representative sample of settings for care of patients and therefore not meet with some occupational therapy practitioners.

Function Interviews

For several interviews the surveyors gather an interdisciplinary group of the organization's staff who have important responsibilities relative to a given function or an aspect of it. The interviews follow up on issues identified in the document review and also reflect observations made by surveyors during their visits to various settings for care of patients. Issues addressed during the interviews include how the organization measures and assesses its performance of the functions and, when appropriate, improves its performance. Some function interviews relevant to occupational therapy include the patient and family education interview, the human resources interview, the information management interview, and the performance improvement interview.

---

3. *A complete list of the documents appears in* 1995 Hospital Accreditation Services Guidelines for Survey, *which is sent to each hospital.*

Review of the Organization's Processes for Competence Assessment

In a review of the organization's processes for competence assessment, surveyors assess the organization's efforts to establish qualifications for staff with specific responsibilities, to provide education and training pertinent to those responsibilities (or to see that staff with such responsibilities have all the necessary education and training), and to evaluate staff specific to their responsibilities.

Feedback Sessions

Because of the nature of organization-wide functions, surveyors cannot reach a final score on compliance until they have visited all the scheduled settings for care of patients and conducted all the other survey interviews and activities. However, after the first day of the survey, surveyors communicate their observations in briefings at the beginning of each day.

Public Information Interviews

Anyone who has information about an organization's compliance with the accreditation standards may request a *public information interview.* During a triennial survey, the Joint Commission requires a hospital to provide an opportunity for presentation of information by consumers and the public, as well as by staff of the organization undergoing the survey.

The Accreditation Decision Process and Other Issues

At the end of the on-site survey, the surveyors enter their findings into a laptop computer, print a draft copy of their report, and present it to the organization. They then send their findings electronically to the Joint Commission's central office for analysis and review. Professional staff internally review these results, reach an accreditation decision, and define any necessary follow-up requirements. If the decision falls within established parameters, staff directly notify the organization of the accreditation decision. Accreditation findings that raise specific concerns are reviewed by the Joint Commission's Accreditation Committee, which then reaches a final decision.

Approximately 11 weeks after the survey, the organization is sent the official accreditation decision and a report detailing the surveyors' findings. This report contains any *type I recommendations,* pertaining to unsatisfactory compliance with a standard that requires correction within a specified time period; *supplemental recommendations,* pertaining to unsatisfactory compliance with a standard that must be corrected by the time of the next full survey; the accreditation decision; and the Accreditation Decision Grid, a tabular representation of cumulative functional scores. Type I recommendations generate either a *focused visit,* in which one or more surveyors return to check progress toward compliance, or a request for a *written progress report*, in which the organization sends the Joint Commission written evidence of compliance. Most accredited organizations receive one or more type I recommendations (each of which requires either a visit or a progress report) and supplemental recommendations. For example, if an organization demonstrates good performance in a given area but does not have the essential policies and procedures in place to support this performance over time, it might receive a score of 2 or 3, resulting in a supplemental recommendation indicating the need to address this issue in the future. If the organization has adequate policies and procedures in place in another area but its performance does not measure up, it might receive a score of 4 or 5, resulting in a type I recommendation.

Organizations undergo a full survey every three years. After being surveyed, they receive one of the accreditation decisions described in table 13-3. The only exception is home care agencies seeking *deemed status* (recognition of Joint Commission accreditation for the purpose of Medicare reimbursement). Such agencies receive visits by Joint Commission surveyors annually. Each annual visit addresses Medicare requirements; every third visit also addresses Joint Commission requirements.

Organizations that are denied accreditation have the right to appeal before a final accreditation decision is made. All other organizations may request a revision of specific recommendations and the accreditation decision within 30 days of receiving the survey report (with the accreditation decision).

Unannounced Surveys

In July 1993 the Joint Commission began conducting annual unannounced one-day surveys at a small, randomly selected sample of accredited organizations at the approximate mid-points of their three-year accreditation cycles. Conducted by a single surveyor, the survey is limited to the five performance areas and underlying standards that survey data for the previous year have identified as being most problematic in accredited organizations. The surveyors are not provided with any information concerning the organization's past or current accreditation. Unannounced survey results may lead to new type I recommendations and may even cause a change in the organization's accreditation status. There is no direct charge to organizations selected for random unannounced surveys.

Table 13-3
Accreditation Decisions of the JCAHO

Decision	Basis
Accreditation with commendation	Organization that receives aggregate score of 90 or above on Accreditation Decision Grid and meets other specified criteria, including no type I recommendations.
Accreditation	Organization that receives aggregate score of 90 or above on Accreditation Decision Grid but receives one or more type I recommendations, or type I recommendations and supplemental recommendations. To maintain accreditation, it must achieve resolution of type I recommendations within specified period.
Conditional accreditation	Organization that is not in substantial compliance with Joint Commission standards but files acceptable plan of correction within specified period. Follow-up survey is scheduled within six months of decision, at which time, to become fully accredited, organization must demonstrate that it has achieved major improvements in compliance with standards.
Provisional accreditation	Most commonly, organization that is newly operational and elects to use Early Survey Policy. Under this option, Joint Commission conducts two surveys. First survey assesses organization's basic structural capabilities (e.g., existence of policy manuals). If organization meets initial requirements, it receives provisional accreditation. Second survey, conducted about six months later, is full survey. After it, organization may qualify for any of other accreditation decisions.
	New track creates alternative mechanism for hospitals and home health agencies seeking initial certification under Medicare program. Organization must have been in actual operation for at least one month and be caring for at least 10% of its average anticipated volume of patients. It undergoes two surveys: initial full accreditation survey and follow-up survey six months later to address track record requirements as well as type I recommendations resulting from initial survey.
Not accredited	Organization that fails to meet Joint Commission standards. It may appeal decision.

The rationales for unannounced surveys are as follows:

1. To provide for continuing interaction between the Joint Commission and accredited organizations

2. To tell the public a highly positive story about the willingness and the ability of health care organizations to maintain good performance on their own cognizance

3. To validate the self-sustaining improvement capabilities of continuous quality improvement approaches

Performance Reports

For surveys conducted as of January 1994, the Joint Commission makes Performance Reports, organization-specific accreditation information, available to the public. This access and the information itself have both symbolic and substantive meaning in the new health care environment. Each Performance Report contains an overview of the organization; the accreditation date and the accreditation decision, including areas with recommendations for improvement, if appropriate; the organization's evaluation level in performance areas reviewed during its survey; and a comparison of the organization's evaluation level with that of other organizations. Also included is a two-page commentary from the organization. Each time an organization's Performance Report is requested, the organization is notified of who made the request and when.

USE OF OUTCOMES AND OTHER PERFORMANCE MEASURES BY THE JOINT COMMISSION

The third initiative of the Joint Commission's Agenda for Change focuses on incorporating outcomes and other performance measures into accreditation. This is essential to the credibility of any modern evaluation activity for health care organizations. Outcomes and other performance measures supplement and guide the standards-based survey process by providing a more targeted basis for the regular accreditation survey, a basis for monitoring between surveys, and a basis for guiding and stimulating continuous improvements.

The Joint Commission will satisfy this commitment by accrediting organizations that participate in recognized performance measurement systems around the country. Recognition of measures will be given by an independent blue-ribbon task force established by the Joint Commission. The Joint Commission has requested that leading measurement systems as well as other organizations submit their measures for consideration. The Joint Commission has been developing a national indicator-based performance measurement system of its own called the Indicator Measurement System (IMSystem). Participation in the IMSystem will be sufficient to meet the performance outcomes measurement requirements of accreditation. However, participation in the IMSystem will not be required; participation in another measurement system endorsed by the task force will also be acceptable. The Joint Commission has invited AOTA to submit any performance measures that it may have for consideration.

It will be feasible to incorporate data and information derived from the use of performance measures into Joint Commission Performance Reports. Participants in alternative recognized measurement systems will be compared in Performance Reports as *cohorts;* that is, their performance will be portrayed in relation to that of other participants in the same system. The Joint Commission believes that incorporating this approach to performance measurement into accreditation decisions will be possible as early as 1997.

The Joint Commission is in the initial stages of creating a National Library of Healthcare Indicators (NLHI). NLHI is a comprehensive indicator catalog that includes performance measures judged by content experts to have face validity for application to various types of health care organizations. It recognizes the wide array of.activities to develop measures and represents an effort to organize available and credible measures into a practical framework that purchasers and health care organizations can easily use. The system classifies the performance indicators into three broad categories: (1) priority clinical conditions arrayed against domains of performance, (2) functional health status arrayed against domains of performance, and (3) satisfaction from the perspectives of patients/ enrollees, practitioners, and purchasers.

SUMMARY OF PART 1

The Joint Commission is the largest and oldest private agency involved in voluntary accreditation in health care. Its mission is to improve the quality of health care provided to the public by developing state-of-the-art performance standards, providing accreditation services for the full range of health care organizations, ensuring the availability of educational and consultative support for organizations seeking accreditation, incorporating outcomes and other performance measures into the accreditation process, and publicly disclosing organization-specific performance information to interested parties. Joint Commission accreditation is available for seven fields: (1) hospitals, (2) health care networks, (3) home care agencies and organizations, (4) long-term-care facilities, (5) behavioral health care, including mental health, chemical dependency, and mental retardation/developmental disabilities services, (6) ambulatory health care providers, and (7) clinical and pathology laboratories. For each field there is a manual containing standards (volume 1) and a set of scoring guidelines (volume 2), and for some fields there is a comprehensive manual.

The publication of the 1995 and 1996 versions of the standards manuals as well as changes in the survey process represent the achievement of a significant milestone in the Joint Commission's Agenda for Change. This agenda includes three major initiatives: (1) revision of the standards to focus on the processes and the functions that most significantly influence care, to emphasize doing the right things and doing them well, and to give more attention to what, less to how and who; (2) redesign of the survey process to focus on assessment of actual performance of the processes and the functions that most significantly influence care; and (3) use of outcomes and other performance measures to capture the results of implemented processes and functions in the survey and to provide comparative information.

PART 2

CARF, The Rehabilitation Accreditation Commission

Christine M. MacDonell, BSOT

HISTORY, MISSION, AND DOMAIN

CARF was created in 1966 by the rehabilitation industry. Two national trade associations, the Association of Rehabilitation Centers and the National Association of Sheltered Workshops and Homebound Programs, recognized the need for an organization independent of the providers to become a standard-setting and accrediting body. This body's mission would be to establish and maintain a national set of standards that would ensure quality programming for persons with disabilities.

That mission continues today, expanded to encompass not just persons with disabilities but others in need of rehabilitation. It is reflected in the organization's statements of vision, purposes, and values:

VISION

- We see ourselves in a dynamic environment as a catalyst for improving the quality and cost-efficiency of services provided by rehabilitation organizations.

- We see ourselves as a major source on rehabilitation outcomes measurement and management.

- We see ourselves as an organization respected internationally for accreditation research and information dissemination.

- We see ourselves as having a vital presence in selected international markets.

- We see ourselves as a responsive advocate in the development of public policy that addresses the needs and concerns of people with disabilities and others in need of rehabilitation.

- We see ourselves as an organization recognized for its responsiveness to the needs of diverse rehabilitation organizations.

(CARF, 1995a, p. v; 1995b, p. v; 1995c, p. vii)

PURPOSES

- To improve the quality of services delivered to people with disabilities and others in need of rehabilitation.

- To identify to consumers, providers, purchasers, and the general public those organizations that meet internationally recognized standards for rehabilitation services.

- To develop and maintain current state-of-the-art standards that organizations can use to assess and improve the quality of their programs.

- To provide an independent, impartial, and objective system of total organizational review and assessment using a peer review approach.

- To conduct a program of accreditation research emphasizing outcomes measurement and management and to disseminate information on common program strengths as well as on areas that have been identified as in need of improvement.

- To provide education and training that enhance the performance of our various constituencies.

- To provide an organized forum in which consumers, providers, purchasers, and others in the field can participate in standards setting to improve program quality.

(CARF, 1995a, p. v; 1995b, p. v; 1995c, p. vii)

VALUES

- We believe in the continuous improvement of both organizational management and service delivery.

- We believe in conducting accreditation, research, and education with the utmost integrity.

- We believe people served by rehabilitation organizations should be treated with dignity and respect.

- We believe in the empowerment of people with disabilities and others in need of rehabilitation services.

- We believe that people with disabilities should have access to quality programs and services that achieve optimal outcomes.

- We believe in being cognizant of the needs of all constituents, including consumers, providers, purchasers, and others in the field.

- We believe in the value of diversity and cultural sensitivity to the constituents we serve.

- We believe programs and standards should be cost effective.

- We believe in treating all staff members and surveyors with respect and dignity.

(CARF, 1995a, p. vi; 1995b, p. vi; 1995c, p. viii)

THE STRUCTURE OF CARF

CARF is an international not-for-profit agency financed by fees from accreditation surveys, sales of publications, fees from seminars, grants, and contributions from sponsoring and associate members. Sponsoring and associate members are organizations that support the goals of accreditation and represent a broad range of expertise (see table 13-1).

CARF is governed by a board of trustees composed of one person appointed by each of 23 sponsoring members, and 20 at-large trustees. The sponsoring-member representatives of the board of trustees appoint the at-large trustees from nominations by the field, on the basis of their expertise, experience, and perspective in matters of importance to CARF. The board of trustees has full authority and responsibility for adopting or modifying standards, awarding or withholding accreditation, and approving basic policies and fiscal matters governing the operation of CARF.

THE CARF STANDARDS

DEVELOPMENT

The present standards have evolved over 29 years with the active support and involvement of providers, consumers, and purchasers of services across the United States and Canada. The standards were originally established and have been maintained as *national consensus standards,* as compared with standards derived from a research base. Truly reflecting the national consensus at any given time, they define the expected inputs, processes, and outcomes in services for persons with disabilities.

REVISION

CARF recognizes and accepts its responsibility to assess and review the continuing applicability and relevance of its standards. It convenes national advisory committees each year to review each section of the standards systematically. Composed of persons with acknowledged expertise, these committees make recommendations to CARF and the board of trustees concerning the adequacy and the appropriateness of standards.

The work of the national advisory committees is a starting point rather than an ending point in the development and the revision of standards. Recommendations from a committee are disseminated for a complete field review by accredited organizations, consumers, surveyors, national professional groups, consumer groups, third-party purchasers, users of services, and others. Usually about 10,000 people have the opportunity to read and comment on proposed standards. Input from the field is carefully scrutinized by CARF and the national advisory committees and has always resulted in changes in the standards before their submission to CARF's board of trustees for final review.

— The time frame for the annual revision of standards is as follows:

January–March	Review by national advisory committees
March–May	Field review
June–July	Review by staff and again by national advisory committees
August	Review by board of trustees' Standards Committee and then by full board, with board adoption following

DISSEMINATION

Once new or revised standards are adopted, they are published the following January in the appropriate source: the *Standards Manual and Interpretive Guidelines for Behavioral Health,* the *Standards Manual and Interpretive Guidelines for Employment and Community Support Services,* or the *Standards Manual and Interpretive Guidelines for Medical Rehabilitation.* They become effective on July 1, the six-month interval providing organizations with time to incorporate changes into operations.

The three sets of manuals and interpretive guidelines are published to fulfill a variety of needs and to accomplish several purposes:

- To provide a means for ongoing self-evaluation and improvement of programs.

- To provide an authoritative source of materials for use in a voluntary program of survey and accreditation.

- To establish and give structure to definitions and standards on a level consistent with current knowledge and experience.

- To provide a source of guidelines and interpretations for the planning and organization of new programs and the orientation of personnel and the designated authority(ies).

- To provide an educational resource for the inservice training of administrative and program personnel as well as students enrolled in educational programs.

(CARF, 1995a, p. v; 1995b, p. v; 1995c, p. vii)

CARF ACCREDITATION PRINCIPLES, CRITERIA, AND CONDITIONS

All organizations are required to be in conformance with Accreditation Principles, Criteria, and Conditions to be eligible for, obtain, or retain accreditation by CARF. These are statements and actions that demonstrate an organization's commitments to the persons whom it serves and to the community. The principles address human rights; the involvement of the persons served in their rehabilitation process; the promotion of independence, self-sufficiency, and productivity in the persons served; and coordination, individualization, and goal orientation in all programs. The criteria represent actions and plans in which an organization should have continuing involvement: input from the persons whom it serves; accessibility; safety; outcomes requirements; and financial stability. The conditions state than an organization will have a track record of at least six months in using the standards. They also state that the organization will release information for the surveyors to review and that consumers will be available to interview during the survey.

CONTENT AND FORMAT OF THE CARF STANDARDS

The standards are organized into sections that address the administration and management practices of the organization; the rehabilitation process (e.g., orientation, assessment, and individual program planning); outcome measurement and management; and specific programs or services. Currently CARF promulgates program standards in the areas indicated in table 13-4.

THE SEVEN STEPS IN THE CARF ACCREDITATION PROCESS

The CARF accreditation process involves seven steps, and within these, two major components: a self-study and an on-site survey. The self-study engages an organization's personnel in examining the organization based on objective standards and criteria; the survey entails the organization's being surveyed on site by peer reviewers. The place of these components in the overall process is evident in the following description of the seven steps:

1. The organization conducts its self-study using the appropriate *Standards Manual and Interpretive Guidelines* (CARF, published annually). To assist the organization in this process, a Self-Study Questionnaire and other documents are available from CARF.

2. The organization completes and submits an Application for an Accreditation Survey at least two full months before the dates requested for the survey. An application fee, which is nonrefundable, must accompany the application.

Table 13-4

Areas Encompassed in CARF Program Standards

Behavioral Health	Alcohol and Other Drug Programs
	• Detoxification Services
	• Outpatient Services
	• Residential Treatment Programs
	Mental Health Programs
	• Inpatient Psychiatric Programs
	• Partial Hospitalization Programs
	• Residential Treatment Programs
	• Community Housing Programs
	• Outpatient Therapy Programs
	• Emergency Crisis Intervention Programs
	• Mental Health Case Management Programs
	Psychosocial Rehabilitation Programs
Employment and Community Support Services	Employment Services
	• Community Employment Services
	• Job Placement
	• Occupational Skill Training
	• Vocational Evaluation
	• Work Adjustment and/or Work Services
	Community Support Services
	• Personal, Social, and Community Supports and Services
	• Family Supports and Services
	• Host Family Supports and Services
	• Respite Supports and Services
	• Living Supports and Services
	Early Intervention and Preschool Developmental Programs
Medical Rehabilitation	Comprehensive Inpatient Categories One, Two, and Three (acute and subacute rehabilitation)
	Spinal Cord Rehabilitation System of Care
	Comprehensive Pain Management Programs
	• Acute Pain Management
	• Chronic Pain Management
	• Cancer Related Pain Management
	Brain Injury Programs
	• Medical Inpatient Programs
	• Community Integrated Programs
	Outpatient Medical Rehabilitation Programs
	Home- and Community-Based Programs
	Occupational Rehabilitation Programs
	• Acute Programs
	• Work-Specific Categories One and Two (outcome-oriented interdisciplinary programs that use real or simulated work)

3. CARF identifies an appropriate survey team and notifies the organization of the dates and the names of surveyors at least 30 days before the survey. Surveyors are peers from the field. They work in CARF-accredited organizations and have administrative and clinical backgrounds. Currently over 50 occupational therapists are CARF surveyors.

4. CARF's survey team conducts the survey, then reports its findings to CARF. The typical survey is two days with two surveyors. If an organization has multiple programs seeking accreditation or is very large, CARF may send more than two surveyors, or the surveyors may stay longer than two days.

5. CARF staff and the Accreditation Committee of the board of trustees evaluate the Survey Report and render an accreditation outcome four to eight weeks after the survey.

6. The organization is notified of the accreditation outcome and receives a written report that describes its strengths and makes specific recommendations for improvement.

7. Within 90 days the organization submits to CARF a Quality Improvement Plan outlining the actions that have been or will be taken in response to the recommendations.

CARF ACCREDITATION OUTCOMES

To be accredited by CARF, an organization should meet each of the Accreditation Principles, Criteria, and Conditions and should demonstrate through a site survey that it is in conformance with the standards established by CARF and the field. Although an organization may not be in full conformance with every applicable standard, the accreditation decision is based on the balance of the organization's strengths against the areas in which the organization needs improvement. Four outcomes are possible: three-year accreditation, one-year accreditation, provisional accreditation, and nonaccreditation. CARF's staff members, surveyors, and trustees use the following guidelines in determining the outcome:

THREE-YEAR ACCREDITATION

An organization that receives three-year accreditation meets each of the Accreditation Principles, Criteria, and Conditions and shows substantial fulfillment of the standards. Its programs and practices are designed and implemented to benefit the persons with disabilities whom it serves. Further, its programs, personnel, and documentation clearly indicate that present conditions represent an established pattern of total operation and that these conditions are likely to be maintained or improved in the foreseeable future.

ONE-YEAR ACCREDITATION

An organization that receives one-year accreditation meets each of the Accreditation Principles, Criteria, and Conditions. It has deficiencies in relation to the standards, but there is evidence of its capability of and commitment to correcting the deficiencies, and evidence of progress toward their correction. On balance the program is benefiting the persons whom it serves, and there is apparent protection of their health, welfare, and safety.

An organization may be considered to be functioning between the three- and one-year levels because of certain conditions. In this instance, accreditation for one year is awarded.

PROVISIONAL ACCREDITATION

An organization that receives provisional accreditation meets each of the Accreditation Principles, Criteria, and Conditions. It has deficiencies in relation to the standards, but there is evidence of its capability of and commitment to correcting the deficiencies, and evidence of progress toward their correction. On balance the program is benefiting the persons whom it serves, and there is apparent protection of their health, welfare, and safety.

Provisional accreditation may be awarded only once, for one year, after an organization has received one-year accreditation during the previous site survey. Provisional status requires that the organization be functioning at a three-year accreditation level at the end of the tenure of provisional accreditation or be nonaccredited.

NONACCREDITATION

An organization that is denied accreditation has major deficiencies in several areas of the standards, and there are serious questions regarding the rehabilitation benefits, health, welfare, or safety of its clientele; or the organization has failed over time to bring itself into substantial conformance with the standards; or the organization has failed to meet the Accreditation Principles, Criteria, and Conditions.

SUMMARY OF PART 2

CARF, The Rehabilitation Accreditation Commission, is an international not-for-profit agency created in 1966 by the rehabilitation industry. Its mission is to establish and maintain a national set of standards that will ensure quality programming for persons with disabilities and others in need of rehabilitation.

CARF's standards have evolved over 29 years with the active support and involvement of providers, consumers, and purchasers. Truly reflecting the national consensus at any given time, they define the expected inputs, processes, and outcomes in services for persons with disabilities. CARF convenes national advisory committees each year to review each section of the standards systematically. Recommendations from a committee are disseminated for a complete field review. Input from the field is carefully scrutinized by CARF and the national advisory committees.

Once new or revised standards are adopted, they are published the following January in the appropriate standards manual: one for behavioral health, one for employment and community support services, and one for medical rehabilitation.

The CARF accreditation process involves seven steps, and within these, two major components: a self-study and an on-site survey. To be accredited by CARF, an organization should meet each of the Accreditation Principles, Criteria, and Conditions and should demonstrate through a site survey that it is in conformance with the standards established by CARF and the field.

PART 3

Accreditation Council on Services for People with Disabilities

Nancy MacRae, MS, OTR/L, FAOTA

HISTORY, MISSION, AND DOMAIN

In the mid-1960s, after its completion of the *Standards for Facilities Serving Individuals with Mental Retardation,* the American Association on Mental Deficiency (now the American Association on Mental Retardation) recognized the need for a national accrediting body (Helsel, 1994). At that time, only 27 percent of the agencies that were studied met the criteria for accreditation (Accreditation Council, 1988). With the help of the National Association for Retarded Children (now the Association for Retarded Children), the United Cerebral Palsy Association, and the Council for Exceptional Children, the American Association on Mental Deficiency realized its objective in 1969 when the Joint Commission on Accreditation of Hospitals (now the Joint Commission on Accreditation of Healthcare Organizations) agreed to provide the aegis for a national accrediting body. The Joint Commission (1969) hoped "to broaden the base and concept of voluntary accreditation in the belief that this cooperative approach [would offer] greater stability while being a stimulant for better realization of the stated purpose of health-related service programs." The Accreditation Council for Facilities for the Mentally Retarded (ACFMR), as it was then known, became the first of several accrediting councils within the Joint Commission.

Grant funding from the Rehabilitation Services Administration of the United States Department of Health, Education, and Welfare helped complete the process. ACFMR held its first meeting in July 1969 and published new standards in 1971. The 1972 federal court decision in *Wyatt v. Stickney* required the defendants to comply with these newly developed standards. That requirement signaled the beginning of the improvement and the depopulation of large residential facilities.

In 1979, ACFMR reestablished itself as the Accreditation Council on Services for Mentally Retarded and other Developmentally Disabled Persons (ACMRDD). It became a not-for-profit organization independent of the Joint Commission, continuing its mission of promoting voluntary accreditation. It published standards again in 1984 and 1987. The standards emphasized an interdisciplinary process, individualized program planning, behavior intervention, and promotion of legal rights. Their publication placed the Accreditation Council in a national leadership role of helping to define contemporary practice in design and dissemination of habilitation standards. In fact, the 1973 certification requirements and standards for intermediate care facilities for the mentally retarded were based on the Accreditation Council's 1971 standards, and the 1988 regulations on the Accreditation Council's 1984 standards (Gardner & Campanella, 1995).

In the early 1990s the Accreditation Council expanded its mission to include persons with any disabilities. Thus 25 years after its beginning, the Accreditation Council remains committed to improving the quality of lives for persons with disabilities.

THE STRUCTURE OF THE ACCREDITATION COUNCIL

Today the Accreditation Council is sponsored by nine organizations (see table 13-1). Each organization sends two representatives to serve on the board of directors for staggered three-year terms. The board of directors has ultimate responsibility for the development and approval of outcome measures, policies and procedures, and accreditation decisions. Currently the board is organized into three committees: the Committee on Organization Services, the Committee on Organization Development, and the Committee on Organization Operations. The Accreditation Subcommittee is a subcommittee of the Committee on Organization Development. The board appoints task forces as necessary. Two current ones are dealing with the issues of accreditation alternatives and synthesis of outcomes, both ultimately to contribute to the next generation of outcomes.

AOTA became a sponsoring organization in 1981. Through its representatives it has influenced not only the development of standards but also their ultimate implementation and the refinement processes necessary for implementation to occur successfully.

THE ROLE AND THE FUNCTIONS OF THE ACCREDITATION COUNCIL

The Accreditation Council pursues its goal of improving the quality of services for persons with disabilities through the following activities (Accreditation Council, 1990):

1. Developing and publishing standards, and now outcome measures, as a benchmark for both quality of services and responsiveness to the persons who are served

2. Revising the standards and the outcome measures to incorporate new knowledge, technology, experience, and concepts

3. Encouraging agencies to use Accreditation Council standards and outcomes for self-evaluation and quality enhancement of services

4. Offering training, consultation, and technical assistance

5. Conducting surveys or reviews to assess compliance with standards or responsiveness to outcomes

6. Awarding accreditation to agencies that meet or exceed criteria established by the Accreditation Council

Additionally the Accreditation Council continues to learn about enhancing quality by securing grants to study such issues as developing outcome measures for early intervention services; creating an outcomes database and analyzing the relationship between outcomes and organizational measures of health, safety, and welfare; developing supported employment outcomes; and determining and trying out alternative methods for conducting quality reviews.

THE OUTCOMES APPROACH OF THE ACCREDITATION COUNCIL

As the mission of the Accreditation Council has become more inclusive, its method of achieving its mission has changed. The change is consistent with a service-driven economy and culture in which the definition of quality rests with the consumer of services. Themes of civil rights, empowerment, and self-determination have underscored this trend. Moving from a product to a market focus has led to specific questions about what the client wants. The Accreditation Council broached such questions with persons with disabilities, inquiring about the outcomes that they desired in their lives. This led to the development in 1993 of an outcomes approach to the improvement of quality.

Thus, whereas the Accreditation Council once directed its attention to a program's compliance with standards and the processes involved in achieving them, it now focuses on the individual's determination to accomplish what he or she desires and needs. The transition to an emphasis on outcomes has required an apparently simple but actually complex paradigm shift. Outcomes are not prescriptive, but determined by individuals, with the ultimate challenge being for service and support agencies to figure out ways to help individuals both determine and meet these outcomes. Professionals have the expertise through methodologies and techniques collaboratively to help persons with disabilities meet their desired outcomes.

Individual decision making and choice are fundamental for outcomes to be achieved. For informed choices to be made, three dimensions are necessary: (1) experience with possible options, which provides a basis from which a person can choose; (2) social support throughout the choice process, which helps with the decision making; and (3) creativity in devising contextual alternatives, which aids in the realization of outcomes (Accreditation Council, 1993). To promote informed choices, practitioners must view a person holistically and make an effort to understand his or her motivations. If a person is unable to participate actively in the choice and decision-making processes, there must be attempts to understand his or her preferences. Seeking the help of those who know the person best (i.e., family members and caregivers) allows this determination to be made.

The use of outcomes as standards requires professionals and other agency personnel to get to know the whole person. Behavioral measures may help determine whether an individual's desired outcomes are met, yet behavior must be connected to performance; that is, it must occur in a socially valued context. For example, increasing eye-hand coordination or improving performance of activities of daily living must be directed at the socially valued outcomes of living and working more independently.

Dealing with outcomes also requires scrutiny of the dynamic interrelationships among individual outcomes, and between individual outcomes and organizational processes. Outcomes cannot be realized unless the basic health, safety, and welfare components are addressed. On this solid foundation, work on outcomes can go forward.

Accreditation is no longer the primary focus of the Accreditation Council. It is only one of the ways in which the council enables organizations to improve the quality of their services. *Quality* in this context is defined as an organization's responsiveness to individuals' expectations for outcomes rather than its compliance with organizational processes. When accreditation is used as a procedure for enhancing quality, it is *formative evaluation,* that is, continuous assessment of the ability to strive for and achieve improvement in quality.

THE ACCREDITATION COUNCIL'S OUTCOME-BASED PERFORMANCE MEASURES

The Accreditation Council's current edition of standards (1993) is therefore concerned not with standards per se, but with outcomes for people and with related *outcome-based performance measures,* or outcome measures. The outcome measures assess the presence of "outcomes that people with disabilities want from their support or service programs" (p. v). Some examples of outcome measures are "People choose their daily routine,"

"People choose to participate in the life of the community," and "People are safe." They "can be used with all services and programs—residential, vocational, social or educational—and for people with different disabilities" (p. v).

The outcome measures emphasize that policies, procedures, and organizational processes targeting health, safety, and welfare are a necessary framework for providing services. The measures enable agencies to conduct a self-assessment, that is, to determine the extent to which they are helping people achieve outcomes. Finally, the measures serve as a basis for an on-site review.

DEVELOPMENT

Initial development of the outcome measures occurred with the help of a grant from Illinois's Community Integrated Living Arrangements (CILA) program and with input from people participating in the CILA program. In 1992–93 the Accreditation Council conducted 10 field tests of the measures in the United States and Canada. It used a variety of sites providing a wide range of services and supports to persons of differing disabilities. The field tests demonstrated content validity and interrater reliability. The council continues to collect data on the measures. It will assess construct validity once it has completed an adequate number of surveys for factor analysis (Accreditation Council, 1993).

FORMAT AND CONTENT

There are 30 outcome measures, formulated around a core of 10 outcomes (see table 13-5). Although the outcome measures apply to each person, they do not prescribe a specific result. They "begin with the identification of goals, preferences, experiences, and a range of choices ('People choose personal goals') and conclude with questions concerning satisfaction with services and supports and general state-of-life satisfaction ('People are satisfied with services' and 'People are satisfied with their personal life situations')" (Accreditation Council, 1993, p. 6).

The outcome measures rest on six principles (Accreditation Council, 1993):

1. Individual choice and decision making
2. Rights balanced by responsibility
3. Comprehensive planning—the belief that "a well designed and well managed service process will lead to outcomes for people" (p. 7)
4. Individualization
5. Organizational process and personal outcomes—identification of specific organizational processes that help people realize outcomes

Table 13-5

Outcomes for People and Related Performance Measures

Outcome	Outcome-Based Performance Measure
Personal goals	1. People choose personal goals.
	2. People realize personal goals.
Choice	3. People choose where and with whom they live.
	4. People choose where they work.
	5. People decide how to use their free time.
	6. People choose services.
	7. People choose their daily routine.
Social inclusion	8. People participate in the life of the community.
	9. People interact with other members of the community.
	10. People perform different social roles.
Relationships	11. People have friends.
	12. People remain connected to natural support networks.
	13. People have intimate relationships.
Rights	14. People exercise rights.
	15. People are afforded due process if rights are limited.
	16. People are free from abuse and neglect.
Dignity and respect	17. People are respected.
	18. People have time, space and opportunity for privacy.
	19. People have and keep personal possessions.
	20. People decide when to share personal information.
Health	21. People have health care services.
	22. People have the best possible health.
Environment	23. People are safe.
	24. People use their environments.
	25. People live in integrated environments.
Security	26. People have economic resources.
	27. People have insurance to protect their resources.
	28. People experience continuity and security.
Satisfaction	29. People are satisfied with services.
	30. People are satisfied with their personal life situations.

Note. *From* Outcome-Based Performance Measures *(p. 11), by the Accreditation Council on Services for People with Disabilities, 1993, Landover, MD: Author. Copyright ©1993 by the Accreditation Council on Services for People with Disabilities. Reprinted with permission.*

6. Quality by design—design of services and supports to achieve outcomes

Each outcome measure is based on underlying values. Examples of underlying values are those that support work (see table 13-6). These values should be used to guide meeting the individual's choices about whether or not to work, and where to work. Options may be limited, or be beyond the control of either the individual or the organization. Organization personnel must then take steps to develop the next-best alternative for the individual while they plan ways to address changing the existing circumstances, perhaps through advocating state or community action.

Because outcomes have a different level of importance for each person, the outcome measures are not ranked or weighted. A dynamic relationship exists between each person and the outcomes. Individual differences, preferences, and life stages or circumstances change the importance of each outcome at varying times and reflect the constancy of change in people's lives.

APPLICATION OF THE MEASURES

Before the Accreditation Council reviews an agency, the agency completes an application form providing information about the persons whom it serves and supports, the services that it provides, and the procedures by which it addresses issues concerning health, safety, and welfare. The

---

Table 13-6
Underlying Values Supporting the Outcome Measure,
"People Choose Where They Work"

- For the majority of adults in our society, work provides a significant amount of economic support and self esteem.

- If people have alternative means of support and do not wish to work, it is quite acceptable not to work.

- The same range of options for work that are available to all people should be available to people with disabilities.

- When people are unable to make explicit choices, the organization provides opportunities for different experiences and explores and respects individual preferences.

- People who are of retirement age need access to a variety of post employment options.

Note. *From* Outcome-Based Performance Measures *(p. 25), by the Accreditation Council on Services for People with Disabilities, 1993, Landover, MD: Author. Copyright ©1993 by the Accreditation Council on Services for People with Disabilities. Reprinted with permission.*

length of the review is determined by the number of persons served, the scope of services, and the geographic area covered. To prepare for the review, the agency then conducts a *self-assessment*. That is, it identifies the full scope of individual options and opportunities available to assist in the achievement of desired outcomes. It then makes a determination about the presence or the absence of outcomes. It also assesses its procedures, including specific steps that staff members use to support or maintain outcomes. The agency gathers this information by interviewing three of the persons whom it is serving or persons who know them well. It summarizes the data in a narrative report that indicates whether outcomes are met or present for each person interviewed, provides a brief description of how outcomes are not being met, and identifies both the barriers to their being met and efforts of the organization to diminish or eliminate the barriers. The agency submits this report to the Accreditation Council six to eight weeks before the review.

An *independent quality review* of the agency then occurs. It consists of a site visit during which the review team applies the 30 outcome measures to a representative sample of persons with disabilities whom it has chosen, through observations and interviews. The team also conducts interviews with staff members, family members, and other persons receiving services and supports, in order to gather all the information necessary to determine if outcomes are present.

For each of the outcome measures, the team must obtain answers to two questions:

1. Is the outcome present [for the individual]?

2. Has the organization designed and initiated a process that enables (or will enable) the person to overcome barriers and achieve the outcome? If the answer is yes, what is the organizational process?

(Accreditation Council, 1993, p. 5)

Thus for each outcome measure there is an individual-outcome answer and an organizational-process answer. Both are desired because they demonstrate whether the organization has been deliberately responsive to the individual's preferred outcomes.

Once the review is completed, the reviewers send their draft report to the Accreditation Subcommittee, which the board of directors has empowered to act on its behalf in making decisions on the accreditation status of any given organization. The report describes the sample and summarizes the reviewers' findings for each of the 10 categories of outcomes, grouping comments under commendations or recommendations. The report also recommends a decision.

ACCREDITATION DECISIONS OF THE ACCREDITATION COUNCIL

The Accreditation Subcommittee carefully reviews the draft report and renders a decision based on (1) the number of outcomes present, (2) the number of individual processes present, and (3) the number of overall performance measures present for two-thirds of the sample. Decisions range from accreditation for three years to no accreditation.

The self-assessment and the independent quality review both provide valuable information to an agency. Feedback indicates the extent to which outcomes are present, the persons who are achieving relatively few outcomes, and the outcomes that persons most and least often achieve. Such information allows organizations to identify the organizational processes that contribute to realization of outcomes. This emphasis on outcomes can add energy and resolve to follow-up, and help the organization design a more focused and increasingly responsive agency. Thus the organization can initiate and continue a cycle of formative evaluation that progressively affects quality.

RELEVANCE OF THE ACCREDITATION COUNCIL'S WORK TO OCCUPATIONAL THERAPY

Through its participation in the Accreditation Council, AOTA has helped define and operationalize the quality-enhancement movement that the Accreditation Council has spearheaded. The particular significance of occupational therapy's long involvement with the Accreditation Council is its expertise on such matters as activities of daily living (especially feeding), the use of activities in meaningful programming, and the need for adaptive equipment and environmental adaptations; also its abiding belief that each individual must be viewed as a whole person with unique capabilities and challenges. The Accreditation Council both sought and accepted advice in these areas in development and refinement of the standards and then the outcome measures. Occupational therapy's active role in Accreditation Council meetings and governance and its frequent participation in reviews have made its input and feedback more credible, especially given the depth of occupational therapy's experience with the populations at which the Accreditation Council directs its work.

AOTA's experience with standards showed what institution- and community-based facilities could do to improve both the living and the working/programming conditions that they offered to persons with disabilities. The emphasis on process proved to be crucial in laying the groundwork for responding to what people desired. The new focus assumes a solid process that allows flexibility in helping meet the outcomes desired by each individual.

Experience to date with the outcome measures has found an extremely receptive field. The challenges inherent in meeting individual outcome measures feed the enthusiasm of those who are in the vanguard of facilitating independence, choice, and autonomy for persons with disabilities. Valuing what the individual wants and attempting to meet corresponding outcome measures gives new meaning to understanding the individual and the organizational processes necessary to accomplish the task. Collaboration with the individual, other team members, and community agencies fosters the unique creativity that is key to meeting the outcomes that the individual wants.

For the occupational therapy manager, once the organization for which he or she works has decided to seek accreditation, involvement in the self-assessment is crucial. Ensuring that organizational components such as safety, protection of rights, opportunities for staff training, and continuing evaluation of success in achieving desired outcomes are in place, and that the credentials of occupational therapy personnel are appropriate and up-to-date, are important basic tasks. More pivotal is implementation of the philosophy of helping clients express and meet their desired outcomes—that is, devotion of energy specifically to meeting clients' needs for occupational therapy services and documenting clients' satisfaction with them. This core value is consistent with occupational therapy's philosophy and may simply require reconceptualizing how to identify desired outcomes and how to measure progress toward them. Working toward efficaciously delivering occupational therapy services to meet clients' desired outcomes ultimately requires clarification of both methods and measurement, and reinforces the importance of learning about and communicating with clients. Collaboration with clients adds immeasurably to the final results of what can be achieved.

As more is learned, more can be expected, both of persons with disabilities and of the habilitation and rehabilitation fields' ability to help such persons express and meet their needs. Collaborating in meeting the ever-changing and -intensifying demands for quality can only advance what professionals and the Accreditation Council do for persons with disabilities. Extending the Accreditation Council's work internationally (to Canada and soon to Taiwan) will add to the continually expanding knowledge and practice base that the council is committed to strengthening in order to be responsive to the needs of persons with disabilities.

SUMMARY OF PART 3

Created in 1969 as the first of several accrediting councils within the Joint Commission on Accreditation of Hospitals, today the Accreditation Council is an independent not-for-profit agency sponsored by nine organizations. It pursues its goal of improving the quality of services for persons with disabilities by (1) developing and publishing outcome measures as a benchmark for both quality of services and responsiveness to the persons who are served; (2) revising the outcome measures to incorporate new knowledge, technology, experience, and concepts; (3) encouraging agencies to use outcome measures for self-evaluation and quality enhancement of services; (4) offering training, consultation, and technical assistance; (5) conducting reviews to assess responsiveness to outcomes; and (6) awarding accreditation to agencies that meet or exceed criteria established by the Accreditation Council.

The Accreditation Council's current edition of standards (1993) is concerned with 10 outcomes for people and with 30 related *outcome-based performance measures,* or outcome measures. The outcome measures assess the presence of "outcomes that people with disabilities want from their support or service programs" (p. v).

To prepare for a review by the Accreditation Council, an agency conducts a self-assessment. An *independent quality review* of the agency then occurs. It consists of a site visit during which the review team applies the 30 outcome measures to a representative sample of persons with disabilities whom it has chosen, through observations and interviews. The site visit also includes interviews with staff members, family members, and other persons receiving services and supports.

PART 4

Other Accrediting Agencies of Interest to Occupational Therapy

COMMUNITY HEALTH ACCREDITATION PROGRAM

CHAP, established in 1965 and now a fully independent subsidiary of the National League for Nursing, accredits home- and community-based health care organizations of all kinds—voluntary, not-for-profit, proprietary, and publicly financed. Its purpose is to use accreditation to elevate the quality of home care in the United States and to offer the public a sound basis for selection of home care providers and services.

CHAP's standards are based on national consensus. Revised as needed but at least every two years, they address quality of services and products, availability of resources, financial viability, and attention to consumers (CHAP, n.d.). Core standards apply to all organizations seeking accreditation. Specialty standards focus on specific clinical areas: professional services, paraprofessional services, infusion therapy, public health, hospice, pharmacy, and so forth. In recent years, with a grant from a private foundation to conduct the necessary research and development, CHAP has developed outcome measures.

The CHAP board of review, consisting of executives from CHAP–accredited agencies, consumers, and purchasers, makes the final decision about accreditation on the basis of an organization's self-study and the site visit report. With agencies seeking accreditation for the first time, the possible outcomes are full accreditation with or without required actions or recommendations; deferral of initial accreditation for a specified time pending additional information or a focused site visit; or denial of accreditation. With agencies seeking continued accreditation, the options are renewal of full accreditation; formal warning of deficiencies, to be corrected within a specified time; or withdrawal of accreditation.

ACCREDITATION COUNCIL FOR OCCUPATIONAL THERAPY EDUCATION

ACOTE is the nationally recognized accrediting body for all education programs for the occupational therapist and the occupational therapy assistant in the United States, its territories, and commonwealths. ACOTE accredits occupational therapy education programs at two levels using sep-arate sets of standards: *Essentials and Guidelines for an Accredited Educational Program for the Occupational Therapist* (AOTA, 1991a) and *Essentials and Guidelines for an Accredited Educational Program for the Occupational Therapy Assistant* (AOTA, 1991b). The standards address both academic and field-work education. The ACOTE Essentials Review Committee is responsible for periodic revision of both sets of standards.

Approximately every seven years, on a staggered basis, all occupation-al therapy programs in United States colleges and universities are visited to determine whether they continue to meet the education standards. ACOTE manages this process.

Education programs in occupational therapy are the profession's source of supply of prepared practitioners. The two *Essentials* documents provide a mechanism for the profession indirectly to ensure that new prac-titioners have the necessary knowledge and skills to begin practice. Only graduates of accredited programs may take the national certification examination of the National Board for Certification in Occupational Therapy (NBCOT).

REFERENCES

Accreditation Council on Services for People with Developmental Disabilities. (1988). *1990 standards for services for people with developmental disabili-ties, field review edition.* Boston: Author.

Accreditation Council on Services for People with Developmental Disabilities. (1990). *Standards and interpretation guidelines for services for people with developmental disabilities.* Landover, MD: Author.

Accreditation Council on Services for People with Disabilities. (1993). *Outcome based performance measures.* Landover, MD: Author.

American Occupational Therapy Association. (1991a). *Essentials and guidelines for an accredited educational program for the occupational therapist.* Rockville, MD: Author.

American Occupational Therapy Association. (1991b). *Essentials and guidelines for an accredited educational program for the occupational therapy assis-tant.* Rockville, MD: Author.

CARF, The Rehabilitation Accreditation Commission. (1995a; published annually). *1995 standards manual and interpretive guidelines for behavioral health.* Tucson, AZ: Author.

CARF, The Rehabilitation Accreditation Commission. (1995b; published annually). *1995 standards manual and interpretive guidelines for employ-ment and community support services.* Tucson, AZ: Author.

CARF, The Rehabilitation Accreditation Commission. (1995c; published annually). *1995 standards manual and interpretive guidelines for medical rehabilitation.* Tucson, AZ: Author.

Community Health Accreditation Program. (1993a). *Standards of excellence for community/public organizations.* New York: Author.

Community Health Accreditation Program. (1993b). *Standards of excellence for home care.* New York: Author.

Community Health Accreditation Program. (1993c). *Standards of excellence for hospice.* New York: Author.

Community Health Accreditation Program. (n.d.). *CHAP: Here to stay* [Brochure]. New York: Author.

Gardner, J., & Campanella, T. (1995). Beyond compliance to responsiveness: New measures of quality for accreditation. In *WORK: A Journal of Prevention, Assessment and Rehabilitation* (Woburn, MA: Butterworth-Heinemann), *15*(2), 107–14.

Helsel, E. (1994). *Early history of the Accreditation Council and involvement of Professor Herschel Nisonger.* Unpublished synopsis prepared for the Board of Directors of the Accreditation Council.

Joint Commission on Accreditation of Hospitals. (1969). *Bulletin of the Joint Commission on Accreditation of Hospitals,* no. 53. Chicago: Author.

Wilson, F. A., & Neuhauser, D. (1985). *Health services in the United States* (2nd rev. ed.). Cambridge, MA: Ballinger.

Wyatt v. Stickney, 344 F. Supp. 373 (M.D. Ala. 1972).

ADDITIONAL RESOURCES

ORGANIZATIONS

Accreditation Council for Occupational Therapy Education, 4720 Montgomery Lane, P.O. Box 31220, Bethesda, MD 20824-1220, telephone (301) 652-2682

Accreditation Council on Services for Persons with Disabilities, 100 West Road, Suite 406, Towson, MD 21204, telephone (410) 583-0060

CARF, The Rehabilitation Accreditation Commission, 101 North Wilmot Road, Suite 500, Tucson, AZ 85711, telephone (520) 325-1044

Community Health Accreditation Program, 350 Hudson Street, New York, NY 10014, telephone (800) 669-1656, ext. 242

Joint Commission on Accreditation of Healthcare Organizations, One Renaissance Boulevard, Oakbrook Terrace, IL 60181, telephone (630) 792-5000

SECTION 7

Communicating

Chapter 14, the first of two chapters on the manager's role of communicating, addresses basic concepts and principles of effective two-way communication. It interprets communication as a repetitive process, involving verbal and nonverbal exchange, interpretation, feedback, clarification, and verification. The chapter describes factors that facilitate communication and factors that raise barriers to it.

Chapter 15 expands the concept of communication to encompass collaboration, represented in a particular model of practice, consultation. The model is particularly attractive in today's dynamic health care environment, as new and different opportunities open up for occupational therapy personnel. The chapter presents theoretical models of consultation and relates them to various levels of consultation. It describes consultation as occurring in four stages: initiation and clarification, assessment and communication, interactive problem resolution, and evaluation and termination.

CHAPTER 14

Principles of Communication

Catherine Nielson, MPH, OTR/L, FAOTA

Catherine Nielson, MPH, OTR/L, FAOTA, is an associate clinical professor in the Occupational Therapy Division of the University of North Carolina at Chapel Hill. Experienced as both a clinical and an academic administrator, she has been teaching administration, including communication, to graduate students for 11 years. Also, she has conducted numerous workshops for practicing therapists on communication and related topics. She holds an MPH in health policy and administration from the university.

C ommunication is an iterative process. It involves the exchange of words, nonverbal information, and cues; the interpretation of meaning; and a cycle of feedback, clarification, and verification of the intent of the interchange. Clear and accurate communication can be blocked at any point in the process, resulting in a range of problems from simple misperception to complete breakdown in the interaction and the relationship.

It has been estimated that 80 percent of the people who experience problems at work do so because they do not communicate well (Bolton, 1986). Skill in communication, like any learned response, can be improved. Learning to communicate effectively in the workplace requires a valuing of good communication, self-awareness of skills and deficits, and a lifelong commitment to develop and practice good habits and skills.

Communication underlies most management functions. Effective communication skills are the foundation of effective management. For example, successful management of human resources, from interviewing to supervision through disciplinary action, requires careful listening, accurate interpretation and responses, and a clear articulation of meaning and content in all exchanges. Even management activities that are not directly related to people and relationships, such as budget negotiations, marketing presentations, and program planning, depend on good communication skills.

Ultimately the manager's success in many areas of administration depends on an ability to communicate clearly with subordinates, peers, and superiors and, in turn, to interpret messages accurately. Katz (1974) identifies human skill as one of three basic skills of management. Human skill, including both "the understanding [of] what others really mean by their words and behaviors" and equal skill in communicating with others, is essential to effective management at all levels of responsibility (p. 91).

A DEFINITION OF EFFECTIVE COMMUNICATION

Devereaux (1992) defines true communication as comprehension and understanding that has been achieved by both the sender and the receiver through an interactive process. Rakich, Longest, and Darr (1992) describe effective communication as including all verbal and nonverbal methods, including the use of silence, which conveys meaning. In both of these definitions, understanding—conveying accurate meaning—is the critical outcome. Communication depends on a successful blend of the content, or what is said, and the process, or how it is sent, interpreted, refined, and ultimately understood. Effective communication is not simply provision of information, but a dialogue in which parties exchange and process information until they reach a shared meaning.

THE STRUCTURE OF MEANING

Meaning is derived through an interaction of content and context. Although content is the words that the sender actually uses, all communication occurs within layers of context that provide the background for interpretation by the receiver. To understand how meaning evolves, both content and context must be examined.

CONTENT AS A CONTRIBUTOR TO MEANING

Language is inherently ambiguous. Although the sender attempts to select words with specific meanings, words often have several definitions. Haney (as cited in Clampitt, 1991) says that the 500 most commonly used words in the English language have over 14,000 definitions! The use of a given word can result, then, in several outcomes. The recipient may have the same definition as the sender, may have a totally different definition, or may be unable to determine a definition. It is the responsibility of the sender to determine if the words that he or she has chosen for a message are similarly defined by the recipient.

Not only can words have multiple dictionary definitions, but people often form their own unique meanings for words. Clampitt (1991) describes words as containers or stimulators of meaning rather than as consistent and accurate indicators of meaning. Understanding this phenomenon is important for managers in order to avoid the "twisted message" (Walton, 1989, p. 80). According to Walton, a two-way conversation actually contains four messages: (1) what the sender intended to say and thinks that he or she communicated; (2) what the recipient heard; (3) what the recipient then intended to say as a response and thinks that he or she communicated; and (4) what the original sender heard. The twisted message can occur at any of these four points if the two persons define words differently, fill in conversational blanks, or simply "hear what they want to hear." The number of possible messages and the potential for twisting them grow as more people join a conversation.

CONTEXT AS A CONTRIBUTOR TO MEANING

Interpreting meaning solely from content is impossible. The context of each participant in the communication as well as the context of the communication itself must be understood in order for an accurate interpretation of meaning to occur.

Context may be defined as a person's "self-constructed image of the world" (Clampitt, 1991, p. 34). People create context through their life experiences. Family of origin, culture, schooling, social spheres, business experiences, and myriad other factors intertwine to create an internal mechanism for assigning meaning to a given interaction or behavior. Each person carries around a unique view of the world that influences the way in which he or she interprets messages. A common context increases the possibility of understanding. The more alike their background or experience, the more likely two persons are to attribute the same meaning to a message.

A common context can develop through familiarity and repeated contacts. Multiple exposures to and discussions of people's roles, circumstances, and settings allow people to see and talk about similarities and differences in life experiences and understand how they lead to varying interpretations of meaning. The informal or social aspect of the workplace is an important vehicle for developing a shared context within a work group. As co-workers share stories, they more clearly understand individual contexts, they create a common context, and they enhance communication among themselves. It is important that the manager participate in this process. The shared context should incorporate management's values and perspectives. The manager must understand staff members' individual contexts in order to anticipate and avoid possible misinterpretations.

EFFECTS OF EMOTION, STRESS, AND THREAT

Although content and context are primary contributors to meaning in communication, other factors can influence meaning. Emotion, stress, and threat are among the barriers that may also complicate or obscure accurate interpretation of meaning. Still other barriers or roadblocks to effective communication are discussed later in the chapter.

Clinically, occupational therapy practitioners well understand the importance of work; managers of occupational therapy services should also understand it. Positive work experiences contribute to self-esteem and self-identity. Pragmatically, work is a source of financial security. Work satisfies both basic and high-level needs for people. It should not be surprising, then, that communication in the workplace is susceptible to emotional influences. A manager and a staff member are engaged in a hierarchical relationship in which the manager has control over the continuation of a vital source of security and self-worth for the staff member. Any communication from the manager is at risk of being interpreted through the emotional screen caused by inherent differences in power and authority.

Stress is another intrinsic aspect of the workplace that can influence a person's sending and interpretation of a message. Staff members and managers bring personal stress into the work setting. The workplace contributes additional stressors such as daily requirements for productivity and accountability, regular fluctuations in volume and intensity of caseloads, and annual performance appraisals. Stress can affect both the manager and the staff member, creating a high-risk communication environment in which both content and context can be misunderstood and the message miscommunicated. During periods of stress a person simply cannot process as much information as accurately or as easily as he or she can in times of low demand.

The highly emotional and potentially stressful nature of workplace communications can result in real or perceived threats to a staff member. A staff member who feels threatened increases his or her self-protection and raises barriers. Rather than prompting a search for common meaning and understanding, stress and emotion often result in negative behaviors that break communication down. Resistance, rebellion, arguments, noncompliance, and submissive behavior may all indicate that a staff member did not receive the intended meaning of a communication but did perceive a threat (Bolton, 1986). At such times it is imperative that the manager look at the communication from the perspective of the staff member to identify possible explanations for the reaction. The manager then has a basis for further exploration of the intended message with the person.

TWO-WAY COMMUNICATION

One of the most effective means of avoiding misinterpretation is to embrace the attitudes, practice the skills, and develop the habits of two-way communication. Effective communication is based on holding attitudes of respect for others, demonstrating empathy, being honest about one's feelings and ideas, and listening as well as speaking for clarity (Bolton, 1986).

Communication is a cycle of reciprocal speaking, listening, responding, clarifying, and verifying. Effective communication between a manager and a staff member should be considered a give-and-take conversation in which both parties strive for clarity and use listening and feedback as insurance for an accurate exchange. The manager ultimately cannot force understanding on a staff member. However, the manager can take steps in communicating to convey the value and the importance of effective communication, to model good skills, and to reinforce the skills demonstrated by the staff member.

OPENING OF THE COMMUNICATION LOOP

Although communication is a shared process, the manager often has the responsibility for initiating the exchange and opening up and maintaining the process for the staff member's participation. To create a positive environment for two-way communication, the manager should be aware of some aspects of communication that are unique to the workplace.

Communication between managers and staff members is affected by *position power,* the power associated with a position. In management communications the position often "speaks" rather than the person in the position. In other words, when a manager approaches a staff member to initiate a conversation, the staff member reacts primarily to the authority and the power that the position represents, not to the individual. This may make it quite difficult for some staff members to engage in a give-and-take conversation. Position power also carries a credibility tag that "determines to a large extent how that message will be treated" (Clampitt, 1991, p. 97). Although credibility is associated with individual competence at any level of an organization, an assumed credibility attaches to communications from a manager because of the position's access to information and authority to take action. Communication that initiates with the manager can have a different effect than the same message originating with another source because of position power. A manager's recognition of this and sensitivity to the staff member's point of view can aid in opening the communication loop.

SPEAKING WITH CLARITY

As the person responsible for initiating interactions with staff members, the manager has the opportunity to craft his or her approach. The manager can think through the proposed conversation, focus clearly on the message, and choose words that accurately convey his or her meaning. This kind of preparation not only eases the initial phase of the conversation but provides the manager with practice in formulating concise and accurate messages. The skill will ultimately carry over to spontaneous interchanges.

THE NEED TO KNOW AND TIMING

In many organizations, information is equated with power. In truth the power of information lies in how the information is communicated and used. Sharing information with staff members, initiating a dialogue, developing understanding among staff members, and encouraging an open communication loop are powerful management tools. To maximize the effectiveness of two-way communication, the manager must use these tools judiciously.

First, the manager is in the best position to distinguish information from communication. Information is factual—for example, data, news, or announcements. "Communication deals with factors such as feelings, values, expectations, and perceptions, which demand that the individual believe or do something or become a particular kind of person" (Devereaux, 1992, p. 264). The manager must correctly decide if the situation calls for information sharing or a dialogue among staff members.

Second, the manager must determine if the communication need is urgent, important, or both. Urgent matters call for a rapid response. Important issues are those that clearly relate to the mission and the purpose of the organization. When a rapid response is necessary, the manager may take action and then inform staff members of the action and the rationale for it. With important issues the manager should communicate with staff members to ensure a common understanding of the issues and possible actions. When issues are both urgent and important, the manager must judge and balance the need to act quickly and inform staff members against the need to discuss the issues. An accurate assessment of the nature of the situation will ensure that communication with staff members is efficient and effective.

Finally, the manager must determine the timing of multiple pieces of information. Urgency and importance may overlap in such a way that the manager must communicate simultaneously on several issues. At other times, communication may occur sequentially. In either instance the manager should attempt to choose the optimal timing to ensure open communication. In all situations the primary communication objective is to keep staff members adequately informed and appropriately involved in issues, but not overwhelmed by a volume of unnecessary information at the wrong time.

USE OF ANOTHER'S SYSTEM AND LANGUAGE

Effectiveness in communication often depends on knowing the recipient and targeting communication to the recipient (see also chapter 4, "Marketing," and chapter 5, "The Targeting of Communications"). In a sense, communication takes on aspects of marketing. Two-way communication is more likely to occur when the manager identifies the staff member's needs and perspectives and addresses them through the communication. This is similar to understanding the staff member's context or taking on the staff member's point of view, discussed earlier. With such information the manager can incorporate relevant language, examples, stories, and analogies into the exchange. Approaching the communication at the staff member's level also enables the manager to acknowledge communication differences among staff members and determine the most appropriate channel or method of communication for a given person. When a manager is individualizing communication, it is important that his or her use of language and the staff member's perspective be genuine and sensitive, not patronizing or condescending.

COMMUNICATION ON THE SAME EMOTIONAL LEVEL

Communication in the workplace is a blend of social, emotional, and intellectual exchanges (Walton, 1989). Although the emphasis of most work-related communication is intellectual, people use social overtones in initiating conversation and establishing rapport in all settings. Moreover, communicating at an emotional level is a part of many work relationships, not only among colleagues but between the manager and the staff member. Just as the manager should individualize communication in terms of language and perspective, so should the manager keep his or her emotional tone parallel to that of the recipient. Empathy and respect for the emotional effect of a message are fundamental concerns of effective communication. In employment settings, emotional concerns are heightened because of the inherent threat and emotional risks present for many staff members when communicating with the boss. A manager must be able to listen with compassion to staff members' concerns, respect their fears, and understand their anger. Empathy, consideration, and understanding of emotional content are part of the feedback and clarification process in communication. The manager cannot assume knowledge of either the nature or the intensity of the staff member's emotional reaction. The emotional meaning of the interaction must be uncovered through the cycle of communication. The manager who is not able to respond genuinely to the emotional aspects of a communication will have a difficult time eliciting the full trust and confidence of staff members.

FACILITATION OF COMMUNICATION

Effective communication is an interpersonal relationship that depends on a two-way exchange of information and meaning. Speaking with clarity is an integral component of the exchange, but true communication of accurate meaning may depend more on the nonverbal aspects of the exchange, especially on listening.

All participants maintain the communication loop by *active listening.* Listening is more than hearing. It is an active process encompassing a number of skills that indicate attention, encourage the speaker, and verify meaning. Learning to speak is encouraged and lauded as an important developmental milestone, but learning to listen is poorly understood and infrequently taught.

THE SKILLS AND THE ART OF LISTENING

Many experts in communication have studied listening and offer suggestions for developing and improving listening skills. There are similarities and basic good advice in all their work. The skills of listening can be summarized as (1) using verbal and nonverbal cues to indicate attention; (2) helping or encouraging the speaker; and (3) doing something with (e.g., responding to and verifying) what is heard.

Bolton (1986) breaks listening into three clusters of skills: attending, following, and reflecting. He focuses on clusters, or small groups of related skills, to improve listening so that the learner gradually acquires and integrates the skills. *Attending skills* are those that indicate careful attention to the speaker. Primarily nonverbal, these skills involve use of eye contact, body motion, and posture, and control of environmental distractions. *Following skills* are those that encourage the speaker to talk but do not allow the listener to interrupt. Good following includes the use of verbal cues (such as nonthreatening invitations to talk and neutral verbal responses of one or two words), *paraverbal language* (voice cues, such as tone or volume), and nonverbal cues (such as gestures or silence). *Reflecting skills* involve asking questions, paraphrasing content, suggesting meaning, and periodically summarizing both content and meaning. Good listeners use all the skills together to create a comfortable communication environment.

Walton (1989) offers additional observations about listening. To improve attention, he advocates adopting a positive attitude toward all communication, monitoring oneself for lapses in concentration and correcting them, searching out the interesting aspects of any exchange, and avoiding a hurry-up-and-get-this-over style. He does not identify specific techniques to encourage the speaker, but reinforces the notion that the listener must adopt the point of view of the speaker in order to understand the message. He describes active listening as "bouncing" the message around to search for ideas, to identify the feelings that are being expressed, and to focus on the central thought. At this point in listening, Walton advocates questioning as a way not only to clarify and obtain feedback but also to focus the conversation, indicate interest, and build rapport with the speaker.

Ultimately, learning to listen requires an accurate assessment of current abilities, including both a self-assessment and input from others. Developing skills is then a dedicated process of practice, feedback, and more practice. The art of listening evolves as skills are slowly integrated into and used naturally in all communication.

NONVERBAL LANGUAGE

Listening is basically a nonverbal skill with delicate verbal undertones. Throughout the communication cycle, meaning is transmitted in both verbal and nonverbal modes. To understand communication fully, then, the listener must be able to read nonverbal language. Facial expression, posture, movement, and gestures are all common physical indicators of underlying feeling and emotion. A note of caution is needed in interpreting these cues. There are cultural and individual differences in the meaning of body language. The listener cannot assume an accurate interpretation without verification from the speaker. The same is true of paraverbal language (Walton, 1989). Voice tone and volume, rate of speech, and other voice cues can provide hints to emotional state, but again, because of cultural or individual variations, these hints should be cautiously considered until verified. In interpreting nonverbal and paraverbal language, the listener is looking for both congruence with and discrepancies between it and the speaker's verbal language. At times a speaker will purposely use body language or voice cues that are at odds with his or her true feelings in order to mask or disguise a particularly difficult or painful reaction.

THE FEELING BEHIND THE WORDS

Because words are only containers of meaning, listening for feeling behind the words is a critical contributor to understanding what a speaker is trying to convey. In conversations, particularly in workplace communications, it is very easy and decidedly more comfortable to focus on content rather than feeling and to verify understanding only at that level. Listening for feeling and reflecting feeling back for verification represent a much more personal level of communication and are much riskier for the listener and the speaker. Good listeners allow and even encourage speakers to share their feelings. Acknowledging emotional reactions and clarifying the feelings facilitates the development of a common context for the two persons and moves the level of understanding along farther and faster. "Feelings are often the energizing force that helps us sort our data, organize it, and use it effectively as we shape and implement our action steps" (Bolton, 1986, p. 54).

Clinically this skill is referred to as *interactive reasoning, therapeutic use of self,* or *establishing rapport.* Clinicians regularly use it to understand a client as a unique individual and to feel the effect that the client's condition has had on his or her everyday life. As clinicians, occupational therapy practitioners naturally look beyond a client's spoken word to other sources, again nonverbal and paraverbal ones, to form a complete picture of the depth of a client's reaction. The occupational therapy practitioner in a manager role can transfer this skill from the clinic to the manager's office by acknowledging overt expressions of feeling, paying attention to more subtle cues such as word choice or body language, and admitting his or her own emotional responses.

THE ENVIRONMENT OF COMMUNICATION

Although many of the skills of communication in management are applications of clinical communication skills, the context of communication shifts dramatically when an occupational therapy practitioner makes a transition from the clinician role to the manager role. Suddenly there are multiple environments in which he or she must interact. The facility or the organization as a whole becomes a primary environment for communication along with the clinic or treatment environment.

The communication environment or external context has a substantial influence on communication. As the practitioner transverses roles to the manager, many things change. There are more people with whom to communicate. The language spoken changes to include financial, human resource, legal, and administrative jargon. Communication is no longer within a single discipline or even with related disciplines, but with all the diverse disciplines and employment groups within the facility. Communication occurs at more and different levels in the organizational hierarchy and with persons of greater power and influence. At the same time the manager has to continue to speak the language of the practitioner and attend to the communication environment at the departmental level. The successful communicator becomes multilingual and adept at translating from one language to another.

THE CULTURE OF AN ORGANIZATION

Becoming multilingual is not a component of the manager's formal education or orientation program. The manager's ability to span communication boundaries comfortably develops parallel to the manager's knowledge of and comfort with the organization's culture and the roles that informal and formal communication play within that culture. *Organizational culture* is a shared sense of values, beliefs, and customs that defines acceptable behavior, establishes norms, and fixes rules for employees' conduct at all levels of an organization. Culture not only celebrates but sanctions behavior. In a large organization there is often a generic prevailing culture and numerous subcultures that have transformed broader organizational standards into unique sets of expectations, rewards, and punishments for a distinct working group. Organizational culture is both overtly and symbolically communicated as life within an organization unfolds. Cues to reading the culture lie in myths and stories that circulate among the employees, celebrations and rituals, and communication patterns, styles, and rules. The multilingual manager in a large organization must also be multicultural to avoid violating norms and standards in his or her communication across the organization.

An example of the relationship between organizational culture and communication is the existence of implicit rules that regulate communication in a work setting. These informal rules govern conditions of communication such as who can initiate and terminate a conversation, what are appropriate topics, and what are appropriate circumstances (Clampitt, 1991). Clampitt notes that the rules vary from setting to setting and that the effective communicator must be aware of the special rules of each setting at the personal, departmental, and organizational levels. The manager plays a crucial role in orienting staff members to the rules that govern workplace communications so that communications are open and staff members are aware of their rights and responsibilities as communicators. Understanding the communication rules prevents cultural mishaps that can close off communication.

FORMAL AND INFORMAL COMMUNICATION

Culture prescribes both formal and informal communications in an organization. The cultural norms and habits of an organization determine what is communicated through formal lines versus what is fed through or initiated in the informal system. Formal communication uses the chain of command and authority lines within the organization. It follows the traditional top-to-bottom and bottom-to-top flow of information and is often restricted to a specific work group or unit within the organization. Informal communication occurs across both hierarchical and departmental lines. Personal power and influence have more impact than formal authority and power. The informal network, or grapevine, rapidly spreads information through the organization; formal communication often proceeds slowly.

The astute manager learns quickly how to tap into the informal system and how to assess the truth and the value of information that arrives by way of it. Often, informal communication relates the emotional effect of and response to formal communication. A combination of formal and informal communication can provide the manager with the clearest interpretation of meaning. The facts are contained in the formal communiqué, while the affect is in the informal system. Together a complete message is transmitted.

The manager also attends to the formal and informal communication systems within his or her own department and makes choices regarding how and when to use each system. Attention to and use of informal communication methods and contacts allow the manager to work with the informal system and not be caught off guard by rumors or inaccurate interpretations of information.

CHANNELS OF COMMUNICATION

Communication methods or channels are conduits for messages. Increasingly the manager has to consider multiple mechanisms for communicating, from low to high technology. It is not uncommon for a manager to employ a mix of communication channels for a single message, depending on the content and the intent of the message and the number and the types of intended recipients.

Selecting the most appropriate communication method requires an examination of (1) the message, (2) the recipient, and (3) the method. Qualities of each influence the final choice. In regard to the message, the sender should evaluate factors such as the need for confidentiality or privacy; the need for dialogue; the importance, the length, the complexity, and the urgency of the message; and the need for a permanent record of the communication. Considerations relative to the recipient include his or her preferred method of communication, his or her skill and comfort with various communication channels, the hierarchical relationship between the sender and the recipient, the familiarity of the sender and the recipient, and the proximity of the recipient. Finally, the sender should evaluate the channel in terms of reliability, cost in time and money, access, confidentiality, and the skill needed to use it.

Today's manager has multiple means available for communication. The growth in the communication industry is both overwhelming and exciting. A manager can thoughtfully consider and choose the most effective method of communication for any situation from an array of traditional and technologically advanced channels.

TRADITIONAL CHANNELS OF COMMUNICATION

Traditionally most management communication has occurred face-to-face or in writing. Face-to-face communication takes place in either a one-on-one or a group context with corresponding degrees of privacy and personal contact and dialogue. Written communication is often equated with more formal communication for situations when a permanent record is necessary. However, written communication is certainly not restricted to those situations, circulating memos and staff member newsletters being examples of less formal uses of written communication channels. Written communication has advanced significantly with the advent of word processing and copy machines. Both have increased the ease and decreased the cost of disseminating written information to large groups.

The telephone is another conventional form of communication. It retains the informality and personal contact of face-to-face communication, but increases the distance that can exist between sender and recipient. Conference calls offer the same ease in long-distance communication to a group. In general, traditional communication channels are lower in cost and widely available across public and private employment settings.

THE INFLUENCE OF TECHNOLOGY

Technology is advancing at such a rapid rate that what is considered advanced today will not be in six months. Workplace communication has changed dramatically with the advent of the facsimile machine, voice mail, and electronic mail. Computer networks and teleconferencing open up opportunities for real-time communication between persons at great distances from one another. The exchange of information and dialogue can occur immediately. Confidentiality and privacy, however, are not guaranteed. Higher-technology communication methods are the most costly and often require additional skills and training for the communicator to be efficient in their use.

Face-to-face communication will never be replaced as the primary method used between the manager and the staff member. Alternative methods can supplement personal contact, but still require the same degree of attention to communication basics in order to be effective tools. Many of the problems that occur in face-to-face communication take place in alternative channels, where they can be more difficult to diagnose and correct.

BARRIERS TO EFFECTIVE COMMUNICATION

Communication is a complex activity. With all the dimensions involved in communicating effectively, problems inevitably occur and communication is blocked. Both environmental factors and personal factors can cause problems (Rakich, Longest, & Darr, 1992). Environmental factors include conditions in both the physical setting and the organizational culture. A chaotic and distracting environment will obviously slow down or sidetrack a dialogue. A formal room arrangement can reinforce power and authority and intimidate some speakers. An organization with many rules governing communication can stifle the free exchange of ideas and information. Personal factors range from motivation to actual skill in expressing ideas or listening effectively. A high degree of stress can alter a communication. Poor communication skills or inappropriate communication methods can cloud meaning and damage the process. Differences in personal communication styles and conflicting personal motives can produce barriers.

Ideally the manager recognizes the potential for communication breakdowns and uses good communication skills for prevention of them. This is not always a realistic expectation. Therefore the manager must also be able to recognize that a communication breakdown has occurred, diagnose the problem, and take corrective action. Being aware of the more common types of communication barriers is the first step in being able to address the problem. They are roadblocks, information overload, distortion, hidden agendas and messages, and gender differences in communication styles.

ROADBLOCKS

Roadblocks to effective communication are responses that may block the message from being communicated. These are the red flags that should alert the manager to a potential for breakdown. A negative effect is not a given, but roadblocks are high-risk responses. Either the sender or the receiver can throw out a roadblock, intentionally or unintentionally. Bolton (1986) identifies three categories of roadblocks: judging, sending solutions, and avoiding the other's concerns. *Judging* involves evaluating and approving or disapproving the content and the message of the interaction. *Sending solutions* includes offering advice, orders, or threats without fully listening to the exchange. *Avoiding* occurs when the listener somehow diverts the conversation.

These responses are considered barriers because they can all potentially "block conversation, thwart the other person's problem-solving efficiency, and increase the emotional distance between people" (Bolton, 1986, p. 17). All three types of responses are communication shortcuts that seek to assume meaning prematurely and end the communication without completing the process of listening and seeking clarity and accuracy.

INFORMATION OVERLOAD

More is not always better. Although each person has a unique capacity for information, all people have a saturation point beyond which they are unable to listen, process, and respond. They have an acquired communication dysfunction that shuts down the useful exchange of ideas and information. With effective screening of the timing, the amount, and the type of communication demands, the manager can control information overload to an extent. Because information overload is a personal response, the manager must recognize the signs of saturation in each staff member.

DISTORTION

Communication distortion is a natural phenomenon. The likelihood of distortion increases as distance increases between the originator of a message and the recipient. Distortion increases if messages have to pass through multiple hierarchical layers in an organization. Distortion occurs when a message is passed along "because people have different responsibilities, beliefs and concerns. Details are omitted. Some are highlighted.

Inferences become fact . . . Priorities shift. Nuances are lost" (Clampitt, 1991, p. 95). Distortion in an organization is like the childhood game of gossip. As the message circulates through the players, each child hears a different version. By the end of the game, the final message usually bears no resemblance to the original. Although the game results in laughter and enjoyment, distortion at the organizational level can create serious problems. With important communication issues the manager must go to the original source of the communication to avoid the effects of distortion. The manager should also recognize that even at the departmental level, distortion can occur as messages circulate among staff members.

HIDDEN AGENDAS AND MESSAGES

In a communication the possibility exists that one participant will abuse the situation with overt dishonesty or concealed motives. People may purposely distort and bias messages to achieve their own goals, meet their needs, or have their point of view dominate. Often it is not immediately apparent that this is occurring. It becomes obvious that there are discrepancies between the words, the actions, and the behaviors of a person only after repeated attempts to clarify the meaning of a communication. Such strategies not only impose an immediate block to communication but can result in permanent damage to a relationship and to future communication because the person has violated the trust base necessary for open communication.

GENDER DIFFERENCES IN COMMUNICATION STYLES

One aspect of internal context that has received increased attention recently is gender differences, particularly in communication. Gender is a powerful influence on context because men and women continue to have different life experiences that shape their use and definition of words and the implied meanings. Deborah Tannen (1994) is well-known for her study of male and female communication styles and the breakdown that can occur because of these differences. Tannen characterizes male communication in the workplace as bantering, teasing, and avoiding the "one-down" position. Women, Tannen contends, communicate to get the job done without using force and are sensitive to the effect that communication has on others. Although Tannen acknowledges both ways of speaking as equally valuable, she emphasizes that problems can occur when men and women take each other literally. The result can be insulting or confusing and definitely nonproductive.

This issue has great significance in a female-dominated field such as occupational therapy. Female occupational therapy managers often deal with males at higher levels in the organization. Male occupational therapy managers supervise staffs of primarily females. At the staff level, males are a minority presence. In all three applications, differences in the ways that men and women relate can break down or delay effective communication.

THE ETHICS OF COMMUNICATION

Many communication barriers pose ethical dilemmas for the manager. Every communication has an ethical dimension as the speaker decides what information, motives, or feelings to disclose. Clampitt (1991) illuminates this concern with his position that the single measure of communication effectiveness is whether the communicator has met his or her goals. A person's goals can be either ethical or unethical. Clampitt maintains that whether the intention was positive (understanding, clarifying, informing) or negative (deceiving, misleading, confusing), effective communication occurs when the sender's goals are met.

Confidentiality is another dimension of ethical communication. Confidential information is often conveyed in workplace communication. Staff members' compensation and performance are examples of issues that the manager must hold in confidence. When a staff member shares personal information, the manager must be an ethical listener. Staff members who come to the manager with personal concerns are taking a risk. The manager should respect that risk. He or she should first decide whether or not to accept the responsibility of receiving the personal information. If the manager decides to accept the information, he or she must consider it privileged. If the manager decides not to engage in a personal exchange, then he or she has a human responsibility to direct the staff member to appropriate support systems.

When staff members share personal information that affects their work, the ethical issues for the manager increase. The manager is in the position of balancing a staff member's needs and rights against his or her own responsibilities to the organization. As in most situations that raise ethical issues, there is no right answer. The manager should approach ethical issues in communication just as he or she would approach other ethical issues. A systematic exploration and analysis of the problem can generate options and identify the risks of taking each option. The manager's final decision should be the choice that seems to do the most good with the least amount of harm. (For a more detailed discussion of ethics, see chapter 18, "Ethical Dimensions of Occupational Therapy.")

COMMUNICATION OF A PROFESSIONAL IMAGE

A manager may put communication principles to use in other ways. Words, nonverbal language, and paraverbal language convey meaning. In addition, the physical appearance of the speaker conveys meaning. Physical appearance is not limited to tangibles such as dress and grooming but includes intangibles such as poise and confidence. Standards of professional dress are environmentally determined, an aspect of the organization's culture. New managers, in particular, may need to attend to this component of the culture as they make the transition to the manager role.

Clinical dress codes that blend the image of a competent practitioner with comfort and safety are quite different from administrative dress codes. Administrative dress standards are set to project an aura of business competence and to pave the way for a manager to interact across hierarchical lines within an organization and with key players outside the organization. Clinical dress codes are overtly stated. Administrative dress codes are rarely published, but are adhered to and valued by most participants. The traditional code of professional dress—for men, dark suit, white shirt, and tie—has given way to greater individual expression and choice. Still, the manager who strays too far from the organizational norm may have to work harder to have his or her message taken seriously.

Professional image permeates all communication channels. A manager's written communication should be well organized, properly formatted, and free of spelling and typographical errors. Telephone communication should be based on the principles of clear speaking and active listening. Any interaction has the potential to communicate meaning. The manager must broadly define communication. The same standards for comprehension and understanding should apply to all exchanges and channels.

SUMMARY

Communication involves the exchange of words, nonverbal information, and cues; the interpretation of meaning; and a cycle of feedback, clarification, and verification of the intent of the interchange. Clear and accurate communication can be blocked at any point in the process. Learning to communicate effectively in the workplace requires a valuing of good communication, self-awareness of skills and deficits, and a lifelong commitment to develop and practice good habits and skills.

Communication underlies most management functions. Ultimately the manager's success in many areas of administration depends on an ability to communicate clearly with subordinates, peers, and superiors and, in turn, to interpret messages accurately.

Meaning is derived through an interaction of content and context. Language is inherently ambiguous. It is the responsibility of the sender to determine if the words that he or she has chosen for a message are similarly defined by the recipient. *Context* may be defined as a person's "self-constructed image of the world" (Clampitt, 1991, p. 34). A common context increases the possibility of understanding.

Other factors can influence meaning. Work satisfies both basic and high-level needs for people, so it should not be surprising that communication in the workplace is susceptible to emotional influences. Stress can also create a high-risk communication environment. Further, the highly emotional and potentially stressful nature of workplace communications can result in real or perceived threats to a staff member.

One of the most effective means of avoiding misinterpretation is two-way communication. To create a positive environment for two-way communication, the manager should be aware of some aspects of communication that are unique to the workplace: (1) Communication between managers and staff members is affected by the power associated with a position. (2) As the person responsible for initiating interactions with staff members, the manager has the opportunity to craft his or her approach. (3) Sharing information with staff members, initiating a dialogue, developing understanding among staff members, and encouraging an open communication loop are powerful management tools. (4) Two-way communication is more likely to occur (a) when the manager identifies the staff member's needs and perspectives and addresses them through the communication and (b) when the manager keeps his or her emotional tone parallel to that of the recipient of the communication.

All participants maintain the communication loop by *active listening*. The skills of listening can be summarized as (1) using verbal and nonverbal cues to indicate attention; (2) helping or encouraging the speaker; and (3) doing something with (e.g., responding to and verifying) what is heard.

When an occupational therapy practitioner makes a transition from the clinician role to the manager role, he or she must suddenly interact in multiple environments. The manager's ability to span communication boundaries comfortably develops parallel to the manager's knowledge of and comfort with the organization's culture and the roles that informal and formal communication play within that culture.

It is not uncommon for a manager to employ a mix of communication channels for a single message. Selecting the appropriate communication methods requires an examination of variables related to (1) the message—for example, the need for confidentiality or privacy and the need for dialogue; (2) the recipient—for example, his or her preferred method of communication and his or her skill and comfort with various communication channels; and (3) the method—for example, reliability and cost in time and money.

Today's manager has multiple means available for communication. Traditional channels, low in cost and widely available, include face-to-face communication, written communication, and the telephone. Modern channels, costly and requiring some training to use, comprise the facsimile machine, voice mail, electronic mail, computer networks, and teleconferencing.

Both environmental factors and personal factors can block communication (Rakich, Longest, & Darr, 1992). Environmental factors include conditions in both the physical setting and the organizational culture. Personal factors range from motivation to actual skill in expressing ideas or listening effectively. Being aware of the more common types of communication barriers is the first step in being able to address the problem. They are roadblocks (judging, sending solutions, and avoiding), information overload, distortion, hidden agendas and messages, and gender differences in communication styles.

Every communication has an ethical dimension as the speaker decides what information, motives, or feelings to disclose. A person's goals in communicating can be either ethical or unethical. Confidentiality is another dimension of ethical communication. Further, when staff members share personal information that affects their work, the manager is in the position of balancing their needs and rights against his or her own responsibilities to the organization.

Physical appearance also conveys meaning—not just tangibles such as dress and grooming but intangibles such as poise and confidence. Clinical dress codes are quite different from administrative dress codes.

Professional image permeates all communication channels. The same standards for comprehension and understanding should apply to all exchanges and channels.

REFERENCES

Bolton, R. B. (1986). *People skills: How to assert yourself, listen to others, and resolve conflicts* (2nd ed.). New York: Simon & Schuster.

Clampitt, P. G. (1991). *Communicating for managerial effectiveness.* Newbury Park, CA: Sage.

Devereaux, E. (1992). Principles of communication. In J. Bair & M. Gray (Eds.), *The occupational therapy manager* (Rev. ed., pp. 261–73). Rockville, MD: American Occupational Therapy Association.

Katz, R. L. (1974, September-October). HBR classic: Skills of an effective administrator. *Harvard Business Review, 52,* 90–102.

Rakich, J. S., Longest, B. B., Jr., & Darr, K. (1992). *Managing health services organizations* (3rd ed.). Baltimore: Health Professions Press.

Tannen, D. (1994). *Talking from 9 to 5.* New York: Morrow.

Walton, D. (1989). *Are you communicating?* New York: McGraw Hill.

ADDITIONAL RESOURCES

Adair, J. (1984). *The skills of leadership.* Aldershot, Hants, England: Gower.

Bartolome, F. (1993). *The articulate executive.* Boston: Harvard Business School.

Miyake, S., & Trostler, R. J. (1987). Introducing the concept of a corporate culture to the hospital setting. *American Journal of Occupational Therapy, 41,* 310–14.

Pozgar, G. D. (1986). On the grapevine. *The Health Care Supervisor, 4*(2), 39–49.

CHAPTER 15

Consultation: A Collaborative Approach to Change

Cynthia F. Epstein, MA, OTR, FAOTA
Evelyn G. Jaffe, MPH, OTR, FAOTA

KEY TERMS

Client. The person or the system seeking help.

Consultant roles. Multiple sets of behaviors that may be performed by a consultant in the course of a consultation: adviser, helper, facilitator, outsider, change agent, evaluator-diagnostician, clarifier, trainer, planner, extender.

Consultation. The interactive process of helping others solve existing or potential problems by identifying and analyzing issues, developing strategies to address problems, and preventing future problems from occurring.

Consultation process. A facilitative process in which a client receives help from a consultant through an interactive, egalitarian relationship based on mutual respect.

Environment. A complex of internal and external conditions or factors that surround an individual or a community and influence behavior or organizational structure.

This chapter is based in part on chapter 2, "Theoretical Concepts of Consultation" (pp. 15–54), and chapter 4, "Approaches to Consultation" (pp. 86–117), by E. G. Jaffe, 1992; chapter 5, "Preparation for Consultation" (pp. 118–34), chapter 6, "The Process of Consultation" (pp. 135–66), chapter 7, "Occupational Therapy Consultation Practice: An Overview" (pp. 167–87), chapter 42, "Toward a Theoretical Model of Occupational Therapy Consultation" (pp. 676–713), chapter 43, "Summary" (pp. 714–21), and appendix A, "Glossary" (pp. 722–31), by E. G. Jaffe and C. F. Epstein, 1992; and chapter 41, "Marketing: A Continuous Process" (pp. 650–74), by C. F. Epstein, 1992; in E. G. Jaffe and C. F. Epstein (Eds.), Occupational Therapy Consultation: Theory, Principles, and Practice, St. Louis, MO: Mosby–Year Book. Copyright ©1992 by Mosby–Year Book, Inc. Adapted with permission.

External consultant. An independent agent, outside the organization, with whom the client contracts to provide consultation services.

Internal consultant. An employee of the client system who is asked to provide consultation services within the organization.

Levels of consultation. A conceptualization of consultation as occurring on three possible levels: case centered (targeted on a specific person), educational (targeted on a specific client group), and program and/or administrative (targeted on a specific system).

Models of consultation. A conceptualization of consultation as having nine possible foci, each calling for different strategies on the part of the consultant: clinical model, collegial model, behavioral model, educational model, organizational development model, process management model, program development model, social action model, and systems model.

Preventive outcomes. The results achieved through consultation activities.

Cynthia F. Epstein, MA, OTR, FAOTA, is the president and the executive director of Occupational Therapy Consultants, Inc. in Bridgewater, New Jersey. She has over 30 years of experience as a consultant, practicing in such diverse areas as vocational rehabilitation research and program development, adult day treatment, wheelchair management, school-based programming, and long-term care. She earned her master's degree in vocational rehabilitation at New York University.

Evelyn G. Jaffe, MPH, OTR, FAOTA, is an assistant professor at Samuel Merritt College. She has been a consultant in occupational therapy for over 35 years, specializing in community mental health, high-risk infants, school-age parents, and primary prevention in the workplace. She earned her master's degree in the School of Public Health at the University of Michigan.

Consultation as a model of service delivery continues to develop a presence in occupational therapy practice (AOTA, 1990). Responding to significant changes in the health care marketplace, many of today's practitioners and their clients seek a collaborative approach to resolving problems that occur at varied levels of health care and across diverse practice settings. Consultation supports this approach, expanding the potential for development of successful outcomes for clients.

The changing nature of health and human service delivery has also created challenges for today's practitioner. Stringent criteria for approval of services, coupled with time-limited appropriations, fixed payments per patient, and increasing competition among disciplines for the same funds, call for practitioners who are knowledgeable, skilled, and able to respond quickly. They must not only diagnose the functional problems of individuals but understand and effectively address the organizational and process problems of systems. In this regard there is an increasing need to understand and use principles of consultation in all areas and at all levels of occupational therapy practice.

Every occupational therapy practitioner may be called on to provide consultation within the context of his or her job. Experienced practitioners possessing particular expertise may provide consultation as their primary role (AOTA, 1993). Whether consultation is a secondary or primary role, the practitioner must understand how to use principles of consultation to meet clients' needs.

Consultation is the interactive process of helping others solve existing or potential problems by identifying and analyzing issues, developing strategies to address problems, and preventing future problems from occurring. Key elements in consultation, in addition to occupational therapy expertise, are an understanding of (1) systems (see chapter 7, "Organizational Effectiveness"), (2) organizational development (see chapter 7), (3) behavior, and (4) the principles of prevention. The consultant must have an ability to listen and communicate effectively, as well as a capacity to diagnose and facilitate resolution of existing or potential problems (Yerxa, 1978).

Occupational therapy consultants provide services in varied settings. These include such traditional environments as hospitals, long-term-care facilities, and schools (Cunninghis, 1992; Rogers & Wood, 1992; Rourk, 1992; Weiss, 1992), and the growing areas of industry, community agencies and services, regulatory agencies, professional organizations, and international health programs (Devereaux, 1992; Izutsu, 1992; Jacobs, 1992; Kauffman, 1992). The services may be requested by individuals, departments, or entire systems, and they may involve a brief intervention or an extended relationship. Services are delivered using a client-centered approach that emphasizes an interactive relationship between consultant and client (AOTA, 1995).

A consultant may be from a private practice or from another type of organization outside the system that is requesting help. Alternatively a consultant may be an employee of the organization that is seeking consultation. Any occupational therapy practitioner might, then, receive a request to provide consultation to a department or a staff of his or her organization. The *client,* the person or the system seeking help, uses consultation to improve planning and interaction with colleagues, consumers, or employees (Lippitt & Lippitt, 1986; Ulschak & SnowAntle, 1990). The consultant helps the client mobilize internal and external resources that will facilitate change and lead to problem resolution (Lippitt & Lippitt, 1986).

An occupational therapy consultant helps a client consider new or revised elements, information, concepts, perspectives, values, attitudes, and skills in the course of consultation. During this time it is critical that the consultant view problems from a broad, client-centered perspective, with systems, models, and contexts as an integral part of the decision-making process (AOTA, 1993, 1994, 1995; Dunn, Brown, & McGuigan, 1994; Jaffe & Epstein, 1992, chap. 5).

Inherent in occupational therapy practice is enablement of the client through improved occupational performance, thereby allowing the client to perform daily functions successfully and to take charge of his or her life (Yerxa, 1983). The client and the practitioner work collaboratively to design and implement required services (AOTA, 1995). Similarly, occupational therapy consultation requires collaboration between the client and the consultant. The goal of consultation is also enablement of the client. The consultant's task is to develop an environment in which positive change can take place, thereby leading to improved performance by the client.

Jaffe and Epstein (1992, chap. 42) have proposed a theoretical model of consultation that "integrates occupational therapy and consultation concepts within an ecological framework" (p. 709). The model relates the principles, the philosophical assumptions, and the theoretical premises of occupational therapy to those of consultation. It recognizes ecological contexts as a critical factor in goal achievement for both occupational therapy and consultation. AOTA's (1994) "Uniform Terminology for Occupational Therapy" offers support for this perspective.

Relevant theoretical principles on which the consultation model draws include those of systems theory, ecology, occupational therapy, consultation, and health promotion. The model incorporates and acknowledges "the synergetic relationship between occupational therapy, human ecology and consultation" (p. 677).

The model is based on the milieu or *environment* in which the consultative activities occur; the application of the *human ecological perspective* of the client; *collaboration* between the consultant and the client; the *adaptation* or change facilitated by this collaborative approach; and ultimately the *enablement* of the client to achieve *improved function* and maximize his or her *human potential*. Concepts of prevention are basic to this model because the ultimate goal of consultation is to help the client develop skills to prevent future problems. Consultation therefore enables the client to assume a proactive stance, anticipating and forestalling situations that could lead to further problems or dysfunction.

Today's practice environments seek efficient and cost-effective responses to the varied needs of health and human service clientele. Occupational therapy practitioners can offer such responses by furthering their knowledge and understanding of occupational therapy consultation. This chapter provides an overview of consultation concepts and the process of consultation. It discusses important skills and knowledge needed to perform the role of consultant. Also, it addresses marketing and business as they relate to establishing a consultation practice.

AN EXPANDING MARKETPLACE

Changing legislative priorities, economic and social issues, continued advances in technology, and an expanding system of managed care in the provision of health services (see chapter 1 for a discussion of managed care) have profoundly influenced the growing demand for consultation services. Federal legislation, including the Education for All Handicapped Children Act of 1975, the Technology-Related Assistance for Individuals with Disabilities Act of 1988, the Americans with Disabilities Act of 1990, and the Individuals with Disabilities Education Act of 1990, has increased consumer awareness of the need for skilled occupational therapy consultants.

The crisis created by the 1995 budget reform movement has mandated a rethinking of the nation's welfare system as well as its programs for education, housing, and health care (Morrow, 1995). At such a time, planners, managers, and consumers seek consultants with expertise to help them move successfully through the process of change.

Concurrently the global information highway and growing assistive technology have created new and exciting options for persons with disabilities. As a key member of the assistive technology team, the occupational therapy consultant helps initiate and develop technological services for this population (Post, 1992).

The health care environment has changed dramatically from the traditional fee-for-service scheme to a system of managed care. Managed care and many similar plans that emphasize cost containment have been embraced by insurance companies, regulatory agencies, hospitals, and other health agency consortia and provider organizations. In controlling cost and access, systems influence how occupational therapy services are provided. Traditional one-on-one treatment services may not always be feasible or may be severely limited under such systems. Indirect services, including consultation and case management, will be the option of choice for many health care providers. Consultation skills to help consumers, families, employers, and communities assess needs, identify strengths, and develop and coordinate resources are essential for today's practitioner.

The consultant is usually found at the leading edge of practice, initiating occupational therapy services in new markets. For example, recent reforms in welfare have placed able-bodied welfare recipients in public works projects (Carlson, 1995). Implementation of such reforms involves a dramatic role shift for welfare department personnel. As an evaluator, an analyst, and a trainer, the occupational therapy consultant may help identify and resolve specific problems faced by a welfare department, its personnel, and their clients being placed in work programs.

Another concern is the growing number of prisoners with drug-related problems who return to jail after parole. An occupational therapy consultant in California (P. Wilbarger, personal communication, August 1995) participated in a pilot program with recent parolees who were drug addicted. As part of a multidisciplinary consultation team, she evaluated each parolee and shared her findings with project personnel. A major problem that the consultant identified was the great difficulty most of these adults had with sensory processing and sensory modulation. She provided training for project staff to build a common base of understanding of these problems. She then facilitated the development of an appropriate program plan. Consultation of this type helps establish occupational therapy services in new and growing markets.

School systems constitute the largest single practice setting for registered occupational therapists (OTRs) and the second largest for certified occupational therapy assistants (COTAs) (AOTA, 1990). Since the passage of the Education for All Handicapped Children Act in 1975, increasing numbers of children have been identified and referred for school-based occupational therapy services. Initially the focus of referrals was children who were physically and mentally challenged and children with learning disabilities. In recent years, though, there have been growing numbers of children who are HIV infected (Parks, 1994) or affected by prenatal drug exposure (Kelly, Walsh, & Thompson, 1991). This has changed the demographics of children now included in education settings. Occupational therapy consultants with specific expertise in pediatric practice and a knowledge of educational systems must be available to help develop educationally related programs for this diverse population of children.

Current educational programs for children with disabilities emphasize an integrated or inclusive approach, with placement in regular classroom settings. Inclusion has created great resistance on the part of teachers, who feel that they are not trained to work with children with disabilities ("Teachers Union Limits," 1994). However, parents and administrators have given strong support to the concept (McDonnell, McDonnell, Hardman, & McCune, 1991; Peak Parent Center, 1988).

This shift in educational philosophy has had a major effect on related services such as occupational therapy. Educators now appreciate and use occupational therapy services for children with special needs. However, the current mandates for cost containment and educational relevance require a change in how these services are provided. Many occupational therapy practitioners have been providing one-on-one services to children in a separate area of the school. The move to inclusion has increased the demand for therapists to become consultants to teachers. The practitioner-consultant must therefore take his or her knowledge and expertise into the classroom (Dunn, 1985, 1988, 1992; Hanft & Place, 1996; Lifter, 1993; Weiss, 1992). Using a collegial model of consultation (see Models of Consultation, later in this chapter), the consultant can engender a supportive milieu for collaborative problem solving. The expertise of teacher and consultant can be joined for the benefit of both the students with special needs and the classroom as a whole.

There are also increasing needs for consultation at the opposite end of the developmental spectrum. Persons 65 years old or older are an ever-growing constituency. These consumers are primary recipients of services under Medicare and Medicaid, which the budget revolution of the 1995 Congress targeted for major cuts ("Budget Revolution," 1995). As a result, this population is making greater use of community-based services.

The concept of long-term care has expanded. Long-term care is now viewed as a continuum, with the preferred option being to maintain older persons in their home. The need for community-based occupational therapy services will therefore continue to grow. The focus will be at a secondary rather than a tertiary level of prevention (Grossman, 1977).

In adult day care, for example, Partners in Caregiving (1995) projects that 7,000 more centers will be needed in the United States by the year 2000. Occupational therapy consultants will be in demand to help develop programs, provide case consultation, and train staff members (Epstein, 1992; Jaffe & Epstein, 1992, chap. 25).

As older persons age at home, their risk of falling or experiencing other types of accidents increases. Establishing a safe home environment for continued independence and function has always been an important occupational therapy concern (Patterson, 1994). Often the clinician is called in after the accident. Reaching the older person at risk is more of a challenge. Consultation provides greater opportunities for reaching this segment of the population.

A significant number of at-risk elderly persons live in retirement communities. A major goal for residents is accident prevention. One successful strategy in this area is a computerized evaluation tool called EASE-2000 (Enhanced Assessment for Senior Environments), developed by an occupational therapist for use by fellow practitioners (Christenson, 1996). The consulting practitioner completes an assessment of a client and his or her home environment with the assistance of this specially designed computer program. The computer quickly sorts the consultant's data input, identifying hazards and generating possible solutions immediately, along with recommendations for adaptive devices that may increase the client's functional independence. Retirement communities working with EASE consultants have been able to customize safer environments for their residents and homeowners (M. Christenson, personal communication, September 1995).

Although funding for Medicare and Medicaid may be decreasing, older persons are becoming more knowledgeable consumers. Maintaining independence is their primary goal. Occupational therapy practitioners who have expertise in evaluating the occupational performance of older adults are the consultants of choice to work with these consumers and those who constitute their support system.

Other growing markets include those related to technology and accessibility. Assistive technology enables many persons with disabilities to achieve greater independence and productivity. Post (1992), Bain (1992), and Grady (1992) describe some activities of occupational therapy consultants with expertise in technology. These include providing extensive technological assistance in seating, positioning, and mobility for clients who are developmentally disabled, consulting on the use of environmental control units for persons who are physically challenged, and facilitating consumers' use of technology through effective communication.

Accessibility issues resulting from the Americans with Disabilities Act of 1990 have created innumerable opportunities for occupational therapy consultation to industries, private and public businesses, and corporations. There is increased demand by city planners, developers, architects, and others involved in designing living space for help in conforming to this landmark legislation ("AOTA Consultant Networks," 1995; Samson, 1992).

Employers and lawyers seek consultation on aspects of the Americans with Disabilities Act concerning employment of persons with disabilities. The occupational therapy consultant is uniquely qualified to help develop reasonable accommodations for job performance and to conduct work capacity evaluations for employees with disabilities (Kornblau, 1992). Additionally, lawyers may seek expert opinions in litigation arising from failure to address legislative mandates, creating yet another market for occupational therapy consultation (Samson, 1992).

As the 21st century begins, opportunities in new markets will continue to emerge. Deregulation and cost-containment legislation have spurred privatization in the health care industry. Occupational therapy consultants and entrepreneurs are now working collaboratively in—even establishing and owning—health clinics, fitness centers, day-care programs, and holistic health centers.

Changes in health care delivery models, combined with younger and older populations that are increasing rapidly as a result of life-sustaining technology, have helped occupational therapy become one of the nation's fastest-growing occupations. Within the profession, survey results show that "about a third of OTRs and a quarter of COTAs consider 'consultation' to be their secondary employment function" (AOTA, 1990, p. 2). The need for practitioners whose primary function is occupational therapy consultation will increase dramatically in future years. Building a core of consultants begins with expanding the knowledge base of prospective consultants. The information presented in this chapter is intended to widen the perspective of occupational therapy students and practitioners with an overview of the basic concepts, process, and practice of consultation.

CONCEPTS OF CONSULTATION

Consultation is a multidimensional, highly complex, dynamic activity. Successful consultation is not happenstance, but the result of knowledge, skill, and grounding in the theoretical foundations of the activity. It requires careful study and understanding of (1) a client's environment, (2) the various models or approaches that a consultant might use, (3) the different roles and styles appropriate to a specific system, and (4) the process of consultation. Before undertaking consultation, a prospective consultant should have a thorough knowledge of the concepts that provide a theoretical framework for consultation.

MODELS AND LEVELS OF CONSULTATION

Models of consultation are drawn from many fields of study, including sociology, psychology, education, medicine, and business. Jaffe and Epstein (1992, chap. 2) identify nine theoretical models (see table 15-1).

Further, they explain that consultation occurs on different levels (see table 15-2), as the situation requires.

Table 15-1
Models of Consultation

Clinical or Treatment Model

Patient-focused model based on diagnosis and recommendations for treatment, frequently in specific case; often considered case consultation

Collegial or Professional Model

Peer-centered model based on egalitarian, problem-solving relationship with professional colleagues; considered collaborative consultation

Behavioral Model

Behavior-focused model based on control, adaptation, modification, or change of learned behavior

Educational Model

Information-centered model with consultant acting as educator and trainer to enhance staff knowledge and skills that can support desired consultation outcomes

Organizational Development Model

Management-focused model based on examination of organizational structure, leadership styles, and interpersonal communication and relationships

Process Management Model

Group-based model focused on process dynamics of client, with consultant acting as catalyst for staff development and building of group skills to manage organizational process more effectively

Program Development Model

Service-centered model focused on development of new programs or modification of existing programs to improve services, involving assessment, design, implementation, and evaluation

Social Action Model

Social reform model focused on social values and policies, with consultant acting as advocate to facilitate social change

Systems Model

Overall system–centered model based on specific values and culture of client (school, corporation, health facility, community agency, etc.); focused on understanding system's mission and goals in order to effect change in system

Note. *From "Theoretical Concepts of Consultation" (chap. 2, pp. 44–46, table 2-1), by E. G. Jaffe, 1992, in E. G. Jaffe and C. F. Epstein (Eds.),* Occupational Therapy Consultation: Theory, Principles, and Practice, *St. Louis, MO: Mosby–Year Book. Copyright ©1992 by Mosby–Year Book. Adapted with permission.*

Table 15-2
Levels of Consultation

Level I: Case-Centered Consultation

Targeted on specific person, with aim of achieving appropriate behavioral or physical change; derived from traditional Clinical or Treatment Model; usually involves specialized assessments to diagnose problem

Level II: Educational Consultation

Targeted on specific client group (staff, clinicians, teachers, administrators, etc.), with aim of improving function, efficiency, and ability; derived from Educational Model; involves in-service training or staff development

Level III: Program and/or Administrative Consultation

Targeted on specific system (school, agency, corporation, health facility, etc.), with aim of promoting institutional change; derived from Systems, Program Development, and Organizational Development models; involves program planning, administrative and management skill development, and strategic planning

Source. *From "Influencing Social Change in Community Mental Health," by S. Nagler and S. Cooper, 1970, in P. E. Cook (Ed.), Community Psychology and Community Mental Health: Introductory Readings, San Francisco: Holden-Day.*

Consultation may involve only one model and one level, as is frequently the case when a consultant is called in as an expert to help resolve a clinical problem. Such a situation usually requires evaluation of a specific patient and the development of recommendations to be carried out by persons on site. For example:

A Scenario, Phase 1:
Adult Day Center Consultation

An adult day center located in a suburban community provides a socialization program for its predominantly older clientele. Center staff members are concerned about a client with rheumatoid arthritis who is experiencing increased difficulty in maintaining independent mobility with an old wheelchair. They ask an occupational therapy consultant to assess the client's need for a new wheelchair that will increase her functional independence at the center and at home.

The consultant shares her findings, recommendations, and suggestions for vendors with the center staff and their client. The information serves as a guide for their deliberations. They identify a medical equipment dealer who is able to fulfill the consultant's specifications, and they make arrangements for him to bring several chairs to the center on a day that the client is present. In this way the client can make a final choice with support from center staff members. The consultant indicates that she is available if needed for a follow-up visit.

In this example the consultant uses the Clinical or Treatment Model, at Level I, Case-Centered Consultation.

At other times a client may ask a consultant to address more complex issues, requiring use of multiple models and levels of consultation. Following are some extensions of the previous example into a more complex consultation in which several models and levels come into play:

A Scenario, Phase 2:
Adult Day Center Consultation

During her visit to the adult day center, the consultant becomes aware of the growing number of clients with Alzheimer's disease who are in early stages of decline. Staff members are finding it difficult to engage them in meaningful activities. This results in disruption of programs for all center clients and increased frustration among staff members.

The consultant mentions her extensive experience in program development for persons with Alzheimer's disease to the center director. The director asks for a proposal to help the center develop more effective programs for the clients with Alzheimer's disease. The consultant submits a proposal, and it is accepted.

The consultant first works with staff members as they implement their existing program. This is an opportunity for her to experience and understand some of the subtle issues related to programming. It also helps her establish a collegial relationship with staff, which forms the basis for collaborative problem solving on program development.

Staff requests for further training arise from the program development meetings. The consultant initiates training sessions to broaden staff members' understanding of Alzheimer's disease and its relationship to clients' behavior. As part of the training, she shares program and behavioral strategies that have been successfully used in similar programs.

Staff members begin discussing their observations and experiences. As the consultant guides them, their negative attitudes and behaviors toward the clients surface as a significant issue. Through role playing and modeling, the consultant helps staff members consider adaptations to and modifications of their behaviors that will elicit positive responses from the clients.

The development of new programs for the clients with Alzheimer's disease then becomes an interactive process. The consultant presents her ideas and strategies. Staff members, using their newly gained insight, consider the consultant's ideas and contribute some of their own. The consultant facilitates problem solving. The outcome is a revised program structure agreed on by all concerned.

On her reentry into the center, the consultant is operating on Level III, Program Consultation. Her work with staff members then evolves to the Collegial Model. Her goal is to see the existing program as they see it and to establish working relationships with them. This approach creates a foundation for collaborative problem solving using the Program Development Model. From this effort come requests for training, which prompt the consultant to activate the Educational Model and concurrently to move to Level II, Educational Consultation. At this juncture she uses both the Educational Model and the Behavioral Model. These help her to plan effective training programs for staff members and concurrently to develop strategies to assist staff members in examining their attitudes and behaviors related to the clients with Alzheimer's disease. Once staff members are ready to create new programs, the consultant is back to Level III, Program Consultation.

A Scenario, Phase 3:
Adult Day Center Consultation

During one of the consultant's sessions with the center director and the director's assistant, they share a new problem. Outside funding is becoming more limited. To maintain and expand the program, the center's board of directors has begun negotiations with the state Division of Developmental Disabilities to include 12 young adults with multiple handicaps in the program. There are two empty rooms at the center, which can house the new clients. Two very influential members of the board are pushing for this change, even though the board members know very little about the requirements for serving such a population or the effect that such a group might have on service to the older adults currently in the program.

The center director has visited several programs serving young adults with multiple handicaps. She feels that this population will require more intensive staffing and extensive staff training, and she is concerned that the new group might have a negative effect on the current clientele. She suggests to the board members that they introduce a medical day-care component into the social program. This would require a Certificate of Need from the Department of Health. Having experienced some very negative feedback from this department earlier in the center's history, the board does not respond positively to the director's suggestion.

The director feels that the board needs an outside expert to help the members look at options before they make a final decision. She knows that the consultant has experience with both medical day care and adults with multiple handicaps, so she asks the consultant to submit another proposal. The director and the board review the document and hire the consultant for a third phase.

Program expansion and a more diverse client base would bring change in the organizational structure. The consultant identifies forces that would impede or facilitate the desired goal of expansion. She analyzes the overall organization and its environment to help the board consider the effects of such change on the system.

Her first task is to help the board look at the pros and the cons of expansion in regard to the two populations under discussion. The consultant has a pool of broad-based resources available through her involvement in state and national organizations representing persons with developmental disabilities and the aging population. She arranges an educational program for the board. She uses the meeting both to educate and to begin examining the process dynamics of the board and its relationship to the whole organization. The meeting generates discussion and strategy building to study the two options further. There are some strong advocates in both camps, but about half the board is neutral. Three task groups are formed: group 1 to look at the young adults, group 2 to consider medical day care, and group 3 to analyze funding sources for each. At the consultant's suggestion, one or more members of the executive board join each task group. The consultant herself works with each group. She also uses the opportunity to help the executive board understand how to work with the whole board and its support staff more efficiently and effectively.

The three-month process generates some unexpected outcomes. Working in their task groups and as a group of the whole, board members become more aware of all the needs for day programming in their community. They also identify some young adults with physical disabilities who are looking for a barrier-free environment for weekly evening activities. This group cannot afford to pay for space.

The consultant helps each task group analyze its findings and generate recommendations for the whole board to consider. When the whole board meets, with the consultant acting as a facilitator, the members realize that they need to revise their mission and goals before making any final decisions. As they work through this process, it becomes clear that their mission is to serve older adults and the support systems of older adults. Using the recommendations of the medical day-care group and the findings of the funding group, they put together a plan of action. Their plan will bring in the needed moneys and add staff members such as occupational and physical therapy practitioners who can benefit both the social and the medical clients.

The consultant feels that the board's new mission statement opens the door for greater center involvement in community needs for adults. Realizing that the evening program sought by the young adults with physical disabilities is a perfect way for the center to support community needs at a minimal cost, she meets with the director to share her observations and the benefits that can be derived from such a move. Together they generate a proposal to the board recommending incorporation of the evening program into center activities, once medical day care is under way. The board likes the concept and agrees to review the proposal.

As the consultant begins to work with the board, she employs the Educational Model and works at Level II, Educational Consultation. Through her training programs, board members' knowledge and understanding expand, and their problem-solving abilities increase. The consultant knows, however, that there are many conflicts within the group, and significant communication gaps, which will impede continued movement. She therefore turns to the Process Management Model and concurrently moves to Level III, Program Consultation. Operating at both Level II and Level III, the consultant shifts between the Process Management and Organizational Development models, supporting the work of the task groups, on the one hand, and helping the executive board work with the whole board and the staff, on the other hand. These activities lead logically to the board's clarification of mission, calling for a Systems Model of consultation. The Social Action Model then comes into play as the consultant becomes an advocate for the young adults with physical disabilities.

A Scenario, Phase 4: Adult Day Center Consultation

The board requests that the consultant stay on to help the center obtain its Certificate of Need. Additionally, board members ask that the consultant help them as they interview the first medical day-care clients. They value her expertise and want to make sure that the program can meet these new clients' needs.

In staying on to help the center obtain its certificate, the consultant will employ the Collegial Model, operating at Level II, Educational Consultation. Finally, when she helps the board interview prospective clients, she will come full circle, returning to Level I, Case-Centered Consultation, using the Clinical Model.

These models and levels provide an organizing framework for analyzing, planning, and implementing any given consultative experience.

PRINCIPLES OF PREVENTION

The ultimate goal of consultation is to help clients assume a proactive stance, enabling them to anticipate or forestall problems that otherwise could lead to dysfunction. Concepts of prevention are therefore inherent in all consultation. They are also inherent in occupational therapy practice. Many authors have discussed the principles of prevention (Epstein, 1979; Grossman, 1977; Jaffe, 1980, 1986; Jaffe & Epstein, 1992, chap. 2; West, 1969; Wiemer, 1972). Jaffe and Epstein (1992, chap. 2) describe three types:

1. *Primary prevention:* activities undertaken before the onset of a problem to avoid occurrence of malfunction or disability in a population potentially at risk

2. *Secondary prevention:* early diagnosis, identification, and detection of populations at risk to prevent chronic dysfunction or permanent disability

3. *Tertiary prevention:* rehabilitation and remediation of a problem or illness to prevent further problems, loss, or disability

(pp. 48–49)

PREVENTIVE OUTCOMES

As a consultant, the occupational therapy practitioner must understand basic prevention principles and use them to achieve *preventive outcomes.* Related to the three levels of consultation, these are the results achieved through consultation activities. For instance:

1. *Tertiary preventive outcome:* Modification of the behavior of a specific client through change and maintenance, occurring at Level I, Case-Centered Consultation. In the earlier example the new wheelchair will increase the client's functional activities of daily living (behavior), and center staff members are knowledgeable about the equipment's maintenance needs.

2. *Secondary preventive outcome:* Modification of behavior through process management and skill development, occurring at Level II, Educational Consultation. In the example, staff members develop more effective programming for and behavioral approaches to clients with Alzheimer's disease.

3. *Primary preventive outcome:* Transformation of an institution or a system through program development and organizational restructuring, occurring at Level III, Program and/or Administrative Consultation. In the example the board of directors is able to expand its client base to meet growing community needs.

Enablement of the client is an inherent goal for occupational therapy practitioners. Merging the concepts of prevention with occupational therapy consultation practice at various levels assures the client and the consultant of a proactive approach that acknowledges the important relationship between client, consultant, and environment.

ENVIRONMENTAL AND SYSTEMS ANALYSIS

Successful consultation outcomes begin with careful analysis and planning. An environmental and systems analysis is an important preliminary step. The *environment* is a complex of internal and external conditions or factors that surround an individual or a community. These factors influence behavior or organizational structure. The *external environment* includes political, economic, social, demographic, cultural, and physical factors; the *internal environment* includes personal and organizational goals, resources available, power and control, organizational structure, the physical environment, and more. Analysis of these factors helps the consultant determine the consultation frame(s) of reference.

The systems in which occupational therapy consultation may take place include health care facilities, schools, social agencies, the community, industry, regulatory agencies, and political arenas. The consultant's systems analysis should ascertain the state of the system through study and evaluation of all the internal and external environmental factors that may influence it. This will help the consultant determine the goals of the consultation and identify the strategies.

THE CONSULTATION PROCESS

Consultation brings to mind such words as *diagnosis, analysis, advice, articulation, opinion, counsel, recommendation, communication, suggestion,* and *help.* The consultant may be thought of as a change agent, a counselor, a reflector, a health advocate or agent, a professional adviser, or a facilitator. Although consultation includes all these activities and functions, more than anything else, consultation is a process. Occupational therapy consultation is a facilitative process in which a client receives help through an interactive, egalitarian relationship based on mutual respect. Problem solving is a key component, involving identification of issues, analysis of issues, and resolution of problems. Consultants use a systems perspective to develop an environmental analysis and interactive communication. Consultants also identify available internal and external resources.

Consultation occurs in four stages: (1) initiation and clarification, (2) assessment and communication, (3) interactive problem resolution, and (4) evaluation and termination. Within these stages are eight basic steps: entry into the system, negotiation of a contract, diagnostic analysis leading to problem identification, goal setting and planning through establishment of trust, maintenance, evaluation, termination, and possible renegotiation (Jaffe & Epstein, 1992, chap. 6; Lippitt & Lippitt, 1986). The consultation may be a short-term problem-specific intervention, be provided at predetermined intervals, or occur on a continuing basis as needed. Prime examples of organizations that may need continuing consultation are community-based ones such as school systems, community mental health centers, nursing homes, and adult day centers. In some of these settings, occupational therapy services may be mandated by law. The direct service provider may be a certified occupational therapy assistant, a nurse, a teacher, an aide, an activities coordinator, a volunteer, or another caregiver, and the occupational therapy consultant may provide help and recommendations to the service provider. The consultation process, however, is the same as outlined in the following sections.

INITIATION AND CLARIFICATION

The initial identification of a need or a problem may precipitate a request for consultation services. On the other hand, the consultant may see a need within a particular system and present a proposal. In early meetings with the client, the consultant delineates his or her knowledge and experience. The client presents an overview of the system and enumerates the desired outcomes of the consultation. During these interactions there is an opportunity to clarify roles, expectations, and goals, leading to a formal contract.

Entry into the System

Entry into the system or the organization is the first step in the consultation process and may develop in one or more of four ways. The entry is based on exploration of the potential for consultation in the system (Jaffe & Epstein, 1992, chap. 6).

1. *Planned entry*—The individual develops a strategy and presents a proposal.

2. *Opportunistic entry*—The situation arises spontaneously and the individual seizes the moment.

3. *Uninvited entry*—The individual perceives a need and attempts to enter the system.

4. *Invited entry*—The individual is invited because of specific skills.

(p. 136)

In the earlier example the client initially invites the consultant because she has specific clinical expertise that the client requires. The consultant's subsequent involvement occurs opportunistically. Ultimately, though, at each phase of the consultation, the client invites the consultant to enter the system. Planned, opportunistic, and uninvited entry are only methods to obtain a foothold for demonstrating that a client would benefit from consultation.

During the entry step the consultant should consider certain factors:

1. *The potential for a mutual relationship.* The consultant and the client must determine if there is the potential to develop a working relationship that includes mutual respect and trust.

2. *Initial assessment of needs.* The consultant may want to do some preliminary fact-finding, explore the needs and the issues that may be creating problems within the system, and provide a tentative diagnosis of the situation.

3. *Readiness for change.* The consultant should explore the client's readiness to devote the necessary time and effort to problem identification, and assess the system's ability to accept change.

This initial step also provides the opportunity for both potential client and consultant to explore possible consultation activities before entering into a formal contract.

Negotiation of a Contract

Clear communication and understanding are essential in establishing a collaborative relationship. This stage culminates in the drawing up of a contract, which both parties sign. The formal document defines the purpose of the consultation, describes the qualifications of the consultant, identifies the obligations and the expectations of both parties, and delineates procedures, time constraints, and the method and the amount of compensation.

ASSESSMENT AND COMMUNICATION

Once the consultant has formalized a contract and established open communication with the administrator or another source of power within the system, he or she begins to assess the problem. The consultant draws on professional knowledge, experience, and resources in conjunction with an in-depth study of the client's competence and knowledge. Additionally the consultant becomes familiar with the special terminology and procedures used in the setting, to ensure effective communication and accurate identification of the problem or the needs of the client. The consultant also considers external sources of power such as regulatory agencies, funding sources, and community consumer groups, for they may have a direct influence on the system and the problem at hand.

Diagnostic Analysis Leading to Problem Identification

Preliminary diagnostic work in the entry phase prepares the consultant to perform a more intensive diagnosis of the system, which is essential to the success of any consultation. Study must include an environmental and systems analysis that reveals the organizational structure, the internal and external trends and resources that have an effect on the system, and the corporate culture, mission, and goals. During data collection the consultant should identify both forces that impede movement and forces that facilitate progress (Lewin, 1951).

Goal Setting and Planning Through Establishment of Trust

In addition to helping the consultant identify the needs and the problems of the system, the diagnostic process provides the framework for the next step in consultation, collaborative goal setting and planning. This step aids the consultant in establishing the mutual respect necessary to a successful consultation. It is essential for the consultant to develop a good working relationship with the client in order to identify the desired outcomes of the consultation. Knowledge of formal and informal lines of communication, system politics, key power figures, and the ways in which decision making occurs in the system will enhance the planning phase.

INTERACTIVE PROBLEM RESOLUTION

After thoroughly studying the situation and carefully analyzing the data that he or she has gathered, the consultant begins the process of interactive problem resolution. First, the consultant shares the data with the client. Decisions, though, remain the province of the client. Therefore, if the consultant wishes to help effect change in the system, he or she must collaborate with the client. Interactive problem resolution demonstrates the consultant's commitment to helping the client effect change through collaborative strategy development. This collaborative strategy development has a basis in the consultant's role as a trainer, a facilitator, an educator, a communicator, and a resource person. Participative decision making allows the consultant to facilitate identification of multiple strategies for consideration. The consultant must also demonstrate a commitment to confidentiality and an adherence to professional ethics (see chapter 18, "Ethical Dimensions in Occupational Therapy"). The consultant and the client build a relationship of mutual trust and respect, establishing an open environment in which the client can consider change strategies, using the perspective and the suggestions offered by the consultant.

Maintenance

Implementation of the plans that emerge from the consultation is the maintenance phase. During this phase an internal and external communication network or feedback system is developed that facilitates a review of observations, perceptions, and progress. Through communication and sharing of knowledge, the client and other members of the system develop greater understanding and appreciation of the consultant's occupational performance perspective. During data gathering, the consultant meets and works with a variety of persons who are concerned with the problem at hand. These occasions provide further opportunities to observe the system in action and consider possible solutions. The consultant must be constantly aware of the needs of the persons working in the system and the difficulties that they face when the system is considering change.

During this stage the consultant should identify sources for feedback and reflection. If the consultant is an outsider, he or she may not always perceive and interpret actions and information accurately. Using a variety of techniques—interviews, surveys, group discussions, documentation, and so forth—the consultant should verify information.

EVALUATION AND TERMINATION

The final stage of the consultation process is evaluation and termination. An exit or summary conference usually occurs between the consultant and the client to provide an opportunity for clarification, feedback, evaluation, and discussion of any remaining areas of concern. The consultant prepares a final report containing the following information: dates of service, individuals/departments involved, plan of action and methodology used, findings, assessment, collaborative strategy development, and recommendations, including possible follow-up to allow an avenue for further communication as needed.

Evaluation

The feedback network provides information for evaluation of the consultation. Throughout the consultation activities the consultant monitors and evaluates the outcomes of the intervention. "The evaluation process is an integral part of planning and implementation," providing the data necessary "to clarify goals, refine or revise intervention strategies, and develop future plans" (Jaffe & Epstein, chap. 6, pp. 147–48). Similar to the data gathering performed during the diagnostic phase, evaluation includes both formal and informal methods of assessment. Informal evaluation occurs during the consultant's periodic observations of and feedback from the client, either independently or in collaboration with the client. "Formal evaluation consists of data collection and analysis based on the specific outcome objectives desired from the consultation" (Jaffe & Epstein, 1992, chap. 6, p. 149).

Termination

The consultant and the client should prepare for termination during development of the initial contract when they establish preliminary goals and time frames. Termination may occur at any time during the consultation. The following factors should be considered in the termination phase:

1. *Early or premature termination:* dissatisfaction with the consultation and the consultant-client relationship

2. *Obstacles to termination:* development of mutual dependency in the consultant-client relationship, stability of income for the consultant with the current work, and the client's not being willing to assume the responsibilities generated by the consultation

3. *Easing of termination:* initial delineation of (a) objectives, (b) the limits of the consultation, and (c) the consultant's and the client's responsibility for decision making and implementation

Possible Renegotiation

Contracts may include the possibility of renegotiation at any time in the consultation to allow for changes in or expansion of the goals of the consultation. On termination of the original contract, the parties may decide to renegotiate if the client requests additional help.

Regardless of the setting, the four stages and the eight basic steps provide the foundation for all consultation. An understanding of these stages and steps in the consultation process will help clarify the roles and the functions of the consultant and assist the consultant in providing successful consultation activities.

CONSULTANTS' ROLES

There are many dimensions to the actual role of the consultant. Natural role shifts occur at various stages of consultation as relationships develop, new information becomes available, and the consultant facilitates change. The consultant may be an internal consultant, employed within the system, or an external consultant, brought in from outside the system. He or she may assume a singular role or, more usually, take on multiple roles as the consultation progresses, providing a variety of services depending on the needs and the setting of the client.

Although a setting may call for variations, in current practice the consultant performs the following roles:

1. An *adviser,* a *helper,* a *facilitator* with occupational therapy expertise, who is invited into a system

2. An *outsider,* therefore an external consultant, with no formal
   authority in a system

3. A *change agent,* using knowledge of the system, its goals, and its
   objectives to effect positive change

4. An *evaluator-diagnostician,* identifying problems

5. A *clarifier,* helping a client analyze and understand a problem
   objectively

6. A *trainer,* providing opportunities to learn skills that will aid in the
   development of short- and long-term goals

7. A *planner,* collaborating with the client to develop or modify
   long-range plans

8. An *extender,* providing occupational therapy assessment and
   developing maintenance programs to be carried out by the client
   when direct treatment services are not feasible or appropriate

EXTERNAL VERSUS INTERNAL CONSULTATION

The way in which the consultant perceives a client and is perceived by
the client depends to a large extent on whether the consultant is inside the
system or outside it. An *internal consultant* is an employee of the client system who is asked to provide consultation services within the organization.
An *external consultant* is an independent agent, outside the organization,
with whom the client contracts to provide consultation services.

Role expectations for both the client and the consultant, the consultant's behavior, the consultant's frames of reference, and the consultant's
choice of roles are directly related to the consultant's relationship with the
system. It is important for the consultant to understand this. As an employee, the internal consultant is an integral part of the system, with knowledge of the corporate culture and the strengths and the weaknesses of the
organization. This may or may not be considered an advantage, depending on the needs of the organization. The outsider, or external consultant,
may have a fresh, objective perspective. Each type of consultant has advantages and disadvantages. Administrators should base their choice of an
internal or an external consultant on the specific problems and the needs
of the system.

THE NONDIRECTIVE-DIRECTIVE CONTINUUM

Lippitt and Lippitt (1986) have described the consultant's roles as dynamic components of the consultant's work. They present the multiple roles
of the consultant as occurring along a continuum from nondirective to
directive (see figure 15-1). In a *nondirective role* the consultant collects and
provides data as a guide for problem solving by the client, whereas in a

directive role the consultant provides active leadership in directing activities to enhance the client's skills. Frequently the consultant begins a relationship in a nondirective role, during the diagnostic phase of environmental and systems analysis. As the consultation progresses, he or she may shift to a more directive position of educating and training clients. The consultant must be aware when the need for change arises and adjust the role accordingly. Change efforts will be effective only if the consultant is aware of when and how to shift and is proficient in the behavioral characteristics of the particular role required in a situation.

Occupational therapy practitioners are familiar with many of the roles of the consultant and have used them in practice. In a therapeutic relationship the practitioner appropriately assumes a more active role in problem resolution. In a consultative relationship the consultant collaborates with the client to help define and clarify the problem, consider options, and establish a course of action.

The consultant does not make decisions; the client does. This is true even when the consultant assumes a more directive role, such as that of trainer/educator. Here the consultant trains the client, who assumes the active role after gaining information from the educational process.

Another example is the provision of consultation in the role of information specialist. Using their expertise, occupational therapy consultants provide special knowledge, as is evident in the example previously presented. In such a situation the consultant assumes a more directive role, but the client remains in control, defining the problem and the objectives of the consultation.

Rogers and Wood (1992) illustrate the more directive roles in their description of consultation in an acute psychiatric hospital. Bachner (1992) discusses performance of the more directive roles in a consultation on a client with developmental disabilities residing in a group home. Donna Weiss (1992), a consultant to a regional special services school commission, explains important strategies that she used with preschool teachers and staff while performing the more directive roles of joint problem solver, educator and trainer, and information specialist. The commission engaged her services to help ensure effective incorporation of sensorimotor learning into the preschool classroom routine.

ROLE PREPARATION

In any given consultation experience the consultant may need to assume several roles. The consultant must be knowledgeable with regard to the various role possibilities and should develop a role repertoire that fits his or her individual style and personality, as well as the specific needs of the client.

Figure 15-1
Multiple Roles of the Consultant

Objective Observer	Process Counselor	Fact Finder	Identifier of Alternatives and Linker to Resources	Joint Problem Solver	Trainer/ Educator	Information Specialist	Advocate
Raises questions for reflection	Observes problem-solving process and raises issues mirroring feedback	Gathers data and stimulates thinking	Identifies alternatives and resources for client and helps assess consequences	Offers alternatives and participates in decisions	Trains client	Regards, links, and provides policy or practice decisions	Proposes guidelines, persuades, or directs in the problem-solving process

Client   Consultant

Nondirective ← Level of Consultant Activity in Problem Solving → Directive

Note. *Adapted from* The Consulting Process in Action *(2nd ed., p. 61), by G. Lippitt and R. Lippitt. Copyright ©1986 by Pfeiffer & Company, San Diego, CA. Used with permission.*

The varied environments in which consultants practice call on them to use flexibility and creativity as part of their role. To meet today's pressing demands for occupational therapy service and to respond to continued growth in demand, greater numbers of practitioners will need to assume consultant roles. As they do, they may find it helpful to recall Mazer's (1969) action model of consultation: "Community consultation in occupational therapy must mean using professional expertise to enable people to grow and heal other people more effectively" (p. 420).

CONSULTATION SKILLS AND KNOWLEDGE

The occupational therapy philosophy of helping others do for themselves carries over naturally into consultation. Knowledge and professional competence in occupational therapy and an understanding of professional ethics and behavior (see chapter 18, "Ethical Dimensions in Occupational Therapy") help provide a sound foundation for developing consultation skills. So do education and training in such areas as human development and group process. Professional experience as a supervisor and a manager adds to a consultant's qualifications, as does an expanded knowledge base.

Numerous authors have identified areas of knowledge critical in consultation. These include systems theory and behavioral sciences; developmental theory as it applies to individuals, groups, organizations, and communities; education and training methodologies, including problem solving and role playing; human personality, attitude formation, and change; and self-knowledge (Gallessich, 1982; Gilfoyle, 1992; Jaffe & Epstein, chaps. 5, 6; Lippitt & Lippitt, 1986).

"A mutually supportive and synergistic relationship can exist between direct treatment roles and indirect consultation approaches" (Jaffe & Epstein, 1992, chap. 42, p. 683). In both cases there is recognition and appreciation of the environment as a critical factor. Principles of human ecology apply as well. "Understanding and effectively utilizing these approaches help reinforce the important role of the environment for both therapist/consultant and patient/client. Thus the occupational therapy treatment/consultation interaction bonds these processes together" (p. 683). Figure 15-2 illustrates the similarity between these two processes, while acknowledging their uniquenesses.

Key skills that the consultant must possess are communicating, educating, diagnosing, and linking. To employ these skills successfully, the consultant must also be able to establish effective interpersonal relationships. Attitudes and attributes such as flexibility, creativity, maturity, and self-confidence help the consultant move successfully in varied environments.

COMMUNICATING

Communicating is a primary consultation skill. It encompasses more than verbal and written abilities. Body language, role modeling, use of analogies, reflection, and confrontation may all be incorporated into it. Similarly the ability to listen to what is—and is not—said, and to how it is presented, provides valuable insight. The consultation environment communicates too. A working space with walls covered by lists of rules, regulations, and procedures conveys a very different message from one whose walls and shelves contain interesting artwork and growing plants.

Written and oral communication must take into consideration differences in language usage in the consultation setting. In school settings, industry, and day-care centers, for example, catchphrases or special terms may be used as part of the communication process. Outsiders unfamiliar with this language may feel cut off from meaningful dialogue. Occupational therapy personnel also use special terms and phrases that may not be understood in community environments. When consultants use professional terminology, they must define their terms in the client's language.

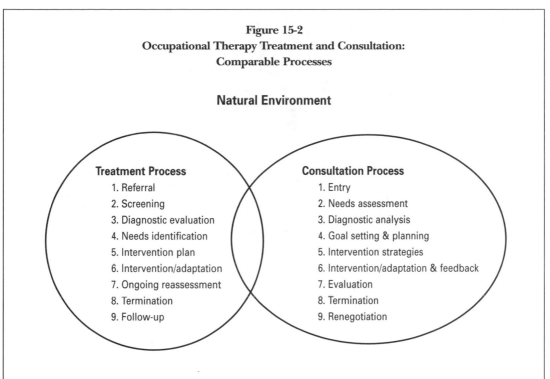

Figure 15-2
Occupational Therapy Treatment and Consultation:
Comparable Processes

Natural Environment

Treatment Process
1. Referral
2. Screening
3. Diagnostic evaluation
4. Needs identification
5. Intervention plan
6. Intervention/adaptation
7. Ongoing reassessment
8. Termination
9. Follow-up

Consultation Process
1. Entry
2. Needs assessment
3. Diagnostic analysis
4. Goal setting & planning
5. Intervention strategies
6. Intervention/adaptation & feedback
7. Evaluation
8. Termination
9. Renegotiation

Note. *From "Toward a Theoretical Model of Occupational Therapy Consultation" (chap. 42, p. 684), by E. G. Jaffe and C. F. Epstein, 1992, in E. G. Jaffe and C. F. Epstein (Eds.),* Occupational Therapy Consultation: Theory, Principles, and Practice, *St. Louis, MO: Mosby–Year Book. Copyright ©1992 by Mosby–Year Book. Adapted with permission.*

EDUCATING

Training and educating are basic components of consultation. The consultant may use a variety of methods to help broaden the client's skills and further develop his or her abilities to effect change independently. Designing and leading workshops is one such method (Cunninghis, 1992; Ellexson, 1992; Izutsu, 1992; Jacobs, 1992; Jaffe & Epstein, 1992, chap. 28). Using this approach, the consultant is able to present new material, and the client is able to participate actively through experiential learning. Special audiovisual materials and computerized instructional programs may be used, allowing the client to proceed at a comfortable pace, with built-in opportunities for feedback and discussion (Weiss, 1992). The materials must be clearly presented and relevant for the client.

DIAGNOSING

Occupational therapy practitioners are most familiar with assessment technology as it pertains to diagnosis and treatment of persons who are dysfunctional. Consultation calls for a more global perspective. Moving into a dysfunctional system, the consultant must gather data from a variety of sources in collaboration with the client. As the consultant reviews and assesses data, he or she obtains feedback, which helps in verification and clarification before the consultant reaches a final diagnosis or conclusion. The consultant must have the ability to diagnose problems; to locate sources of help, power, and influence; to understand the client's values and culture; and to determine readiness for change (Lippitt & Lippitt, 1986).

LINKING

Linking is a skill that comes naturally to occupational therapy practitioners. As proponents of adaptation, they constantly identify resources and alternative methods to help achieve a particular goal. The consultant links the client to appropriate resources both within and outside the consultation environment. A consultant, for example, may learn about new and competitive sources for equipment and supplies when consulting with one organization. He or she may link these resources to another client, when appropriate.

ESTABLISHING EFFECTIVE INTERPERSONAL RELATIONSHIPS

Establishing effective interpersonal relationships requires an understanding of the client's value system and attitudes, and the external and internal pressures on the system. These all have a bearing on the capacity to change. For example, pressured by time and environment, an aide finds it quicker, easier, and less frustrating to feed a child who is able to eat independently with adaptive equipment. Yet the aide also wants to further the child's independence. The consultant's task is to help the aide and other team members understand the importance of self-care so that it becomes a first priority. The consultant's task also involves working with the aide's supervisors so that they will find methods of modifying time and environmental constraints and thus foster change in the aide's behavior. To develop such a collaborative relationship, the consultant must have a sincere interest in the client and must gain the client's confidence and respect.

EXHIBITING CERTAIN ATTITUDES AND ATTRIBUTES

Consultation requires a high degree of self-direction, comfort with taking risks, and ease in working without a formalized support system. Satisfaction for a job well done comes through the success achieved by the client. This indirect type of gratification necessitates a strong sense of security and self-confidence on the part of the consultant.

Maturity, flexibility, a sense of humor, and a sense of timing are also important. At times a crisis shunts the original consultation problem aside. The consultant may come prepared to deal with one problem and find the system's priority to be quite different. At such a moment no one is amenable to considering lesser issues, and the consultant must help resolve the more pressing problem.

The consultant must make a realistic appraisal of his or her limitations and abilities. Everyone cannot be an expert at everything. When additional skills are required, the consultant should have the confidence to acknowledge this and to suggest other resources, one of which may be the client.

ON BECOMING A CONSULTANT

When forging into new and less secure settings, consultants should follow the Scout motto, "Be prepared." They should consider current and future consultation environments. They should create a marketing plan based on careful study of economic factors (see chapter 4, "Marketing"). Further, they should develop and use resources appropriately. The "business of being in business" can then become a reality.

CURRENT AND FUTURE CONSULTATION ENVIRONMENTS

Occupational therapy consultants can be found in private practices, in public and private school systems, in industry, in occupational therapy departments of hospitals and rehabilitation centers that have community outreach programming, and in schools of occupational therapy whose faculty members provide community- and campus-based consultation. A small number serve as administrative consultants for state and federal governments, national health organizations, insurance companies, accrediting agencies, and other national groups concerned with health issues.

They provide services in unusual and familiar settings. Some of the more unusual settings include prisons, Native American reservations, programs dealing with abuse of children and elderly persons, and women's crisis centers. The most familiar settings for occupational therapy consultants are school systems, community mental health centers, and nursing homes. Consultants also advise architects and designers, and analyze the occupational performance of employees to help plan more appropriate and efficient work environments.

Current health planning has finally moved toward firm support of a health promotion model of care. The emphasis on primary prevention can be seen in the growing use of health maintenance organizations (HMOs) and other managed care plans that provide all necessary medical care, including routine health screenings and other preventive measures, for a fixed yearly fee, or *capitation*. Capitation has reduced referrals to health professionals, requiring many to change from a direct service model to a consultation model. Limitations require prioritization of services, especially for practitioners in acute care settings. The emerging hospital model views the practitioner as a consultant who assesses the patient and makes recommendations regarding individual needs for services that will be provided after discharge (Marmer, 1995a).

Grady (1995) predicts that occupational therapy practice in the 21st century will be in the community. It will require a collaborative practice model in which practitioner, client, family, and close community members communicate effectively on behalf of the individual consumer of occupational therapy services. This perspective supports the growth of occupational therapy consultation in current and new markets. Growing community-based areas of concern will include poverty, advocacy, and independent living (Marmer, 1995b).

Today's technologically oriented information society requires occupational therapy consultants to be more knowledgeable regarding the use of robotics and computers (Post, 1992; Struck, 1994). Their expertise in using occupation as a health determinant and their understanding of the effect that activity—or lack of it—has on health will be important assets in the society of the future. The occupational therapy consultant's unique perspective will also help persons experiencing deficits in occupational performance related to living and working in space, underground, or undersea.

MARKETING OF CONSULTATION SERVICES

Success at consultation is intimately related to successful marketing (see chapter 4, "Marketing"). Using a marketing perspective, the consultant performs an in-depth analysis of both the market that he or she has targeted and the ability of the business to be responsive. Establishing an effective marketing mix, the consultant identifies a needed consultation service (a product) in a particular market; prices this service competitively; provides a persuasive proposal to a potential client; and uses creative promotional strategies to build a referral base. Recognizing the value of marketing, the consultant dedicates time, energy, and money to this aspect of business.

Having defined an area of competence and potential practice environments, and having readied a marketing plan, the consultant is ready to develop a promotion plan (see chapter 5, "The Targeting of Communications"). This requires knowing the target market and the potential for acceptance of the service. It also means identifying all possible activities that can generate referrals or recommended clients. For example:

1. Promoting one's services through such tools as professional brochures, letters, business cards, and yellow page listings

2. Networking with fellow practitioners, professionals in allied fields, and former clients and agency personnel who are advocates of one's competence

3. Doing research, drawing on health planning reports, economic indicators of growing health services, local health classified ads, and state department of health listings of potential user agencies and organizations

The potential consultant must be willing to contribute time and energy to community activities that focus on health concerns. Providing free lectures, assisting in planning and running special programs, and participating in committees and on boards not only heighten a consultant's visibility but expand his or her knowledge base and resource network.

Using a sales promotion technique, the consultant might offer free information on a subject of interest to potential clients. An example might be current information on new rulings pertaining to the Americans with Disabilities Act. Public relations strategies are important. These include news releases, articles published by the consultant, and lectures at meetings where potential clients gather.

Personal selling is the core promotional tool for the consultant. "Marketing makes the task of selling easier; it sets expectations, it informs, it educates" (Shenson, 1990, p. 6). The consultation literature indicates that personal referral is the most effective sales strategy (Holtz, 1988; Schrello, 1990; Shenson, 1990).

Consultation is a service product. It is intangible, directly related to the consultant providing the service. As such, it is also inseparable from the consultant's perspective and his or her interactions with the client. Consultation services are perishable. If a limited or fluctuating market exists, the consultant can be without work. Therefore, marketing must be a continuous process for the consultant. Indeed, the consultant must integrate consistent and meaningful marketing into his or her management of the consultation practice.

DEVELOPMENT AND USE OF RESOURCES

Developing the competence necessary to provide consultation services means devoting time, money, and creative energy to building up a "hip-pocket necessity"—resources. Not only are resources important in a given consultation setting; they also provide a natural support system for the consultant, who often practices in isolation. Included in this category are people, places, literature, educational experiences, and political and economic concerns.

One often hears, "It is not *what* you know, but *whom* you know." This statement needs modification for the consultant: "It is *what and whom* you know that help make you successful." Experience alone, within a sheltered setting, will not expand the consultant's knowledge base for consultation. Meeting other professionals within and outside occupational therapy helps broaden the consultant's perspective, heighten the consultant's awareness of important trends, and alert the consultant to changes affecting health care practice.

Networking through local and national professional organizations is a method for the consultant to build a natural support system. It also helps the consultant develop a roster of experts who can provide needed information, advice, or direction on a specific problem. Membership in community and other professional organizations, and participation in meetings and committees extend the resource network. Field visits also stimulate information sharing and networking, and help provide perspective on geographic and socioeconomic differences that influence the responses of a given system.

Continuing education for the consultant includes extensive review of professional and related literature, and attendance at occupational therapy and multidisciplinary conferences and workshops. As well as maintaining and improving the consultant's competence, these activities help the consultant stay abreast of changes, trends, and emerging issues affecting the health care market. They also increase the consultant's familiarity with differences in language usage and terminology, thus enhancing his or her communication skills.

Economics and politics play major roles in shaping the delivery of today's health care. Pending legislation, newly enacted laws, changes in reimbursement methodologies, and revised guidelines for service provision all have significant implications. Continuing review of current publications and special newsletters aids the consultant in staying up-to-date.

Judicious use of resources helps maintain a broad and well-rounded knowledge base. This expanded perspective, with its related support system, encourages creativity and flexibility. A commitment to continued development of resources allows the consultant and the client to draw from a comprehensive and current pool of information.

THE BUSINESS OF BEING IN BUSINESS

A decision to own and operate a business is a significant step for any practitioner. The considerations and the complexities of entrepreneurship require major commitments of time, energy, and money. Self-education, risk-taking abilities, and organizational and management skills are important prerequisites.

Today's entrepreneur-practitioner may be a self-employed person, a partner in a group practice, or an owner or a part-owner of a corporation. Each of these options has particular legal, economic, and tax considerations. Each also has different practice benefits with regard to sharing responsibilities, caseloads, resources, and support systems.

Forms of Business

Self-Employment

In a solo practice the practitioner is responsible for all the work performed and has full control of the business. As a sole proprietor, he or she must keep detailed records of any and all income and expenses. The sole proprietor must also pay estimated taxes to cover income tax and Social Security obligations. He or she may set aside a portion of earnings in a retirement plan.

Developing a fee structure requires that the prospective consultant consider labor costs (his or her current salary and benefits), overhead (business costs), the area's going rate for consultation services, and a reasonable profit. The prospective consultant then divides this sum by the number of hours or days that he or she expects to work, plus those usually allocated for sick time, vacations, professional development, and marketing. For example:

> Ann Jones, OTR, is establishing a consultation business. She currently earns $60,000 per year. This includes all holidays and other leave days for a total of 260 paid days per year. Her compensation is therefore approximately $230 per day. Ann knows that she will need many unpaid days to establish and market her new business. She estimates that she will be able to bill a total of 180 days to clients. Therefore she must charge approximately $330 per day to maintain her salary level. Ann estimates her overhead, her other cost, at $36,000 per year, or $200 per billable day. She thus calculates that she needs a minimum of $530 per day for her billable days. Consultants in her region charge anywhere from $450 to $650 per day. Ann decides to charge $550 per day, keeping herself in the middle of the market pricing.

Although it is appropriate for a consultant to research the current market value of a service in the geographic area that he or she has targeted, the antitrust laws prohibit competitors from fixing prices for services. Occupational therapy practitioners in consultation or private practice are in competition under the antitrust laws and must be cautious about how they obtain their information.

Many tax deductions are possible in maintaining a business. A consultant must itemize and document any that he or she takes. Malpractice insurance, which is necessary to protect the consultant from liability, is an important deduction. A room in his or her home that a consultant uses solely for business may qualify for an office-in-home deduction. Other possible deductions include travel expenses when away overnight, a per-mile rate for an automobile used to conduct business, professional dues, the cost of subscriptions to professional journals, fees and expenses for continuing education, the cost of uniforms, and child care expenses.

A self-employed practitioner may hire other people. These people become employees, and the employer is responsible for making timely payroll deductions, providing benefits, and establishing written policies and procedures for the business.

Practicing alone offers the consultant great freedom and control. It means developing support systems and backup arrangements, though, for the times when the consultant cannot meet an obligation.

Partnership

In a group practice the consultant participates as a partner. Partners share some expenses, such as overhead, whereas they bear other expenses, such as transportation, as individual partners. Partners allocate income according to a formula on which they agree. In general, the rules for individual proprietorships apply to partnerships.

Professionally a partnership can have many rewards. It fosters mutual support, facilitates a sharing of ideas and expertise, builds in a backup system, and, by virtue of its size, offers expanded visibility and marketability.

Incorporation

Some consultants choose incorporation. Those who incorporate expect to generate a large volume of work and usually employ others. A major advantage of a corporation is that it is considered a legal entity. If the business goes under or a client sues, the corporation takes responsibility, not the officers. (This does not preclude the need for practitioner-owners to hold professional liability insurance.) If money must be borrowed to set up the corporation or expand it, the corporation is the legally responsible party.

Some advantages of a corporation include expanded pension and other fringe benefits, such as health insurance, continuing education, and limited personal liability. The company can also reimburse officers and employees for expenses incurred as part of the business, rather than their having to deduct the expenses from their income.

Planning

The world of business may be a new and unfamiliar place for the occupational therapy practitioner. Stepping into it requires research, in-depth planning, and professional advice. A broad array of books, periodicals, and organizations are available as resources to practitioners contemplating this step. Specific books, pamphlets, and articles detailing occupational therapy private practice should be reviewed during the preliminary planning period (Hertfelder & Crispen, 1990; Jaffe & Epstein, 1992; Ryan, 1988).

The prospective consultant should develop a business plan to provide an overall framework for the practice and a basis for decision making. It should include an assessment of the consultation market being targeted; a statement of mission and goals; a business concept; and an organizational plan. The aspiring entrepreneur should seek guidance from financial and legal advisers. At this important juncture their knowledge will be critical in making final decisions regarding such issues as self-employment versus partnership or incorporation, and in developing contract formats for use with potential clients.

Being in business for oneself can be an exciting and rewarding experience. Although there are many risks, numerous frustrations, and extensive commitments, this model of practice is attracting increasing numbers of practitioners. The satisfaction of building a business, the opportunities offered in new markets, and the freedom of self-direction are among the many dividends.

CONCLUSION

Consultation is a rapidly expanding area of occupational therapy practice. As the pool of experienced practitioners increases and as settings diversify and proliferate, consultants are playing major roles in shaping future practice.

Practitioners at every level of practice should take advantage of daily opportunities to build their consultation skills. With greater experience they can attempt more complex consultation tasks. As occupational therapy practitioners increase their visibility, they must expand their knowledge of consultation, the health care system, and the issues and the trends that affect the system's growth. Maintaining and improving professional competence and quality improvement in service delivery are critical factors for the successful practice of occupational therapy consultants. Experience and competence are hallmarks of the community consultant, who will continue to forge new roles and directions for the profession.

Consulting has emerged as a major force in the health care arena, the business world, and society in general. Occupational therapy's role in prevention of disability and promotion of health will continue to grow with the expansion of consultation services. The consultant model presented in this chapter is based on a human ecology perspective. These concepts will help prepare the practitioners of today and tomorrow to function in a world of rapid change.

SUMMARY

Consultation is the interactive process of helping others solve existing or potential problems by identifying and analyzing issues, developing strategies to address problems, and preventing future problems from occurring. The *client*, the person or the system seeking help, uses consultation to improve planning and interaction with colleagues, consumers, or employees (Lippitt & Lippitt, 1986; Ulschak & SnowAntle, 1990).

Jaffe and Epstein (1992, chap. 42) have proposed a theoretical model of consultation that "integrates occupational therapy and consultation concepts within an ecological framework" (p. 709). The model is based on the milieu or *environment* in which the consultative activities occur; the application of the *human ecological perspective* of the client; *collaboration* between the consultant and the client; the *adaptation* or change facilitated by this collaborative approach; and ultimately the *enablement* of the client to achieve *improved function* and maximize his or her *human potential*.

Changing legislative priorities, economic and social issues, continued advances in technology, and an expanding system of managed care in the provision of health services have profoundly influenced the growing demand for consultation services. As the 21st century begins, opportunities in new markets will continue to emerge.

Models of consultation are drawn from many fields of study. Jaffe and Epstein (1992, chap. 2) identify nine theoretical models. Further, they explain that consultation occurs on different levels, as the situation requires.

Concepts of prevention are inherent in all consultation. Jaffe and Epstein (1992, chap. 2) describe three types: primary, secondary, and tertiary. As a consultant, the occupational therapy practitioner must understand basic prevention principles and use them to achieve *preventive outcomes*. Related to the three levels of consultation, these are the results achieved through consultation activities.

Successful consultation outcomes begin with careful analysis and planning. An environmental and systems analysis is an important preliminary step.

Consultation occurs in four stages and, within them, eight basic steps: (1) initiation and clarification, including (a) entry into the system and (b) negotiation of a contract; (2) assessment and communication, including (a) diagnostic analysis leading to problem identification and (b) goal setting and planning through establishment of trust; (3) interactive problem resolution, including (a) maintenance; and (4) evaluation and termination, including (a) evaluation, (b) termination, and (c) possible renegotiation.

In current practice the consultant performs many roles: adviser, helper, facilitator, outsider, change agent, evaluator-diagnostician, clarifier, trainer, planner, and extender. The way in which the consultant perceives a client and is perceived by the client depends to a large extent on whether the consultant is inside the system, an internal consultant, or outside it, an external consultant. Lippitt and Lippitt (1986) present the multiple roles of the consultant as occurring along a continuum from nondirective to directive. In any given consultation experience the consultant may need to assume several roles.

Areas of knowledge critical in consultation include systems theory and behavioral sciences; developmental theory; education and training methodologies; human personality, attitude formation, and change; and self-knowledge. Key skills that the consultant must possess are communicating, educating, diagnosing, and linking. The consultant must also be able to establish effective interpersonal relationships. Attitudes and attributes such as flexibility, creativity, maturity, and self-confidence help the consultant move successfully in varied environments.

When forging into new and less secure settings, consultants should follow the Scout motto, "Be prepared." They should consider current and future consultation environments. They should create a marketing plan based on careful study of economic factors. A critically important activity is developing resources through such endeavors as networking, membership in other organizations, continuing education, and the monitoring of current economic and political developments.

Today's entrepreneur-practitioner may be a self-employed person, a partner in a group practice, or an owner or a part-owner of a corporation. Each of these options has particular legal, economic, and tax considerations. Each also has different practice benefits with regard to sharing responsibilities, caseloads, resources, and support systems.

A decision to own and operate a business is a significant step for any practitioner. The considerations and the complexities require major commitments of time, energy, and money. Being in business for oneself can be an exciting and rewarding experience, however.

Consulting has emerged as a major force in the health care arena, the business world, and society in general. Occupational therapy's role in prevention of disability and promotion of health will continue to grow with the expansion of consultation services.

REFERENCES

American Occupational Therapy Association. (1990). *1990 member data survey.* Rockville, MD: Author.

American Occupational Therapy Association. (1994). Uniform terminology for occupational therapists (3rd ed.). *American Journal of Occupational Therapy, 48,* 1047–54.

American Occupational Therapy Association. (1995). Concept paper: Service delivery in occupational therapy. *American Journal of Occupational Therapy, 49,* 1029–31.

American Occupational Therapy Association Occupational Therapy Roles Task Force. (1993). Occupational therapy roles. *American Journal of Occupational Therapy, 47,* 1087–99.

Americans with Disabilities Act of 1990, Pub. L. No. 101–336, 104 Stat. 327.

AOTA consultant networks go worldwide. (1995, December 7). *OT Week,* p. 4.

Bachner, S. (1992). Occupational therapy consultation in developmental disabilities. In E. G. Jaffe & C. F. Epstein (Eds.), *Occupational therapy consultation: Theory, principles, and practice* (chap. 24, pp. 408–18). St. Louis, MO: Mosby–Year Book.

Bain, B. K. (1992). Environmental control unit consultation. In E. G. Jaffe & C. F. Epstein (Eds.), *Occupational therapy consultation: Theory, principles, and practice* (chap. 36, pp. 575–80). St. Louis, MO: Mosby–Year Book.

The budget revolution: Special report. (1995, May 22). *Time,* pp. 30–41.

Carlson, M. (1995, September 25). Mother's work. *Time,* p. 30.

Christenson, M. (1996). Adaptations for vision changes in the elderly. *Occupational Therapy Practice, 1*(1), 30–33.

Cunninghis, R. N. (1992). Activities consultation in long-term care settings. In E. G. Jaffe & C. F. Epstein (Eds.), *Occupational therapy consultation: Theory, principles, and practice* (chap. 12, pp. 254–62). St. Louis, MO: Mosby–Year Book.

Devereaux, E. B. (1992). Occupational therapy consultation in health care consortiums: Systems/program consultation. In E. G. Jaffe & C. F. Epstein (Eds.), *Occupational therapy consultation: Theory, principles, and practice* (chap. 19, pp. 338–52). St. Louis, MO: Mosby–Year Book.

Dunn, W. (1985). Therapists as consultants to educators. *Sensory Integration Special Interest Section Newsletter, 8*(1), 1–2.

Dunn, W. (1988). Models of occupational therapy service provision in the school system. *American Journal of Occupational Therapy, 42,* 718–23.

Dunn, W. (1992). Occupational therapy collaborative consultation in schools. In E. G. Jaffe & C. F. Epstein (Eds.), *Occupational therapy consultation: Theory, principles, and practice* (chap. 9, pp. 210–36). St. Louis, MO: Mosby–Year Book.

Dunn, W., Brown, C., & McGuigan, A. (1994). The ecology of human performance: A framework for considering the effect of context. *American Journal of Occupational Therapy, 48,* 595–607.

Education for All Handicapped Children Act of 1975, Pub. L. No. 94–142, 89 Stat. 773.

Ellexson, M. T. (1992). Industrial consultation as an internal consultant. In E. G. Jaffe & C. F. Epstein (Eds.), *Occupational therapy consultation: Theory, principles, and practice* (chap. 27, pp. 445–60). St. Louis, MO: Mosby–Year Book.

Epstein, C. F. (1979). Directions in long-term care. *Gerontology Specialty Section Newsletter, 2*(4), 1, 4.

Epstein, C. F. (1992). Long term care. In H. L. Hopkins & H. D. Smith (Eds.), *Willard and Spackman's Occupational therapy* (8th ed., pp. 816–21). Philadelphia: Lippincott.

Gallessich, J. (1982). *The profession and practice of consultation.* San Francisco: Jossey-Bass.

Gilfoyle, E. M. (1992). Future directions: Vital connections. In E. G. Jaffe & C. F. Epstein (Eds.), *Occupational therapy consultation: Theory, principles, and practice* (epilogue, pp. 777–83). St. Louis, MO: Mosby–Year Book.

Grady, A. P. (1992). Technology adoption: Linking through communication. In E. G. Jaffe & C. F. Epstein (Eds.), *Occupational therapy consultation: Theory, principles, and practice* (chap. 37, pp. 581–90). St. Louis, MO: Mosby–Year Book.

Grady, A. (1995). Building inclusive community: A challenge for occupational therapy [1994 Eleanor Clarke Slagle Lecture]. *American Journal of Occupational Therapy, 49,* 300–10.

Grossman, J. (1977). Preventive health care and community programming [Nationally Speaking]. *American Journal of Occupational Therapy, 31,* 351–54.

Hanft, B., & Place, P. (1996). *The consulting therapist: A guide for physical and occupational therapists in schools.* Tucson, AZ: Therapy Skill Builders.

Hertfelder, S. D., & Crispen, C. (Eds.). (1990). *Private practice: Strategies for success.* Rockville, MD: American Occupational Therapy Association.

Holtz, H. (1988). *How to succeed as an independent consultant* (2nd ed.). New York: Wiley.

Individuals with Disabilities Education Act of 1990, Pub. L. No. 101–476, 104 Stat. 1142.

Izutsu, S. (1992). Program consultation to agencies in developing countries. In E. G. Jaffe & C. F. Epstein (Eds.), *Occupational therapy consultation: Theory, principles, and practice* (chap. 34, pp. 548–56). St. Louis, MO: Mosby–Year Book.

Jacobs, K. (1992). Occupational therapy consultation in business and industry. In E. G. Jaffe & C. F. Epstein (Eds.), *Occupational therapy consultation: Theory, principles, and practice* (chap. 26, pp. 434–44). St. Louis, MO: Mosby–Year Book.

Jaffe, E. G. (1980). The role of the occupational therapist as a community consultant: Primary prevention in mental health programming. *Occupational Therapy in Mental Health, 1*(2), 47–62.

Jaffe, E. G. (1986). Prevention, "an idea whose time has come": The role of occupational therapy in disease prevention and health promotion. *American Journal of Occupational Therapy, 40,* 749–52.

Jaffe, E. G., & Epstein, C. F. (Eds.). (1992). *Occupational therapy consultation: Theory, principles, and practice.* St. Louis, MO: Mosby–Year Book.
Chap. 2, Theoretical concepts of consultation (pp. 15–54), by Jaffe.
Chap. 5, Preparation for consultation (pp. 118–34), by Jaffe.
Chap. 6, The process of consultation (pp. 135–66), by Jaffe & Epstein.
Chap. 25, Adult day-care consultation in a rural community (pp. 419–30), by Epstein.
Chap. 28, Health education consultation in the workplace (pp. 461–77), by Jaffe.
Chap. 42, Toward a theoretical model of occupational therapy consultation (pp. 676–713), by Jaffe & Epstein.

Kauffman, S. H. (1992). Occupational therapy consultation for adult rehabilitation program standards and regulations. In E. G. Jaffe & C. F. Epstein (Eds.), *Occupational therapy consultation: Theory, principles, and practice* (chap. 31, pp. 504–18). St. Louis, MO: Mosby–Year Book.

Kelly, S., Walsh, J., & Thompson, K. (1991). Birth outcomes, health problems and neglect with prenatal exposure of cocaine. *Pediatric Nursing, 17,* 130–36.

Kornblau, B. (1992). Legal issues in occupational therapy consultation. In E. G. Jaffe & C. F. Epstein (Eds.), *Occupational therapy consultation: Theory, principles, and practice* (chap. 38, pp. 594–621). St. Louis, MO: Mosby–Year Book.

Lewin, K. (1951). *Theory in social science.* New York: Harper.

Lifter, K. (1993). Implementation of the consultative approach in the classroom in support of related services: Guidelines for special service providers. *Special Services in the Schools, 7,* 145–66.

Lippitt, G., & Lippitt, R. (1986). *The consulting process in action* (2nd ed.). San Diego: University Associates.

Marmer, L. (1995a, February 13). Prioritizing care: Necessary for low staffed, high volume clinics. *Advance for Occupational Therapists,* p. 19.

Marmer, L. (1995b, May 9). Community-based OTs: Short on needed skills? *Advance for Occupational Therapists,* pp. 11, 50.

Mazer, J. L. (1969). The occupational therapist as consultant. *American Journal of Occupational Therapy, 23,* 417–21.

McDonnell, A., McDonnell, J., Hardman, M., & McCune, G. (1991). Educating students with severe disabilities in their neighborhood school: The Utah Elementary Integration Model. *Remedial and Special Education, 12*(6), 34–45.

Morrow, L. (1995, December 25). Newt's world. *Time,* pp. 50–51.

Parks, R. A. (1994). Occupational therapy with children who are HIV positive. *Developmental Disabilities Special Interest Section Newsletter, 4*(1), 5–6.

Partners in Caregiving. (1995). *Life after diagnosis: Adult day services in America.* Winston-Salem, NC: Wake Forest University, Bowman-Gray School of Medicine.

Patterson, V. (1994, December 8). Caution: Home safety hazards ahead. *OT Week,* p. 16.

Peak Parent Center. (1988). *Strategy ideas for supporting students in regular classes: Discover the possibilities.* Colorado Springs, CO: Author.

Post, K. M. (1992). Technology consultation: The leading edge. In E. G. Jaffe & C. F. Epstein (Eds.), *Occupational therapy consultation: Theory, principles, and practice* (chap. 35, pp. 560–74). St. Louis, MO: Mosby–Year Book.

Rogers, J. C., & Wood, W. (1992). Consultative models in geriatric psychiatry. In E. G. Jaffe & C. F. Epstein (Eds.), *Occupational therapy consultation: Theory, principles, and practice* (chap. 16, pp. 293–310). St. Louis, MO: Mosby–Year Book.

Rourk, J. D. (1992). The occupational therapist as a state education agency consultant. In E. G. Jaffe & C. F. Epstein (Eds.), *Occupational therapy consultation: Theory, principles, and practice* (chap. 8, pp. 195–209). St. Louis, MO: Mosby–Year Book.

Ryan, M. C. (1988). Getting started in private practice. *American Occupational Therapy Association Administration and Management Special Interest Section Newsletter, 4*(2), 1–3.

Samson, L. (1992). Consultancy issues concerning accessibility. In E. G. Jaffe & C. F. Epstein (Eds.), *Occupational therapy consultation: Theory, principles, and practice* (chap. 22, pp. 385–94). St. Louis, MO: Mosby–Year Book.

Schrello, D. M. (1990). *The complete marketing handbook for consultants.* San Diego: University Associates.

Shenson, H. L. (1990). *Shenson on consulting.* New York: Wiley.

Struck, M. (Ed.). (1994). Assistive technology in the schools [Special issue]. *School System Special Interest Section Newsletter, 1*(3), 1–4.

Teachers union limits "inclusion" in policy on special-needs pupils. (1994, July 7). *Star Ledger* (Newark, NJ), p. 15.

Technology-Related Assistance for Individuals with Disabilities Act of 1988, Pub. L. No. 100–407, 102 Stat. 1044.

Ulschak, F. L, & SnowAntle, S. M. (1990). *Consultation skills for heath care professionals.* San Francisco: Jossey-Bass.

Weiss, D. (1992). Program development consultation for the classroom. In E. G. Jaffe & C. F. Epstein (Eds.), *Occupational therapy consultation: Theory, principles, and practice* (chap. 10, pp. 237–43). St. Louis, MO: Mosby–Year Book.

West, W. L. (1969). The growing importance of prevention. *American Journal of Occupational Therapy, 23,* 226–31.

Wiemer, R. B. (1972). Some concepts of prevention as an aspect of community health. *American Journal of Occupational Therapy, 26,* 1–9.

Yerxa, E. J. (1978). The occupational therapist as consultant and researcher. In H. L. Hopkins & H. D. Smith (Eds.), *Willard and Spackman's Occupational therapy* (5th ed., pp. 689–93). Philadelphia: Lippincott.

Yerxa, E. J. (1983). Audacious values: The energy source for occupational therapy practice. In G. Kielhofner (Ed.), *Health through occupation: Theory and practice in occupational therapy* (pp. 149–62). Philadelphia: F. A. Davis.

SECTION 8

Payment, Regulatory, and Ethical Issues

The final section of *The Occupational Therapy Manager,* containing three chapters, treats major issues that affect the practice of occupational therapy. Chapter 16, "Evolving Health Care Systems: Payment for Occupational Therapy Services," summarizes the provisions of three federally administered health insurance programs, Medicare, the Civilian Health and Medical Program of the Uniformed Services, and the Federal Employees Health Benefit Program; and four state-administered programs, Medicaid, workers' compensation, the Individuals with Disabilities Education Act, and civil rights protection of persons with disabilities. The chapter covers private insurance plans as well, the traditional indemnity type like Blue Cross/Blue Shield and integrated systems like health maintenance organizations and preferred provider organizations.

"State Regulation and Specialty Certification of Practitioners," chapter 17, describes state governments' mandatory processes for establishing and applying standards to individual practitioners, and nongovernmental voluntary processes for doing the same. The chapter summarizes provisions of the North American Free Trade Agreement pertaining to the movement of professionals across the borders of Canada, the United States, and Mexico.

The last chapter, "Ethical Dimensions in Occupational Therapy," identifies and explains eight moral principles that form the basis for ethical behavior. It describes a three-step process of ethical reasoning and addresses the role of the occupational therapy manager in facilitating ethical decision making. The chapter concludes with five open-ended scenarios in which circumstances raise ethical issues for occupational therapy practitioners.

CHAPTER 16

Evolving Health Care Systems: Payment for Occupational Therapy Services

V. Judith Thomas, MGA

KEY TERMS

Capitation. A payment system under which the provider is paid prospectively, usually on a monthly basis, for each member of a specific population (e.g., members of a health plan or Medicaid beneficiaries), regardless of whether any covered health care service is delivered.

Diagnosis codes. Codes that describe the patient's condition or the medical reason for the patient's requiring services.

Fee for service. A payment system under which the provider is paid on the basis of some type of rate per unit of service (e.g., a procedure code or a per diem).

Procedure codes. Codes that describe specific services performed by health care professionals.

Prospective rate. A formula that aggregates payment for groups of services necessary for a patient's care for a specific type of injury or illness or over a specific duration of time (e.g., per case or per episode).

Risk sharing. Distribution, at the end of a year, of unused funds in a "risk pool" on the basis of a predefined reward formula, to providers who meet the targeted utilization and cost goals.

V. Judith Thomas, MGA, is the director of the Reimbursement Policy Program in AOTA's Government Relations Department. In previous positions she managed a health care policy branch in the Health Care Financing Administration's Office of Payment Policy and provided systems analysis support in the development of a managed health care administrative system. She earned her master's degree at the University of Maryland.

Occupational therapy practitioners are paid for their services in a variety of ways, often depending on the setting in which they work. They may be employees of, or have contractual arrangements with, a large health care provider, a school system, or another organization. Alternatively they may be in private practice; if so, they receive direct payment for specific services or groups of services either from insurers, or from patients who are uninsured or who purchase occupational therapy services not covered under the patients' own insurance contracts. Regardless of payment method, it is important for occupational therapy managers and practitioners to understand the scope of benefits offered by the major public and private health plans in their area. An understanding of payers' rules, coverage limitations, and billing practices allows occupational therapy practitioners to assist their patients and families with care decisions, as well as to develop more effective treatment plans in conjunction with other health care professionals. This knowledge also provides a common ground for managers' discussions and negotiations with payers, often leading to reduced claim denials and better contract provisions.

Public funds for occupational therapy services are typically available through either insurance or grant programs. Federal and state insurance programs such as Medicare, Medicaid, and workers' compensation generally have structured guidelines specifying which services are covered, in what settings, and by whom. Grant programs such as the Individuals with Disabilities Education Act (1990), the Community Mental Health Centers Act (1963), the Older Americans Act (1965), and Social Security Title XX, the Social Services Block Grant Program (part of the Omnibus Budget Reconciliation Act of 1981), include occupational therapy as part of an overall program for a specific population. Grant programs are more flexible, allowing private, state, or local entities to provide specially designed programs as long as they meet broad national goals.

Under private insurance plans, services are usually provided to groups of individuals through benefit programs offered by employers or other organizations. However, individuals may purchase policies directly from companies, such as Blue Cross/Blue Shield, commercial insurers, and managed care organizations.

This chapter examines the major sources of payment that have historically been available for occupational therapy services. Also, it discusses some of the changes occurring in the United States health care delivery system that may affect future provision of occupational therapy services.

FEDERALLY ADMINISTERED SYSTEMS

MEDICARE

Established by Congress in 1965 as Title XVIII of the Social Security Act, Medicare is by far the largest single payer for occupational therapy services. It provides health insurance coverage for about 14 percent of the total population, including nearly all the nation's elderly (65 years of age and older), over 4 million disabled persons, and over 200,000 persons with end-stage renal disease (Vladeck & King, 1995). With the anticipated increase in the elderly population, it is projected that Medicare will cover nearly 20 percent of the population by 2030 (U.S. Bureau of the Census, 1994). Occupational therapy practitioners provide services to Medicare beneficiaries in a wide range of settings—hospital inpatient and outpatient facilities, physicians' offices, skilled nursing facilities, comprehensive outpatient rehabilitation facilities, hospices, rehabilitation agencies, and clinics—and through home health agencies and private practice. Recent administrative policy and payment changes in the Medicare program are altering both the distribution of occupational therapy practitioners and the decisions that managers and practitioners must make in the provision of care.

The Medicare program, which is administered by the Health Care Financing Administration (HCFA), consists of the Hospital Insurance Program (Part A), which pays for hospital inpatient, skilled nursing facility, home health, and hospice care, and the Supplementary Medical Insurance Program (Part B), which covers hospital outpatient, physician, and other professional services, including occupational therapy services performed by independent practitioners. Table 16-1 explains the basis for Medicare payment to various types of providers.

Generally, occupational therapy is considered a Medicare-covered service under the following circumstances. Services must be—

1. Prescribed by a physician and furnished according to a written plan of care approved by the physician.

2. Performed by a qualified occupational therapist, or by an occupational therapy assistant under the general supervision of an occupational therapist.

3. Reasonable and necessary for the treatment of the person's illness or injury.

There are no restrictions on diagnoses (i.e., they may be physical or psychiatric or both; no specific diagnosis will automatically prevent payment). There is only the requirement of "an expectation that the therapy will result in a significant practical improvement in the individual's level

Table 16-1
Medicare Payment Methods in Specific Provider Settings

Provider Type	Payment Method
Hospital, acute care	*Inpatient:* DRG (exceptions: psychiatric, alcohol/drug, rehabilitation, distinct-part psychiatric, and long-term care) *Outpatient:* cost, subject to limits
Hospital exempt from Medicare prospective payment system	Cost, subject to limits
Skilled nursing facility	Cost, subject to limits
Home health agency	Cost, subject to per-visit limits
Hospice	Cost-related prospective payment, subject to aggregate limit
Prepaid health care organization (health maintenance organization, preferred provider organization, etc.)	*Risk-based:* Prospective per capita payment *Cost:* Interim per capita payment with cost settlement
Rehabilitation agency; outpatient occupational therapy, physical therapy, or speech-language therapy	Cost
Rural health clinic	All-inclusive rate per visit; occupational therapy covered as "incident to a physician's service"
Comprehensive outpatient rehabilitation facility	Cost; after deductible reduction, lesser of (1) 80% of reasonable cost or (2) reasonable cost minus 20% of reasonable charges
Independent practice	80% of RBRVS[a] fee, subject to $900 yearly limit
Physician's office	80% of RBRVS[a] fee paid as incident to physician's service

a. RBRVS stands for Resource Based Relative Value Scale. See text under section Medicare Supplementary Medical Insurance Program (Part B).

of functioning within a reasonable period of time" (HCFA, Pub. 13, sec. 3101.9). Medicare manuals containing specific coverage information for each delivery setting are available through the Government Printing Office.

Medicare Hospital Insurance Program (Part A)

Occupational therapy services are covered under Part A when they are provided to eligible beneficiaries who are inpatients of hospitals or skilled nursing facilities or patients receiving services under the Medicare home health or hospice benefits. Since October 1993, acute care hospitals have received a *prospective,* or predetermined, rate per inpatient discharge based on established *diagnosis-related groups* (DRGs). This per-case rate covers all inpatient services, including occupational therapy. Individual hospitals determine the mix of services that is appropriate for each patient. Specialty hospitals, such as those offering psychiatric, rehabilitation, pediatric, and long-term care, are at present exempt from the prospective payment system (PPS) applicable to acute care hospitals, as are psychiatric and rehabilitation units of acute care general hospitals. These facilities and units continue to be paid retrospectively on a reasonable-cost basis for all covered services, including occupational therapy. Occupational therapy services are provided to inpatients of psychiatric hospitals or units based on a provision of Part A that requires hospitals to have a sufficient number of "qualified therapists, support personnel, and consultants" to provide comprehensive therapeutic activities for psychiatric inpatients (Public Health, 1986b).

Occupational therapy is also a covered service under Medicare's skilled nursing facility and home health benefits. Patients who receive skilled nursing care must require either skilled nursing or skilled rehabilitation (i.e., occupational therapy, physical therapy, or speech-language therapy) on a *daily basis*, defined in Medicare policy as at least five days a week. To qualify under the Part A home health benefit, a homebound patient must need intermittent skilled nursing care, physical therapy, or speech-language therapy before receiving occupational therapy. However, Medicare patients may continue to receive occupational therapy under the home health benefit after their need for skilled nursing, physical therapy, or speech-language therapy ends (HCFA, Pub.13, sec. 3132).

Hospice care is a special Part A benefit for eligible Medicare beneficiaries whom a physician has certified as *terminally ill*, defined in the regulations as a medical prognosis of fewer than six months to live. A patient who elects to receive hospice benefits must waive inpatient Medicare benefits during the election period. Hospice services may be provided by public agencies or private organizations that are primarily engaged in providing care to terminally ill people.

Medicare regulations for hospices mandate that four core services be available to patients 24 hours a day: counseling, nursing, physicians' services, and social services. The hospice must also provide, as needed, occupational therapy, physical therapy, speech-language therapy, home health aides, homemaker services, and medical supplies, either directly or under a contractual arrangement. Occupational therapy may be provided to control a patient's symptoms or to enable a patient to maintain activities of daily living and basic functional skills. All hospice employees and all providers of additional services, such as occupational therapists, must be licensed, certified, or registered in accordance with applicable state laws. Hospice benefits are paid on a prospective basis. The rates, which are updated annually, are based on four primary levels of care corresponding to the degree of illness and the amount of care required.

Medicare Supplementary Medical Insurance Program (Part B)

Occupational therapy services are covered as Part B outpatient services when furnished by or under arrangements with any Medicare-certified provider (i.e., a hospital, a skilled nursing facility, a home health agency, a rehabilitation agency, a clinic, or a public health agency). A provider may furnish outpatient occupational therapy services to a beneficiary in the home or in the provider's outpatient facility, or, under certain circumstances, to a beneficiary who is an inpatient in another institution. Outpatient occupational therapy services are also covered under Part B as comprehensive outpatient rehabilitation facility (CORF) services. A CORF is a public or private institution that is primarily engaged in providing (by or under the supervision of physicians) diagnostic, therapeutic, and restorative services on an outpatient basis for the rehabilitation of injured, sick, or disabled persons. When occupational therapy is provided by or for a certified facility provider, the facility usually bills for the services. (When occupational therapy is provided by a rehabilitation agency under contract to another provider, the agency may do the billing under some circumstances.)

Part B outpatient occupational therapy services may also be furnished to beneficiaries by a Medicare-certified occupational therapist in independent practice (OTIP) when the services are provided by the therapist or under the therapist's direct supervision in his or her office or in the patient's home. OTIPs are paid according to the codes billed (see the later section Billing and Coding for Services). The amount of payment is derived from the Medicare Physicians' Fee Schedule, also known as the Resource Based Relative Value Scale (RBRVS). This fee schedule is used to pay for all physicians' services billed to Medicare. Beginning in 1995, payment for outpatient occupational therapy services furnished by a Medicare-certified OTIP is limited to $900 in incurred expenses annually per beneficiary. (This limit has been increased twice since January 1, 1990.)

Outpatient occupational therapy services are also covered under Part B of Medicare as incidental to a physician's services when rendered to beneficiaries in a physician's office or a physician-directed clinic. The occupational therapist or therapy assistant providing the services must be employed (either full- or part-time) by the physician or the clinic, and the services must be furnished under the physician's direct supervision (i.e., the physician must be on the premises). The services must be directly related to the condition for which the physician is treating the patient, and they must be included on the physician's bill to Medicare.

Partial-hospitalization services connected with the treatment of a beneficiary with a psychiatric diagnosis (in a hospital-affiliated or community mental health center psychiatric day program) are also covered under Part B of Medicare, but only if the beneficiary would otherwise require inpatient psychiatric care. Under this benefit, Medicare covers occupational therapy services if they are reasonable and necessary for the diagnosis or the active treatment of the beneficiary's condition. They must be reasonably expected to improve or maintain the beneficiary's condition and functional level and to prevent relapse or hospitalization. The course of treatment must be prescribed, supervised, and reviewed by a physician.

Durable Medical Equipment, Prosthetics, and Orthotics

Expenses incurred by a beneficiary for the rental or the purchase of durable medical equipment (e.g., a wheelchair or a walker) are reimbursable under Part B if the equipment is used in the patient's home and if it is necessary and reasonable to treat an illness or an injury or to improve the functioning of a "malformed body member." Medicare defines *durable medical equipment* as that which can withstand repeated use, is primarily and customarily used to serve a medical purpose, and generally is not useful to a person in the absence of illness of injury. An example is oxygen-assistance breathing equipment. Raised toilet seats, bathtub grab bars, and most types of adaptive equipment are not covered because they are not considered medically necessary.

Certification of Providers as Meeting Medicare's Conditions of Participation

All Medicare institutional providers (e.g., hospitals and home health agencies) and individual providers (e.g., OTIPs and physicians) must be certified as meeting Medicare conditions of participation as well as complying with all relevant state and local laws and regulations. Before Medicare issues a provider number, providers must either be surveyed by state health agencies and certified using HCFA guidelines, or receive *deemed status* by previously meeting the accreditation standards of a recognized accrediting organization, such as the Joint Commission on Accreditation of Healthcare Organizations or the American Osteopathic Association.

Although in all health care settings, occupational therapy personnel must meet specific state licensure, certification, or other applicable state regulatory requirements, Medicare conditions of participation related to the provision of occupational therapy services differ for various provider settings. For example, in a hospital setting, occupational therapy personnel must meet qualifications "specified by a facility's medical staff that are consistent with state law" (Public Health, 1986a). In home health agencies and comprehensive outpatient rehabilitation facilities, Medicare regulations require that occupational therapy services be provided by occupational therapists or occupational therapy assistants who are eligible for certification by the National Board for Certification in Occupational Therapy (NBCOT), formerly the American Occupational Therapy Certification Board (see chapter 17, "State Regulation and Specialty Certification of Practitioners").

Medicare Managed Care

The Health Care Financing Administration (HCFA) certifies and awards *cost* or *risk* contracts to health maintenance organizations (HMOs) and other competitive medical plans (CMPs) to provide all Part A and Part B Medicare services (except hospice care) to Medicare enrollees. HCFA pays HMOs and CMPs that participate on a cost basis under a retrospective, reasonable-cost methodology. HCFA pays those that participate under risk contracts a monthly *capitated* amount (an amount per enrolled beneficiary) for each class of Medicare beneficiary. As of February 1996, over 190 plans participated in the Medicare program under risk contracts (HCFA, 1996).

Medicare managed care plans typically cover all preventive, acute, and subacute health services. They must be able to deliver with "reasonable promptness" all medically necessary services that Medicare beneficiaries are entitled to receive and that are available to Medicare beneficiaries who are living in the same geographic area but are not enrolled in a managed care plan (Public Health, 1985). In addition, most plans offer other health care benefits (e.g., coverage of preventive care and prescriptions) that are not included in traditional Medicare coverage. The standard Medicare Part B premium is always required. Although additional cost-sharing levels vary according to policies established by each plan, the beneficiary is often required to pay a supplemental premium for *Medigap* insurance—coverage of Medicare deductibles, Medicare coinsurance, and services not covered by Medicare. Medicare first gave its beneficiaries the option of enrolling in an HMO in 1982. However, fewer than 10 percent had opted for managed care plans by the end of 1995 (Brick, 1996).

HCFA is experimenting with provision of other types of managed care through waivers and demonstration projects, which may be written into future legislation or regulation. For example, in 1995, HCFA announced a new Medicare *point-of-service* insurance option permitting its HMO enrollees to seek care outside the HMO's provider network, typically at higher cost-sharing levels than those for "in-network" care. HCFA does not mandate that the plan make selected services or providers available outside the network. Instead, each plan specifies the providers and the services that Medicare enrollees may access outside the HMO provider network.

THE CIVILIAN HEALTH AND MEDICAL PROGRAM OF THE UNIFORMED SERVICES

The Civilian Health and Medical Program of the Uniformed Services (CHAMPUS) is a United States Department of Defense program of health care for the dependents of active-duty members of the armed forces and for retired members. It shares the cost of medical and other health care that eligible beneficiaries receive from civilian sources. For dependents, CHAMPUS is considered secondary to any other health care plan in which a person is enrolled. CHAMPUS, like Medicare, contracts with private health insurers such as Blue Cross/Blue Shield for claim-processing and utilization review services. CHAMPUS regulations provide for a basic health care program and a special program of rehabilitative benefits.

Basic Program

Under the basic program, CHAMPUS beneficiaries may obtain both inpatient and outpatient medical and mental health care from civilian sources. To qualify for payment, occupational therapy services must be deemed medically necessary by a supervising physician and must be intended to help the patient overcome or compensate for disability resulting from illness, injury, or the effects of a CHAMPUS–covered condition. The occupational therapist or therapy assistant must be an employee of a CHAMPUS–authorized provider and must render the services in connection with CHAMPUS–authorized care in an organized inpatient or outpatient rehabilitation program. The employing institution must bill for the services. In 1995 the Department of Defense published a notice proposing to authorize direct payment for occupational therapy services delivered by self-employed therapists and therapy services provided by freestanding corporations or foundations (including outpatient rehabilitation facilities) that provide outpatient care, home health, and technical diagnostic procedures. At this writing, final regulations and the effective date of these changes have not been published.

CHAMPUS Managed Care

In November 1995, CHAMPUS implemented a new program for members called TRICARE, which incorporates options and incentives for managed care benefits. Under the TRICARE Prime option, CHAMPUS beneficiaries obtain services through an HMO network. Under TRICARE Standard, a continuation of the old CHAMPUS benefit, enrollees may use either the HMO network providers, or choose non-network CHAMPUS providers at a higher out-of-pocket cost. Plans that contract under the TRICARE Prime option may offer benefits beyond the standard CHAMPUS options. Occupational therapists (only therapists will receive direct payment under CHAMPUS) who want to deliver care to CHAMPUS beneficiaries must meet requirements as both CHAMPUS–authorized providers (when coverage becomes available) and TRICARE contractors.

Special Program of Rehabilitative Benefits

The special program of rehabilitative benefits available under CHAMPUS is for seriously physically handicapped and moderately or severely mentally retarded spouses and children of active-duty members. It provides coverage on an inpatient and outpatient basis with a small deductible. However, the qualifying requirements are extremely stringent. CHAMPUS provides a handbook with specific details about this benefit (see Additional Resources for the address and the telephone number of CHAMPUS).

FEDERAL EMPLOYEES HEALTH BENEFIT PROGRAM

The Federal Employees Health Benefit Program, which is administered by the Office of Personnel Management, covers federal government employees, retirees, and their dependents. The federal law and regulations governing the scope of benefits that must be offered specify only broad categories, such as hospital, surgical, and medical services. Therefore coverage of individual types of service, such as occupational therapy, and the settings in which they may be provided is determined by each of the large number of private plans with which the government contracts to administer health care services.

The Federal Employees Health Benefit Program has historically included such insurers as Blue Cross/Blue Shield, Aetna, the Government Employees Hospital Association, and a number of postal worker plans (e.g., the Postmasters Benefit Plan and the Mail Handlers Plan). Over the past few years the Office of Personnel Management has contracted with a greater number of national and local managed care organizations (e.g., Kaiser Permanente, Principal Health Care, and Healthplus). Most managed care organizations contend that occupational therapy is covered in some settings; however, the scope of coverage is generally restricted, and outpatient visits are usually limited in number and duration. When the Federal Employees Health Benefit Program–Blue Cross/Blue Shield plan expanded coverage of outpatient occupational therapy in 1993, it concurrently imposed a limit of 50 (high option) or 25 (low option) visits yearly, which applies to all outpatient rehabilitation (i.e., occupational therapy, physical therapy, and speech-language therapy) visits.

With the advent of provider networks, occupational therapists often face impediments to participation, such as arbitrary limits on types of providers included in the network or misconceptions about the scope of occupational therapy or the relationship between occupational therapy and physical therapy. In pure managed care plans (e.g., HMOs), use of nonaffiliated providers results in a total denial of payment for services, regardless of medical necessity.

Many traditionally fee-for-service plans have introduced managed care options into their packages. For example, the Federal Employees Health Benefit Program–Blue Cross/Blue Shield plan introduced a nationwide preferred provider network in 1993. It did not include occupational therapists until 1996. Use of this network results in lower out-of-pocket costs for federal subscribers.

STATE-ADMINISTERED PROGRAMS

MEDICAID

Medicaid, Title XIX of the Social Security Act (originally enacted in the Social Security Amendments of 1965, amended in the Social Security Amendments of 1971), is a federal-state program that provides health care to the poor and the *medically indigent*. States have great flexibility in the definition of medically indigent and in the makeup and the administration of the program, so benefits vary significantly from state to state. States must include all recipients of Aid to Families with Dependent Children and most beneficiaries of Supplemental Security Income. Not all states provide Medicaid coverage for the medically needy. Some states have a spend-down provision under which families with moderately high incomes may become eligible for Medicaid when their medical expenses reduce their income below the state standard.

Medicaid services fall into two categories, mandatory and optional. Mandatory services are ones that a state must provide to qualify for federal matching funds. They include hospital services; laboratory work and X-rays; skilled nursing facility services; physicians' services; early and periodic screening, diagnosis, and treatment (EPSDT) for persons under 21 years of age; and family planning. States must provide certain services, including occupational therapy, that are necessary to treat a condition identified during EPSDT. Coverage of these services is required even if they are not normally covered under the state's Medicaid program. Occupational therapy provided as a freestanding discipline is considered an optional service, along with physical therapy, speech-language therapy, drugs, psychiatric care, and others. Nursing home reforms adopted by Congress in 1987 require Medicaid nursing facilities to provide skilled rehabilitation services, including occupational therapy, to patients who require them.

In 1988, Congress approved legislation to allow school systems to bill Medicaid for certain related services, including occupational therapy, provided to children in schools. Implementation of this rule has resulted in the development of various state methods to determine responsibility and pay for occupational therapy services provided to school-age children. The seemingly overlapping language of education and Medicaid laws governing the provision of care for school-age children has given rise to the question of whether services to individual children should be funded as education or health care.

Medicaid Managed Care

To administer the Medicaid program more efficiently, state governments may apply to the federal government for *waivers*, which allow states flexibility in the types of services and delivery methods that they provide to some or all Medicaid recipients. Most state waivers require that enrollment in managed care plans or use of provider networks be approved by the state. A Section 1915(b) waiver (of the Social Security Act) allows a state to restrict a beneficiary's choice of provider and is often limited to selected geographic regions within a state. A Section 1115 waiver is a more extensive research-and-demonstration project that is usually granted for five years. Under Section 1115, states are allowed to test major changes in how Medicaid services are delivered. Under most Section 1115 waivers, the existing benefit packages, including occupational therapy benefits, that were available before the waiver was approved continue to be available through a managed care plan contractor. However, the risk of having services limited is increased when authority for case management, coverage decisions, and utilization review is transferred from the state government to a managed care plan.

To date, most state waivers have focused enrollment in managed care plans on the Aid to Families with Dependent Children population, which primarily comprises women and children with routine care needs, rather than the Supplemental Security Income population, which is primarily made up of disabled beneficiaries with more-expensive chronic care needs. According to a recent major study, "States have been cautious about extending managed care to [Supplemental Security Income] populations, in part because relatively few managed care organizations have developed expertise in managing special needs of these populations" (Lewin–VHI, 1995, p. ES-2). Information on Medicaid coverage of occupational therapy may be obtained from state offices of medical assistance (Medicaid).

WORKERS' COMPENSATION

Workers' compensation programs, developed to compensate employees who have job-related injuries or illnesses, are financed jointly by individual employers or groups of employers and state governments.[1] Each state has a workers' compensation governing board or commission that develops policies regulating whether an employer is required to participate, what the financial responsibility of the employer is, what benefits are provided, which workers are covered, and how the insurance is administered. Workers' compensation insurance may be administered through private insurance plans under contract with the state or through individual employers or groups of employers that administer their own programs (known as *self-insuring*).

Workers' compensation programs consist of two components, cash benefits and medical benefits. Although the growth of total workers' compensation costs has slowed since 1990 to less than 3 percent a year, medical benefit costs have grown at a rapid rate, leading to initiation of a variety of cost-containment strategies in states.

Limits on Choice of Providers

States have adopted a number of restrictions on an employee's ability to select an initial provider of care or to change providers during treatment. According to the Workers' Compensation Research Institute (as cited in Burton, 1996), as of January 1995, fourteen states allowed an unrestricted initial choice, four states mandated selection from an employer or insurer network, and thirteen required use of a managed care organization.

Use of Medical Fee Schedules

As of 1995, forty states had adopted some type of fee schedule that prescribed payment amounts for all services performed by health care practitioners for workers' compensation patients. Fee schedules vary in which services are included, what coding scheme is required (see the later section Billing and Coding for Services), what formulas are used to calculate the actual dollar amounts, which state entity develops and controls the use, and how and how often they are updated. A relative value system is used in most jurisdictions, but wide state-to-state variances exist in the compensation for individual procedures.

Regulation of Hospital Rates

States have adopted various methods (e.g., fee schedules and discounted charges) to regulate workers' compensation hospital expenditures, often in conjunction with *all-payer* systems that affect payments to all hospitals. Although some states use the DRG–based Medicare system, many of the DRGs do not apply to the workers' compensation population.

---

1. *This section is based on "Workers' Compensation, Twenty-Four-Hour Coverage, and Managed Care," by J. Burton, 1996, January–February,* Workers' Compensation Monitor, 9(1), 11–21.

Utilization Controls

Because cost and pricing controls alone do not curtail use of services, some states have incorporated various means to address the provision of "unnecessary or inappropriate care." These include retrospective claim review, precertification of services, and case management programs.

Workers' Compensation Managed Care

Another approach to controlling costs by states and employers that self-insure has been to contract with HMOs and preferred provider organizations (PPOs) to provide workers' compensation medical care. In this way, workers' compensation programs can take advantage of existing cost-containment strategies used by HMOs, such as case management, utilization review protocols, and return-to-work programs, without having to make incremental changes in state policy.

To date, the few research projects designed to determine whether these strategies actually reduce the cost of care are inconclusive. A more comprehensive approach to the reform of the workers' compensation system is *24-hour coverage*. According to Burton (1996), this term describes "efforts to reduce or eliminate the distinctions between the medical benefits, income benefits, and disability management services provided to disabled workers for work-related injuries and diseases and . . . [those] provided to disabled workers for non-work-related injuries and diseases" (p. 17). These attempts to coordinate medical, income, and disability benefits from different payment sources vary greatly in configuration and structure. Additional information may be obtained from individual state workers' compensation boards or commissions or the International Association of Industrial Accident Boards and Commissions (see Additional Resources for an address and a telephone number).

EDUCATION PROGRAMS AFFECTING CHILDREN WITH DISABILITIES

Individuals with Disabilities Education Act

The Education for All Handicapped Children Act (often called Public Law Number 94-142), reenacted in 1990 as the Individuals with Disabilities Education Act (IDEA), provides federal grants to states to ensure that eligible children with disabilities have access to a "free, appropriate public education." This statute has been amended over the years to include preschool-aged children (Education of the Handicapped Amendments of 1986) and additional services such as assistive technology and transition planning (Education of the Handicapped Amendments of 1990). At present it consists of a number of parts that determine the scope of services that states must provide to infants and children with disabilities.

Part B of IDEA requires that public school systems and other state agencies involved in educating children with disabilities (ages 3–21) make available "a free appropriate public education that includes special education and related services to meet their unique needs" (Education, 1977). Under this program, occupational therapy is considered a *related service*, playing a supportive role in helping children benefit from special education (AOTA, in press).

Part H of IDEA authorizes grant moneys to states "to develop and implement a statewide, comprehensive, coordinated, multidisciplinary, interagency program of early intervention services for infants and toddlers with disabilities and their families" (Education, 1989). Under this early intervention program, for children newborn through two years of age, occupational therapy is considered a *primary service*. Under Part B and Part H of IDEA, occupational therapy services must be provided according to an individualized education program (IEP) and an individualized family service plan (IFSP), respectively, by a qualified therapist (as defined by state law).

The Rehabilitation Act of 1973 (Section 504) and the Americans with Disabilities Act (ADA) of 1990

Congress enacted the Rehabilitation Act of 1973 (Section 504) and the Americans with Disabilities Act (ADA) of 1990 to protect the rights of persons with disabilities. These civil rights laws may be used to ensure nondiscrimination against students who do not qualify for services under IDEA but need educational support (Copenhaver, 1995). Section 504 includes all institutions that receive federal funding and, with the passage of the ADA, "private institutions" (that is, private schools) with 15 or more employees. There are no federal funding provisions under these acts. Individual states have designated various agencies to administer them.

In 1995, over one-third of all registered occupational therapists (OTRs) in the United States reported that they worked with children in a variety of settings. School systems were the number one employers (either by salary or by contract) of OTRs, and the number two employers of certified occupational therapy assistants (COTAs) (Phyllis Burchman, director of research, AOTA, personal communication, March 1996). Because administrative responsibility for all the programs developed under the IDEA resides with the state governments, occupational therapy practitioners in school settings must work closely with local and state education officials on issues related to funding, human resources, and regulation of services.

PRIVATE INSURANCE AND MANAGED CARE PLANS

Although it is possible to specify the number of private companies offering some type of health insurance, it is impossible to delineate all the variations of plan options offered in the United States. Insurers, especially large companies such as Blue Cross/Blue Shield plans, Aetna, MetLife, and Prudential, have many product lines of health insurance (PPOs, point-of-service plans, indemnity, etc.), including managed care options, and often will negotiate unique benefit and premium configurations for a single employer. Therefore a practitioner can never make assumptions about a person's coverage by plan name alone.

Because there are no federally mandated requirements for benefits or payment, each state determines the extent of control that it wants to impose on the insurance companies operating within its borders. Also, because employers that self-insure health care benefits are governed not by state insurance codes but by the Employee Retirement Income Security Act (ERISA), there are widely divergent practices across the country. Consistently, traditional indemnity insurers, in addition to administrators of managed care organizations [e.g., HMOs, PPOs, and physician-hospital organizations (PHOs)], are introducing managed care principles into their plans. The following management techniques are often implemented in conjunction with cost-controlling payment strategies, such as use of discounted or capitated rates and preferred provider networks to manage costs and quality more effectively:

1. *Case management.* Especially for long-term or high-cost cases, insurers use case managers, often employed outside the plan, to oversee and designate which group of services will yield the best outcome. Frequently this decision-making power allows a case manager to approve treatments that a plan might not normally cover. Some insurers use the terms *case management* and *managed care* synonymously.

2. *Precertification* or *preauthorization.* The requirement that specific tests, surgical procedures, or categories of services (e.g., mental health) be authorized before they are allowed gives the insurer the opportunity to deny "unnecessary" treatment or substitute lower-cost services.

3. *Mandatory second opinion.* Insisting on a second opinion before approval of any or specific types of surgical procedures serves as a check on a physician's decision regarding the need for surgery. It presents an opportunity for another physician to suggest an alternative, less costly treatment.

4. *Third-party administrator.* To obtain the best economies, insurers contract with a private company that specializes in management of various administrative functions (e.g., claims) and managed care responsibilities (e.g., utilization review) of a plan or an employer (if self-insured).

Because state laws and plan philosophies differ, practitioners must research on a very local level the environment in which private insurers operate. Following are questions that occupational therapy managers and practitioners should ask about their patients' health care coverage before providing service. They should also ask these questions about their own policies.

1. What specific types of inpatient and outpatient health care services does the plan cover?

2. Are there limitations in number of visits, sites at which services may be received, or yearly costs for specific services?

3. Is there a network of providers from whom patients must obtain services? Can a patient "opt out" of the network, and if so, what financial disincentives exist?

4. What copayments, deductibles, or other out-of-pocket expenses exist for using non-network providers? Under what circumstances?

5. Does the plan offer case management services for some conditions?

This type of information is essential for practitioners to provide the optimal covered care and to assist patients in making decisions about continuing care that their insurance may not cover. It also provides a basis for managers and practitioners to evaluate the benefits of joining a health plan provider panel or a preferred provider network.

BILLING AND CODING FOR SERVICES

Payment for services provided by both facility and individual providers is usually predicated on proper coding and completion of claim forms. Two common billing forms are (1) the Uniform Bill (UB-92; HCFA-1450), used by institutional providers such as hospitals and home health agencies, for Medicaid, CHAMPUS, and Medicare (for most Part A service billing); and (2) the HCFA-1500 claim form, primarily used by private practitioners such as physicians and occupational therapists in independent practice,[2] for Medicare, CHAMPUS, Medicaid, and workers' compensation in most states.

---

2. Insurers generally do not recognize occupational therapy assistants for direct payment because they require supervision and do not perform evaluations.

Public and private payers usually require health care facilities and practitioners to represent their services in terms of diagnosis and procedure codes. Not all payers cover the same range of services or permit use of the same codes. In addition, state regulations or payer policies may establish limitations on the amount paid for a specific code or combination of codes.

DIAGNOSIS CODES

Diagnosis codes describe the patient's condition or the medical reason for the patient's requiring services. They are critical to obtaining a favorable determination of coverage. ICD-9-CM (*International Classification of Diseases, 9th Revision, Clinical Modification,* 1993, updated annually) is the most frequently used diagnosis-coding system in the United States. Under the ICD coding system, diseases are categorized primarily by anatomical systems. Also, ICD contains supplementary classifications covering (1) factors influencing health status and (2) external causes of injury and poisoning. An additional volume provides a listing of ICD surgical and medical procedures, which are mainly used to code inpatient hospital services. Figure 16-1 offers tips for using diagnosis codes effectively.

Figure 16-1
Tips for Using Diagnosis and Procedure Codes

Using Diagnosis Codes (ICD-9-CM)

- Use the most current version of the ICD-9-CM manual, which is updated in October of each year.
- Remember that the patient's condition is key to a medical necessity determination. Justify the care provided by presenting the essential information to assist the payer in determining the need for care.
- Always code as principal diagnosis (the first diagnosis referenced in item 21 on the HCFA-1500 claim and item 67 of the UB-92) the current condition that prompted the patient's visit. Code other conditions or a chronic condition when applicable to the present treatment.
- Relate each service, procedure, or supply to an ICD-9 code. Make sure the ICD-9 codes on your bill reflect the reasons for each service provided.

Using Procedure Codes (HCPCS)

- Always review the most recent codes and definitions for new code numbers and modified descriptions of services. Level I (CPT) and II HCPCS codes are updated each January.
- Be specific. Always select the code(s) that most closely describe the service(s) provided. Avoid using "unlisted procedure" codes.
- Most CPT codes in the Physical Medicine and Rehabilitation section are defined in 15-minute segments. When coding more than one [15-minute] unit for a single service, indicate the number of units (item 24 G on the HCFA-1500 form). Do not list the same code multiple times.
- List the CPT code and units, where necessary, for each modality and procedure performed. For example, where a modality is used as a precursor to therapy, both the modality and the treatment code can be billed.
- Use modifiers when appropriate with HCPCS codes to describe when a procedure or service has been altered by some specific circumstance but not changed in its definition or code. The modifier indicates to the insurance carrier that the procedure should be manually priced. A complete list of modifiers is contained in the CPT and Level II HCPCS manuals; however, check with the payer to determine local policy in using modifiers.
- Use CPT special service codes (i.e., 99000 to 99199) when appropriate along with the primary procedure code.

Note. *From "Code It Right" (p. 14) by V. J. Thomas, 1996, February 8,* OT Week.

PROCEDURE CODES

Procedure codes describe specific services performed by health care professionals. One of the most widely used procedure-coding systems is the HCFA Common Procedure Coding System (HCPCS), which includes the American Medical Association's (updated annually) *Physicians' Current Procedural Terminology* (CPT),[3] referred to as Level I HCPCS; the HCFA–developed alphanumeric codes, referred to as Level II HCPCS; and local codes, referred to as Level III HCPCS, created by Medicare and other carriers as needed, when other HCPCS codes do not suffice. Level II HCPCS also contains codes for durable medical equipment, prosthetics, orthotics, and supplies (DMEPOS) and some procedures not found in the CPT system. Figure 16-1 also offers tips for using procedure codes effectively.

Current Procedural Terminology

Since 1990, HCFA has contracted with the American Medical Association to use the CPT coding system as the basis for the Medicare Physicians' Fee Schedule (as noted earlier, also known as the Resource Based Relative Value Scale, RBRVS) and to assist with the development of *relative work values* (RVWs) for each code. In May 1993 the American Medical Association invited nine nonphysician practitioner associations to participate in the CPT Editorial Panel and Relative Value Scale Update Committee processes by forming a Health Care Professionals Advisory Committee. AOTA was included in this initial group, along with the American Academy of Physician Assistants, the American Nurses Association, the American Optometric Association, the American Physical Therapy Association, the American Podiatric Medical Association, the American Psychological Association, the American Speech-Language-Hearing Association, and the National Association of Social Workers. In 1995 the American Chiropractic Association joined the committee. These associations, individually and as a group, make recommendations to the annual update of CPT and the relative work values.

The coding system, which is updated annually by the American Medical Association, provides a uniform terminology for each of thousands of medical procedures. Occupational therapists in independent practice use CPT codes to bill Medicare and most other public and private insurers. Although occupational therapists most often use codes in the Physical Medicine section of CPT, under American Medical Association guidelines, physicians and nonphysician practitioners should select the codes that most accurately identify the services performed. Other than the requirement that the service be within the scope of practice of the practitioner,

---

3. *CPT five-digit codes and two-digit modifiers are copyrighted by the American Medical Association.*

there are no CPT restrictions for use of codes in any section. Occupational therapists should request information on allowable codes, service definitions, and documentation policies before billing a new insurer.

EVOLVING PAYMENT METHODOLOGIES

FEE FOR SERVICE

Traditionally, providers have been paid on the basis of *fee for service*, some type of rate per unit of service (e.g., a procedure code or a per diem). This rate may be based on a fee schedule or may be a negotiated discounted rate for a specific treatment or specific groups of treatments. Generally under fee for service, a practitioner is paid for each code or service billed and has no incentive to limit procedures and tests or to examine lower-cost types of treatment. In a fee-for-service system the insurer assumes the primary risk because under the contractual provisions with the employer or another consumer, the insurer must pay for all covered care. For this reason, payers often use cost-saving techniques such as preset service limitations or post-payment utilization reviews to identify overuse by providers.

PROSPECTIVE RATE

Most *prospective rate* formulas are designed to aggregate payment for groups of services necessary for a patient's care for a specific type of injury or illness or over a specific duration of time (e.g., per case or per episode). The Medicare DRG payment is a prospective rate that includes all surgical and medical services (except physicians') required to treat a patient with a specific diagnosis during a specific hospital inpatient stay. Under a prospective payment system, providers have greater flexibility in determining mix of services. However, because a prospective rate is based on the average expense for a particular condition, the provider is at risk for ensuring that costs in the aggregate do not exceed payments.

CAPITATION

In a *capitation* payment system the provider is paid prospectively, usually on a monthly basis, for each member of a specific population (e.g., members of a health plan or Medicaid beneficiaries), regardless of whether any covered health care service is delivered. This prospective rate is termed *per member per month* and is customarily based on the past claim experience of the specific capitated population. Under capitation the provider has the benefit of a predictable revenue source, but is at greater financial risk because more service equals less profit. For a provider the per-member-per-month amount is the most important factor in determining the profitability, or even the feasibility, of a capitated contract.

Capitation provisions are primarily found in HMO contracts because this type of managed care organization is the most homogeneous in terms of administrative and utilization controls. However, legal affiliations and payment relationships among hospitals, clinics, laboratories, and other types of health care providers are continually evolving, and other types of networks are using forms of capitated payment. Capitation rates were initially developed for payment of primary care physicians. This payment method is more easily (and equitably) calculated for primary care physicians, who as gatekeepers have the most patient interaction and the most control of services. Additionally, it is easier to project service cost and therefore to set a valid per-member-per-month rate.

PPOs and many HMOs continue to pay specialists—whether physicians, therapists, or other provider types—on a fee-for-service basis. As provider chains and multispecialty organizations continue to grow, however, it becomes easier to estimate statistically the amount of treatment that a prospectively set per-member-per-month rate should cover without the risk of catastrophic loss to the provider. When physicians, independent practice associations, specialty rehabilitation groups, and hospitals are capitated, therapy services are sometimes subcontracted to another entity that may be paid under a different method.

In addition to the per-member-per-month amount, providers should consider all aspects of a contract in evaluating the viability of a capitation arrangement. Table 16-2 presents some of these factors.

Table 16-2

Factors to Consider in Evaluating the Viability of a Capitation Arrangement

Factor	Consideration
Number of members in capitated population	The greater the number of members, the higher the overall prospectively paid monthly rate from that plan will be.
Member profile	Risk (i.e., use of services) is statistically determined by age, sex, and health care factors relative to type of service provided.
Specific details of plan that affect members' access to and incentives to use services	Benefit package, member deductibles and copayment amounts, referral requirements (e.g., requirements that care be referred by primary care physician), or high copayment for therapy will reduce demand for services. For example, provider may require higher capitation rate to offset low copayment.
Numbers of other similar providers in network	Generally, if there are few providers offering similar services, per-member-per-month rate must be high enough to cover cost of expected large number of referrals.

RISK SHARING AND RISK POOLS

The concept of *risk sharing* and the construction of *risk pools* are critical issues for providers in deciding whether or not to join a capitated network. Risk adjustments can also exist in noncapitated contractual arrangements. A risk pool of dollars is created from a designated amount of money withheld from payments to providers throughout the year, and it is used to meet specified expenses of the pool. On the basis of a predefined "reward" formula, unused funds in the pool are distributed at the end of the year to providers who meet the targeted utilization and cost goals. The design of the pool (e.g., specialties of providers and number per pool) and the way in which it is used during the year determine the risk (i.e., whether there is any money in the pool by the end of the year). An infinite number of arrangements and formulas can be created under the guise of risk sharing. Providers should understand the details of each contract to which they commit.

CONCLUSION

Payment resources for all health care services are shrinking. Federal and state policymakers are seeking ways to redefine essential services and to provide them at minimal cost. The administrative control of health benefits is gradually shifting to state and local levels and private health insurers. In most states, public programs and private plans are relying on preferred provider networks and managed care strategies to lower costs. With the growth of managed care, the separation between provider and insurer is narrowing as mergers create new health care entities.

For occupational therapy managers and practitioners, these trends argue for better articulation of the value of occupational therapy and development of practice methods that demonstrate more cost-effective ways to provide quality rehabilitation services. For independent practitioners, changing funding methods may require affiliation with larger provider entities that can better negotiate with the health care payers of the future.

SUMMARY

Public funds for occupational therapy services are typically available through either federal or state insurance programs, which generally have structured guidelines specifying which services are covered, in what settings, and by whom; and grant programs, which include occupational therapy as part of an overall program for a specific population. Under private insurance plans, services are usually provided to groups of individuals through benefit programs offered by employers or other organizations. However, individuals may purchase policies directly from companies.

Medicare is by far the largest single payer for occupational therapy services. The Medicare program consists of the Hospital Insurance Program (Part A), which pays for hospital inpatient, skilled nursing facility, home health, and hospice care; and the Supplementary Medical Insurance Program (Part B), which covers hospital outpatient, physician, and other professional services, including occupational therapy services performed by independent practitioners. Generally, occupational therapy is considered a Medicare-covered service if it is (1) prescribed by a physician and furnished according to a written plan of care approved by the physician; (2) performed by a qualified occupational therapist, or by an occupational therapy assistant under the general supervision of an occupational therapist; and (3) reasonable and necessary for the treatment of the person's illness or injury.

The Civilian Health and Medical Program of the Uniformed Services (CHAMPUS) is a United States Department of Defense program of health care for the dependents of active-duty members of the armed forces and for retired members. It shares the cost of medical and other health care that eligible beneficiaries receive from civilian sources. CHAMPUS regulations provide for a basic health care program and a special program of rehabilitative benefits.

The Federal Employees Health Benefit Program covers federal government employees, retirees, and their dependents. Coverage of individual types of services and the settings in which they may be provided is determined by each of the large number of private plans with which the government contracts to administer health care services.

Medicaid is a federal-state program that provides health care to the poor and the medically indigent. Medicaid services fall into two categories: (1) mandatory services, which a state must provide to qualify for federal matching funds; and (2) optional services. Mandatory services include hospital services; laboratory work and X-rays; skilled nursing facility services; physicians' services; early and periodic screening, diagnosis, and treatment (EPSDT) for persons under 21 years of age; and family planning. Occupational therapy provided as a freestanding discipline is considered an optional service.

Workers' compensation programs, developed to compensate employees who have job-related injuries or illnesses, are financed jointly by individual employers or groups of employers and state governments. Each state has a workers' compensation governing board or commission that develops policies regulating whether an employer is required to participate, what the financial responsibility of the employer is, what benefits are provided, which workers are covered, and how the insurance is administered. Workers' compensation programs consist of two components, cash benefits and medical benefits.

The Education for All Handicapped Children Act, reenacted in 1990 as the Individuals with Disabilities Education Act (IDEA), provides federal grants to states to ensure that eligible children with disabilities have access to a "free, appropriate public education." Part B of IDEA requires that public school systems and other state agencies involved in educating children with disabilities (ages 3–21) make available "a free appropriate public education that includes special education and related services to meet their unique needs" (Education, 1977). Under this program, occupational therapy is considered a *related service*. Part H of IDEA authorizes grant moneys to states "to develop and implement a statewide, comprehensive, coordinated, multidisciplinary, interagency program of early intervention services for infants and toddlers with disabilities and their families" (Education, 1989). Under this program, occupational therapy is considered a *primary service*. Under Part B and Part H of IDEA, occupational therapy services must be provided according to an individualized education program (IEP) and an individualized family service plan (IFSP), respectively.

The Rehabilitation Act of 1973, Section 504, and the Americans with Disabilities Act (ADA) of 1990 may be used to ensure nondiscrimination against students who do not qualify for services under IDEA but need educational support (Copenhaver, 1995).

Private insurers have many product lines and will often negotiate unique benefit and premium configurations for a single employer. Four management techniques are often implemented in conjunction with cost-controlling payment strategies: (1) case management, (2) precertification or preauthorization, (3) mandatory second opinion, and (4) third-party administrator.

Payment for services provided by both facility and individual providers is usually predicated on proper coding and completion of claim forms. Two common billing forms are (1) the Uniform Bill (UB-92; HCFA-1450); and (2) the HCFA-1500 claim form.

Public and private payers usually require health care facilities and practitioners to represent their services in terms of diagnosis and procedure codes. *Diagnosis codes* describe the patient's condition or the medical reason for the patient's requiring services. *Procedure codes* describe specific services performed by health care professionals.

The concept of risk sharing and the construction of risk pools are critical issues for providers in deciding whether or not to join a capitated network.

REFERENCES

American Medical Association. (updated annually). *Physicians' current procedural terminology.* Chicago: Author.

American Occupational Therapy Association. (in press). *Guidelines for occupational therapy practice under the Individuals with Disabilities Education Act.* Bethesda, MD: Author.

Americans with Disabilities Act of 1990, Pub. L. No. 101–336, 104 Stat. 327.

Brick, L. L. (1996, February). Medicare HMOs to expand role of rehab, subacute. *Continuing Care, 15*(2), 18–19.

Burton, J. (1996, January-February). Workers' compensation, twenty-four-hour coverage, and managed care. *Workers' Compensation Monitor, 9*(1), 11–21.

Community Mental Health Centers Act of 1963, Pub. L. No. 88–164, Title II, 77 Stat. 290.

Copenhaver, J. (1995). *Section 504: An educator's primer.* Logan, UT: Mountain Plains Regional Resource Center. (Address: 1780 North Research Parkway, Suite 112, Logan, UT 84322-9620.)

Education, 34 C.F.R. § 300.1 (1977), redesignated at 45 Fed. Reg. 77368 (1980).

Education, 34 C.F.R. § 303.1 (1989), as amended at 56 Fed. Reg. 54688 (1991).

Education for All Handicapped Children Act of 1975, Pub. L. No. 94–142, 89 Stat. 773.

Education of the Handicapped Amendments of 1986, Pub. L. No. 99–457, 100 Stat. 1145.

Education of the Handicapped Amendments of 1990, Pub. L. No. 101–476, 104 Stat. 1103.

Employee Retirement Income Security Act of 1974, Pub. L. No. 93–406, 88 Stat. 829.

Health Care Financing Administration. (1996, February). *Medicare prepaid health plans report.* Baltimore: Author.

Health Care Financing Administration. (updated continually). *Medicare intermediary manual.* Baltimore: Author.

Individuals with Disabilities Education Act Amendments of 1991, Pub. L. No. 102–119, 105 Stat. 587.

Individuals with Disabilities Education Act of 1990, Pub. L. No. 101–476, Section 901, 104 Stat. 1103.

International classification of diseases, 9th revision, clinical modification (ICD-9-CM). (1993; updated annually). Salt Lake City, UT: Med-Index Publications; Bethesda, MD: National Center for Health Statistics (Vols. 1–2); Baltimore: Health Care Financing Administration (Vol. 3).

Lewin–VHI, Inc. (1995). *States as payers: Managed care for Medicaid popula-tions.* Washington, DC: National Institute for Health Care Management.

Older Americans Act of 1965, Pub. L. No. 89–73, 79 Stat. 218, as amended.

Omnibus Budget Reconciliation Act of 1981, Pub. L. No. 97–35, 95 Stat. 357.

Public Health, 42 C.F.R. § 417.414 (1985), amended at 58 Fed. Reg. 38062 (1993), 60 Fed. Reg. 45673, 45677 (1995).

Public Health, 42 C.F.R. § 482.56 (1986a).

Public Health, 42 C.F.R. § 482.62(g)(2) (1986b).

Rehabilitation Act of 1973, Section 504, Pub. L. No. 93–112, 87 Stat. 355.

Social Security Amendments of 1965, Title XVIII, Medicare, Pub. L. No. 89–97, 79 Stat. 286, as amended.

Social Security Amendments of 1971, Title XIX, Medicaid, Pub. L. No. 92–223, 85 Stat. 802, as amended.

United States Bureau of the Census. (1994). *Current population reports, 1994.* Washington, DC: Government Printing Office.

Vladeck, B. C., & King, K. M. (1995). Medicare at 30: Preparing for the future. *Journal of the American Medical Association, 274,* 259–62.

ADDITIONAL RESOURCES

CHAMPUS Information Office, Aurora, CO 80045-6900, telephone 303/361-1000

Health Care Financing Administration, 7500 Security Boulevard, Baltimore, MD 21244-1850, telephone 410/786-3000

International Association of Industrial Accident Boards and Commissions, 1575 Aviation Center Parkway, Suite 512, Daytona Beach, FL 32114, telephone 904/252-2915

Office of Personnel Management, Theodore Roosevelt Federal Building, 1900 E Street NW, Washington, DC 20415, telephone 202/606-1000

Workers' Compensation Research Institute, 101 Main Street, Cambridge, MA 02142, telephone 617/494-1240

State Regulation and Specialty Certification of Practitioners

Barbara Winthrop Rose, BSOT, OTR, CVE, CWA, CHT, FAOTA

KEY TERMS

Certification. The process by which an agency grants a person permission to use a certain title if that person has attained entry-level competence; may be mandatory or voluntary, as determined by state law; may also be nongovernmental.

Credentialing. A generic term for the processes described in this chapter; derived from *credentials,* "a predetermined set of standards, such as licensure or certification, establishing that a person or institution has achieved professional recognition in a specific field of health care" (*Mosby's,* 1994, p. 409).

Licensure. "The process by which an agency of government grants permission to an individual to engage in a given occupation upon finding that the applicant has attained the minimal degree of competence required to ensure that the public health, safety, and welfare will be reasonably well protected" (U.S. Department of Health, Education, and Welfare, 1977, p. 17).

Registration. The process by which an agency grants a person permission to use a certain title if that person has registered with the agency; may be mandatory or voluntary, as determined by state law; may also be nongovernmental.

Regulation. The process "through which laws are implemented" (Scott & Acquaviva, 1985, p. 1).

Specialty certification. The voluntary process by which a profession recognizes persons who have achieved advanced-level competence.

Title control (sometimes called a *trademark act*). The process by which an agency grants a person permission to use a certain title if that person has attained entry-level competence.

Barbara Winthrop Rose, BSOT, OTR, CVE, CWA, CHT, FAOTA, is a co-owner of Functional Hand Therapy Alliance, Inc. of Houston, Texas. She has served on the American Occupational Therapy Political Action Committee as a member, as the secretary, and as the chair. In 1994 she received the Lindy Boggs Award from AOTA in recognition of her significant contributions to occupational therapy through political activity. She did her undergraduate work in occupational therapy at the University of Kansas.

The objectives of this chapter are (1) to give an overview of regulation of the occupational therapy profession as mandated in state laws and regulations on licensure, certification, title control, and registration; and (2) to explain the role of private-sector organizations in nongovernmental certification and registration of occupational therapy practitioners. Like voluntary accreditation, discussed in chapter 13, these are mechanisms for setting and applying standards of education and practice. Unlike accreditation, however, which pertains to organizations and programs, these mechanisms pertain to individuals. They strongly affect the practice of occupational therapy, determining who enters the profession, under what terms, who may use professional titles, and so forth. Discussion of them illustrates the important influence that state legislative and regulatory bodies have on the occupational therapy profession. It also serves to inform the occupational therapy manager about the legal and nongovernmental frameworks for credentialing. *Credentialing*, a generic term for the processes described in this chapter, is derived from the word *credentials*, defined in health care as "a predetermined set of standards, such as licensure or certification, establishing that a person or institution has achieved professional recognition in a specific field of health care" (*Mosby's*, 1994, p. 409).

The chapter also addresses state regulation of practitioners in the special context of the North American Free Trade Agreement (NAFTA). This agreement allows Canadian and Mexican occupational therapists to work in the United States on a temporary basis if they meet certain requirements, including applicable state standards.

STATE REGULATION

In government, *regulation* is the process "through which laws are implemented" (Scott & Acquaviva, 1985, p. 1).[1] Legislation typically undergirds regulation: Legislators, elected officials, enact a law, and regulators, appointed officials, translate the law's provisions into regulations. Both kinds of officials make decisions that directly and indirectly affect occupational therapy managers and practitioners. The decisions include setting of professional standards, coverage and reimbursement for occupational therapy services, funding for higher education, and awarding of research grants.

---

1. *This section is based in part on "Regulation and Standard Setting" (pp. 342–44), by S. B. Fine, J. Bair, S. P. Hoover, and J. D. Acquaviva, 1992, in M. Gray and J. Bair (Eds.), The* Occupational Therapy Manager *(Rev. ed.), Rockville, MD: American Occupational Therapy Association. Copyright ©1992 by the American Occupational Therapy Association, Inc.*

In the United States the earliest evidence of state regulation of professions was the Virginia medical practice act of 1639. State licensure activity did not begin in earnest, however, until the late 1800s. "By 1900 most states had licensed attorneys, dentists, pharmacists, physicians, and teachers. Between 1900 and 1960, most states also granted licensure to 20 additional groups, including accountants, nurses, real estate brokers, barbers, chiropractors, and funeral directors" (Shimberg & Roederer, 1994, pp. 1–2). The profession of occupational therapy resisted licensure until the 1970s (Quiroga, 1995), when Florida and New York became the first states to license occupational therapists and occupational therapy assistants.

Today, state regulation of occupational therapy practitioners takes several forms: licensure, mandatory certification, title control, mandatory registration, and voluntary certification and registration. Each form is authorized by state law. As mechanisms of the state, all these processes are meant to protect the public from harm. Table 17-1 presents them in decreasing order of restrictiveness, summarizing their major features and differentiating them according to (1) the level of protection that they afford the public, (2) requirements for practice, and (3) oversight agency. As of June 1996, all 50 states, the District of Columbia, Guam, and Puerto Rico regulate occupational therapists. With the exception of Colorado, Rhode Island, and Virginia, all states, the District of Columbia, Guam, and Puerto Rico regulate occupational therapy assistants. The form of regulation in 39 states, the District of Columbia, Guam, and Puerto Rico is licensure; in 5 states (Indiana, Missouri, Vermont, Virginia, and Wisconsin), mandatory or voluntary certification; in 3 states (Kansas, Michigan, and Minnesota), registration; and in 3 states (California, Colorado, and Hawaii), title control (AOTA, 1996).

Licensure, the most restrictive form of state regulation, is "the process by which an agency of government grants permission to an individual to engage in a given occupation upon finding that the applicant has attained the minimal degree of competence required to ensure that the public health, safety, and welfare will be reasonably well protected" (U.S. Department of Health, Education, and Welfare, 1977, p. 17). The law undergirding this process, a *licensure law,* defines the scope of practice. A licensure law is therefore often referred to as a *practice act.* Figure 17-1 presents AOTA's Model Practice Act Definition of Occupational Therapy.

Mandatory certification and *title control* are processes by which a government agency grants a person permission to use a certain title if that person has attained entry-level competence. The laws undergirding these processes are a *certification law* and a *title act* (sometimes called a *trademark*

Table 17-1
Major Types of State Regulation of Occupational Therapy Practitioners

Type of Regulation	Description	Requirements for Practice[a]	Oversight Agency
Licensure	Provides highest level of public protection by prohibiting unlicensed persons from practicing occupational therapy or referring to themselves as occupational therapists or occupational therapy assistants. Licensure laws reserve certain scope of practice to those who are issued license.	Mandates entry-level competency.	State health department usually delegates authority to occupational therapy board or advisory board, consisting of occupational therapy practitioners, consumers, and/or other health professionals.
Mandatory Certification[a] (certification as granted by occupational therapy regulatory board or advisory board/council, to be distinguished from nongovernmental certification granted to persons passing AOTCB exam)	Protects public by prohibiting noncertified persons from referring to themselves as occupational therapists or occupational therapy assistants, although they may practice under certain circumstances if they do not refer to their services as occupational therapy. Certification laws may provide for definition of occupational therapy.	Mandates entry-level competency.	Government agency maintains registry of individuals who successfully complete eligibility requirements.
Title Control (sometimes called *trademark act*)	Prohibits noncertified persons from referring to themselves as occupational therapists or occupational therapy assistants, although they may practice under certain circumstances if they do not refer to their services as occupational therapy.	Mandates entry-level competency.	Government agency maintains registry of individuals who successfully complete eligibility requirements.
Mandatory Registration[a]	Protects public by prohibiting nonregistered persons from referring to themselves as occupational therapists or occupational therapy assistants, although they may practice if they do not refer to their services as occupational therapy.	Competency standards may be required by government agency maintaining register.	Government agency maintains registry of persons who successfully complete eligibility.
Voluntary Certification or Registration (sometimes called *nongovernmental title control*)	Does not protect either title or practice. State does not have legal authority to prohibit noncertified or nonregistered persons from practicing occupational therapy unless they have violated certain standards of care.	There are usually no state requirements for practice. However, practitioner's professional association may advise on entry-level competency. Practitioners are subject to entry-level competency requirements for reimbursement by third-party insurers, private investors, and Medicare.	Other than state's constitutional authority to govern health, safety, and welfare, there are usually no express requirements for governance of profession.

Note. *From* Major Types of State Regulation for Occupational Therapy Practitioners *[Fact sheet], by American Occupational Therapy Association, Government Relations Department, 1994, July, Bethesda, MD: Author.*

a. *The terms* certification *and* registration *are often used interchangeably. It is important to understand individual state provisions and protections of each type of regulation, rather than assume that certain provisions are automatically included.*

Figure 17-1
Definition of Occupational Therapy Practice for State Regulation

Occupational therapy is the use of purposeful activity or interventions designed to achieve functional outcomes which promote health, prevent injury or disability and which develop, improve, sustain or restore the highest possible level of independence of any individual who has an injury, illness, cognitive impairment, psychosocial dysfunction, mental illness, developmental or learning disability, physical disability or other disorder or condition. It includes assessment by means of skilled observation or evaluation through the administration and interpretation of standardized or nonstandardized tests and measurements.

Occupational therapy services include but are not limited to:

1. the assessment and provision of treatment in consultation with the individual, family or other appropriate persons; and

2. interventions directed toward developing, improving, sustaining or restoring daily living skills, including self-care skills and activities that involve interactions with others and the environment, work readiness or work performance, play skills or leisure capacities or enhancing educational performances skills; and

3. developing, improving, sustaining or restoring sensorimotor, oral-motor, perceptual or neuromuscular functioning; or emotional, motivational, cognitive or psychosocial components of performance; and

4. education of the individual, family or other appropriate persons in carrying out appropriate interventions.

These services may encompass assessment of need and the design, development, adaptation, application or training in the use of assistive technology devices; the design, fabrication or application of rehabilitative technology such as selected orthotic devices; training in the use of orthotic or prosthetic devices; the application of physical agent modalities as an adjunct to or in preparation for purposeful activity; the application of ergonomic principles; the adaptation of environments and processes to enhance functional performance; or the promotion of health and wellness.

Approved by the Representative Assembly July 1994

Note. *From* Definition of Occupational Therapy Practice for State Regulation *[Fact sheet], by American Occupational Therapy Association, Government Relations Department, 1994, July, Bethesda, MD: Author. Copyright ©1994 by the American Occupational Therapy Association, Inc.*

act), respectively. The states treat mandatory certification and title control differently, so further generalization about them is difficult.

Mandatory registration is the process by which a government agency grants a person permission to use a certain title if that person has registered with the agency. The agency may or may not require the person to meet a standard of entry-level competency. Shimberg and Roederer (1994) argue that this form of regulation is appropriate "when the threat to life, health, safety and economic well-being is relatively small and other forms of legal redress are available to the public" (p. 5).

Voluntary certification and *voluntary registration* are processes by which a government agency acknowledges that a person meets certain qualifications associated with a title (which may or may not be equivalent to a standard of entry-level competency) but does not protect either the title or a related scope of practice. Under these types of state regulation, a noncertified or nonregistered person may also legally practice in the profession, assuming that he or she meets the requirements of third-party payers. (*Note:* Noncertification in this instance does not refer to certification as granted by the National Board for Certification in Occupational Therapy [NBCOT].)

Occupational therapy managers and practitioners should be careful not to confuse mandatory and voluntary certification, which are state mechanisms, with nongovernmental certification, which is a private-sector mechanism. Likewise, they should be careful not to confuse mandatory and voluntary registration with the counterpart in the private sector, nongovernmental registration. (See the later discussion under Nongovernmental Certification and Registration.)

REGULATORY OR ADVISORY BOARDS

In the health care professions the agency of government granting the permission under the various types of regulation is typically the state department of health. Under a licensure system, that department usually delegates its authority to administer regulations to a board consisting of (1) members of the profession being regulated, (2) consumers, and (3) representatives of related professions. Across the states and across the professions, regulatory boards operate on a continuum from full autonomy, to a strictly advisory role or no board at all, with a centralized agency responsible for administration (Shimberg & Roederer, 1994).

Table 17-2 lists the characteristics that scholars of occupational licensing believe regulatory entities should have. The most broad-reaching power of regulatory boards is that of writing rules and regulations, which have the force of law. Boards may establish rules and regulations for (1) issuance of a license or a certificate, or granting of registry status; (2) supervision of assistants and unlicensed occupational therapy personnel; and (3) continuing competency requirements when specified by law.

In occupational therapy an example of an autonomous board is the North Dakota licensure board. It is fully responsible for implementing the licensure law. Board members write regulations, send out applications, collect fees, issue licenses, and hear complaints. They purchase clerical, printing, legal, or investigative services as needed, usually from other state agencies. In occupational therapy, most states have regulatory boards or advisory councils that are essentially autonomous but receive administrative services, review, and funding from a central agency. In a few states a central agency administering regulatory laws maintains complete

---

Table 17-2

Recommended Characteristics of Regulatory Entities

1. Appropriate professional expertise in the decision making process;

2. Input from the public who are ultimately impacted by any regulatory decision;

3. Fiscal accountability to the citizens of the state;

4. Decisions made with the public's interest, as opposed to the profession's interest, in mind;

5. Avoidance of unnecessary bureaucratic "red tape" for current or future licensees as well as the public;

6. Staffing that includes individuals with the relevant expertise to handle the administrative details of regulation;

7. Avoidance of political pressure and influence in decision making;

8. Appropriate checks and balances included in the overall operations;

9. Automation of administrative functions, as appropriate;

10. Impartial review and resolution of jurisdictional disputes;

11. Clear delegation of authority from the executive and legislative branch to the regulatory body;

12. Timely and appropriate orientation of new board members as to their role and responsibilities;

13. Timely investigations of complaints;

14. Timely and appropriate disciplinary action taken against licensees who violate the law or rules; and

15. Periodic assessment of the regulatory law and rules.

Note. *From* Questions a Legislator Should Ask, *by B. Shimberg and D. Roederer (2nd ed., K. Schmitt, Ed.) (pp. 18–19), 1994, Lexington, KY: Council on Licensure, Enforcement and Regulation. Copyright ©1994 by Council on Licensure, Enforcement and Regulation. Reprinted with permission.*

---

authority. This is true, for example, in New York, where the occupational therapy board only advises the Board of Regents within the Department of Education.

Renewal

A common but not universal feature of state licensure, certification, and registration systems is a requirement that the practitioner renew his or her credential every so often. Typically, to qualify for renewal, the practitioner must fulfill a continuing education requirement—for example, a certain number of contact hours or continuing education units—and pay a renewal fee. The assumption underlying this requirement is that by participating in continuing education, the practitioner will maintain his or her competence. Scholars of licensing point out that there is no strong research to support this assumption (Shimberg & Roederer, 1994).

As of September 1995, of the 39 states with occupational therapy licensure laws, 25 had a continuing education requirement, to be met every year in some states, every second year in others. The District of Columbia and Puerto Rico also had such requirements. Of the 5 states with occupational therapy certification laws, only two had continuing education requirements; and of the 3 states with occupational therapy registration laws, only one did (AOTA, 1995).

In a few states that have no continuing education requirement, a movement is afoot to create one. Also, other regulatory agencies may require that staff members of health care facilities participate in continuing education—for example, the Joint Commission on Accreditation of Healthcare Organizations and CARF, The Rehabilitation Accreditation Commission (see chapter 13, "Voluntary Accrediting Agencies").

Disciplinary Action

Boards protect the public by providing consumer information, monitoring regulated practitioners, and investigating complaints. They have the power to discipline practitioners using a variety of sanctions, ranging from a reprimand to revocation of a license, a certificate, or registered status. The latter removes the practitioner's right to practice in that state and is thus used only in extreme cases. Less harsh methods may include such actions as peer review of records, educational meetings, supervision with or without a mentor, continuing education, and suspension of a license, a certificate, or registered status. When a complaint is filed with both a licensure board and NBCOT, some licensure boards await the outcome with NBCOT before investigating the complaint.

THE FUTURE OF STATE REGULATION

Many have viewed state regulation of health care professionals critically. Reform has taken the form of appointment of public members to licensing boards, creation of umbrella agencies to oversee licensing boards, passing of sunset laws (requiring termination of the enabling legislation by a specific date unless the legislature renews it) and sunrise laws (requiring that professions meet certain criteria before licensing is initiated), and rulings by the Federal Trade Commission on the anticompetitive aspects of some licensing laws (Young, 1987). Some critics have proposed a system that would encourage consumers to rely on information and their own judgment regarding the preparation of health care professionals. Others have proposed programs to modify the state regulatory structure.

The most recent proposal for reform of the state regulatory structure relating to the health care workforce, published in late 1995 by the Taskforce on Health Care Workforce Regulation of the Pew Health Professions Commission, would alter that structure significantly. Citing the many transformations in the nation's health care system, the task force characterizes the existing regulatory system as "out of step with today's health care needs and expectations" (n.p.). It calls for a system that would be "*standardized* where appropriate; *accountable* to the public; *flexible* to support optimal access to a competent workforce; and *effective* and *efficient* in protecting and promoting the public's health, safety and welfare" (n.p.). The targets of standardization would be regulatory terms (e.g., *licensure* to denote state regulation, *certification* to denote private-sector regulation) and entry-level competencies. Accountability would take the form of (1) interdisciplinary regulatory boards with a majority of public members, consolidated around related health professions or health service areas; (2) board responsibility for educating consumers about practitioners' competence; (3) continuing assessment of practitioners' competence; (4) reform of the disciplinary process; and (5) evaluation of the regulatory system's effectiveness. Flexibility would come into play in allowance for overlapping scopes of practice. Effectiveness and efficiency would be sought in (1) some of the measures to achieve accountability, just mentioned; (2) collection of data on the health care workforce, to support planning; and (3) public-private partnerships to streamline regulation. The prospects of the task force's recommendations being adopted by any states are unknown at this writing.

NONGOVERNMENTAL CERTIFICATION AND REGISTRATION

Nongovernmental certifying organizations such as NBCOT recognize persons who have attained entry-level competence in broad areas of responsibility of their profession through the mechanism of *certification* or *registration*. A person completing the certification or registration process, which is voluntary, is granted a certificate and may also become entitled to use a special designation with his or her name, such as *certified* or *registered*.

Professional organizations such as AOTA recognize persons who have attained advanced-level competence through *specialty certification*. This too is a voluntary process.

CERTIFICATION OF OCCUPATIONAL THERAPY PRACTITIONERS AT THE ENTRY LEVEL

In the mid-1930s AOTA initiated a program of nongovernmental certification for occupational therapists, which it then administered for over 50 years.[2] The association introduced a similar program for occupational therapy assistants in the early 1960s. In the mid-1980s, concern arose in AOTA governing bodies about the appearance of a conflict of interest between the association's mission to promote the growth of the profession and its obligation to protect the public against unqualified professionals. This concern led to the founding in 1986 of an independent organization, NBCOT, and the transfer of the certification program from AOTA to NBCOT (Madelaine Gray, first executive director of NBCOT, personal communication, January 24, 1996).

The goal of NBCOT is to promote public health, safety, and welfare by establishing, maintaining, and administering standards, policies, and programs for certification and registration of occupational therapy practitioners.[3] An indication of NBCOT's commitment to protection of the public is the composition of its governing board: six public members, five OTRs, three COTAs, and NBCOT's executive director (a nonvoting member). NBCOT's bylaws stipulate that at least one-third of the members be public members.

NBCOT certifies qualified persons as *registered occupational therapists* (OTRs) or *certified occupational therapy assistants* (COTAs). Certification by NBCOT indicates to the public that the OTR or the COTA has met all of NBCOT's educational, fieldwork, and examination requirements.

Basis for Certification

NBCOT certifies occupational therapy practitioners on the basis of separate examinations for therapists and assistants. The examinations are objective measures of entry-level competence, each consisting of 200 items in a multiple-choice format.

NBCOT's Certification Examination Development Committee, a group of content experts (OTRs and COTAs) drawn from a wide variety

---

2. *In the early years AOTA called the program for occupational therapists* registration *and granted the designation* registered *to applicants who successfully completed the education, fieldwork, and examination requirements. In later years the program became known as a* certification and registration *program.*

3. *The remainder of this section is based on* About AOTCB, *1995, April;* Questions Most Frequently Asked by Students About Certification, *1992, July; and various forms and handouts; Gaithersburg, MD: National Board for Certification in Occupational Therapy. Adapted with permission.*

of work settings and geographic regions, develops the examinations with assistance from other OTRs and COTAs who have expertise in specific practice areas and are trained item writers. NBCOT contracts with a testing company for psychometric guidance in developing and administering the examinations.

A candidate who has passed the NBCOT examination receives a certificate, which he or she may show to employers and regulatory boards. NBCOT reissues the certificate every five years to indicate that it has not withdrawn or revoked certification because of disciplinary action.

Approximately 66,000 occupational therapists and 23,000 occupational therapy assistants have been certified since the 1930s. In 1995 about 4,700 new occupational therapists and 2,450 new occupational therapy assistants were certified (Edna Wooldridge, director of evaluation and research, NBCOT, personal communication, March 14, 1996). The examinations are administered twice a year nationwide and around the world.

Requirements for Eligibility to Take the Examination

Persons Trained in the United States

To take the examination for certification, persons who were trained in the United States, its territories, or commonwealths must meet the following requirements:

For Certification as an OTR

1. Be a graduate of an occupational therapist education program accredited by AOTA's Accreditation Council for Occupational Therapy Education (ACOTE)

2. Have successfully completed all therapist-level fieldwork required by the education program (but not less than six months)

For Certification as a COTA

1. Be a graduate of an occupational therapy assistant education program accredited/approved by AOTA's ACOTE

2. Have successfully completed all assistant-level fieldwork required by the education program (but not less than 440 hours or 12 weeks)

Persons Not Trained in the United States

Persons who were not trained in the United States must meet different requirements. Current information on these requirements is available directly from NBCOT (see Additional Resources for an address and a telephone number).

Currently the established foreign test centers are in Australia, Canada, Hong Kong, India, Israel, the Philippines, South Africa, Taiwan, and the United Kingdom. An applicant can arrange with NBCOT to take the test in a nonestablished foreign test center.

The examination is in English. Therapists who were not trained in the United States are required to pass English-language proficiency examinations before being approved to take the examination for certification as an OTR.

Relationship to State Regulation, Private or Public Employment, and Third-Party Reimbursement

NBCOT certification is independent of state regulation. All the states that regulate occupational therapy practitioners use NBCOT's certification requirements as a part of the basis for determining a person's eligibility for state regulation. Individual states may have other requirements. It is essential that practitioners contact the regulatory agency in the states in which they want to practice for information about the legal requirements for working in those states.

NBCOT certification is not a legal requirement for public or private employment unless a state mandates it as a condition of licensure, certification, or registration. Individual employers and third-party payers may require NBCOT certification.

Disciplinary Action

An essential part of NBCOT's responsibility is disciplinary action. The purpose of the agency's disciplinary action program is to protect the public from persons whose behavior reflects incompetence, a breach of ethics, or impairment. OTR, COTA, and public members of the governing board sit on the Disciplinary Action Committee, and one of the public members chairs it. Final actions of the committee are published in a quarterly newsletter, *NBCOT Information Exchange*. NBCOT's disciplinary actions are independent of disciplinary actions by AOTA's Commission on Standards and Ethics and state regulatory boards or agencies.

For further information on application procedures, deadlines, processing information, specific examinations, and other matters, the prospective applicant should contact NBCOT (see Additional Resources for an address and a telephone number).

SPECIALTY CERTIFICATION FOR OCCUPATIONAL THERAPISTS

Specialty certification in occupational therapy by the AOTA is of fairly recent origin, AOTA's Representative Assembly having authorized the first program in 1989.[4] AOTA is the sole sponsor of this specialty certification program. A Specialty Certification Board consisting of five OTRs oversees the program.

Specialty certification is currently available in two areas, neurorehabilitation and pediatrics. The certification is voluntary in that a person need not have it to work as an OTR. The award of specialty certification indicates that a therapist has met predetermined standards and criteria in the designated area.

The objectives of specialty certification are as follows:

1. To support quality health care by promoting the development of specialized knowledge in the practice of occupational therapy

2. To assist consumers and others in the health care community in identifying therapists with expertise in specific areas of practice

3. To promote the continued development of the art and the science underlying the practice of the profession

4. To facilitate and respond to the future development of best practice, education, and research in occupational therapy

5. To provide assistance and support to the career development of occupational therapy practice specialists

Basis for Certification

AOTA awards specialty certification on the basis of practitioners' having met specific experiential and professional development criteria and their having successfully completed a 225-item multiple-choice examination. An advisory committee developed the professional criteria, building on work submitted by the Steering Committee of the Special Interest Sections. AOTA then contracted with the American College Testing Company to provide expert guidance in development and implementation of the examinations. An overview of the examination development process is available from AOTA.

Requirements for Eligibility to Take the Examination

To take the examination, persons must meet three requirements:

1. Certification as an OTR by NBCOT

2. Five or more years of clinical experience (a minimum of 4,160 hours) since initial certification in the specialty area (neurorehabilitation or pediatrics, as appropriate), 1,040 hours of which

---

4. *This section is based on various forms and handouts published by AOTA's Practice Division.*

must have been obtained within the last five years (which may be in a combination of treatment, monitoring, consultation, supervision, and clinical research)

3. Completion within the last five years of 5 professional development activities from a list of 13 possible activities available from the Specialty Certification Program office

Renewal

An OTR must renew his or her specialty certification every five years from the date on which he or she took the examination. Recertification requires professional activities in a combination of the selected areas of practice, including clinical practice, teaching, continuing education, and clinical research.

Grounds for Revocation

Participation in any of the following will result in the revocation of specialty certification: (1) falsification of the application; (2) falsification of any information requested by the Specialty Certification Board; (3) revocation of certification or licensure as an occupational therapist; or (4) cheating on the examination.

CROSS-BORDER TRADE IN SERVICES UNDER THE NORTH AMERICAN FREE TRADE AGREEMENT

The North American Free Trade Agreement (NAFTA), which became effective on January 1, 1994, is designed to eliminate barriers to trade in goods and services among Canada, Mexico, and the United States of America, which together represent over 650 million consumers. Among other effects, the agreement promotes relatively free movement of professional service providers like occupational therapy practitioners across the borders of the three countries. [Furthermore—but not the subject of this chapter—companies may now market occupational therapy devices and products across national boundaries without excessive tariffs (Joe, 1993).]

DEFINITION AND SCOPE OF CROSS-BORDER TRADE IN SERVICES

The pertinent part of NAFTA in terms of the subject of this chapter is Chapter 12, "Cross-Border Trade in Services," and Annex 1210.5, "Professional Services" (NAFTA, 1993). Chapter 12, Article 1213, defines *cross-border trade in services* as "the provision of a service: (a) from the territory of a Party [a party to the agreement—that is, Canada, Mexico, or the United States] into the territory of another Party, (b) in the territory of a Party by a person of that Party to a person of another Party, or (c) by a national of a Party in the territory of another Party" (pp. 12-6, -7). Chapter 12, Article 1201, identifies the scope of coverage of the chapter, stating that it applies to measures that Canada, Mexico, and the United States adopt or maintain relating to cross-border trade in services by service providers. Among the measures are those "affecting (a) the production, distribution, marketing, sale and delivery of a service; (b) the purchase or use of, or payment for, a service; . . . [and] (d) the presence in its territory of a service provider of another Party" (p. 12-1). This clearly encompasses state and professional regulation of occupational therapy practitioners.

GENERAL PRINCIPLES

Chapter 12, Articles 1202–1205, of NAFTA apply several general principles of free trade to cross-border trade in services. First, under the principle of national treatment, each of the three countries, including all states or provinces within them, must accord to service providers of the other two countries "treatment no less favorable than it accords, in like circumstances, to its own service providers" (p. 12-2). Second, under the principle of most-favored-nation treatment, each of the three countries must accord to service providers of the other two countries "treatment no less favorable than that it accords, in like circumstances, to service providers" of any other country, a party to the agreement or not (p. 12-2). Third, the standard of treatment in any given circumstance must be the better of national treatment or most-favored nation treatment. Finally, any of the three countries may not require a "local presence" by a service provider of the other two countries (p. 12-2); that is, it may not require the provider to establish or maintain an office or an enterprise in its territory, or to reside there, as a condition of cross-border trade in services.

PROVISIONS RELATING TO LICENSING AND CERTIFICATION

Chapter 12, Article 1210, specifically addresses licensing and certification, recognizing that these mechanisms may unnecessarily restrain trade. The article requires the three countries to strive to ensure that any related measure they adopt or maintain meets three standards:

(a) [It] is based on objective and transparent criteria, such as competence and the ability to provide a service;

(b) [It] is not more burdensome than necessary to ensure the quality of a service; and

(c) [It] does not constitute a disguised restriction on the cross-border provision of service.

(pp. 12-4, -5)

In annex 1210.5, the chapter sets forth general provisions relating to *professional services,* defined elsewhere in the chapter as "services, the provision of which requires specialized postsecondary education, or equivalent training or experience, and for which the right to practice is granted or restricted by a Party" (p. 12-7). The general provisions of the annex fall into four categories, three of which are of particular interest to this discussion: processing of applications for licenses and certifications; development of professional standards; and temporary licensing. The processing provision calls for action on applications within a reasonable time. The standards provision requires the three countries to "encourage the relevant bodies in their respective territories to develop mutually acceptable standards and criteria for licensing and certification of professional service providers and to provide recommendations on mutual recognition to the Commission [the body established by NAFTA to oversee implementation]" (p. 12-8). The standards may address education, examinations, experience, conduct and ethics, professional development and recertification, scope of practice, knowledge of local factors like laws and language, and consumer protection. The temporary licensing provision requires each country to encourage relevant bodies in its territory to develop procedures for the temporary licensing of professional service providers from the other two countries.

IMMIGRATION PROVISIONS AND PROCEDURES

Under NAFTA a Canadian or Mexican citizen *who has a job offer in the United States* in any of a number of professions, including the medical and allied health professions, may be granted one-year multiple-entry Trade NAFTA (TN) status.[5] Currently TN status is renewable indefinitely on an annual basis. Occupational therapists may qualify for the TN-1 nonimmigrant (i.e., temporary visa) option, which is available to academic professionals. Table 17-3 presents the requirements and the procedures. NAFTA treats citizens from the two countries differently (Shusterman, 1994), as the table indicates.

---

5. *The information about TN status, the TN-1 nonimmigrant option, and the availability of other options is based on "Immigration Options and Procedures for Advanced Teaching and Research Professionals" (pp. 10–17), by R. E. Hopper, 1994, in R. P. Deasey, S. M. Borene, L. R. Burgess, D. J. Kartje, D. A. M. Ware, and P. R. Yanni (Eds.),* American Immigration Lawyers Association Guidebook: Immigration Options for Professors and Researchers, *Washington, DC: American Immigration Lawyers Association. That chapter is an abridged version of "Immigration and Higher Education: Procedures and Strategies for the Global Recruitment of Teachers and Scholars," by R. E. Hopper, 93-9* Immigration Briefings *(September 1993). Copyright © 1993 by Federal Publications, Inc. Adapted with permission. Hopper, an attorney in Houston, Texas, is board certified in immigration and nationality law.*

Table 17-3
NAFTA Regulations for Canadian and Mexican Citizens with Job Offers,
Who Apply for Trade NAFTA Status

CANADIAN CITIZENS

Applicant's Responsibility

Citizen may file application for admission for up to one year as TN professional with immigration officer at U.S. Class A port of entry, U.S. airport handling international traffic, or U.S. pre-clearance/pre-flight station. Applicant must present following:

1. Evidence of Canadian citizenship (no passport is required unless applicant is entering U.S. from outside Western Hemisphere).

2. Proof of both engagement in business activities at professional level and applicant's professional qualifications. Such proof may be in form of letter from prospective employer in U.S. Immigration officer may require support in form of licenses, diplomas, degrees, certificates, or membership in professional organization. Degrees, diplomas, or certificates received from educational institution not in Canada, Mexico, or U.S. must be accompanied by evaluation by reliable credential evaluation service. Supporting evidence must also fully affirm following:

   a. Appendix 1603.D.1 profession of applicant

   b. Description of professional activities, including brief summary of daily job duties, if appropriate

   c. Anticipated length of stay

   d. Educational qualifications or other credentials that demonstrate professional status

   e. Arrangements for remuneration for services to be provided

   f. If required by state or local law, Canadian citizen's compliance with all applicable laws and/or licensing requirements for professional activity in which he or she will be engaged

Each U.S. Class A port of entry from Canada has designated INS Free Trade Officer (FTO) to process applicants seeking entry. Because some FTOs prefer to review applications ahead of time, and because some ports may have FTOs available only during certain hours, it is important to call FTO at planned port of entry before applying.

MEXICAN CITIZENS

Limit of 5,500 citizens may be classified as TN nonimmigrants annually. Spouses and children are not counted against this limit.

Employer's Responsibility

1. File I-129 petition with U.S. Immigration and Naturalization Service (INS) Northern Service Center, in Lincoln, Nebraska. Petition must include following:

   a. Certification from Secretary of Labor on Form ETA 9035 that petitioner has filed appropriate documentation with Department of Labor in accordance with Section (D)(5)(b) of Annex 1603 of NAFTA.

   b. Evidence that citizen/applicant meets minimum education requirements or alternative credential requirements of Appendix 1603.D.1 of NAFTA.

   c. Statement from U.S. employer identifying professional category and describing job duties and any state or local licensing requirement. If no license is required, that fact must be stated. U.S. equivalency evaluations of degrees from institutions not located within Mexico, Canada, or U.S. must also be provided. Evidence of experience should consist of letters from former employers or, if applicant was previously self-employed, business records attesting to such self-employment. Copies of any required state or local licenses are also necessary.

2. Immediately notify INS of any changes in employment terms or conditions that affect TN eligibility, or if petitioner no longer employs applicant.

continued

Applicant's Responsibility

Citizen with approved I-129 petition must obtain TN visa at U.S. consular post before entering U.S.

GENERAL INFORMATION

Readmission

Neither Canadian nor Mexican citizen is required to reapply for TN classification to reenter U.S. during petition validity unless he or she is returning to new employer.

Extensions/Change of Employers

Extensions valid for one year each may be obtained for both Canadian and Mexican applicants by filing I-129 petition with INS Northern Service Center. Authorization to change or add employers is obtained in same way.

Self-Employment Prohibited

TN professionals may not engage in self-employment in U.S.

Temporariness

TNs have no statutory exemption from requirement to prove that they are not intending immigrants. INS interim rule specifically states that presumption of immigrant intent in Immigration and Nationality Act, Section 214(b), applies to Canadian and Mexican TN applicants. This could conceivably result in TN applicant being denied entry or extension of status where labor certification or immigrant visa petition has been filed on his or her behalf.

Note. *From "Immigration Options and Procedures for Advanced Teaching and Research Professionals" (pp. 10–17), by R. E. Hopper, 1994, in R. P. Deasey, S. M. Borene, L. R. Burgess, D. J. Kartje, D. A. M. Ware, and P. R. Yanni (Eds.),* American Immigration Lawyers Association Guidebook: Immigration Options for Professors and Researchers, *Washington, DC: American Immigration Lawyers Association. That chapter is an abridged version of "Immigration and Higher Education: Procedures and Strategies for the Global Recruitment of Teachers and Scholars," by R. E. Hopper, 93-9,* Immigration Briefings *(September, 1993). Copyright © 1993 by Federal Publications, Inc. Adapted with permission.*

There are options in addition to TN-1 nonimmigrant status. Any individual or employer seriously considering immigration procedures for occupational therapy practitioners should consult with the United States Immigration and Naturalization Service (see Additional Resources for an address and a telephone number) and an experienced immigration attorney.

Also under NAFTA, United States occupational therapy practitioners may practice in Canada or Mexico.

At present, all state regulatory laws require that occupational therapists not prepared in the United States complete basically the same requirements that occupational therapists educated in the United States must complete for voluntary certification by NBCOT. On passing the NBCOT certification examination, they must then meet the requirements of the state in which they desire to be employed. Thus, taking the NBCOT certification examination would be to the advantage of occupational therapists prepared in Canada or Mexico if they are planning to work in the United States for an extended period.

IMPLEMENTING AGENCIES

Two federal agencies in addition to the Immigration and Naturalization Service are involved in the implementation of NAFTA: the United States Trade Representative, and the Department of Commerce (see Additional Resources for addresses and telephone numbers of these agencies).

NAFTA has been welcomed by employers who need qualified occupational therapy practitioners, particularly in areas with a shortage of occupational therapists. NAFTA's effect on the occupational therapist's practice options is unknown, but it may expand educational opportunities. This may be facilitated through collaboration among universities with occupational therapy programs.

SUMMARY

State regulation of occupational therapy practitioners takes several forms: licensure, mandatory certification, title control, mandatory registration, and voluntary certification and registration. Each form is authorized by state law and meant to protect the public from harm. *Licensure,* the most restrictive form, is "the process by which an agency of government grants permission to an individual to engage in a given occupation upon finding that the applicant has attained the minimal degree of competence required to ensure that the public health, safety, and welfare will be reasonably well protected" (U.S. Department of Health, Education, and Welfare, 1977, p. 17). The law undergirding licensure defines the scope of practice. *Mandatory certification* and *title control* are processes by which a government agency grants a person permission to use a certain title if that person has attained entry-level competence. *Mandatory registration* is the process by which a government agency grants a person permission to use a certain title if that person has registered with the agency. The agency may or may not require the person to meet a standard of entry-level competency. *Voluntary certification* and *voluntary registration* are processes by which a government agency acknowledges that a person meets certain qualifications associated with a title (which may or may not be equivalent to a standard of entry-level competency) but does not protect either the title or a related scope of practice.

In the health care professions the agency of government granting the permission under the various types of regulation is typically the state department of health. Under a licensure system, that department usually delegates its authority to administer regulations to a board consisting of (1) members of the profession being regulated, (2) consumers, and (3) representatives of related professions.

A common but not universal feature of state licensure, certification, and registration systems is a requirement that the practitioner renew his or her credential every so often. Typically, to qualify for renewal, the practitioner must fulfill a continuing education requirement and pay a renewal fee.

Boards protect the public by providing consumer information, monitoring regulated practitioners, and investigating complaints. They have the power to discipline practitioners using a variety of sanctions.

Nongovernmental certifying organizations such as NBCOT recognize persons who have attained entry-level competence in their profession through the mechanism of *certification* or *registration*. The goal of NBCOT is to promote public health, safety, and welfare by establishing, maintaining, and administering standards, policies, and programs for certification and registration of occupational therapy practitioners.

NBCOT certifies qualified persons as *registered occupational therapists* (OTRs) or *certified occupational therapy assistants* (COTAs) on the basis of separate examinations for therapists and assistants. The examinations are objective measures of entry-level competence.

To take the examination for certification, persons who were trained in the United States, its territories, or commonwealths must meet the following requirements: for certification as an OTR, (1) be a graduate of an occupational therapist education program accredited by AOTA's Accreditation Council for Occupational Therapy Education (ACOTE) and (2) have successfully completed all therapist-level fieldwork required by the education program (but not less than six months); for certification as a COTA, (1) be a graduate of an occupational therapy assistant education program accredited/approved by AOTA's ACOTE and (2) have successfully completed all assistant-level fieldwork required by the education program (but not less than 440 hours or 12 weeks). Persons who were not trained in the United States must meet different requirements.

NBCOT certification is independent of state regulation. All the states that regulate occupational therapy practitioners use NBCOT's certification requirements as a part of the basis for determining a person's eligibility for state regulation. Individual states may have other requirements.

AOTA is the sole sponsor of specialty certification. It is currently available in two areas, neurorehabilitation and pediatrics. The award indicates that a therapist has met predetermined standards and criteria in the designated area.

AOTA awards specialty certification on the basis of a 225-item multiple-choice examination. To take the examination, persons must meet three requirements: (1) certification as an OTR by NBCOT; (2) five or more years of clinical experience (a minimum of 4,160 hours) since initial certification in the specialty area, 1,040 hours of which must have been obtained within the last five years; and (3) completion within the last five years of 5 professional activities from a list of 13 possible activities. An OTR must renew his or her specialty certification every five years.

The North American Free Trade Agreement (NAFTA), which became effective on January 1, 1994, is designed to eliminate barriers to trade in goods and services among Canada, Mexico, and the United States of America. The agreement promotes relatively free cross-border trade in services by professional service providers like occupational therapy practitioners.

On the subject of licensing and certification, the agreement requires the three countries to strive to ensure that any related measure they adopt or maintain "(a) is based on objective and transparent criteria . . . ; (b) is not more burdensome than necessary to ensure the quality of a service; and (c) does not constitute a disguised restriction on the cross-border provision of service" (NAFTA, 1993, pp. 12-4, -5).

Under NAFTA a Canadian or Mexican citizen *who has a job offer in the United States* in any of a number of professions may be granted one-year multiple-entry Trade NAFTA (TN) status. Currently TN status is renewable indefinitely on an annual basis. Occupational therapists may qualify for the TN-1 nonimmigrant (i.e., temporary visa) option. There are options in addition to TN-1 nonimmigrant status. At present, all state regulatory laws require that occupational therapists not prepared in the United States complete basically the same requirements that occupational therapists educated in the United States must complete for voluntary certification by NBCOT. On passing the NBCOT certification examination, they must then meet the requirements of the state in which they desire to be employed.

REFERENCES

American Occupational Therapy Association, Government Relations Department. (1996, June). *Compilation of occupational therapy state regulatory information* [Fact sheet]. Bethesda, MD: Author.

Joe, B. (1993, December 16). NAFTA opens new doors for OT practitioners. *OT Week,* p. 10.

Mosby's medical, nursing, and allied health dictionary (4th ed.). (1994). St. Louis, MO: Mosby.

The North American Free Trade Agreement Between the Government of the United States of America, the Government of Canada, and the Government of the United Mexican States. (1993). Washington, DC: Government Printing Office. Pub. L. No. 103–182, 107 Stat. 2057, codified at 19 U.S.C. §§ 3301 *et seq.*

Pew Health Professions Commission, Taskforce on Health Care Workforce Regulation. (1995, September). *Reforming health care workforce regulation: Policy considerations for the 21st century* [Brochure]. San Francisco: Pew Health Professions Commission.

Quiroga, V. A. M. (1995). *Occupational therapy: The first thirty years, 1900–1930.* Bethesda, MD: American Occupational Therapy Association.

Scott, S. J., & Acquaviva, J. D. (1985). *Lobbying for health care: A guidebook for professionals and associations.* Rockville, MD: American Occupational Therapy Association.

Shimberg, B., & Roederer, D. (1994). *Questions a legislator should ask* (2nd ed., K. Schmitt, Ed.). Lexington, KY: Council on Licensure, Enforcement and Regulation.

Shusterman, C. (1994, April 7). NAFTA stimulates the flow of goods and professionals. *OT Week,* p. 10.

United States Department of Health, Education, and Welfare, Public Health Service. (1977). *Credentialing health manpower* [Publication No. (OS) 77-50057]. Bethesda, MD: Author.

Young, S. D. (1987). *The rule of experts: Occupational licensing in America.* Washington, DC: Cato Institute.

ADDITIONAL RESOURCES

ORGANIZATIONS

American Occupational Therapy Association, Practice Division, Neurorehabilitation and Pediatric Specialty Certification Programs, 4720 Montgomery Lane, P.O. Box 31220, Bethesda, MD 20824-1220, telephone 301/652-2682

National Board for Certification in Occupational Therapy, Inc., 800 South Frederick Avenue, Suite 200, Gaithersburg, MD 20877-4150, telephone 301/990-7979

Office of the United States Trade Representative, Office of the Western Hemisphere, 600 17th Street NW, Washington, DC 20508, telephone 202/395-3412—*for information about trade policy issues*

United States Department of Commerce, Office of NAFTA/Room 3022, 14th and Constitution Avenue NW, Washington, DC 20230, telephone 202/482-0305—*for information about export of goods and services*

United States Immigration and Naturalization Service, Attention: Office of Adjudications, 425 I Street NW, Washington, DC 20536, telephone 202/514-5014—*for information about qualifications for Trade NAFTA (TN) status*

PUBLICATIONS

American Occupational Therapy Association, Government Relations Department. (1995, November). *Definition of occupational therapy for state regulation* [Fact sheet]. Bethesda, MD: Author.

American Occupational Therapy Association, Government Relations Department. (1995, November). *Definitions of occupational therapy and requirements for practice by state* [Fact sheet]. Bethesda, MD: Author.

Thomson, L. K., & Thomson, N., for the Commission on Practice. (1995). *Report on NAFTA: The impact on occupational therapy in the United States of America.* Bethesda, MD: American Occupational Therapy Association.

CHAPTER 18

Ethical Dimensions in Occupational Therapy

Karin J. Opacich, MHPE, OTR/L, FAOTA

KEY TERMS

Autonomy. Self-governance.

Beneficence. Actions that benefit others, including but not limited to acts of mercy, kindness, and charity.

Confidentiality. The obligation not to disclose personal information without authorization.

Ethical reasoning. A process involving three steps: recognizing ethical tensions in practice; becoming conversant in the language of ethics and ethical principles; and establishing a strategy for conducting the conversations that will lead to ethical resolution.

Ethical tensions. Feelings that all is not morally right.

Fidelity. Promise keeping or faithfulness.

Justice. Equity and fairness.

Nonmaleficence. Doing no harm.

Privacy. Respect for a person's right to limit access to his or her personal sphere.

Veracity. The obligation to tell the truth.

"The failure of the health care professions to take human values as seriously as they should has led to a range of institutional responses, from holistic medicine to ethics committees. Each in its own way is a response to the problem of putting health care in the context of human values. Both bioethics and professional ethics reflect a concern to put health care within the perspective of human values, as well as to develop means for mastering that perspective, for critically reexamining it and refashioning it. There has been a recognition that we must reclaim our role as custodians of human values in health care if technology is to serve us well in the future."

● ●

(Engelhardt, 1986, p. 40)

Karin J. Opacich, MHPE, OTR/L, FAOTA, is an assistant professor and the education coordinator in the Department of Occupational Therapy at Rush University, and an instructor in the university's Department of Religion, Health, and Human Values. She is also a doctoral student in the School of Public Health at the University of Illinois and a member of AOTA's Accreditation Council for Occupational Therapy Education. She maintains a small community-based practice in pediatric occupational therapy.

Ancient and contemporary philosophers have contemplated the human condition throughout the ages, wrestling with such metaphysical questions as What is good? What is fair? What is right? What are the duties and the obligations of human beings to one another? What are their obligations to safeguard nonhuman resources? The accumulated contemplations of moral philosophers can assist humans with the ethical quandaries that they face in their personal and professional lives.

Occupational therapy practitioners espouse the values and the commitments of their field. Philosophical statements embedded in the profession's historical documents and literature guide practitioners in the provision of occupational therapy, serving as their professional and moral consciences. These statements help them define the ethical obligations of occupational therapy.

In professional preparation, educators expend much effort teaching and refining clinical reasoning. They pay less attention to ethical reasoning. Ethical reasoning parallels clinical reasoning, influencing the decisions that occupational therapy practitioners make as clinicians, managers, educators, or researchers. Recognizing the effect of ethical legacy on the practice of occupational therapy, the *Essentials and Guidelines for an Accredited Educational Program for the Occupational Therapist* (AOTA, 1991a) specifically state that the following content pertaining to professional ethics must be included in occupational therapy curricula:

II. B. 6. Professional ethics

>   a. AOTA standards and ethics policies and their effect on the therapist's conduct and patient treatment.

>   b. Functions of national, state, and local occupational therapy associations, and other professional associations and human service organizations.

>   c. Recognition of the necessity to participate in the promotion of occupational therapy through educating other professionals, consumers, third party payers, and the public.

>   d. Individual responsibility for planning for future professionaldevelopment in order to maintain a level of practice consistent with accepted standards.

II. B. 7. Fieldwork education . . .

>   c. Level II Fieldwork shall be required and designed to promote clinical reasoning and reflective practice, to transmit the values and beliefs that enable the application of

ethics related to the profession, to communicate and model professionalism as a developmental process and a career responsibility, and to develop and expand a repertoire of occupational therapy assessments and treatment interventions related to human performance.

(p. 6)

The *Essentials and Guidelines for an Accredited Educational Program for the Occupational Therapy Assistant* (AOTA, 1991b) also address issues of ethics as integral parts of approved curricula:

II. B. 3. Occupational therapy principles and practice skills . . .

h. Develop values, attitudes, and behaviors congruent with:

(1) The profession's standards and ethics.

(2) Individual responsibility for continued learning.

(3) Interdisciplinary and supervisory relationships within the administrative hierarchy.

(4) Participation in the promotion of occupational therapy through involvement in professional organizations, government bodies, and human service organizations.

(5) Understanding of the importance of and the role of the occupational therapy assistant in occupational therapy research, publication, program evaluation, and documentation of services.

(p. 6)

Not only should this language provide impetus for conveying ethical reasoning to aspiring occupational therapy practitioners, but it should serve as an incentive for practicing professionals to revisit and articulate their professional ethics.

RECOGNITION OF ETHICAL TENSIONS

Affective cues commonly alert health care professionals to ethical tensions. A practitioner may feel conflicted, have an intuitive moral response to a situation, or sense a threat to personal integrity. In short, when faced with an ethical challenge, the practitioner may feel on some level that all is not right. Recognizing the symptoms, the practitioner must then sort out psychological and social sensitivities from ethical tensions. This requires identifying the source from which the tension emanates. The descriptions of ethical tensions developed by Jameton (see table 18-1) may help clarify the sources of ethical tensions.

Table 18-1
Descriptions of Ethical Tensions

Ethical uncertainty	Being unsure of what moral principles apply or if a problem is indeed a moral problem
Ethical distress	Knowing the "right" course of action but feeling constrained to act by institutional rules
Ethical dilemma	Facing two or more equally unpleasant alternatives that are mutually exclusive

Source. *Based on information in* Nursing Practice: The Ethical Issues *(pp. 6, 157), by* A. Jameton, 1984, Englewood Cliffs, NJ: Prentice-Hall.

MORAL PRINCIPLES APPLICABLE TO HEALTH CARE

When a source of tension seems to be related to ethics, further analysis is required. By connecting the ethical tensions in a real-life scenario to the existing literature on moral reasoning, practitioners and managers can benefit from the experience and the interpretations of others. The literature expounding on moral principles is vast and continually growing. *Principles of Biomedical Ethics* (Beauchamp & Childress, 1994) provides basic definitions and comprehensive explanations of moral principles in health care. Major ethical principles are autonomy, beneficence, nonmaleficence, justice, and several that govern relationships. They are briefly summarized in the following sections. Readers should become familiar with these moral principles and the issues related to them. Professional codes of ethics establish rules of conduct based on these principles. The *Occupational Therapy Code of Ethics* (see appendix 18-A) represents the professional association's effort to guide and regulate the ethical practices of its members. Policy-making bodies within AOTA, such as the Commission on Standards and Ethics, generate related statements and position papers. An article entitled "Core Values and Attitudes of Occupational Therapy Practice" (see appendix 18-B) is an example of commentary on the moral content of occupational therapy.

Professionals are usually regulated both by their associations and by law. On the national level the American Occupational Therapy Certification Board has a well-defined mechanism for dealing with ethical complaints about occupational therapy practitioners. State licensure is an example of legal regulation; licensure boards may reflect ethical dimensions if they review complaints about professional conduct.

AUTONOMY

Autonomy is the principle of self-governance. It pertains to liberty rights, the right to privacy, the right to individual choice, and generally the right to self-determination. In health care, autonomy is at issue in discussions of competency, informed consent, disclosure of information, and acceptance or refusal of medically indicated treatment. Autonomy becomes more complicated and requires further clarification when the practitioner is dealing with children, pregnant adults or adolescents, persons with mental impairments or cognitive deficits, and persons unable to speak for themselves for any reason. Many states have enacted legislation addressing autonomy. For instance, in the event that a medical condition impairs a person's autonomy, a law might authorize a health care agent to make decisions on the person's behalf. It is important for health care professionals to be aware of the laws and the provisions of the states in which they practice. Because occupational therapy practitioners are involved in team discussions and decisions, they may be called on to contribute observations or other data that reflect a patient's understanding of his or her condition and associated treatment options. In some instances occupational therapy practitioners may participate on or be official members of institutional ethics committees (Kyler-Hutchison, 1994). Managers can prepare staff members for these experiences by addressing principles, legislation, and protocol related to aspects of autonomy.

BENEFICENCE

Beneficence refers to actions that benefit others, including but not limited to acts of mercy, kindness, and charity. It implies both actively doing good and considering the potential harm of an action. *Paternalism,* the presumption that health care professionals know what is best for a patient by virtue of their expertise, frequently arises as an issue in medicine in connection with beneficence. Particularly in today's climate, a patient's participation in the selection of medical alternatives and in pursuit of health care is preferred. Regarding the balancing aspect of beneficence, the analysis of options must consider both risk with respect to cost, and benefit in consideration of burden. Ultimately choices are made based on their value to the recipients of service. Of particular importance for occupational therapy is recognition that efficacy studies can attest to the outcomes and the potential benefit of therapy. Such evidence can assure practitioners of the opportunity to do good on behalf of the patient (Beauchamp & Childress, 1994).

NONMALEFICENCE

Nonmaleficence is inextricably related to beneficence. Taken from the Hippocratic tradition, it means "doing no harm." Although there is frequently debate about the extent to which anyone is obligated to prevent or remove harm, it is generally accepted that a health care practitioner ought to refrain from inflicting harm. The concept of nonmaleficence is debated in relation to withdrawal of treatment, hastening of death, passive and active euthanasia, and other decisions that affect the length or the quality of life. Quality in living is historically an important notion in occupational therapy.

JUSTICE

Justice is a complex principle that generally relates to issues of equity and fairness. Two major aspects of justice are *distribution* and *retribution*. Distributive justice pertains to the rationing of goods and services. This principle helps determine who is entitled to what. Retributive justice guides decisions about reallocating goods and services that have been distributed unfairly. When commodities or resources are limited, allocation becomes a critical issue. When individuals or groups have been wrongfully deprived, making restitution becomes an issue. The concepts of human rights, equality, and fair opportunity are all facets of justice (Beauchamp & Childress, 1994). For example, the demand for occupational therapy currently exceeds the supply. The principle of justice helps occupational therapy managers assign priorities in providing services. Fees for services rendered support occupational therapy in medical, community, educational, industrial, and other settings. Consumers' access to occupational therapy may be limited by their ability to pay; persons of lesser means who need occupational therapy services may not have access to them in the prevailing health care delivery system.

PRINCIPLES GOVERNING RELATIONSHIPS

No less important are several principles governing relationships. Critical to creating trust, these principles form the basis for the covenant between patient or client and health care provider (May 1995). *Veracity* refers to the obligation to tell the truth in a relationship. *Fidelity* pertains to promise keeping or faithfulness. *Privacy* refers to respecting a person's right to limit access to his or her personal sphere. *Confidentiality* pertains to authorized disclosure, or nondisclosure, of personal information.

ETHICAL PERSPECTIVES

In any situation that raises ethical questions, several principles may apply simultaneously. Once a practitioner has identified the applicable stakes, he or she must determine which will take priority in developing options to resolve the moral problems at hand. Specific theories and frameworks of ethical problem solving may clarify issues, just as conceptual models and congruent tests and measures help to illuminate human performance problems.

Pojman, in his 1989 anthology *Ethical Theory: Classical and Contemporary Readings,* divides the study of ethical theory into 13 categories: (1) what ethics is, (2) ethical relativism, (3) ethical egoism, (4) values, (5) utilitarianism, (6) Kantian and deontological systems, (7) virtue-based ethical systems, (8) fact/value definition, (9) moral realism, (10) morality and self-interest, (11) ethics and religion, (12) justice, and (13) rights. Most college graduates have encountered a few of these perspectives in philosophy courses. The categorization does not include all existing perspectives and theories, but it should give occupational therapy practitioners an appreciation of the breadth of literature that can be helpful to them when they face ethical quandaries. Each theory within a category provides a distinct perspective from which to make ethical decisions that are internally consistent. A serious student of ethics will study, compare, and contrast the characteristics of ethical theories and apply them to support moral argument, just as occupational therapists use social and scientific theories to develop treatment interventions. Most occupational therapy practitioners have less facility with moral theory than with social or scientific theory, but that does not preclude their participation in health care conversations concerning moral reasoning.

THE PROCESS OF ETHICAL REASONING

Recognizing ethical tensions in practice is the first step in the process of ethical reasoning. Becoming conversant in the language of ethics and ethical principles is the second step, enabling one to articulate ethical tensions and develop cogent arguments when ethical concerns are part of a health problem.

A third step is to establish a strategy for conducting the conversations that will lead to ethical resolution. Teresa Savage, a nurse-ethicist, has developed a protocol (see table 18-2) that health care professionals can use to facilitate ethical dialogue. Savage has also done extensive work on moral authority and the ethics of caring. Her generic model allows incorporation of any specific ethical theory. It is clear from the model that team communication and mutual respect are critical components of the ethical reasoning process. It is also clear that a range of acceptable options is more likely to emerge than a single course of action.

Because personal values and traditions differ, what the major stakeholders consider to be the best option may not be what all team participants perceive as the best option. Occupational therapy has at its core a tradition of honoring patients' or clients' values and choices, so occupational therapy practitioners can understand the ambivalence inherent in ethical decision making. It is important to remember that an ethical action is not necessarily a psychological balm. Simply stated, virtue can be

---

Table 18-2
The Savage Facilitation Model of Ethical Contemplation

1. Ascertain facts, impressions, rumors about situation at hand.
2. Verify information with key players.
3. Identify problems to be solved.
4. Sort decisions to be made (e.g., medical, legal, ethical, educational).
5. Identify range of options.
6. Identify ethical ramifications of those options (e.g., morally obligatory, morally permissible, and morally prohibited).
7. Participate in team discussion to plan conference with parties of interest. (*Parties of interest* means those who have investment in outcomes of situation. Parties of interest may include patient, relatives, significant others, health care providers, administrators, etc.)
8. Discuss and resolve team conflict, and designate representatives to speak for team.
9. Discuss options with parties of interest.
10. Evaluate ethical soundness of decision.
11. Implement decision; assist or abide by decision.
12. Reevaluate decision and process by which decision was made.
13. Provide support and respect for parties involved.
14. Reflect on your own involvement in process; incorporate positive aspects into your decision-making process.

Note. *From* The Unrecognized Role of the Nurse in Ethical Decision-Making, *by T. Savage, 1990, October, Paper presented at the University of Illinois College of Medicine Symposium, "A Time to Live . . . A Time to Die: Medical Ethics in the 90's," Rockford, IL. Copyright 1990 by T. Savage. Adapted with permission.*

---

painful. To illustrate dramatically, how might an occupational therapist feel if she considered a patient under her care with newly acquired quadriplegia to have good rehabilitation potential, but the patient had decided to withdraw from medical treatment in order to hasten death? Although the patient would be exercising autonomy, which the therapist would defend professionally, the therapist might think that this course of action was a terrible option.

THE ROLES OF THE OCCUPATIONAL THERAPY MANAGER IN ETHICAL PROBLEM SOLVING

Effective managers are both responsive and visionary. They have a broad perspective, and they use resources and develop strategies in light of that perspective. In health care settings, situations often arise that require consideration of ethical content. Both formal and informal consultations occur among patients, physicians, nurses, other health care professionals, administrators, and legal counsel concerning ethical dimensions of health care. It behooves occupational therapy managers to be aware of ethical tensions and dialogue in their particular settings as well as in the larger health care arena.

Although the law and ethics are not synonymous, managers must be alert to the effect of the law on both clinical and moral decisions. Specific legislation may determine the conditions of compliance or noncompliance with codified social ethics, but it may not be as helpful in identifying ethical priorities for individuals. In light of the complexities of ethical problem solving, the *Occupational Therapy Code of Ethics* (see appendix 18-A) provides a broad foundation for building ethical solutions specific to the practice of occupational therapy.

The remainder of this section explores the duty of occupational therapy managers in four particular managerial functions: (1) facilitation of ethical clinical decision making, (2) professional gatekeeping, (3) allocation of limited resources, and (4) enhancement of the organization's and employees' integrity. Each of these functions calls for a familiarity with the standards and the practices associated with them and an understanding of the ethical tensions inherent in them.

FACILITATION OF ETHICAL CLINICAL DECISION MAKING

With enhanced technology to save lives and ameliorate disease and disability have come ethical tensions for the health care community.[1] Health care professionals, including occupational therapy practitioners, must be prepared to facilitate ethical clinical decision making. Between acute medical crises there is need for reflection on values and the meaning of the illness experience for the individual. This insight, especially when shared with the health care team, can support the patient or the client and his or her family in making ethical decisions that accompany illness. Addressing the issue of competency in the delivery of medical care, Wright (1987) advocates considering values and finding the critical balance between moral and technical issues:

> Since all medical decisions will entail some value commitment or other, the more conscious the understanding of those values the more likely it is that the care given will be appropriate to the patient. In some cases, the choice will be very difficult. Competency, therefore, can be defined not simply as an ability to master and manipulate technological means of providing cures, but also the capacity to relate those technologies to the needs of individual patients, through some method of relating moral and scientific values. (p. 140)

---

1. *This section is based on* Window of Opportunity: Facilitation of Clinical Ethical Decision-Making, *by K. Opacich and T. Savage, 1994, April, Paper presented at the World Federation of Occupational Therapy Conference, London, England. Copyright ©1994 by K. Opacich and T. Savage. Adapted with permission.*

Applying these principles, occupational therapy managers have a duty to ensure clinical competency and to foster competency in ethical reasoning to enhance the care of patients and clients.

An occupational therapy practitioner can support health care decision making by moving the patient or the client through the processes of seeking and clarifying information, assessing values, identifying options, understanding the related consequences, and articulating the ethical ramifications of the choices. The dialogue may entail speculation regarding the effect of decisions on quality of life for a patient or client. An astute practitioner gauges the accuracy of the information on which the patient or client is basing decisions and gently challenges the decisions with questions that help the person address what-if circumstances.

Managers must support practitioners in developing their abilities to address the ethical tensions and concerns that are inevitable in service provision. Managers have a duty to encourage staff members to explore their own value systems and to broaden the scope of their ethical insights by reading and engaging in meaningful dialogue with people representative of a spectrum of cultures and beliefs. Ethical contemplation and clinical application entail perception, understanding, and sensitivity.

PROFESSIONAL GATEKEEPING

Gatekeeping has frequently been used to refer to the responsibility of health care providers to determine who has legitimate access to health care services.[2] Pellegrino (cited in Monagle & Thomasma, 1988) addressed this aspect of gatekeeping even before health care providers experienced the demands of medical insurance reform. Although professional autonomy has been dramatically limited in terms of service provision, gatekeeping as it relates to aspiring practitioners is still largely within the purview of the respective professions. Because occupational therapy practitioners enter into covenantal relationships with people who are by circumstance vulnerable, the profession must accept a duty to determine the worthiness of those who endeavor to provide care.

Gatekeeping safeguards the integrity of a profession and ensures the worthiness of candidates for inclusion. In the health-related professions it is the responsibility of the members of the field. Gatekeeping occurs at several points along the career continuum, beginning with admission to a program of study and extending to retirement from professional life. Each juncture poses a unique set of obligations and tensions relative to one

---

2. *This section is based on* Moral Obligations and Tensions in Professional Gatekeeping, *by K. Opacich, 1994, July, Paper prepared for Ethics of Professional Development, University of Illinois, Chicago. Copyright ©1994 by K. Opacich. Adapted with permission.*

or more of the following: (1) accreditation of academic programs, (2) admission of qualified students, (3) supervision of field experiences, (4) monitoring of academic progression, (5) maintenance of professional registration and/or licensure, (6) monitoring of continuing professional competency, and (7) upholding of standards of practice. By tacit agreement, occupational therapy managers have a duty to attend to gatekeeping by providing fieldwork supervision, ensuring maintenance of professional credentials by staff members, seeking opportunities for staff members to enhance their clinical competency, and ensuring quality services.

Providing Fieldwork Supervision

Preparation for virtually all the health-related professions includes periods of supervised practice. Although beneficence is the guiding principle in both supervision of students and care of patients, the occupational therapy manager must also consider the potential for harm to the student or to the recipient of care in any supervisory arrangement. This issue has been repeatedly and poignantly raised in occupational therapy, which at this time has no formal mechanism for credentialing fieldwork supervisors. The rapidly increasing demand for fieldwork sites has encouraged the use of all viable locations. As a result, there is great variability in commitment and skill among fieldwork supervisors. Managers must assume ultimate responsibility for the quality and the consistency of clinical education programs implemented by staff members. Even if fieldwork supervisors are well intended, fieldwork supervision is essentially an educator's role, and the occupational therapy manager must commit resources to prepare and support staff members who wish to fulfill the role.

Ensuring the Maintenance of Professional Credentials

Professional registration and licensure are other mechanisms established to attest to the competency of practitioners. Occupational therapy practitioners who earn these credentials enjoy the status of full-fledged membership in the field. A profession's insistence on its practitioners' maintaining the appropriate credentials sends a message to the public that the practitioners are trustworthy and accountable. Responsibility for keeping staff members' credentials in good order falls to the occupational therapy manager.

Seeking Opportunities for Staff Members to Enhance Their Clinical Competence

The first line of responsibility for maintaining and advancing professional competence lies with the individual practitioner. Managers have a duty to create opportunities for practitioners to grow and cultivate expertise. When self-monitoring does not occur, professional peers and supervisors must reflect on their duty to their colleagues and their consumers. A review of the deliberations of the American Occupational Therapy Certification Board, which are periodically published in *OT Week*, suggests that most ethical tensions related to competence are resolved long before disciplinary action is unavoidable. Nevertheless, as proposed by May (1975), "In professional ethics, the test of moral seriousness may depend not simply upon personal compliance with ethical principles, but upon the courage to hold others accountable" (p. 32).

Ensuring Quality Services

Ultimately managers are accountable for the quality of services provided by clinicians. Continuous quality management entails establishing and monitoring indicators that address standards and improvements reflective of high-quality occupational therapy practice. Standard setting and regulation are more specifically addressed in previous chapters of this book. It is important to reiterate that both individual and programmatic activities pertaining to accreditation, certification, and licensure communicate earnest commitment to standards of practice. Adherence to these standards is a professional duty addressing the principle of fidelity, and failure to fulfill this duty has both individual and programmatic consequences.

ALLOCATION OF LIMITED RESOURCES

More than ever before in occupational therapy's history, the demand for services exceeds the supply. As long as these conditions prevail, occupational therapy may be considered a scarce resource that must be distributed fairly and equitably. Consequently decisions that might under other circumstances be regarded as purely business choices are today likely to include an ethical component. Decisions regarding access to service become another form of gatekeeping.

Institutions and agencies generate mission statements that embody values and priorities to guide the macro-allocation of resources. At the managerial level, decisions are made that must translate the values and the priorities into micro-allocations. For example, if an institution commits considerable resources to community outreach, the expectation is likely to be that program initiatives within an occupational therapy department will reflect this commitment. Given a choice between establishing a hospital-based hand clinic or a community-based program for developmental screening, a manager might find supporting the latter program more philosophically consistent. In making programmatic decisions, a manager may feel that business considerations are overshadowing ethical considerations. Probably the most dramatic example of competing business and ethical agendas in recent history was the ill-fated Health Security Act of 1993 spearheaded by Hillary Rodham Clinton. The ethical goal of universal access to health care conflicted with the business goal of cost containment, and attempts at health care reform have been diminished to attempts at insurance reform.

Following are some of the ethical questions that might be raised regarding allocation of resources:

1. What is the potential benefit (good) of the program in light of the costs (monetary and psychological)?

2. Which program initiative would result in the greatest good for the greatest number of recipients?

3. Which program addresses the greatest social inequity?

4. Would the organization be morally remiss in *not* providing the service?

5. What alternatives are available to the potential recipients of the service?

6. Which program has the greatest potential for success in promoting better health for the populace?

On a smaller scale, individual practitioners make daily decisions about which patients or clients most need their services. Because occupational therapy practitioners cannot see everyone with a performance deficit, it is important for both managers and clinicians to articulate the rationale that they will use to allocate practitioners' time and expertise to best advantage. To make such determinations solely on the basis of reimbursement trends would be unfortunate. The distress that practitioners are experiencing in relation to this issue is reflected in the literature (Andrews, 1989a; Burke & Cassidy, 1991; Howard, 1991). As Engelhardt (1986) aptly observes,

> We are at present committed to providing (1) the best of care (2) equally to all, while (3) maintaining provider and receiver choice, though at the same time (4) engaging in cost containment. It should be clear that one cannot pursue all four goals at the same time. (p. 40)

ENHANCEMENT OF THE ORGANIZATION'S AND EMPLOYEES' INTEGRITY

In his book *Ethics in Practice: Managing the Moral Corporation,* Andrews (1989b) emphasizes the influence that leaders can have on the moral outlook and the subsequent actions of a company. He contends that traditional ethics has generally been segregated and removed from its application in the real world. Managers are consequently not exposed or attracted to ethical contemplation until they are confronted with real conflict in the workplace. Referring to moral judgment, Andrews (1989a) states,

> Developing it in business turns out to be partly an administrative process involving: recognition of a decision's ethical implications; discussion to expose different points of view; and testing the tentative decision's adequacy in balancing self-interest and consideration of others, its import for future policy, and its consonance with the company's traditional values. (p. 100)

Andrews goes on, "Ethical dereliction, sleaziness, or inertia is not merely an individual failure but a management problem as well" (p. 101). He characterizes managers as powerful influences in implementing the espoused ethics of an organization. To maintain a moral organization, he believes, managers must consciously develop, communicate, and apply ethics along with economic strategies. "The personal values and ethical aspirations of the company's leaders, though probably not specifically stated, are implicit in all strategic decisions," he notes (p. 101).

Another contemporary business ethicist, Marvin T. Brown (1991), has compiled a book of case studies and analyses that reflect the gamut of ethical tensions experienced in the world of work. Some of the examples are specific to health care and are immensely helpful in illustrating the relationship between business agendas and moral decision making. Brown also addresses the duties of employees to an organization and the obligations of an organization to its employees.

Especially in this era of disorganization and uncertainty in health care, it is important for managers, including occupational therapy managers, to keep sight of the ideals and the moral commitments inherent in their professions. Although business acumen is an essential ingredient in the delivery of health care, economic goals can too easily overshadow noble intentions. Managers must safeguard noble intentions and temper business decisions with ethical conscience. Burke and Cassidy (1991) refer to competing values between reimbursement-driven practice and the humanistic values of occupational therapy. Their points underline the need to keep ethical commitments at the forefront of management decisions.

THE ETHICAL ENTERPRISE IN OCCUPATIONAL THERAPY

Enterprise is defined by *Webster's* (1986) as "an undertaking that is difficult, complicated or has a strong element of risk; readiness to attempt or engage in what requires daring and energy" (p. 757). To engage in ethical contemplation, occupational therapy practitioners must become comfortable with the language and the principles associated with ethics in the context of their own work. This section presents five scenarios that might arise in occupational therapy. They may be used as group or individual exercises in conducting ethical inquiry and argument. (It is sometimes less threatening to begin to examine ethical dilemmas outside one's own sphere of control.) In reality, ethical problems most often occur couched in "static." Articulating the specific ethical problem(s) requires willingness, skill, and practice. Each of the scenarios highlights a different aspect of occupational therapy: clinical practice, administration of a clinic, clinical education, clinical research, and consultation. The following set of questions might be helpful in identifying the greatest good in each situation. Additionally managers should take the opportunity to contemplate their roles in resolving identified ethical tensions, whether they are directly or indirectly involved in the situations described.

1. What are the good intentions in conflict in the scenario?

2. What facts, beliefs, and assumptions must be elicited to clarify the situation?

3. Does the scenario pose ethical problems?

4. What moral principles apply to the case? What should be their order of priority?

5. What rules, guidelines, or norms are pertinent to the situation and potentially helpful in resolving the problem(s)?

6. What are the options for resolving the identified problem(s)?

7. Which, if any, of these options are morally prohibited? Morally obligatory? Morally permissible?

8. Which is the best option, and why?

Scenario 1: Ethical Dimensions in Clinical Practice

Marisol is a staff occupational therapist with 10 months of work experience. For the first 6 months of employment, she rotated through the adult rehabilitation and outpatient service programs in the department. For the last 4 months she has been assigned to the gerontology unit. Both her supervisor and her patients have expressed pleasure with her warmth and commitment. For the past 4 weeks Marisol has been working with a 72-year-old woman with a diagnosis of right parietal cerebrovascular accident. Because of the patient's history of transient ischemic attacks, she was living with her daughter, son-in-law, and three young grandsons for the six months preceding her stroke. Her discharge plan is to return to that environment with home health services (occupational therapy, physical therapy, and nursing). She has made good progress, but her performance is inconsistent, and she is moderately dependent in activities of daily living and transfers.

One week before her scheduled discharge date, the patient begins to sob in occupational therapy. Marisol attempts to console her and to determine why she is crying. The patient confides that she is very apprehensive about going home because before her stroke, her daughter began physically abusing her when no one else in the family was present. When the patient calms herself, she adamantly admonishes Marisol not to mention this to anyone because she really has no place else to go. She expresses dismay at not having any friends living in the area and at not having means of her own other than her deceased husband's small Social Security benefits. She also states that she would rather die than go to a nursing home. Marisol does not wish to betray the patient's trust, but is very concerned about the patient's welfare. She reports the incident to her immediate supervisor, who is also uncomfortable with the situation. Both therapists decide to approach the department manager for assistance.

What are the duties and the moral obligations of the manager in this scenario? How can the manager assist Marisol in ethical problem solving? What challenges might the manager face in this role? What options might he or she consider?

Scenario 2:
Ethical Dimensions in Administration of a Clinic

Like most medical centers, Good Faith Community Hospital is attempting to diversify and expand its services to the community. It is a 500-bed training facility in an ethnically diverse, inner-city environment. Among the services it offers is occupational therapy. The department consists of 18 practitioners: 4 full-time equivalents (FTEs) in rehabilitation, 3 FTEs in general medicine/surgery, 3 FTEs in work assessment and work rehabilitation, 2 FTEs in hand therapy, 2 FTEs in home health contracts, 2 FTEs in school contracts, 1 FTE in oncology, and 1 FTE in pediatric outpatient service. At present the department has two vacancies, one in general medicine and the other in oncology, and a practitioner in rehabilitation is on a three-month maternity leave. The workload is usually heavy and the pace hectic, and now staff members are feeling even more stressed.

Top managers have apprised the occupational therapy manager of a stringent institutional cost-containment initiative. Simultaneously top managers are expecting departments to generate new revenue-producing programs. It has been decided that no new positions will be approved in the next fiscal year. Furthermore, each department has been advised to develop a plan for cutting departmental costs by at least 10 percent. Some other allied health services have proposed eliminating positions to achieve this objective. The occupational therapy manager faces some difficult staffing decisions.

Meanwhile an ad hoc committee of occupational therapy practitioners and other health care personnel has been working on a program proposal focusing on adolescent mothers and maternal-child issues. This group hopes to justify another full-time occupational therapist to staff the program within the next three months.

Additionally the Department of Medicine has requested 1.5 FTEs for a 20-bed transdisciplinary cardiac rehabilitation program that the department has proposed. (This is the first time that the Department of Medicine has included occupational therapy services in a new program initiative.)

Further, the Department of Psychiatry has asked that prevocational assessments be conducted before discharge on every psychiatric inpatient between the ages of 15 and 50. The department intends to use this information to support discharge planning and to support disability funding requests for patients with chronic mental impairments who cannot perform remunerative work.

In light of all this, the occupational therapy manager must decide whether to reconfigure the staff, refuse to provide service to new programs altogether, or identify some other mechanism for determining program and staffing priorities.

How can the manager satisfy the business objectives while promoting the best-possible health care? How might he or she compute costs to reflect the value as well as the price of occupational therapy services?

Scenario 3:
Ethical Dimensions in Clinical Education

Michael, a bachelor's-level occupational therapy student from State University, is in the midst of his second three-month Fieldwork II placement. He is eager to complete his education because he has signed an agreement with a rural health care center, which has paid for his last year of schooling in return for a two-year nonnegotiable employment agreement. The site of his Fieldwork II placement is an occupational therapy clinic that primarily serves acute medical and surgical patients, although there are some ambulatory care programs for patients with certain disorders (e.g., multiple sclerosis, head injury, and cerebrovascular accident). Michael, requiring much more intense supervision than most students, has had considerable difficulty adapting to the pace and the diversity of this clinic, which is staffed by five therapists.

Michael's supervisor for the first six weeks had been in the field for five years and had supervised four other occupational therapy students in that time. She had contacted State University for assistance during the third week of Michael's experience and had carefully established learning contracts that Michael was meeting, though not without extraordinary effort. At the mid-term evaluation this supervisor was both critical and encouraging, and Michael decided to proceed with the fieldwork.

During week 7, however, Michael's supervisor broke her leg in a skiing accident and had to be hospitalized for surgery. Her physicians recommended a long period of immobilization following the surgery. Michael was assigned to a new supervisor. The second supervisor is a competent clinician who has pursued occupational therapy as a second career. This is her first occupational therapy job, and she has been at the facility for 11 months. Of the other three therapists in the department, one is a new graduate hired three months ago; the second already has a student; and the third is primarily a pediatric therapist working in both outpatient and community-based programs.

Michael was somewhat apprehensive about the change but felt that he was well enough established in the setting to complete his fieldwork successfully. He has begun to receive increasingly negative feedback, however, and has been told in the 11th week of fieldwork that in all likelihood, he will fail. The clinical supervisor has contacted the academic fieldwork coordinator at State University and invited him to a meeting involving the occupational therapy manager, the second supervisor, and Michael.

What perspective can the manager contribute to this discussion? How have managerial decisions contributed to the problem at hand? How can the manager facilitate ethical problem solving at the meeting? What policies and procedures might be affected by the situation now and in the future?

Scenario 4:
Ethical Dimensions in Clinical Research

Metropolitan County Hospital has been experiencing a dramatic rise in the number of babies born to drug-dependent mothers. Although the literature pertaining to efficacy of treatment with these babies is controversial, the occupational therapy practitioners feel strongly that their services would benefit the infants. Access to the population is strictly limited in the facility, but the neonatal unit is amenable to reviewing a proposal that would empirically demonstrate the value of occupational therapy and other early interventions.

A group of therapists has reviewed the literature and the tests and the measures pertinent to the problem. The eager investigators have generated a proposal for the medical staff and the internal review board. They have selected an instrument and are proposing the following methodology:

> On the third day after birth, all babies identified as drug affected will be assessed using a standardized instrument to detect the presence of neurosensory processing dysfunction. Of those manifesting dysfunction, neonates who are eligible for occupational therapy services by virtue of their funding will be offered the services. The infants of parents or guardians who accept services will be enrolled for six months. At the end of six months, all drug-affected subjects will be retested through the neonatal follow-up clinic. The scores of those who have received occupational therapy will be compared with the scores of those who have not received it.

At present, no external funding is available for this project. The two major public funding agencies do not currently approve occupational therapy for this population because they assume that occupational therapy is not a medical necessity for drug-affected neonates. They sometimes allow up to 12 visits if an infant has physical anomalies or identified neurological disorders. Some, but not all, third-party payers do reimburse for occupational therapy services. Most of the drug-affected babies treated at this facility are born to mothers who rely on public aid.

What feedback can the manager provide to the novice researchers? Which ethical principles are called into question, and what are the stakes? What ethical tensions and implications are embodied in this clinical research protocol?

Scenario 5:
Ethical Dimensions in Consultation

Rebecca has been an occupational therapist for six years. At present she works half-time in a hospital-based outpatient clinic as the outpatient manager, and half-time as a consultant to three long-term-care facilities owned by an investment group. At these facilities she screens new patients, assesses feeding and positioning needs for specified patients, supervises a certified occupational therapy assistant (COTA), and occasionally provides direct treatment to patients with good rehabilitation potential. She spends one-half to one day a week in each of these settings.

The fiscal manager of the long-term-care facilities has approached Rebecca with a request to enroll all patients in feeding groups to be conducted by the COTA. The fiscal manager has expressed the rationale that all patients, no matter how debilitated, can benefit from a feeding program as long as they can be transported from their rooms. Rebecca suspects that the underlying reason is the financial benefit to the agency. Rebecca knows that a recommendation from her, as the registered occupational therapist at the facilities, is necessary for inclusion of residents and ultimately for reimbursement for direct treatment provided by her or the COTA. The reality is that to meet her financial obligations, Rebecca needs the income from her consultancy; it is considerably higher than that from her hospital-based position. Rebecca senses that refusal to comply with the fiscal manager's request will have consequences for her continued employment. She confides in an occupational therapist who is a manager and a friend.

What might Rebecca do to maintain her integrity in this situation? What are the implications of her actions for the COTA who is employed by the facility? What options might the manager friend identify as incurring the least harm and providing the most good?

SUMMARY

Practitioners can glean ethical direction in the practice of occupational therapy from the philosophical statements embedded in the profession's historical documents and literature. These serve as the cornerstones and the moral conscience by which practitioners can determine their moral obligations and respond consistently with professional values.

When practitioners face an ethical challenge, they are likely to experience some intuitive dissonance, which they must differentiate from other sources of tension. If the tensions are ethical in nature, practitioners must analyze them to clarify the moral content. There are many valid approaches to ethical analysis. It helps to identify the ethical frame(s) of reference to be applied. Ethical debate has been documented since the time of Aristotle, so resources for ethical reasoning abound. Principle-driven ethical reasoning is common, but other approaches (e.g., the ethics of caring) may be just as useful.

Recognizing ethical tensions in practice is the first step in the process of ethical reasoning. Becoming conversant in the language of ethics and applying ethical theories and principles is the second step. A third step is to establish a strategy for conducting the conversations that will lead to ethical resolution.

Occupational therapy managers have ethical duties in four particular managerial functions: (1) facilitation of ethical clinical decision making, (2) professional gatekeeping (ensuring the competence of practitioners), (3) allocation of limited resources, and (4) enhancement of the organization's and employees' integrity.

This chapter merely begins to examine the ethical enterprise in occupational therapy. Using the tools and the time-honored traditions of ethical dialogue, occupational therapy practitioners strive to promote meaningfulness in living for the recipients of service. The principles, the examples, the commentary, and the resources included in the chapter are intended to be used as springboards for further examination of practice and professional values so that practitioners can best preserve the integrity of occupational therapy.

It behooves occupational therapy managers to be aware of ethical tensions and dialogue in their particular settings as well as in the larger health care arena. The founders of the profession articulated and demonstrated moral consciousness and established ethical traditions. Upholding those traditions and armed with courage and creativity, occupational therapy managers must be prepared to deal with the ethical dimensions and challenges of contemporary occupational therapy.

REFERENCES

American Occupational Therapy Association. (1991a). *Essentials and guidelines for an accredited educational program for the occupational therapist.* Rockville, MD: Author.

American Occupational Therapy Association. (1991b). *Essentials and guidelines for an accredited educational program for the occupational therapy assistant.* Rockville, MD: Author.

Andrews, K. R. (1989a, September-October). Ethics in practice. *Harvard Business Review,* pp. 99–104.

Andrews, K. R. (1989b). *Ethics in practice: Managing the moral corporation.* Cambridge, MA: Harvard Business School Press.

Beauchamp, T. L., & Childress, J. F. (1994). *Principles of biomedical ethics* (4th ed.). New York: Oxford.

Brown, M. T. (1991). *Working ethics: Strategies for decision making and organizational responsibility.* San Francisco: Jossey-Bass.

Burke, J. P., & Cassidy, J. C. (1991). Disparity between reimbursement-driven practice and humanistic values of occupational therapy. *American Journal of Occupational Therapy, 45,* 173–76.

Englehardt, H. T., Jr. (1986). The importance of values in shaping professional direction. In *Proceedings of Occupational Therapy Education: Target 2000* (p. 40). Rockville, MD: American Occupational Therapy Association.

Health Security Act of 1993, H.R. 3600, S. 1757, 103rd Cong., 1st Sess.

Howard, B. S. (1991). How high do we jump? The effect of reimbursement on occupational therapy. *American Journal of Occupational Therapy, 45,* 875–81.

Kyler-Hutchison, P. (1994, December 15). Issues in ethics: The role of ethics committees. *OT Week,* pp. 9–10.

May, W. F. (1975). Code and covenant or philanthropy and contract? *Hastings Center Report, 5*(6), 29–38.

Monagle, J. F., & Thomasma, D. C. (1988). *Medical ethics: A guide for health professionals.* Rockville, MD: Aspen Publishers.

Pojman, L. P. (Ed.) (1989). *Ethical theory: Classical and contemporary readings.* Belmont, CA: Wadsworth.

Webster's third international dictionary (Unabridged). (1986). Springfield, MA: Merriam-Webster.

Wright, R. A. (1987). *Human values in health care: The practice of ethics.* New York: McGraw-Hill.

ADDITIONAL RESOURCES

American Occupational Therapy Association. (1995). Statement on nondiscrimination and inclusion regarding members of the occupational therapy professional community. *American Journal of Occupational Therapy, 49,* 1009.

Bailey, D. M., & Schwartzberg, S. L. (1995). *Ethical and legal dilemmas in occupational therapy.* Philadelphia: F. A. Davis.

Gilligan, C., Ward, J. V., & Taylor, J. M. (Eds.). (1988). *Mapping the moral domain.* Cambridge, MA: Harvard University Press.

Hansen, R. A. (Ed.). (1988). Ethics [Special issue]. *American Journal of Occupational Therapy, 45,* 276–435.

Hasselkus, B. R. (1991). Ethical dilemmas in family caregiving for the elderly: Implications for occupational therapy. *American Journal of Occupational Therapy, 45,* 206–12.

Hasselkus, B. R., & Stetson, A. S. (1991). Ethical dilemmas: The organization of family caregiving for the elderly. *Journal of Aging Studies, 5,* 99–110.

Hastings Center Report (published six times a year). Hastings-on-Hudson, NY: Institute of Society and Ethics and Life Sciences.

Holmes, H. B., & Purdy, L. M. (Eds.). (1992). *Feminist perspectives in medical ethics.* Bloomington, IN: Indiana University Press.

Jonsen, A. R., Siegler, M., & Winslade, W. J. (1992). *Clinical ethics* (3rd ed.). New York: McGraw-Hill.

Keith-Spiegel, P., & Koocher, G. P. (1985). *Ethics in psychology: Professional standards and cases.* New York: McGraw-Hill.

Monagle, J. F., & Thomasma, D. C. (1994). *Health care ethics: Critical issues.* Gaithersburg, MD: Aspen Systems.

Purtillo, R. (1993). *Ethical dimensions in the health professions* (2nd ed.). Philadelphia: Saunders.

Veatch, R. M. (1989). *Medical ethics.* Boston: Jones & Bartlett.

Welles, C. (1988). Ethical and professional liability considerations for the administrator: Incidents and principles. *Occupational Therapy in Home Care, 5*(1), 119–34.

APPENDIX 18-A

Occupational Therapy Code of Ethics

The American Occupational Therapy Association's *Code of Ethics* is a public statement of the values and principles used in promoting and maintaining high standards of behavior in occupational therapy. The American Occupational Therapy Association and its members are committed to furthering people's ability to function within their total environment. To this end, occupational therapy personnel provide services for individuals in any stage of health and illness, to institutions, to other professionals and colleagues, to students, and to the general public.

The Occupational Therapy Code of Ethics is a set of principles that applies to occupational therapy personnel at all levels. The roles of practitioner (registered occupational therapist and certified occupational therapy assistant), educator, fieldwork educator, supervisor, administrator, consultant, fieldwork coordinator, faculty program director, researcher/scholar, entrepreneur, student, support staff, and occupational therapy aide are assumed.

Any action that is in violation of the spirit and purpose of this Code shall be considered unethical. To ensure compliance with the Code, enforcement procedures are established and maintained by the Commission on Standards and Ethics. Acceptance of membership in the American Occupational Therapy Association commits members to adherence to the *Code of Ethics* and its enforcement procedures.

Principle 1. Occupational therapy personnel shall demonstrate a concern for the well- being of the recipients of their services. (beneficence)

    A. Occupational therapy personnel shall provide services in an equitable manner for all individuals.

    B. Occupational therapy personnel shall maintain relationships that do not exploit the recipient of services sexually, physically, emotionally, financially, socially, or in any other manner. Occupational therapy personnel shall avoid those relationships or activities that interfere with professional judgment and objectivity.

C. Occupational therapy personnel shall take all reasonable precautions to avoid harm to the recipient of services or to his or her property.

D. Occupational therapy personnel shall strive to ensure that fees are fair, reasonable, and commensurate with the service performed and are set with due regard for the service recipient's ability to pay.

Principle 2. Occupational therapy personnel shall respect the rights of the recipients of their services. (e.g., autonomy, privacy, confidentiality)

A. Occupational therapy personnel shall collaborate with service recipients or their surrogate(s) in determining goals and priorities throughout the intervention process.

B. Occupational therapy personnel shall fully inform the service recipients of the nature, risks, and potential outcomes of any interventions.

C. Occupational therapy personnel shall obtain informed consent from subjects involved in research activities indicating they have been fully advised of the potential risks and outcomes.

D. Occupational therapy personnel shall respect the individual's right to refuse professional services or involvement in research or educational activities.

E. Occupational therapy personnel shall protect the confidential nature of information gained from educational, practice, research, and investigational activities.

Principle 3. Occupational therapy personnel shall achieve and continually maintain high standards of competence. (duties)

A. Occupational therapy practitioners shall hold the appropriate national and state credentials for providing services.

B. Occupational therapy personnel shall use procedures that conform to the Standards of Practice of the American Occupational Therapy Association.

C. Occupational therapy personnel shall take responsibility for maintaining competence by participating in professional development and educational activities.

D. Occupational therapy personnel shall perform their duties on the basis of accurate and current information.

E. Occupational therapy practitioners shall protect service recipients by ensuring that duties assumed by or assigned to other occupational therapy personnel are commensurate with their qualifications and experience.

F. Occupational therapy practitioners shall provide appropriate supervision to individuals for whom the practitioners have supervisory responsibility.

G. Occupational therapists shall refer recipients to other service providers or consult with other service providers when additional knowledge and expertise are required.

Principle 4. Occupational therapy personnel shall comply with laws and Association policies guiding the profession of occupational therapy. (justice)

A. Occupational therapy personnel shall understand and abide by applicable Association policies; local, state, and federal laws; and institutional rules.

B. Occupational therapy personnel shall inform employers, employees, and colleagues about those laws and Association policies that apply to the profession of occupational therapy.

C. Occupational therapy practitioners shall require those they supervise in occupational therapy related activities to adhere to the *Code of Ethics.*

D. Occupational therapy personnel shall accurately record and report all information related to professional activities.

Principle 5. Occupational therapy personnel shall provide accurate information about occupational therapy services. (veracity)

A. Occupational therapy personnel shall accurately represent their qualifications, education, experience, training, and competence.

B. Occupational therapy personnel shall disclose any affiliations that may pose a conflict of interest.

C. Occupational therapy personnel shall refrain from using or participating in the use of any form of communication that contains false, fraudulent, deceptive, or unfair statements or claims.

Principle 6. Occupational therapy personnel shall treat colleagues and other professionals with fairness, discretion, and integrity. (fidelity, veracity)

A. Occupational therapy personnel shall safeguard confidential information about colleagues and staff.

B. Occupational therapy personnel shall accurately represent the qualifications, views, contributions, and findings of colleagues.

C. Occupational therapy personnel shall report any breaches of the *Code of Ethics* to the appropriate authority.

Author: Commission on Standards and Ethics (SEC)
Ruth Hansen, PhD, OTR, FAOTA, Chairperson
    Approved by the Representative Assembly: 4/77
    Revised: 1979, 1988, 1994
    Adopted by the Representative Assembly: 7/94

Note. *This document replaces the 1988* Occupational Therapy Code of Ethics, *which was rescinded by the 1994 Representative Assembly.*

APPENDIX 18-B

Core Values and Attitudes of Occupational Therapy Practice

INTRODUCTION

In 1985, the American Occupational Therapy Association (AOTA) funded the Professional and Technical Role Analysis Study (PATRA). This study had two purposes: to delineate the entry-level practice of OTRs and COTAs through a role analysis and to conduct a task inventory of what practitioners actually do. Knowledge, skills, and attitude statements were to be developed to provide a basis for the role analysis. The PATRA study completed the knowledge and skills statements. The Executive Board subsequently charged the Standards and Ethics Commission (SEC) to develop a statement that would describe the attitudes and values that undergird the profession of occupational therapy. The SEC wrote this document for use by AOTA members.

The list of terms used in this statement was originally constructed by the American Association of Colleges of Nursing (AACN) (1986). The PATRA committee analyzed the knowledge statements that the committee had written and selected those terms from the AACN list that best identified the values and attitudes of our profession. This list of terms was then forwarded to SEC by the PATRA committee to use as the basis for the Core Values and Attitudes paper.

The development of this document is predicated on the assumption that the values of occupational therapy are evident in the official documents of the American Occupational Therapy Association. The official documents that were examined are: (a) Dictionary Definition of Occupational Therapy (AOTA, 1986), (b) The Philosophical Base of Occupational Therapy (AOTA, 1979), (c) Essentials and Guidelines for an Accredited Educational Program for the Occupational Therapist (AOTA, 1991a), (d) Essentials and Guidelines for an Accredited Educational Program for the Occupational Therapy Assistant (AOTA, 1991b), and (e) Occupational Therapy Code of Ethics (AOTA, 1988). It is further assumed that these documents are representative of the values and beliefs reflected in other occupational therapy literature.

A value is defined as a belief or an ideal to which an individual is committed. Values are an important part of the base or foundation of a profession. Ideally, these values are embraced by all members of the profession and are reflected in the members' interactions with those persons receiving services, colleagues, and the society at large. Values have a central role in a profession and are developed and reinforced throughout an individual's life as a student and as a professional.

Actions and attitudes reflect the values of the individual. An attitude is the disposition to respond positively or negatively toward an object, person, concept, or situation. Thus, there is an assumption that all professional actions and interactions are rooted in certain core values and beliefs.

SEVEN CORE CONCEPTS

In this document, the core values and attitudes of occupational therapy are organized around seven basic concepts—altruism, equality, freedom, justice, dignity, truth, and prudence. How these core values and attitudes are expressed and implemented by occupational therapy practitioners may vary depending upon the environments and situations in which professional activity occurs.

Altruism is the unselfish concern for the welfare of others. This concept is reflected in actions and attitudes of commitment, caring, dedication, responsiveness, and understanding.

Equality requires that all individuals be perceived as having the same fundamental human rights and opportunities. This value is demonstrated by an attitude of fairness and impartiality. We believe that we should respect all individuals, keeping in mind that they may have values, beliefs, or life-styles that are different from our own. Equality is practiced in the broad professional arena, but is particularly important in day-to-day interactions with those individuals receiving occupational therapy services.

Freedom allows the individual to exercise choice and to demonstrate independence, initiative, and self-direction. There is a need for all individuals to find a balance between autonomy and societal membership that is reflected in the choice of various patterns of interdependence with the human and nonhuman environment. We believe that individuals are internally and externally motivated toward action in a continuous process of adaptation throughout the life span. Purposeful activity plays a major role in developing and exercising self-direction, initiative, interdependence, and relatedness to the world. Activities verify the individual's ability to adapt, and they establish a satisfying balance between autonomy and societal membership. As professionals, we affirm the freedom of choice for each individual to pursue goals that have personal and social meaning.

Justice places value on the upholding of such moral and legal principles as fairness, equity, truthfulness, and objectivity. This means we aspire to provide occupational therapy services for all individuals who are in need of these services and that we will maintain a goal-directed and objective relationship with all those served. Practitioners must be knowledgeable about and have respect for the legal rights of individuals receiving occupational therapy services. In addition, the occupational therapy practitioner must understand and abide by the local, state, and federal laws governing professional practice.

Dignity emphasizes the importance of valuing the inherent worth and uniqueness of each person. This value is demonstrated by an attitude of empathy and respect for self and others. We believe that each individual is a unique combination of biologic endowment, sociocultural heritage, and life experiences. We view human beings holistically, respecting the unique interaction of the mind, body, and physical and social environment. We believe that dignity is nurtured and grows from the sense of competence and self-worth that is integrally linked to the person's ability to perform valued and relevant activities. In occupational therapy we emphasize the importance of dignity by helping the individual build on his or her unique attributes and resources.

Truth requires that we be faithful to facts and reality. Truthfulness or veracity is demonstrated by being accountable, honest, forthright, accurate, and authentic in our attitudes and actions. There is an obligation to be truthful with ourselves, those who receive services, colleagues, and society. One way that this is exhibited is through maintaining and upgrading professional competence. This happens, in part, through an unfaltering commitment to inquiry and learning, to self-understanding, and to the development of an interpersonal competence.

Prudence is the ability to govern and discipline oneself through the use of reason. To be prudent is to value judiciousness, discretion, vigilance, moderation, care, and circumspection in the management of one's affairs, to temper extremes, make judgments, and respond on the basis of intelligent reflection and rational thought.

SUMMARY

Beliefs and values are those intrinsic concepts that underlie the core of the profession and the professional interactions of each practitioner. These values describe the profession's philosophy and provide the basis for defining purpose. The emphasis or priority that is given to each value may change as one's professional career evolves and as the unique characteristics of a situation unfold. This evolution of values is developmental in nature. Although we have basic values that cannot be violated, the degree to which certain values will take priority at a given time is influenced by the specifics of a situation and the environment in which it occurs. In one instance dignity may be a higher priority than truth; in another prudence may be chosen over freedom. As we process information and make decisions, the weight of the values that we hold may change. The practitioner faces dilemmas because of conflicting values and is required to engage in thoughtful deliberation to determine where the priority lies in a given situation.

The challenge for us all is to know our values, be able to make reasoned choices in situations of conflict, and be able to clearly articulate and defend our choices. At the same time, it is important that all members of the profession be committed to a set of common values. This mutual commitment to a set of beliefs and principles that govern our practice can provide a basis for clarifying expectations between the recipient and the provider of services. Shared values empowers the profession and, in addition, builds trust among ourselves and with others.

REFERENCES

American Association of Colleges of Nursing. (1986). *Essentials of college and university education for professional nursing.* Final report. Washington, DC: Author.

American Occupational Therapy Association. (1979). Resolution C, 531–79: The philosophical base of occupational therapy. *American Journal of Occupational Therapy, 33,* 785.

American Occupational Therapy Association. (1986, April). Dictionary definition of occupational therapy. Adopted and approved by the Representative Assembly to fulfill Resolution #596-83. (Available from AOTA, 4720 Montgomery Lane, PO Box 31220, Bethesda, MD 20824-1220.)

American Occupational Therapy Association. (1988). Occupational therapy code of ethics. *American Journal of Occupational Therapy, 42,* 795–96.

American Occupational Therapy Association. (1991a). Essentials and guidelines for an accredited educational program for the occupational therapist. *American Journal of Occupational Therapy, 45,* 1077–84.

American Occupational Therapy Association. (1991b). Essentials and guidelines for an accredited educational program for the occupational therapy assistant. *American Journal of Occupational Therapy, 45,* 1085–92.

Prepared by Elizabeth Kanny, MA, OTR, for the Standards and Ethics Commission (Ruth A. Hansen, PhD, OTR, FAOTA, Chairperson).

Approved by the Representative Assembly June 1993. Previously published and copyrighted by the American Occupational Therapy Association, Inc., in the *American Journal of Occupational Therapy, 47,* 1085–86.

Index

A

Accelerated depreciation, 73

Accounting, 71–75
  accrual basis, 72–73
  concepts, 71–75
  defined, 63, 71

Accounts payable, 79, 97–98

Accounts receivable, 79
  management, 96–97

Accreditation
  defined, 459
  importance, 467–469
  occupational therapy manager's role, 466–467
  process, 466

Accreditation Council for Occupational Therapy Education, 505–506

Accreditation Council on Services for People with Disabilities, 494–503
  accreditation, 464
  accreditation decisions, 502
  development of standards, 464
  domain, 464, 494–495
  functions, 495–496
  history, 494–495
  mission, 494–495
  outcome measures
    application, 500–501
    content, 498–500
    development, 498
    format, 498–500
  practices, 464
  relevance to occupational therapy, 502–503
  role, 495–496
  sponsors, 464
  structure, 495

Accrediting body, quality improvement, 417–418

Accrued expenses, 79–80

Accrued liabilities, 79–80, 98

Accumulated depreciation, 79

Active listening, 518
  defined, 511

Administrator
  career development, 382
  key performance area, 361–362
  major function, 361
  qualifications, 362–363
  role description, 361–363
  scope of role, 361
  supervision, 363

Adult day center, consultation, 543–548

Advisory board, 609–611

Age Discrimination in Employment Act, 321

Alternative delivery system, 19–22

Altruism, 656

American Public Health Association, 22

Americans with Disabilities Act, 319–320, 591

  consultation, 540–541

Annual report, 128, 131

Asset, use limited, 79

Assistive technology, consultation, 540

Authority, 167

  organizational structure, 331

Autonomy, 632, 652

  defined, 627

Avoidable costs, 89

B

Balance sheet, 78–80

  defined, 63, 78

  sample, 78

Beneficence, 632, 651–652

  defined, 627

Billing, payment, 593–596

Book value, 79

Break-even analysis, 91

Budgeting, 83–84

  philosophies, 91

  process, 85

C

Capability analysis

  change, 198

  defined, 191

Capital aset, 73

Capital budget, 84

Capital budgeting, 94–95

  defined, 63

  steps, 95

Capitation, 598–599

defined, 3, 577

Career, 335

  career choices, 341–343

  defined, 327

Career development, 375–390

  administration, 382

  assessment, 379–380

  clinical specialist, 385–386

  defined, 327

  department personnel system, 389

  education, 382

  entry-level certified occupational therapy assistant, 384–385

  environmental scanning, 380–381

  experienced certified occupational therapy assistant to adult day-care coordinator, 387–388

  goal planning, 379–380

  lateral movement across settings, 342

  master clinician to assistant professor, 388–389

  maturation within role, 342–343

  practice administrator to curriculum director, 386

  preparing through education, 381

  preparing through experience, 381

  process, 379–381

  research, 382

  role, 335–343

  role transition, 377–379

  student to practitioner-registered occupational therapist, 383–384

  supervisor, 385–386

  vertical movement within setting, 342

Career mobility, 167

CARF

  The Rehabilitation Accreditation Commission

    accreditation, 463

    accreditation outcomes, 491–492

      nonaccreditation, 492

one-year accreditation, 492

provisional accreditation, 492

three-year accreditation, 491

accreditation principles, 489

accreditation process, 489–491

conditions, 489

criteria, 489

development of standards, 463

domain, 463, 485–487

history, 485–487

mission, 485–487

national consensus standards, 487

practices, 463

purposes, 486

quality improvement, 417

sponsors, 463

standards, 487

content, 489, 490

development, 487

format, 489, 490

revision, 487–488

structure, 487

values, 486–487

vision, 485

The Rehabilitation Accreditation Commission program evaluation model, 403–409

admission criteria, 404

measures, 406

patient descriptors, 408

performance expectancies, 408–409

program goal statements, 404

program structure, 404

purpose statement, 403–404

relative importance of objectives, 409

services provided, 405

statement of objectives, 405–406

time of application of measures, 407

types of patients served, 405

Case conference, 128, 130

Case management, 592

Case manager, 34–35

Cash, 79

Cash budget, 84

Cash equivalent, 79

Cash on hand management, 96

Certification, 612–617, 618–619

certified occupational therapy assistant

certification basis, 613–614

disciplinary action, 615

examination eligibility requirements, 614–615

private or public employment, 615

state regulation, 615

third-party reimbursement, 615

defined, 603

disciplinary action, 611

entry level occupational therapy practitioners, 613–615

registered occupational therapist

certification basis, 613–614

disciplinary action, 615

examination eligibility requirements, 614–615

private or public employment, 615

state regulation, 615

third-party reimbursement, 615

renewal, 610–611

Certification law, 606–608

Certified occupational therapy assistant, 35–36

certification

certification basis, 613–614

disciplinary action, 615

examination eligibility requirements, 614–615

private or public employment, 615

state regulation, 615

third-party reimbursement, 615

defined, 262

distribution across practice settings, 29–30

growth in numbers, 27

job description, 287, 307–314

key performance area, 355–356

major junction, 355

performance review, 307–314

performance standard, 267

qualifications, 356

role, 349–371

  description, 355–356

  scope, 355

school system, 538–539

staffing, 263

supervision, 247–248, 356

Chain of command, organizational structure, 331

Change, 181–182

  assuming responsibilities, 202

  capability analysis, 198

  creating, 201–205

  defined, 191

  enlisting and maintaining commitment, 202

  ensuring authority, 202

  generating awareness, 194–198

  integrating, 205

  interpersonal dynamics, 204–205

  letting go, 198–201

  management, 191–208

  planning, 202–204

  process, 194–205

  resistance, 199

  resistance management, 198–200

    communicating, 199, 201

    explaining, 199, 200

    grieving, 199, 200

    incremental change, 199, 201

    inspiring, 199, 200

  involving, 199, 201

  resource allocation, 204

  surveillance

    clinical practice surveillance, 196

    consumer and market surveillance, 196–197

    environmental surveillance, 197

    organizational surveillance, 196

    personal-professional surveillance, 195

  visioning, 198–200, 201–202

Chart of accounts, 74

Chief financial officer, 68–70

Children with disabilities, education, 590–591

Civil Rights Act Title VII, 321

Civil Service Reform Act, 321

Civilian Health and Medical Program of the Uniformed Services (CHAMPUS), 585–586

  basic program, 585

  managed care, 585–586

  special program of rehabilitative benefits, 586

Client, defined, 533

Clinical integration, 180–181

Clinical specialist

  career development, 385–386

  role transition, 385–386

Close supervision, defined, 248

Closed system, 170

Coding for services, payment, 593–596

Collaboration, 36

Commercial bank loan, 98

Commercial paper, 98

Communication, 117–140, 511–530. See also Specific type

  barriers, 524–527

  channels, 523–524

  clarity, 516

communication loop opening, 515–516

communication objectives identification, 120

components, 118–119

confidentiality, 527

consultation, 551–552, 558

defined, 117, 511, 512

distortion, 525–526

emotional level, 517–518

environment, 521–522

ethical issues, 527

facilitation, 518–520

formal communication, 522

gender, 526–527

hidden agendas, 526

informal communication, 522

information contrasted, 516–517

information flow, 345

information overload, 525

message definition, 123–125, 126

method assessment, 128

method selection, 125–135

methods, 127–135

need to know, 516–517

organizational culture, 521–522

organizational structure, 157

personal visits, 128, 134–135

power, 516

of professional image, 527–528

program development, 120–135
  case study, 136–139

program evaluation, 135

program implementation, 135

target group definition, 120–123

technology, 524

timing, 516–517

two-way, 515–518

use of another's system and language, 517

Communication skills, 343–344

Communication vehicle, defined, 117

Community Health Accreditation Program, 505

Community Mental Health Centers Act, 578

Community newsletter, 128, 130–131

Competition, 38–39, 52
  health care environment, 65–67

Comprehensive Accreditation Manual for Hospitals, 475

Conditions of participation, Medicare, 583–584

Conference presentation, 128, 134

Confidentiality, 633, 652
  communication, 527
  defined, 627

Consensus building, organizational structure, 156–157

Conservatism, 72

Consistency, 72

Consultant
  key performance area, 363
  major function, 363
  qualifications, 364
  role
    defined, 533
    description, 363–364
    scope, 363
  supervision, 364

Consultation, 533–569
  adult day center, 543–548
  Americans with Disabilities Act, 540–541
  assessment, 551–552
  assistive technology, 540
  attitudes and attributes, 560–561
  becoming a consultant, 561–567
  business aspects, 564–567
  business forms, 565–566
  clarification, 550–551

communication, 551–552, 558

concepts, 541–549

consultants' roles, 363–364, 533, 554–557

  preparation, 556–557

consultation environments, 561–562

contract negotiation, 551

  renegotiation, 554

defined, 533

development and use of resources, 563–564

diagnosis, 559–560

diagnostic analysis leading to problem identification, 552

entry into system, 550–551

environmental analysis, 549

evaluation, 553

expanding marketplace, 537–541

  causes, 537–541

external consultation, 555

geriatric practice, 539–540

goal setting, 552

incorporation, 566

initiation, 550–551

interactive problem resolution, 552–553

internal consultation, 555

interpersonal relationships, 560

levels, 541–549

  defined, 534

linking skill, 560

long-term care, 539–540

marketing, 562–563

models, 541–549

  defined, 534

nondirective-directive continuum, 555–556

partnership, 566

planning, 552, 566–567

preventive outcomes, 548–549

principles, 536–537

process, 549–554

  defined, 533

school system, 538–539

self-employment, 565–566

services, 535

skills and knowledge, 557–561

stages, 549–550

systems analysis, 549

technology, 540

termination, 553, 554

theoretical model, 536

training, 559

treatment roles compared, 558, 559

trust, 552

Consumer satisfaction, quality improvement, 415

Consumer service, quality improvement, 415–416

Context, defined, 511, 513

Continuing education, 278

Continuous quality improvement, 183

  defined, 163

Contract negotiation, consultation, 551

  renegotiation, 554

Contribution, 80, 82

Contribution margin, 91

Controllable costs, 89

Controllership, 68

Controlling, 170–172

  manager, 236

Copayment, 31

Corporation, 75

Cost accounting, 86

Cost center, 74, 86

Cost classification, 87–91

Cost containment, 34–37

Cost finding, 87

Cost of goods sold, 82

Cost valuation, 72

Cost-volume-profit analysis, 91

Creating, defined, 191

Credentialing, defined, 603

Criterion measure, 406
  defined, 395

Cross-border trade in services, North American Free Trade Agreement, 617–622
  agencies, 622
  certification, 618–619
  definition, 617–618
  immigration, 619–622
  licensing, 618–619
  principles, 618
  scope, 617–618

Cross-training, 39
  defined, 3

Current asset, 79

Current liabilities, 79, 97–98

Current maturities of long-term debt, 80

Current Procedural Terminology, 595–596

Customer departmentalization, organizational chart, 333, 334

Cycles of events, 175–176
  defined, 163
  qualities, 175

D

Decision making
  causes of faulty, 234–235
  leader, 231–235
  manager, 231–235
  process, 232–233
  techniques, 233–234

Decoding, defined, 117

Deductions from revenue, 73, 81–82

Deficit, 80

Departmentalization
  defined, 327
  organizational chart, 332

Depreciation, 73–74

Developmental Disabilities Assistance Act and Bill of Rights Act, 322

Diagnosis code, 594
  defined, 577

Diagnosis-related group, 12, 580

Dignity, 657

Direct costs, 87

Direct mail, 128, 132

Directing, manager, 236

Disability, trends, 32

Discharge summary, documentation, 431

Disciplinary action, 275–276

Discretionary costs, 89

Disease, trends, 32

Documentation, 36, 424–433. See also Specific type
  defined, 395
  discharge summary, 431
  functional goal, 427
  historical perspectives, 424–425
  long-term goal, 427–428
  monthly summary, 429–430
  patient evaluation, 426
  progress notes, 429–430
  short-term goal, 427–428
  treatment, 429
  treatment planning, 426
  weekly summary, 429–430

Donor-restricted fund, 74

Double-entry bookkeeping, 72, 77

Durable medical equipment, Medicare, 583

E

Earnings, 80

Earnings statement, 80

EASE-2000, 540

Economics, 31

Education

  career development, 382

  children with disabilities, 590–591

  ethical issues, 629–630

  leadership, 215–216

  manager, 215–216

  team, 215–216

  trends, 32–33

Education for All Handicapped Children Act, 590–591

Educator

  key performance area, 357–358

  major function, 357

  qualifications, 358

  role description, 357–358

  scope of role, 357

  supervision, 358

Effectiveness

  defined, 163, 395

  efficiency, relationship, 166

  management, 166

  quality improvement, 416–417

Efficiency

  defined, 163, 395

  effectiveness, relationship, 166

  management, 166

  quality improvement, 416–417

Electronic communication, 344

Emotion

  listening, 520

  meaning, 514–515

Employee newsletter, 127, 128

Empowerment, 330

  defined, 327

Encoding, defined, 117

Entity, 71

Entrepreneur

  key performance area, 370–371

  major function, 370

  qualifications, 371

  role description, 370–371

  scope of role, 370

  supervision, 371

Environment, defined, 533

Environmental assessment

  defined, 101

  marketing, 109–110

    market data sources, 110

Environmental scanning, career development, 380–381

Equality, 656

Equity, 80

Ergonomics, 40

Ethical issues, 8–9, 627–648

  communication, 527

  education, 629–630

  principles governing relationships, 633

Ethical problem solving, roles of occupational therapy manager, 635–641

Ethical reasoning, 629

  defined, 627

  process, 634–635

  Savage facilitation model, 634, 635

Ethical tensions

  defined, 627

  recognition, 630, 631

Evaluation, consultation, 553

Evaluation form, samples, 288–289, 290–292

Excess of revenue over expenses, 80, 82

Expectancy model, 264–265

Expectancy theory, defined, 253

Expense, 73

revenue, matching, 73

Expense variance, 94

Explicit responsibilities, 158–159

External case manager, 34–35

External communication, 130–135
  defined, 130
  methods, 130–135

External consultant, defined, 534

F

Faculty
  key performance area, 366–367
  major function, 365
  qualifications, 367
  role description, 365–367
  scope of role, 365
  supervision, 367

Federal Employees Health Benefit Program, 586–587

Federal government
  health care construction, 9–10
  health planning, 11–12
  human resources legislation, 10–11

Federal legislation, on employment, 319–322

Federally administered system, 579–587

Fee for service, 598
  defined, 577

Fidelity, 633, 654
  defined, 627

Fieldwork coordinator
  key performance area, 364–365
  major function, 364
  qualifications, 365
  role description, 364–365
  scope of role, 364
  supervision, 365

Fieldwork educator
  major junction, 358
  qualifications, 359–360

role description, 358–360
  scope of role, 358
  supervision, 360

Fieldwork supervision, occupational therapy manager, 638

Financial accounting, 71
  defined, 63

Financial analysis, defined, 63

Financial forecasting, 83–91
  concepts, 85–91
  defined, 63
  steps, 84
  terms, 85–91

Financial management, 63–99
  evolution, 67–70

Financial planning, strategic planning, 69

Financial statement, 76–83. See also Specific type
  analysis, 91–94
  defined, 63
  flows, 76
  levels, 76

Finding employment, 316
  employment agreement, 317
  financial considerations, 318
  questions to ask recruiters, 317–318
  recruiter, 315–318
  recruiting company credentials, 317
  working conditions, 317

First-line manager, 166

Fixed asset, use limited, 79

Fixed costs, 87, 88

Formal supervision, types, 352

Formative evaluation, 497
  defined, 459

Freedom, 656–657

Full disclosure, 72

Full-time equivalent
  defined, 253

staffing, 256–257

Function, defined, 459

Functional departmentalization, organizational chart, 332–333

Functional goal, 427
  documentation, 427
  formulation, 427

Functional integration, 180–181

Functional job description, 266–267
  defined, 266
  development, 266–267

Fund accounting, 74

Fund balance, 80

G

Gender, communication, 526–527

General accounting, 71
  defined, 63

General fund, 74

General supervision, defined, 248

Generally accepted accounting principles (GAAP), 71

Generating awareness, defined, 191

Geographic departmentalization, organizational chart, 333–334

Geriatric practice, consultation, 539–540

Goal setting, consultation, 552

Goodwill, 79

Gross patient revenue, 81

Group-model health maintenance organization, 20

H

Health care
  assessment, 65–71
  challenges, 165
  competition, 65–67
  costs, 5, 6, 7, 65, 66
  federal government's role, 9–12
  moral principles, 631–633

occupations, 13–16

opportunities, 67–70

organizations providing care, 17–22

recognition for occupational therapy, 41–42

reimbursement system change, 65

threats, 65–67

trends, 32

vertical system, 18–19

Health care construction, federal government, 9–10

Health Care Financing Administration (HCFA), 579

Health care organization
  key operating indicator analysis, 92–93
  types of, 17

Health care reform, 12

Health fair, 128, 132–133

Health maintenance organization, 20, 22
  defined, 3
  Medicare, 584
  models, 20–21
  open-ended product line, 21

Health network, 19

Health planning, federal government, 11–12

Health Professions Educational Assistance Act, 10

Hill-Burton Act, 9–10

Hospice care, 481

Hospital, vertically organized, 18–19

Human resources, 13–16

Human resources legislation, federal government, 10–11

I

Implicit responsibilities, 159

Improvement measure, 406
  defined, 395

Income from operations, 82

Income statement, 80–82

  defined, 63

  sample, 81

Incorporation, 566

Incremental budgeting, 91

Incremental costs, 89–91

Indemnity, 22

  defined, 3

Independent quality review, defined, 459

Indirect costs, 87

Individual practice association, 21

Individuals with Disabilities Education Act, 578

Information

  communication, contrasted, 516–517

  power, 516

Information flow, 345

Information overload, 525

Innovation, 194

  defined, 191

Inservice training, 128, 129, 278

Institutional licensure, 39

Integrated delivery system, 19–22, 182

  managed care, contrasted, 20

Integrated system, defined, 163

Integrating, defined, 191

Interactive reasoning, 520

Interdisciplinary team, 217

Internal case manager, 35

Internal communication, 127–130

  defined, 127

  methods, 127–130

Internal consultant, defined, 534

Interpersonal dynamics, change, 204–205

Interpersonal relationships, consultation, 560

Interview

  applicant interview analysis, 323

personnel selection, 271–272

  guidelines, 271

Inventory, 79

  management, 97

Investment income, 82

J

Job description, 266–267. See also Functional job description

  certified occupational therapy assistant, 287, 307–314

  defined, 253

  development, 266

  registered occupational therapist, 286, 296–306

Job search. See Finding employment

Job Training Partnership Act, 321

Joint Commission on Accreditation of Healthcare Organizations

  accreditation, 462

  accreditation decision process, 479–480, 481

  Agenda for Change, 473–475

  development of standards, 462

  document review, 477–478

  domain, 462, 470–475

  feedback sessions, 479

  function interviews, 478

  history, 470–475

  hospital survey highlights, 476–482

  interviews with organization's leaders, 478

  mission, 470–475

  newsletter, 473

  organization liaison, 477

  organizational locus, 472

  outcome measures, 482–483

  performance measures, 482–483

  performance reports, 482

  practices, 462

  preparation for survey, 476–477

professional and technical advisory committee, 471

public information interviews, 479

quality assurance, 413

quality improvement, 418

review of processes for competence assessment, 479

scope, 472

scoring guidelines, 471, 475

sponsors, 462

standards dissemination, 488

standards manual, 471, 472

standards revision, 474–475

survey activities, 477–479

survey planning, 477

survey process redesign, 475–482

surveyor complement, 477

total quality management, 415

types of organizations, 471

unannounced surveys, 480

visits to patient care setting, 478

Justice, 633, 653, 657

defined, 627

K

Key operating indicator, 92–93

Key performance area, 342, 350

administrator, 361–362

certified occupational therapy assistant, 355–356

consultant, 363

educator, 357–358

entrepreneur, 370–371

faculty, 366–367

fieldwork coordinator, 364–365

fieldwork educator, 358–359

program director, 367–368

registered occupational therapist, 353–354

researcher, 369–370

scholar, 369–370

supervisor, 360–361

L

Leader

behaviors of effective leader, 222–227

challenging process, 223

characteristics, 228

decision making, 231–235

enabling others to act, 224–226

encouraging, 227

inspiring shared vision, 223–224

modeling the way, 226

power, 230–231

Leadership

clinical practice, 215

defined, 213, 215

direction, 225

education, 215–216

involvement, 225

management, differences, 227–229

negotiation, 225

persuasion, 225

research, 216

team, relationship, 218

Leadership style, 151–153

Leading, 170–172

Learning organization, 147, 183–186

activities, 183–186

defined, 163

dialogue, 185–186

mental model, 184–185

personal mastery, 184

shared vision, 184

systems thinking, 184

team learning, 185

Ledger, 74

Length of stay, 35

Letting go, defined, 191

Levels of expertise, changes, 378–379

Levels of performance, 350, 351
Licensure, 606, 618–619
  defined, 603
  occupational therapy manager, 638
Liquidity ratio, 91–92
Listening
  emotion, 520
  feeling behind the words, 520
  nonverbal language, 519–520
  skills, 518–519
Long-term care, consultation, 539–540
Long-term goal
  defined, 395
  development, 427–428
  documentation, 427–428
Long-term liability, 80
Loss from operations, 82

M

Managed care, 592–593
  Civilian Health and Medical
  Program of the Uniformed Services
  (CHAMPUS), 585–586
  defined, 3
  inclusion of occupational therapy
  services, 37–38
  integrated delivery system,
  contrasted, 20
  Medicaid, 588
    waivers, 588
  Medicare, 584
  workers' compensation, 590
Management
  defined, 145, 163, 213
  effectiveness, 166
  efficiency, 166
  leadership, differences, 227–229
  roles, 168
Management accounting, 71
  defined, 64

Management level, 166–167
  defined, 164
Management of working capital,
defined, 64
Management role, defined, 164
Management style, 151–153
  collaborative style, 151–152
  competitive style, 151–152
  defined, 145
  situation management, 152
  types, 152–153
Management team, 155
Manager
  average, effective, and successful
  managers compared, 169
  behavior, 235–236
  changing expectations, 205–206
  clinical practice, 215
  controlling, 236
  decision making, 231–235
  directing, 236
  education, 215–216
  functions, 165–170, 235–236
  organizing, 235–236
  planning, 235
  power, 230–231
  research, 216
  responsibilities, 158–159
  roles, 157–158
  time allocation, 168–169
Managerial accounting, 71
  defined, 64
Mandatory certification, 606–608
Mandatory registration, 608
Mandatory second opinion, 592
Market analysis, 110–111
  defined, 101
Market segmentation, 110–111
Marketable securities, management, 96
Marketing, 101–116

case study, 113–114

concepts, 104–106

consultation, 562–563

database creation, 111, 112

defined, 101, 103

environmental assessment, 109–110

  market data sources, 110

organizational assessment, 108–109

  market data sources, 109

place, 105–106

position, 106

price, 105

product, 104–105

promotion, 106

Marketing communication, 112–113

Marketing management, defined, 101, 103

Materiality, 72

Meaning

  content as contributor, 513

  context as contributor, 513–514

  emotion, 514–515

  stress, 514–515

  structure, 513–515

  threat, 514–515

Medicaid, 578, 587–588

  managed care, 588

    waivers, 588

Medical Review guidelines, 439–458

  activities of daily living, 442

  adaptive equipment, 452

  cardiac rehabilitation exercise, 452

  certification, 452–453

  documentation forms, 452

  dysphagia, 454–458

  evaluation, 442–443

  focused Medical Review analysis, 454–458

  functional limitation, 443

  Level I Review, 439–440

  Level II Review, 441–458

  level of complexity of treatment, 449–450

  medical history, 441–442

  Medicare Intermediary Manual, 439

  nonskilled occupational therapy, 450

  occupational therapy availability, 453

  orthoses, 452

  pain, 451

  plan of treatment, 443–444

  progress reports, 444–449

  prostheses, 452

  recertification, 452–453

  reporting on new episode or condition, 450

  safety dependence, 443

  secondary complications, 443

  skilled occupational therapy, 449–450

  therapeutic programs, 451

  transfer training, 452

Medicare, 578, 579–587

  conditions of participation, 583–584

  durable medical equipment, 583

  health maintenance organization, 584

  home health benefits, 581

  managed care, 584

  orthotics, 583

  prosthetics, 583

  provider certification, 583–584

  skilled nursing facility benefits, 581

Medicare Hospital Insurance Program (Part A), 579, 580–581

Medicare Supplementary Medical Insurance Program (Part B), 579, 582–583

Memo, 128, 129–130

Mental model, 184–185

Mentoring, 238–239

  defined, 213

Middle manager, 166

Minimal supervision, defined, 248

Mission, 175
  defined, 164

Mission statement, 175
  defined, 51, 53
  value, 54

Monthly summary, documentation, 429–430

Motivation, 263–266
  content theories, 148–149
  contingency theory, 149
  expectancy model, 264–265
  hierarchy of needs, 149
  motivation-hygiene model, 149
  organizational climate, 149–151
  process theories, 148–149
  theories of, 148–151
  Theory X and Theory Y, 149

Multidisciplinary team, 217

Multiskilled practitioner, 39
  defined, 4

N

National consensus standard, defined, 459

Net patient revenue, 82

Network-model health maintenance organization, 21

Newspaper, 128, 131–132

Noise, defined, 117

Noncertification, 609

Noncurrent liability, 80

Nongovernmental certification and registration, 612–617

Nonmaleficence, 632–633
  defined, 627

Nonoperating gain, 82

Nonoperating revenue, 82

Non-revenue-producing service center, 86

Nonverbal communication, 344

listening, 519–520

Norms, 177
  defined, 164, 177

North American Free Trade Agreement, cross-border trade in services, 617–622
  agencies, 622
  certification, 618–619
  definition, 617–618
  immigration, 619–622
  licensing, 618–619
  principles, 618
  scope, 617–618

Notes payable, 80

O

Occupational therapy
  attitudes, 655–658
  core concepts, 656–658
  demand trends, 27
  ethical enterprise in, 641–647
  evolution, 27–30
  functions, 340
  future trends, 31–41
  growth rate, 27
  integrated education and practice taxonomy, 373
  practice setting distribution, 28–30
  recognition, 41–42
  role, 340, 349–371, 376
  role hierarchy, 373
  supply trends, 27
  uniform terminology, 437
    performance areas, 437
    performance components, 437
    performance contexts, 437
  values, 655–658

Occupational therapy aide, defined, 262

Occupational Therapy Code of Ethics, 9, 631, 651–654

Occupational therapy management, evolution, 70–71

Occupational therapy manager
advancing professional competence, 638–639
allocation of limited resources, 639–640
effect on organization and employee integrity, 640–641
ethical problem solving, 635–641
facilitation of ethical clinical decision making, 636–637
fieldwork supervision, 638
licensure, 638
professional gatekeeping, 637–639
quality, 639
registration, 638

Occupational therapy practitioner
changing expectations of, 206
defined, 262
growth in numbers, 27
supervision, 247–249

Occupational Therapy Roles, 373–374

Occupational therapy student, defined, 262

Older Americans Act, 578

Omnibus Budget Reconciliation Act, 322

Open house, 128, 129

Open system, 170

Operating budget, 84

Operating fund, 74

Operating revenue, 81

Opportunity cost, 91

Oral communication, 344

Organization
defined, 164
as system, 174–177
control, 176
system integration, 176–177
systems as cycles of events, 175–176

Organizational assessment
defined, 101
marketing, 108–109
market data sources, 109

Organizational characteristics, 150–151
climate characteristics, 150
formal characteristics, 150

Organizational chart, 331–335
customer departmentalization, 333, 334
defined, 327
departmentalization, 332
functional departmentalization, 332–333
geographic departmentalization, 333–334
occupational therapy department in hospital, 336, 338
occupational therapy department in university, 336, 337
occupational therapy fieldwork program, 336, 339
process departmentalization, 334–335
product departmentalization, 333

Organizational climate
defined, 145
motivation, 149–151

Organizational culture
communication, 521–522
defined, 511

Organizational design, 331

Organizational effectiveness, 163–188
defined, 164
integrated systems approach, 179–181
organizational goals approach, 178
systems approach, 178–183

Organizational relationships, 343–347

Organizational structure, 153–157, 331
authority, 331
chain of command, 331
communication, 157

consensus building, 156–157

defined, 145, 154, 327

participative management, 156–157

powcr, 331

team, 154–155

unity of command, 331

work and role demands, 155

Organizational theory, 146–147

administrative approach, 146

behavioral science approach, 146

classical school, 146

contingency approach, 147

human relations approach, 146

learning organization, 147

participative management, 146–147

process approach, 147

scientific approach, 146

systems thinking, 147

Organized delivery system, 179–180, 182

defined, 163

Organizing, 170–172

manager, 235–236

Orientation, 273

Orthotics, Medicare, 583

Other operating revenue, 82

Outcome

defined, 459

quality improvement, 414

Outcome measure

Accreditation Council on Services for People with Disabilities

application, 500–501

content, 498–500

development, 498

format, 498–500

defined, 459

Outcome-based performance measure, 497–498

defined, 459

Outcomes management

defined, 395

quality improvement, 416

Overhead, 91

P

Participative leadership, 218

Participative management, 146–147

organizational structure, 156–157

Partnership, 75, 566

Patient evaluation, documentation, 426

Payment, 577–600

additional sources, 39

billing, 593–596

capitation, 598–599

evolving payment methodologies, 596–598

fee for service, 598

prospective rate, 598

risk pool, 598

risk sharing, 598

Peer review, 418–419

Peer review organization, quality improvement, 418–419

Per member per month, 598

Performance, form for "upward" appraisal, 325

Performance evaluation

discussing appraisal, 274–275

documenting performance, 274

establishing performance expectations, 273

personnel management, 273–275

Performance objective, sample, 293–294

Performance review

certified occupational therapy assistant, 307–314

registered occupational therapist, 296–306

Performance standard
  certified occupational therapy assistant, 267
  defined, 253
  development, 267
Personal mastery, 184
Personnel management, 253–282
  forecasting vacancies, 267–268
  performance evaluation, 273–275
  personnel selection, 269–273
  theoretical model, 255–256
Personnel selection, 269–273
  interview, 271–272
    guidelines, 271
  job offer, 272–273
  ranking, 270–271
  reference checking, 272
  screening, 270
Physicians' Current Procedural Terminology, 595
Physician-system integration, 180–181
Place
  defined, 101
  marketing, 105–106
Placement specialist. See Recruiter
Planning, 170–172
  change, 202–204
  consultation, 552, 566–567
  manager, 235
  market-based planning cycle, 107–114
  traditional planning cycle, 107
Point-of-service plan, 21
Policy, 346
  defined, 327
Position
  defined, 101
  marketing, 106
Position power, 516
  defined, 511

Power, 230–231
  communication, 516
  information, 516
  leader, 230–231
  manager, 230–231
  organizational structure, 331
  sources, 230
  types, 230–231
Practice act, 39, 606, 608
Preauthorization, 592
Precertification, 592
Preferred provider organization, 20, 21, 22
  defined, 4
Prepaid expense, 79
Prepaid health care plan, history, 20
Prevention, principles, 548
Preventive outcome
  consultation, 548–549
  defined, 534
Price
  defined, 102
  marketing, 105
Privacy, 633, 652
  defined, 627
Private insurance, 592–593
Pro forma, 83
Problem-solving team, 155
Procedure, 346–347
  defined, 327
Procedure code, 594, 595
  defined, 577
Process
  defined, 460
  quality improvement, 414
Process approach, defined, 164
Process departmentalization, organizational chart, 334–335
Product
  defined, 102

marketing, 104–105

Product departmentalization, organizational chart, 333

Product line forecasting, 84

Product output reporting system, productivity standard, 257–258

Productive days
  defined, 253
  staffing plan, 260–261

Productivity standard
  development, 257–259
  product output reporting system, 257–258
  relative value unit, 257
  treatment unit, 258

Productivity statement, defined, 253

Profession, responsibility, 330–331

Professional and technical advisory committee, Joint Commission on Accreditation of Healthcare Organizations, 471

Profitability ratio, 91–92

Profit-and-loss statement, 80

Program director
  key performance area, 367–368
  major function, 367
  qualifications, 368–369
  role description, 367–369
  scope of role, 367
  supervision, 369

Program evaluation, 395–433
  data gathering, 401
  data processing, 402
  data use, 402
  design development, 400–401
  development process, 400
  gaining awareness, 399
  historical perspectives, 398–399
  justifying use, 399–400
  obtaining involvement, 399
  quality improvement, relationship, 421–422

report form development, 402
  services subject to evaluation, 400
  staff training, 401–402
  steps, 399–403
  system elements, 400
  system purposes, 400
  system review, 402–403
  use, 400

Program evaluation system, defined, 396

Progress notes, 128, 129–130
  documentation, 429–430

Promotion
  defined, 102
  marketing, 106

Property, plant, and equipment, use limited, 79

Prospective payment system, 12, 580–581

Prospective rate, 598
  defined, 577

Prosthetics, Medicare, 583

Provider certification, Medicare, 583–584

Prudence, 657

Public health, voluntary organization programs, 25–26

Public Health Service, 22–24
  programs, 24

Public Law Number 94-142, 590–591

Public speaking, 128, 133–134

Q

Quality, 497
  defined, 460
  occupational therapy manager, 639

Quality assurance, 182
  concepts, 413
  defined, 396
  historical aspects, 413
  Joint Commission on Accreditation of Healthcare Organizations, 413

quality improvement, relationship, 413–414

Quality council, quality improvement, 419

Quality improvement, 183, 411–423
  accrediting body, 417–418
  CARF, The Rehabilitation Accreditation Commission, 417
  concepts, 414–417
  consumer satisfaction, 415
  consumer service, 415–416
  current players, 417–419
  data collection, 419–420
  defined, 396, 411–412
  Donabedian's framework, 414
  driving forces, 417–419
  effectiveness, 416–417
  efficiency, 416–417
  elements, 419–421
  historical perspectives, 412–414
  Joint Commission on Accreditation of Healthcare Organizations, 418
  organizational infrastructure, 419
  outcome, 414
  outcomes management, 416
  overcoming obstacles, 422
  peer review organization, 418–419
  process, 414
  program evaluation, relationship, 421–422
  quality assurance, relationship, 413–414
  quality council, 419
  research, relationship, 421–422
  steps, 419–421
  structure, 414
  tools and techniques, 420–421
  value, 416–417
Quality-circle team, 155

R

Rapport, 520
Ratio analysis, 91–92
Ratio of cost to charges, 91
Recruiter, 315–318
  advantages, 316
  disadvantages, 316
  employment agreement, 317
  financial considerations, 318
  methods, 315–316
  questions to ask recruiters, 317–318
  recruiting company credentials, 317
  working conditions, 317
Recruitment, 267–269
  forecasting vacancies, 267–268
  methods, 268–269
Reengineering, 182
Referral, 121, 122, 124
Registered occupational therapist certification
    certification basis, 613–614
    disciplinary action, 615
    examination eligibility requirements, 614–615
    private or public employment, 615
    state regulation, 615
    third-party reimbursement, 615
  defined, 262
  distribution across practice settings, 29–30
  job description, 286, 296–306
  key performance area, 353–354
  major function, 352
  performance review, 296–306
  qualifications, 354
  role, 349–371
    description, 352–354
    scope, 352
  school system, 538–539
  specialty certification, 616–617

certification basis, 616

examination eligibility requirements, 616–617

grounds for revocation, 617

renewal, 617

staffing, 262–263

supervision, 247–248, 354

Registration, 612–617

defined, 603

disciplinary action, 611

occupational therapy manager, 638

renewal, 610–611

Regulation, defined, 603

Regulatory board, 609–611

Rehabilitation, technological advances, 40–41

Rehabilitation Act, 321, 591

Reimbursement system, health care environment, change, 65

Relationship, 328–335

Relative value unit

defined, 253

productivity standard, 257

Report, 128, 129–130

Research

career development, 382

leadership, 216

manager, 216

quality improvement, relationship, 421–422

team, 216

Researcher

key performance area, 369–370

major function, 369

qualifications, 370

role description, 369–370

scope of role, 369

supervision, 370

Responsibility, profession, 330–331

Responsibility center, 74, 86

Retained earnings, 80

Revenue, 73

expense, matching, 73

Revenue center, 74

Revenue variance, 94

Revenue-producing center, 86

Review, defined, 460

Reviewer, 466

defined, 460

Reward system, 276–277

Right-to-health concept, 5–8

historical aspects, 5

Risk pool, 598

Risk sharing, 598

defined, 577

Role, 177, 328–335

career development, 335–343

defined, 145, 164, 327

descriptions, 350–371

interactive, 329

key performance areas, 341

level of expertise, 341

levels of performance, 342

open system, 329

organizations and role options, 336, 337, 338, 339

perspectives, 329–330

professional role options, 339–341

qualifications, 342

traditional organizations, 329

Role delineation, 36

Role modeling, 158

Role responsibility, 331

defined, 327

Role transition

career development, 377–379

clinical specialist, 385–386

department personnel system, 389

entry-level certified occupational therapy assistant, 384–385 experienced certified occupational therapy assistant to adult day-care coordinator, 387–388

master clinician to assistant professor, 388–389

practice administrator to curriculum director, 386

student to practitioner-registered occupational therapist, 383–384

supervisor, 385–386

Routine supervision, defined, 248

Rules and regulations, 346

S

Sales revenue, 82

Scholar

key performance area, 369–370

major function, 369

qualifications, 370

role description, 369–370

scope of role, 369

supervision, 370

Scholarly article, 128, 133

School system

certified occupational therapy assistant, 538–539

consultation, 538–539

registered occupational therapist, 538–539

Scoring guidelines, Joint Commission on Accreditation of Healthcare Organizations, 471, 475

Screening, personnel selection, 270

Segmentation, defined, 117

Self-assessment, 466

defined, 460

Self-directed education, 278

Self-employment, 565–566

Self-insuring, 589

Self-study, 466

defined, 460

Semifixed costs, 87, 89

Seminar, 128, 129, 132

Semivariable costs, 89, 90

Shared vision, 184

Short-term goal

defined, 396

development, 427–428

documentation, 427–428

Short-term investment, 79

Single proprietorship, 74–75

Situation management, management style, 152

Situation (SWOT) analysis, defined, 51

Social Security Title XX, 578

Social Services Block Grant Program, 578

Society, trends, 33

Sole proprietorship, 74–75

Speakers' bureau, 128, 133–134

Specialty certification, 612

defined, 603

registered occupational therapist, 616–617

certification basis, 616

examination eligibility requirements, 616–617

grounds for revocation, 617

renewal, 617

Speech, 344

Staff development, 277–278

Staff training, program evaluation, 401–402

Staffing

appropriate level, 262–263

certified occupational therapy assistant, 263

full-time equivalent, 256–257

issues, 278–279

qualitative aspects, 262–263

quantification of staffing needs, 256–262

registered occupational therapist, 262–263

support personnel, 263

Staffing pattern. See Staffing plan

Staffing plan
  defined, 253
  development, 259–262
  productive days, 260–261

Staff-model health maintenance organization, 20

Standard operating procedures, 346

Standards manual, Joint Commission on Accreditation of Healthcare Organizations, 471, 472

State department of health, 609

State licensure
  disciplinary action, 611
  renewal, 610–611

State regulation, 605–612
  disciplinary action, 611
  future trends, 611–612
  renewal, 610–611
  types, 607

State-administered program, 587–591

Statement of cash flows, 82, 83

Statement of owners' equity, 83

Statement of retained earnings, 83

Statement of revenue and expenses, 80

Statement of stockholders' equity, 83

Step costs, 87, 89

Strategic plan, defined, 51, 54

Strategic planning, 51–60
  benefits, 57
  case study, 58–59
  defined, 51, 53
  evaluation of results, 56–57
  financial planning, 69
  implementation, 56
  pitfalls, 57–58
  situation analysis, 54–55
  steps, 54–57
  strategy development, 55–56

Stress, meaning, 514–515

Structure, quality improvement, 414

Sunk costs, 89

Supervision, 36, 236–238, 239, 351–352
  administrator, 363
  certified occupational therapy assistant, 247–248, 356
  consultant, 364
  defined, 213
  entrepreneur, 371
  faculty, 367
  fieldwork coordinator, 365
  fieldwork educator, 360
  guide, 247–249
  occupational therapy practitioner, 247–249
  program director, 369
  registered occupational therapist, 247–248, 354
  researcher, 370
  scholar, 370
  supervisor, 361
  types, 247–248

Supervisor, 166
  career development, 385–386
  key performance area, 360–361
  major function, 360
  qualifications, 361
  role description, 360–361
  role transition, 385–386
  scope of role, 360
  supervision, 361

Surplus, 80

Surveillance
  change, 195
    clinical practice surveillance, 196
    consumer and market surveillance, 196–197
    environmental surveillance, 197

organizational surveillance, 196
personal-professional surveillance, 195
defined, 192
Survey, defined, 460
Surveyor, 466
defined, 460
SWOT analysis, 54–55
System, defined, 164
System change, 181–182
System integrationist, 177
Systems approach, defined, 164
Systems theory
defined, 164
origins, 170–174
process approach, 170–172
Systems thinking, 147
defined, 164

T

T-account, 76–77
Target group, 120–123
defined, 117
Target market, defined, 102
Team
behaviors of effective team members, 218–222
clinical practice, 215
defined, 213, 214–215
education, 215–216
evolution, 221–222
intellectual/cognitive characteristics, 219
interpersonal characteristics, 219
leadership, relationship, 218
organizational structure, 154–155
patterns, 220–221
personality characteristics, 219–220
research, 216
stages, 221–222

team skills, 219–222
types, 216–218
Team learning, 185
Technology
communication, 524
consultation, 540
Technology Special Interest Section, 41
Therapeutic use of self, 520
Third-party administrator, 593
Threat, meaning, 514–515
Title act, 606–608
Title control, 606–608
defined, 604
Top manager, 166–167
Total nonoperating revenue, 82
Total operating expenses, 82
Total operating revenue, 82
Total quality management, 183, 413, 414–415
consumer focus, 415–416
defined, 164, 396
Joint Commission on Accreditation of Healthcare Organizations, 415
value, 417
Trademark act, 606–608
defined, 604
Training
consultation, 559
legislation supporting, 10–11
Transaction, 72
Transdisciplinary team, 217
Treasurership, 68
Treatment, documentation, 429
Treatment planning, documentation, 426
Treatment unit
defined, 254
productivity standard, 258
Trust, 633

consultation, 552
Truth, 657

U

Uncontrollable costs, 89
Uniform terminology, 437
  performance areas, 437
  performance components, 437
  performance contexts, 437
Unity of command, organizational
structure, 331
Utilization review, 34

V

Value
  defined, 396
  quality improvement, 416–417
  total quality management, 417
Values, 177, 195
  defined, 164, 177
Variable costs, 87, 88
Variance analysis, 93–94
Veracity, 633, 653, 654
  defined, 627
Virtual team, 155
Vision, defined, 51, 53, 213
Vision statement, 198–199
Visioning
  change, 198–200, 201–202
  defined, 192
Visit, defined, 254
Voluntary accrediting agency, 459–506.
See also Specific type
  domains, 462–464
  historical origins, 465
  practices, 462–464
  sources of income, 465
  sponsors, 465
  sponsorship, 462–464

Voluntary certification, 608–609
Voluntary registration, 608–609

W

Weekly summary, documentation,
429–430
Work quantification, 257–258
Work team, 155
Workers' compensation, 578, 588–591
  hospital rate regulation, 589
  limits on choice of providers, 589
  managed care, 590
  medical fee schedules, 589
  utilization controls, 590
Working capital, 80
  management, 96–98
Work-related injury, 40
Work-related injury prevention, 40
Workshop, 128, 129, 132
Written information, 344

Z

Zero-base budgeting, 91